60399A

INTERVENTIONS WITH INFANTS AND PARENTS

WILEY SERIES IN CHILD AND ADOLESCENT MENTAL HEALTH

Joseph D. Noshpitz, Editor

FATHERLESS CHILDREN *by Paul L. Adams, Judith R. Milner, and Nancy A. Schrepf*

DIAGNOSIS AND PSYCHOPHARMACOLOGY OF CHILDHOOD AND ADOLESCENT DISORDERS *edited by Jerry M. Wiener*

INFANT AND CHILDHOOD DEPRESSION: DEVELOPMENTAL FACTORS *by Paul V. Trad*

TOURETTE'S SYNDROME AND TIC DISORDERS: CLINICAL UNDERSTANDING AND TREATMENT *edited by Donald J. Cohen, Ruth D. Bruun, and James F. Leckman*

THE PRESCHOOL CHILD: ASSESSMENT, DIAGNOSIS, AND TREATMENT *by Paul V. Trad*

DISORDERS OF LEARNING IN CHILDHOOD *by Archie A. Silver and Rosa A. Hagin*

CHILDHOOD STRESS *edited by L. Eugene Arnold*

PATHWAYS OF GROWTH: ESSENTIALS OF CHILD PSYCHIATRY Volume 1: NORMAL DEVELOPMENT *by Joseph D. Noshpitz and Robert A. King*

PATHWAYS OF GROWTH: ESSENTIALS OF CHILD PSYCHIATRY Volume 2: PSYCHOPATHOLOGY *by Robert A. King and Joseph D. Noshpitz*

PSYCHIATRIC INPATIENT CARE OF CHILDREN AND ADOLESCENTS: A MULTICULTURAL APPROACH *edited by Robert L. Hendren and Irving N. Berlin*

INTERVENTIONS WITH INFANTS AND PARENTS: THE THEORY AND PRACTICE OF PREVIEWING *by Paul V. Trad*

INTERVENTIONS WITH INFANTS AND PARENTS

THE THEORY AND PRACTICE OF PREVIEWING

PAUL V. TRAD

A Wiley-Interscience Publication

JOHN WILEY & SONS, INC.

New York   Chichester   Brisbane   Toronto   Singapore

Library of Congress Cataloging-in-Publication Data:

Trad, Paul V.
    Interventions with infants and parents: the theory and practice
of previewing / Paul V. Trad.
        p.   cm.—(Wiley series in child and adolescent mental
health)
    Includes bibliographical references (p.   ) and indexes.
    ISBN 0-471-53229-0
    1. Infant psychiatry.   2. Mother and infant.   I. Title.
II. Series.
RJ502.5.T74   1992
618.92′89—dc20   91-3043

Printed in the United States of America
10 9 8 7 6 5 4 3 2 1

Series Preface

This series is intended to serve a number of functions. It includes works on child development; it presents material on child advocacy; it publishes contributions to child psychiatry; and it gives expression to cogent views on child rearing and child management. The mental health of parents and their interaction with their children is a major theme of the series, and emphasis is placed on the child as individual, as family member, and as a part of the larger social surround.

Child development is regarded as the basic science of child mental health, and within that framework research works are included in this series. The many ethical and legal dimensions of the way society relates to its children are the central theme of the child advocacy publications, as well as a primarily demographic approach that highlights the role and status of children within society. The child psychiatry publications span studies that concern the diagnosis, description, therapeutics, rehabilitation, and prevention of the emotional disorders of childhood. And the views of thoughtful and creative contributors to the handling of children under many different circumstances (retardation, acute and chronic illness, hospitalization, handicap, disturbed social conditions, etc.) find expression within the framework of child rearing and child management.

Family studies with a central child mental health perspective are included in the series, and explorations into the nature of parenthood and the parenting process are emphasized. This includes books about divorce, the single parent, the absent parent, parents with physical and emotional illnesses, and other conditions that significantly affect the parent–child relationship.

Finally, the series examines the impact of larger social forces, such as war, famine, migration, and economic failure, on the adaptation of children and families. In the largest sense, the series is devoted to books that illuminate the special needs, status, and history of children and their families, within all perspectives that bear on their collective mental health.

JOSEPH D. NOSHPITZ

Chesapeake Youth Centers
Cambridge, Maryland

Preface

During the past few decades, the face of psychiatry, psychology, and the other disciplines that probe human behavior has changed dramatically. Just as the earth sciences have sought to analyze that fundamental component of matter, the atom, and the biological sciences have focused attention on exploring the mysteries of the individual cell, so too have the social sciences attempted to describe the primal human relationship that serves as a paradigm for all others in the individual's life—the relationship between caregiver and infant. Researchers now believe that by studying this relationship they can comprehend the puzzle of how the individual personality evolves, either in the direction of adaptability and mastery or toward psychopathology and despair.

Of course, this fascination with the caregiver–infant relationship is not new. Indeed, Freud, the father of psychoanalysis, premised his theories on the notion that the patient must retrace his or her steps and painstakingly return to the domain of childhood conflict to cure the self of turmoil in adulthood. Nevertheless, until quite recently childhood and infancy were approached from the perspective of the adult, who had long since cast off the image of youth. Only in the past few decades have researchers determined that the behavior of infants and young children can be evaluated on its own terms and that intervention in these young populations can result in beneficial changes in the mother–infant relationship.

Among the most prominent and challenging studies are those that seek to ascertain the infant's perception of the brave new world in which he finds himself. Although the infant may lack full-fledged language skills, his ability to sense, through a myriad of capacities the events in the external world as well as the maturational alterations occurring within himself, is enormous and overpowering. These studies have demonstrated that the infant can communicate with the caregiver in a purposeful manner and, if the caregiver possesses sufficient intuitive skill to respond to the infant's cues, that a fairly sophisticated rapport develops within the dyad from the first weeks of life.

Equally compelling is that virtually all caregivers apparently tend to preview or rehearse imminent developmental acquisitions with the infant. Previewing refers to the caregiver's ability to represent the contours of upcoming development on the stage of active consciousness and then to convert these representations into dynamic behavioral exercises that acquaint the infant with the sensation of the imminent developmental attainment and the likely effect of this upcoming accomplishment on the relationship between caregiver and infant. In essence, previewing seeks to convey to the infant a sense of mastery over the changes occurring within his own body, as well as a feeling of control over external events. When the infant validates the previewing experience by the factual attainment of the developmental milestone, a feeling of competence ensues, and with it comes a reinforcement of the potency of the dyadic rapport.

Thus, the psychological prerequisites for ensuring adaptive development and the establishment of a secure and coherent personality have been fairly well articulated. Where an adaptive relationship between caregiver and infant has not occurred—either because of some deficit on the part of the caregiver or because of some constitutional deficiency on the part of the infant—early intervention also can often rectify dysfunction or at least mitigate its effects. Caregivers can, in other words, be taught skills of sensitivity and attunement and can learn how to preview effectively to their infants. Such intervention not only enhances the course of infant development, but also produces a beneficial outcome for the dyadic rapport.

Although a growing body of literature has confirmed these findings, as yet no single volume has proposed comprehensive guidelines for conducting this form of early life intervention. This book seeks to achieve this previously elusive goal. From its first chapters, previewing theory and technique are introduced to the reader in a clear and understandable manner that highlights application to the clinical setting. The clinician is then guided in techniques of observation and inquiry that enhance skills of diagnosis. Throughout the volume, various perspectives are considered, including those of the infant, the caregiver, the dyad as an entity, and the family. Given its emphasis on the practical application of intervention techniques to the clinical setting, the book offers a step-by-step approach to the conduct of dyadic treatment. Part One, for example, introduces previewing as a *developmental paradigm* for interventions with infants and caregivers. Part Two is dedicated to various *assessment techniques.* Part Three elaborates on diverse *intervention techniques,* emphasizing benefits and drawbacks of each strategy. Part Four discusses the various phases of *dyadic intervention* and the treatment strategies appropriate to each phase. The last section of the book, Part Five, elaborates on how previewing may be applied as a principle for intervention within the various therapeutic approaches, ranging from *family* to *group,* from *modeling* to *social networks.*

Throughout this book I have used the traditional pronouns *he* (in referring to the infant) and *she* (in referring to the caregiver). This stylistic convention is for ease of reading only; the information herein refers impartially to both sexes unless the specific content states otherwise.

It is my fervent hope that this volume will offer all those clinicians involved in the psychological treatment of caregiver–infant dyads the guidance necessary to effect positive change. Although the book focuses heavily on the treatment of dysfunctional dyads, the material is also addressed to therapists involved in support services for caregivers who are already interacting well with their babies but who wish to improve. Indeed, one premise of this volume is that virtually any caregiver–infant relationship can be enhanced through the introduction of previewing skills designed to foster developmental competence and mastery as well as an optimal emotional rapport.

I am deeply grateful for the dedication and guidance of a group of individuals who supported me during the process of writing and editing this manuscript. For the past several years, I have been fortunate enough to work with Paulina F. Kernberg, M.D., at Cornell University Medical Center. Dr. Kernberg's skill as a clinician and her support as a teacher and mentor have provided an atmosphere conducive to productivity. My deep appreciation goes to Herb Reich, Editor, John Wiley & Sons, for his sustained encouragement with regard to the manuscript. As ever, Wendy J. Luftig allowed me to share my ideas, motivated me to surpass my current accomplishments, and always kept my spirits high. My heartfelt appreciation to Beth Innocenti, Stephanie Hill, Vernon Bruete, Mary Jeness Raine, Ph.D., and Richard H. White, whose thoughtful commentaries have made the long hours of labor worthwhile and rewarding.

PAUL V. TRAD

New York, New York
September 1991

Contents

The Structure and Function of Previewing: Introduction and
Organization of the Book   1

PART ONE
PREVIEWING AS A DEVELOPMENTAL PARADIGM FOR
INTERVENTIONS WITH INFANTS AND CAREGIVERS

Chapter 1
Previewing: An Interpersonal Paradigm for Enhancing
Infant Development   13

Chapter 2
The Role of Parents in Infant Development   35

PART TWO
ASSESSMENT TECHNIQUES

Chapter 3
Assessing the Interpersonal Status of the Infant   65

Chapter 4
Assessing the Interpersonal Status of the Dyad   101

Chapter 5
Assessing Unconscious Defense Operations Affecting
Dyadic Interaction   135

Chapter 6
Assessing the Role of the Infant in the Development of
Family Relationships   163

Chapter 7
Assessing Parallel Processes: The Caregiver–Therapist
Relationship as a Reflection of the Caregiver–Infant Relationship   191

PART THREE
INTERVENTION TECHNIQUES

Chapter 8
Observation and Other Intervention Strategies   227

Chapter 9
Strategies for Enhancing Previewing Through
Representational Exercises   251

PART FOUR ·
APPLYING PREVIEWING DURING
DYADIC INTERVENTION

Chapter 10
Stages in the Caregiver–Therapist Relationship   283

Chapter 11
Applying the Principles of Dream Interpretation to
Dyadic Intervention   315

Chapter 12
Resistance, Transference, and Countertransference: Mechanisms
That Hinder Previewing Abilities 345

Chapter 13
Applying the Principles of Modeling and Psychoeducation to
Dyadic Intervention 367

PART FIVE
APPLYING PREVIEWING DURING NONDYADIC
APPROACHES TO DYADIC INTERVENTION

Chapter 14
Applying Principles of Family Therapy to
Dyadic Intervention 397

Chapter 15
Applying the Principles of Group Therapy to
Dyadic Intervention 423

Chapter 16
Applying Previewing Exercises During Group Therapy 441

Chapter 17
Applying the Principles of Short-Term Psychotherapy to
Dyadic Intervention 463

Chapter 18
Applying the Principles of Social Support to
Dyadic Intervention 483

References 499

Author Index 541

Subject Index 549

INTERVENTIONS WITH INFANTS AND PARENTS

The Structure and Function of Previewing

*Introduction and Organization
of the Book*

During the past several years, in my work as Director of the Child and Adolescent Outpatient Department at Cornell Medical Center—Westchester Division, I have been integrally involved in the treatment of pregnant women and new mothers. Such patients bring to the therapeutic environment an added dimension that is often lacking in the traditional format of individual therapy. This added dimension consists of the caregiver's unique and distinctive relationship with the infant, which unfolds directly in front of the therapist.

The relationship of the pregnant woman with the unborn infant derives mainly from the caregiver's fantasies and expectations concerning the personality of the infant; this bond emerges from the potent somatic and psychological changes that attend the process of nurturing another human being inside of oneself. For new mothers, this relationship becomes a palpable reality with the act of giving birth. Once the birth has occurred, the caregiver is challenged to continue forging an attachment with the infant, which represents the most intimate relationship individuals experience during their life-span. In either case, however, the interpersonal changes that come to fruition during the pregnancy and early infancy period become the predominant force that colors virtually every other relationship in the lives of the dyadic members.

The overriding importance of the relationship between the caregiver and infant makes therapy involving pregnant women and new mothers different from other forms of treatment; there is a primary difference in the nature of the therapeutic relationship that evolves between the therapist and caregiver. With caregiver–infant therapy, distinctly different processes are at work. The infant's arrival or, in the case of the pregnant woman, the imminence of birth catapults the caregiver into a new relationship that coaxes forth characteristic interactional behavior patterns, even those that have been long suppressed. The caregiver will, in other words, be called on to resurrect her own unique style of interpersonal exchange in forging a rapport with the infant. As a result of the infant's presence, therapists become eyewitnesses to the unfolding of the mother–infant relationship. They can observe firsthand how the caregiver reenacts conflict, transposes it onto the relationship with the infant, and generates maladaptive modes of communication. Dyadic therapy incorporates four significant features that distinguish it from individual therapy:

1. The therapist's immediate observation and interpretation of how the caregiver transfers conflict to the infant facilitates diagnosis of maladaptive interactional patterns.
2. The therapist's role as a supportive observer, rather than as a neutral figure upon whom conflict is displaced, promotes objectivity in both diagnosis and treatment.

3. The therapist can effect change that is immediately enacted in the reproducible context between the caregiver and infant. In this regard, such techniques as previewing, modeling, and guidance used by the therapist during interaction with the infant can be tested by the caregiver in the therapist's presence.

4. The therapist focuses on modulating the caregiver's behavior in order to adapt to the infant's developmental rhythms. Thus, this form of treatment emphasizes future interpersonal outcome between caregiver and infant, rather than merely the resurrection of past conflict. In fact, although earlier conflict can be scrutinized during dyadic therapy, it is resolved within the context of a new and dynamic relationship with the infant. Mastering this new relationship motivates the caregiver to strive for behaviors that will enhance the infant's potential for adaptive development, as well as the caregiver's own sense of predicting imminent development. The therapist participates in a supportive capacity, fostering the caregiver's skill in *previewing* or anticipating the infant's imminent developmental attainments and preparing for them by exploring the implications of such changes.

Caregiver–infant therapy has a further advantage that is best summed up in the word *flexibility*. One example of this flexibility is that sessions can be held with only the caregiver and therapist in attendance, during which the caregiver provides the therapist with her descriptions of infant development and of the type of interaction that is occurring within the dyadic relationship. The therapist can then conduct a session with both the caregiver and the infant to ascertain the accuracy of the caregiver's representation of the infant's maturational trends and to assess how the caregiver responds during interaction. Dyadic therapy thus permits the therapist to consensually validate the patient's point of view in a way that is not feasible with individual therapy.

Caregiver–infant therapy also can be flexible by including fathers and other family members in sessions along with mothers. Moreover, this form of treatment is conducive to group sessions, consisting of several caregivers who share developmental perceptions about their infants. All of these formats are amenable to the one significant factor—the presence of the infant—that makes caregiver–infant therapy a challenging and innovative approach to the diagnosis and treatment of maladaptive behavior patterns between caregivers and their infants.

Dyadic therapy permits the therapist to formulate a global impression of the dynamics of any particular caregiver–infant relationship. This impression is composed of the numerous *microassessments* the therapist performs during any given session. The therapist can evaluate the dynamics of the interaction while observing and continuing a dialogue with the caregiver.

As this bimodal (verbal and behavioral) evaluation proceeds, the therapist can begin to discern the presence or absence of *intuitive* caregiver behaviors that promote adaptive development. Moreover, dyadic treatment provides the therapist with a firsthand view of whether the caregiver is introducing appropriate previewing behaviors into her interaction with the infant. Although the behaviors of the infant should provide a sufficient stimulus to motivate a caregiver response, the caregiver's own behaviors and attributions provide the therapist with insights that can later be validated by observing sequences of dyadic interaction. This occurs both when the therapist engages the infant in play and when the therapist passively observes the caregiver and infant during dyadic exchange. This book discusses numerous phenomena, gleaned from direct observation and from clinical interactions with caregivers, that facilitate the therapist's task in formulating interpretations and achieving diagnostic insight.

Just as the diagnostic implications of dyadic behavior are facilitated during dyadic treatment, so too is the therapist's ability to render effective interventions that will result in more optimal behavior patterns. As with diagnosis, the environment of the caregiver–infant therapy allows administration of treatment techniques at an accelerated pace, and the therapist can observe the treatment's effects almost immediately, as they are revealed during sequences of dyadic interaction. It should be remembered that when the caregiver interacts with the infant, she is offering the therapist palpable segments of life experience and is revealing to the therapist how she perceives the infant's development. Indeed, it may take several sessions before the caregiver feels comfortable sharing these intimate moments in the therapist's presence because they require the caregiver, in effect, to disclose the intrapsychic dynamics of her relationship with the infant.

In the unique situation of dyadic therapy, the therapist's observations, interpretations and recommendations not only will be absorbed by the caregiver intellectually, but such insights will also be immediately woven into the fabric of the dyadic interaction and applied to the communication with the infant. In this respect, the relationship between the infant and caregiver represents a kind of mirror that vividly and palpably transfers the caregiver's alliance with the therapist. Because of this phenomenon whereby the dynamics of the therapist's relationship with the caregiver are juxtaposed with the caregiver's relationship with the infant, the therapeutic relationship assumes a unique and predominant role in dyadic therapy.

An illustration can probably best describe the potency of the therapeutic relationship in dyadic therapy. During one particular session with a caregiver and her 3-month-old infant, I voiced concern about the mother's uncharacteristically disheveled appearance. The mother stared suddenly at the floor, offering no response or even a minor acknowledgment to my queries. Coincidentally, at just that moment the infant began to shift position in his carriage, emitting deep gurgling noises. The mother then turned in the direction of the infant and barked out, "Stop it . . . be quiet!" The sudden and abrupt nature of this response was surprising until I realized that the caregiver was not addressing the message as much to the infant as to me. Nevertheless, the incident created the indelible impression that a therapeutic intervention directed at the caregiver could almost immediately be transferred by the caregiver to the dyadic relationship with both rapid and dramatic effects. As a consequence, it becomes crucial for the therapist engaged in dyadic therapy to monitor continuously the relationship with the caregiver, dispensing interventions and interpretations that can be transferred to the dyadic relationship in an adaptive manner that enhances development.

It is worth mentioning as well that witnessing the effect of a productive intervention almost instantaneously as it is enacted in the caregiver relationship with the infant is enormously gratifying. In contrast to individual treatment, which requires the patient to attain insight and eventually test out newly discovered "truths" in the real world, caregiver–infant therapy enables the patient immediately to experiment with insights by engaging the infant directly in newly developed interactive exchanges. Once the therapist has acquired diagnostic and treatment insights, initiating and monitoring changes in the dyadic relationship becomes an integral aspect of virtually every session.

To assist the therapist in attaining these skills, this book presents examples of typical responses between the caregiver and infant, and between the caregiver and therapist. Each of these responses commonly occurs during dyadic treatment, and each challenges the therapist to formulate a diagnostic explanation and to engage in an appropriate intervention. For convenience, these responses have been divided into those that emanate from the caregiver during interaction with the infant, and those that are initiated by the therapist when interacting with the caregiver and/or infant. A definition, diagnostic outline, example, and interventive technique are provided with each response.

This volume also introduces therapists to the nuances of dyadic interaction by delineating certain core behaviors that are known to occur between infants and caregivers whose relationship conforms to the optimal pathways of adaptation. These core behaviors have been labeled *intuitive* by a variety of researchers, who suggest that intuition is the emblem of an adaptive relationship with the infant. Intuitive behaviors range from particular eye-gazing patterns, to physical holding gestures, to vocalizations the caregiver uses in promoting a pleasurable atmosphere and soothing away distressful experiences. By learning to recognize these intuitive behaviors in any particular caregiver–infant dyad, the therapist will acquire an indispensable guide for assessing the degree of adaptation or, conversely, the level of maladaptation between caregiver and infant.

The following chapters further provide therapists with other diagnostic techniques that probe the effectiveness of dyadic interaction. For example, therapists are tutored in methods designed to detect the degree of overall competence the caregiver brings to interaction and to assess whether an atmosphere of *reciprocity* and *affect attunement* imbues the dyadic relationship. Is the caregiver genuinely sensitive to infant cues, in the sense that all aspects of the infant's regulatory processes—including somatic, socioaffective, cognitive, and motivational processing—are addressed in a synchronous, reciprocal manner that promotes adaptive growth and development? When the dyad manifests such behaviors, both caregiver and infant appear to be communicating their emotional needs on a profound level. In addition, guidelines are given for evaluating whether the caregiver is fostering an adaptive response by offering sufficient stimulation through exposure of the infant to adequate contingent stimuli, and whether the infant's expectations are being met.

A dynamic and innovative technique introduced in this book involves what is referred to here as *previewing.* Previewing entails the caregiver's capacity to anticipate or predict imminent developmental achievement in the infant and subsequently to behave as an "auxiliary supporter" who facilitates the infant's experimentation with the interpersonal implications of the new aspect of maturation. An illustration will demonstrate how previewing works within the dyadic relationship. Assume that the infant has attained the capacity to maintain an erect sitting posture on his own. Shortly thereafter, the infant is likely to begin to display gestures that indicate imminent crawling behavior. These are referred to as precursory behaviors. For example, the infant may begin making thrusting motions with his feet or may begin to crawl for a few steps by supporting himself on his elbows. An alert caregiver will perceive these behaviors and be eager to facilitate the infant's progress. Thus, she will help the infant crawl slowly for a brief interval, providing muscle support for his limbs, and then gradually permit this behavior to recede, as the infant returns to his previous sitting posture. Such a caregiver would be previewing the infant, because she would be demonstrating the capacity to anticipate and represent developmental achievement, to convert these representations into actual exercises with the infant, and to serve as an auxiliary supporter of the infant's inchoate developmental manifestations.

This book contends that previewing represents an index for measuring the level of adaptability present within a caregiver–infant dyad. Indeed, the incidence of previewing behavior is perhaps one of the most effective means for diagnosing whether the caregiver is engaging in an adaptive relationship promoting development or in a maladaptive relationship stifling the potential for autonomy within the infant.

Moreover, observations of interaction among adaptive dyads reveal that the infant is also capable of initiating previewing behaviors. Such behaviors occur when the infant manifests gestures and other behavioral signs of an impending developmental milestone and turns to the caregiver for guidance in exercising the essential skills for attaining the milestone. An infant who is on the developmental brink of crawling, for example, may begin to demonstrate kicking manifestations and then may gaze directly at the caregiver while emitting vocalizations in her direction. These behaviors suggest that the infant possesses some awareness of imminent developmental achievement but has also come to rely on the caregiver as a supportive partner in order to forecast the *continuity* of their rapport. When the therapist witnesses an episode of previewing, it becomes apparent that a distinct form of communication is transpiring within the dyad. This form of communication relies on myriad behavioral signals in the dyadic exchange. For each dyad these signals are unique and personal, highlighting the significant role played by the caregiver in devising these signals and reinforcing them for the infant during interaction. The manner and extent of previewing, therefore, becomes a significant barometer of the level of adaptation within the dyad.

Because, as noted earlier, previewing manifestations appear to permeate the interaction among adaptive dyads and are conspicuously absent in dyads in which maladaptive exchange is evident, one previewing technique in this book involves the enhancement of previewing behaviors. It is important to recognize, however, that the emergence of these behaviors is actually the final outcome of a lengthy internal process of representation and prediction on the part of the caregiver. To be able to preview imminent developmental changes to the infant, the caregiver must first possess some fundamental knowledge about the scope of upcoming maturational achievements and must be able to envision or represent her infant attaining these achievements. The therapist can test this capacity for representational ability during the initial intake process by asking the caregiver to describe what she anticipates for the infant developmentally in the next weeks or months. If the caregiver is able to describe developmental changes with enthusiasm, the therapist should then compare how the caregiver's interaction with her infant reflects the verbal report. That is, does the caregiver transfer her skill in anticipating the infant's maturational trends to actual sequences of interaction? Where the caregiver appears to lack an awareness of the infant's long-term developmental capacity when being interviewed initially, the therapist should also engage in a comparison exercise by observing the type of interaction that actually occurs within such a dyad.

Treatment may then strive to enhance the caregiver's representational skills, on the theory that active positive representation promotes adaptive previewing in both the infant and caregiver, which in turn propels the infant in the direction of developmental autonomy while simultaneously reinforcing the rapport with the caregiver. As will be discussed, there are numerous techniques for encouraging caregivers to represent the infant's upcoming development. Rather than adopting one specific approach, the techniques advocated here reflect an eclectic perspective that strives to acquaint the caregiver with the overall trends of development, while making her sensitive to the unique capacities that apply to her infant. The practitioner is advised to use a wide variety of techniques for fostering more adaptive behaviors within the dyad. Thus, if the therapist senses that traditional psychotherapy will be effective, he or she is directed to help the caregiver delve into past conflict that may have been reawakened within the parenting situation. Caregivers who are amenable to this form of treatment will be urged to free associate with regard to episodes in their own childhoods that may have been traumatic or stressful. The therapist and caregiver will then explore how these previous conflicts have been transferred to the relationship with the infant and how conflict in the dyadic relationship resembles earlier conflicts the caregiver experienced during her own maturation.

Although traditional psychotherapy represents one approach, it is by no means the only technique offered in this book. In fact, by training the therapist in detecting intuitive behaviors and observing instances of previewing during dyadic interaction, the book presents an array of approaches to instill adaptive interaction within any therapeutic framework. For example, both intuitive behaviors and previewing can be instilled in caregivers who are deficient in these skills. In introducing caregivers to these interpersonal skills, therapists can use such aids as modeling and videotaping. Modeling techniques are particularly helpful because, in distinction to other forms of treatment, during dyadic therapy they present the caregiver with a vivid and palpable example of how to improve and enhance interaction in a forceful, persuasive, and direct way. Even caregivers who cannot articulate conflict clearly or who lack sufficient verbal skills for engaging in more sophisticated psychotherapy can benefit from observations of previewing behavior instituted by the therapist in the caregiver's presence. Most caregivers will be able to respond to these techniques effectively and rapidly.

Some caregivers will respond soon after sessions during which the therapist engages in supportive inquiry; in other cases, the therapist may wish to engage in interaction directly with the infant and subsequently ask the caregiver to model the interaction. Caregivers may also benefit from observing videotapes of their own or of others' interactions. From observations of these tapes, the therapist can gradually point to behaviors that appear designed to stimulate responsiveness in the infant, such as gazing behaviors, vocalizations, and specific holding behaviors. Many caregivers can then learn to integrate these manifestations into their interactive sequences with the infant to forge a more adaptive relationship.

This book, then, strives to provide therapists with diagnostic and treatment techniques centered around previewing behaviors that can be used from the inception of dyadic therapy to its termination. The following pages provide the therapist with a full spectrum of interventive techniques designed to isolate conflict that has resulted in maladaptation during the caregiver–infant interaction. These diagnostic guidelines alert the therapist to phenomena that are generally overlooked during more traditional assessments. Rather than adhering to a precise format, the book provides the therapist with a broad spectrum of techniques and guides the professional in the selection of the most effective strategy for enhancing adaptive development and instilling previewing manifestations in a particular caregiver–infant dyad.

PART ONE

Previewing as a Developmental Paradigm for Interventions with Infants and Caregivers

Chapter 1

Previewing

An Interpersonal Paradigm for Enhancing Infant Development

INTRODUCTION

This chapter explores the assessment and therapeutic applications of a developmental phenomenon that helps explain the extraordinarily complex and intricate relationship between mother and infant. The phenomenon, referred to as *previewing,* may be used to interpret a wide variety of interpersonal behaviors emanating from the caregiver that acquaint the infant with upcoming developmental trends. In addition, previewing enhances understanding of how the infant comes to predict and master imminent developmental change, as well as acclimate to the continually changing relationship with the caregiver.

All caregivers engage in previewing to varying degrees—whether the caregiver's relationship with the infant enhances adaptation or is marred by emotional conflict. Of course, virtually all infants appear to be constitutionally primed to engage in particular kinds of behaviors that fulfill maturational potential. But through the previewing process the caregiver infuses the infant's new skills with meaning, purpose, and direction. Moreover, previewing encompasses far more than the overt manifestations of both the caregiver and infant; it also includes the caregiver's diverse subjective representations concerning the interpersonal implications that future developmental changes will precipitate in the relationship. Previewing captures the full texture of the caregiver's ability to make predictions about the infant's development and gradually to share these predictions with the infant as both members of the dyad traverse the developmental journey. From the caregiver's perspective, this journey begins during the planning of the pregnancy and continues throughout the child's life. By using the previewing process, the caregiver communicates with the infant in a highly intimate way designed to enhance rapport in the relationship. This sense of intimacy enables the mother and infant to accommodate the immediate demands sparked by developmental change. Through previewing the caregiver simultaneously validates current and future developmental achievement for the infant.

Considering all of these factors, previewing may be defined as a *self-perpetuating* dyadic process during which the caregiver represents imminent developmental trends and translates these representations into behavioral exchanges that introduce the infant to both the experience of what a future developmental change will be like and to the implications such changes will have on his relationship with the caregiver.

Although composed of a diverse series of interpersonal events, previewing, from the infant's perspective, is a potent force that provides coherence to the continual unfolding of his developmental destiny. During infancy the challenges confronting the infant are formidable. At birth, the infant is a creature ruled, to a large extent, by constitutional urgings. He is dependent on the caregiver for his most basic needs. Lacking the ministrations of a sensitive caregiver, the infant would be unable to integrate the seemingly uncontrollable physiological forces emanating from his own body. As the infant internalizes his interactions with the external world, the experience of control over biological processes becomes preeminent. The caregiver helps the infant coordinate the burgeoning changes that characterize development. From the relationship with the caregiver and, most notably, her ability to assist the infant in integrating future maturational growth, adaptive development evolves. Previewing clarifies this process because it fosters the reconciliation of internal and external perceptions, as well as current and imminent developmental attainment.

This chapter will highlight the three key components of previewing. The first of these components is the caregiver's capacity to represent imminent development. Representation is a reflective state during which perceptions of past, current, and/or future interactions become accessible to consciousness through the generation of images. Because previewing involves not only the caregiver's awareness of the infant's current status, but also her perceptions concerning imminent developmental acquisition, caregiver representations will encompass images derived from memories of past experience, as well as images constructed from anticipations about the future. The second component of previewing involves the caregiver's role as an auxiliary partner for the infant. In adopting this stance, the caregiver devises behavioral exercises that help introduce the infant to upcoming skills and conveys to the infant not only that she will be available to guide and coordinate precursory developmental skills, but also that she is providing a safe haven within which the infant can practice and learn how to predict the future of their relationship. The third and final component of previewing is the caregiver's capacity to sense when the infant has become satiated with the previewing exercise and wishes to return to his previous level of achievement. In fulfilling this role, the caregiver's sensitivity to infant cues and manifestations becomes paramount.

Specific examples of the overt manifestations of previewing are manifold. The caregiver who senses that her infant is ready to crawl or walk and who exercises the infant's limbs so that he is able to practice these functions is exhibiting previewing behavior. So too is the caregiver who guides the hand of an infant who is trying to grasp a small utensil. The typical baby talk engaged in by the caregiver introduces the infant to the rhythms of conversation and is another example of a previewing exercise. Additionally, the entire previewing process is a means for reinforcing the continuity to the dyadic rapport, because the caregiver practices in the present how the relationship with her infant will be transformed by future maturational challenges.

As a result of its myriad effects, previewing offers a bold and innovative way of viewing the mother–infant relationship and the behaviors manifested by each dyadic member. It is reasonable to ask, however, how both caregiver and infant come to formulate representations about one another and how they come to predict the interactions that each will manifest in the future. In other words, how does the infant's somatic and psychological development enhance his ability to respond to caregiver previewing behaviors, enabling him to begin engaging in predictions about his own interactions? Moreover, does research in the area of mother–infant interaction contribute to an understanding of how interpersonal exchanges during episodes of previewing enhance the acquisition of imminent developmental change? This chapter explores these issues and examines empirical data that demonstrate how maternal previewing behaviors exert an overriding influence on the infant's maturational trends.

PREVIEWING INTERPERSONAL OUTCOMES

The Caregiver's Perspective

From Perception to Action.   For quite some time therapists have posited that early intervention can enhance infant development (Fraiberg, Shapiro, & Cherniss, 1980). A number of researchers have also elaborated on the notion that maternal manifestations may be used to stimulate the infant's developmental competence. For example, one concept, *scaffolding,* was coined by Wood, Bruner, and Ross (1976) to explain the caregiver's behavioral strategies designed to compensate at any given maturational level for current deficiencies in the infant's developmental skill. Vygotsky (1978) conceived the notion of a *zone of proximal development* and commented that the competent parent combines supportive behaviors with the challenging goals presented by the environment to assist the infant in achieving skills that lie incrementally beyond his current level of mastery. In Vygotsky's view, the caregiver is sensitive to the next zone of developmental competence and, through supportive encouragement, guides the infant's development in that direction. Another theorist, Kaye (1982), used the word *apprenticeship* to describe the nature of the interactions between mother and infant. For Kaye, the apprenticeship paradigm illustrates how parents, as the more developmentally competent partners, foster the infant's achievement of skills and knowledge by delicately balancing or compensating for the infant's lack of developmental skill, while simultaneously challenging the infant's developmental potential.

These observations of the parental role have been reinforced by several studies that focused on the acquisition of specific developmental milestones after specific interventions were initiated. In one study, Lagerspetz, Nygard, and Strandvik (1971) found that when infants were trained in crawling behavior for 15 minutes daily over a period of 3 weeks, they learned to crawl at a significantly earlier age than might have otherwise been expected. Moreover, these researchers determined that training in a specific motor activity, such as crawling, not only had a developmental effect on the achievement of that particular milestone, but also had a favorable influence on locomotor development in general. These findings have led researchers to hypothesize a possible *transfer* from the acquisition of certain skills to other developmental phenomena. The work of Lagerspetz et al., which involved experimenters, rather than parents, also indicates that infants may demonstrate this form of developmental progression when exposed to specific behavioral manifestations on a regular basis—even if such manifestations are performed by an individual with whom the infant does not have a strong attachment relationship. This finding provides empirical validation for one of the qualities that is associated with previewing: Developmental achievement can be enhanced through intervention that relies on a specific form of interpersonal exchange.

Do parents engage in these behaviors spontaneously, thereby demonstrating an initiative to stimulate developmental achievement? Zelazo, Zelazo, and Kolb (1972) found that the manifestation of infant walking could be accelerated by early parental exercise involving support of the infant in a vertical, weight-bearing posture daily from the 2nd through the 8th week of life. Interestingly, Zelazo et al. reported that some parents appear, on their own initiative, to assist their babies in walking and standing movements during the newborn period. If certain parents spontaneously engage in these forms of behavior with their infants, what kinds of expectations do these parents harbor about their infant's development?

This question has been explored by Hopkins and Westra. These researchers have not only determined that there are cultural differences among the expectations of parents, but also that parental expectations correlate directly with the level of the infant's developmental skills. In one of their studies, Hopkins and Westra (1989) sought to compare the maternal expectations of three cultural groups—mothers of Jamaican, British, and Indian descent, all of whom were living in Great Britain. These researchers were especially interested in comparing the predictive validity of maternal expectations in relation to the cultural background of these mothers. To probe the maternal expectations, the researchers interviewed these mothers when the infants were 1 month old. At that time, mothers were asked to estimate the age in months at which the infant would first achieve the milestones of sitting alone, crawling, and walking. Significantly, the Jamaican mothers voiced predictions of infant sitting and walking behavior that were significantly earlier than both of their counterparts. Moreover, during the interviews the mothers of Jamaican descent expressed difficulty in being able to predict when their infants would begin crawling. It was as if these mothers could not represent crawling behavior. As the researchers continued to follow these dyads, they found that, in fact, the Jamaican infants sat and walked independently at a significantly earlier age than the infants in the other two groups. Furthermore, one quarter of these Jamaican infants progressed from sitting to walking without ever having crawled. This study suggests that the differences in motor development and in the achievement of motor milestones bears a direct relationship to maternal expectations of infant maturation when the infant is only 1 month old. These findings can be related to the work by Ninio (1979), who demonstrated that parental expectations may affect cognitive abilities, and to the studies of Tulkin and Kagan (1972), who have demonstrated that the development of the infant's communicative abilities can be predicted by parental expectations.

Hopkins and Westra (1990) sought further to investigate the mechanism by which maternal expectations affect infant development. These researchers probed the specific behavior manifested by the mothers that signified their expectations about infant development. Significantly, it was determined that a highly discrete kind of behavior, referred to as *formal handling*, was manifested by all of these mothers. Formal handling was defined as a kind of touching and manipulating of the infant's body in a pedagogical manner that served to educate the infant about body function (Hopkins and Westra, 1988). Formal handling, which consists of passive stretching movements along with massaging, becomes evident in the mothers' behavior shortly after birth and appears to facilitate selectively the development of milestones such as sitting and walking.

The researchers found that formal handling acts as a *mediating link* between maternal expectations about motor development and subsequent infant outcome. In particular, the greater the degree of the mother's involvement with the handling routine, the more accurate was the mother's prediction of the age at which her infant would sit and walk alone. Mothers who engaged in formal handling were able to anticipate with far greater precision the ages at which their infants would sit and walk alone relative to other mothers who used only part or none of the handling routine. From these findings, Hopkins and Westra concluded that a system of physical training for infants can act as a mediating link between maternal expectations regarding motor development and the subsequent ages at which the infant attains such milestones.

Taken together, these empirical observations substantiate the value of using *previewing* for understanding the dynamics of developmental changes. First, these studies indicate direct relationships among maternal expectations, maternal behavior, and infant outcome. The relationship of these variables is reinforced by the theory of previewing, which posits that caregivers initially represent imminent developmental change and subsequently convert these representations into interpersonal manifestations. In this way they not only encourage their infants to experience upcoming developmental milestones, but also expose their infants to an arena where they can represent the interpersonal implications of these changes to the dyadic relationship. Hopkins and Westra's work indicates that the predictions of caregivers may be *spontaneously* transformed into manifestations that result in more optimal developmental consequences for the infant.

The work of Hopkins and Westra suggests that a particular form of maternal behavior, characterized by these researchers as formal handling, directly affects the direction of infant maturational achievement. This finding raises the issue of whether caregivers exhibit other naturally occurring manifestations that enhance and promote the consolidation of developmental milestones. Another research team, Tamis-LeMonda and Bornstein (1990), assessed infant habituation and maternal encouragement of attention at 5 months and correlated these findings with toddler language comprehension, language production, and pretend play at 13 months. The researchers found that early maternal encouragement explained unique qualities in the toddler's language comprehension, as well as in the manifestations of their language skills and play behavior. This finding is consistent with other studies that have associated maternal stimulation in the first year with 1-year play competence (Belsky, Goode, & Most, 1980); 1-year vocabulary size (Bornstein, 1985; Ruddy & Bornstein, 1982); 1½-year cognitive competence (Clarke-Stewart, 1973; Yarrow, Morgan, Jennings, Harmon, & Gaiter, 1982); 2-year cognitive/language competence (Olson, Bates, & Bayles, 1984); 4-year intelligence test performance (Bornstein, 1985); and maternal stimulation at 2 and 5 months with infant visual and tactual exploration (Bornstein & Tamis-LeMonda, 1989).

Tamis-LeMonda and Bornstein (1990) focused on a phenomenon referred to as *maternal didactic stimulation* and explored how such behaviors were related to developmental competence. Maternal didactic stimulation was defined as a naturally occurring, caregiver-initiated activity such as attempting to engage the infant's attention by highlighting properties of objects and events in the immediate environment. The caregiver would demonstrate how an object worked, pointing toward the object, naming the object, describing the unique qualities of the object, and so on. Since earlier studies had demonstrated that training parents to behave in a particular fashion correlated with language comprehension, play competence, and attention span, Tamis-LeMonda and Bornstein decided to track four key developmental milestones in their study. These milestones included language production, language comprehension, play competence, and attention span. To examine systematically the interrelations among these four significant areas of development, the researchers assessed developmental status in each of these areas beginning when the infants were 13 months of age. A corollary goal of the study was to consider the role played by maternal didactic stimulation in relation to the development of each of these milestones.

The methodology of the study included home visits to observe free play.

Investigators also administered extensive maternal interviews that probed perceptions in each of the four developmental areas. The study revealed that, on average, mothers engaged their infants through didactic stimulation during approximately 75% of the observed intervals. Some mothers, however, exhibited didactic stimulation during only 33% of the intervals, whereas other mothers manifested didactic behaviors almost 100% of the time. It was also found that maternal didactic stimulation was significantly associated with language comprehension and play competence. In contrast, no similar association was found for language production or attention span. Moreover, the researchers noted that even when maternal didactic stimulation was considered in isolation, infants manifested increased competence over time in each of the developmental areas examined, suggesting an *innate* timetable that might be enhanced by, but was not entirely dependent on, contemporaneous maternal stimulation.

This study provides significant insight for understanding how previewing behaviors may affect maternal and infant developmental trends. First, unlike some of the studies discussed earlier that relied on a form of training, Tamis-LeMonda and Bornstein sought to examine a naturally occurring maternal behavior, more akin to the formal handling manifestations discussed by Hopkins and Westra. Tamis-LeMonda and Bornstein examined how a more all-encompassing form of behavior affected several different domains of infant competence. The findings suggest that caregivers possess particular kinds of naturally occurring skills (e.g., previewing) designed to enhance the infant's development. Another finding that emerged from the study was that virtually all of the mothers examined manifested evidence of didactic stimulation, although they exhibited this skill in varying degrees. This observation suggests a spectrum of maternal didactic behaviors: Although most mothers use didactic stimulation 75% of the time, smaller groups either display these manifestations far less (33%) or more frequently (100%). Finally, this study is significant because it establishes that spontaneous behavior(s) can enhance developmental competence across a wide variety of domains.

Heckhausen (1987) formulated the *one-step-ahead* concept. This model seeks to explain how, to encourage the infant in mastery behaviors, the mother may balance for the infant's weaknesses by intentionally guiding certain actions, as well as by helping the infant master subskills necessary for a particular developmental skill. The caregiver accomplishes this by establishing a specific action goal, sharing this goal with the infant when necessary, breaking the interaction into substeps, and carefully monitoring and guiding the infant's manifestations.

Heckhausen designed a longitudinal study to track intradyadic developmental change. The study focused on the interactions of 12 infants performing various tasks. These dyads were videotaped on five occasions at bimonthly intervals between the infants' 14th and 22nd months. As the infants gained greater mastery over certain tasks, the caregivers gradually withdrew their support. Heckhausen found that mothers adhered to a one-step-method strategy when adapting their instructions to their infant's current level of mastery. Heckhausen noted that throughout the period of the study, the mothers devoted substantial effort to supplementing their infant's actions. Heckhausen concluded that the infant's performance was the product of *joint effort* by mother and infant for the purpose of supplementing the infant's developmental skills.

Through their research, each of these investigators offers confirmation of the notion that most adaptive caregivers tend to engage in some form of instrumental behavior that appears designed to stimulate and enhance the infant's developmental skill. Moreover, these studies suggest that caregiver manifestations in this regard are quite specific. That is, the caregiver appears to possess an intuitive sensitivity to the infant's current developmental level and can precisely predict the scope of imminent attainment.

Nevertheless, these studies omit reference to the dyadic members' subjective processes during the process of developmental acquisition. In particular, caregiver representational skills not only allow the caregiver to formulate an impression of the milestones on the next developmental horizon, but also enable rehearsing imminent interpersonal changes that will occur because of enhanced developmental attainments. The caregiver previews to the infant what the experience of a particular developmental milestone will be like and, significantly, rehearses with the infant how future attainment of the milestone will *change* the relationship they share. This approach provides the infant with a paradigm from which to experience a sense of continuity over emotional experience and controllability over developmental phenomena.

From Action to Representation. Several researchers, including Main, Kaplan, and Cassidy (1985), Benoit, Zeanah, and Barton (1989), Stern (1985, 1989), and George and Solomon (1989), have discussed the evolution of internal representations within the context of the dyadic relationship. These internal representations occur in both caregiver and infant and essentially comprise numerous replications of external experience.

To understand how representations activate and guide interpersonal processes, it is necessary to examine the caregiver's subjective representations, particularly during interaction with the infant. The representation of relational patterns may be viewed as the abstraction of various subjective experiences. For the purposes of the previewing process, internal representations are those mental processes embodying not only previous or current interactions, but also anticipatory predictions concerning future interaction.

Several researchers have suggested that representations are organized in a hierarchical fashion, with more general, global representations superseding specific representational imagery. Stern (1989), for example, has suggested that a sequence of interaction between caregiver and infant is encoded by the caregiver as an *episodic memory*. A group of episodic memories that resemble one another is then abstracted into a *prototype memory* or *representation*. This prototype signifies the lowest level in the representational hierarchy. When the prototype memory represents a group of similar interactive moments or sequences (e.g., feeding, walking, talking, playing), the representation has been *generalized*. More extensive interactive sequences are represented at the next level in the hierarchy, which Stern identifies as a *represented scenario*. This level of representation contains diverse interactive sequences, such as play sequences. The integration of these sequences into a unified whole has been denominated as an *internal working model*, a concept originally coined by Bowlby (1969). This level of representation encodes not only the "content" but also the "nature of the emotions" experienced and the "meaning" attributed to such experiences. At this level of organization, internal working models play an important role in regulating the interpersonal behavior within the dyad.

Interactive moments have also been referred to as *scripts*. Nelson and Gruendel (1981) have indicated that the qualities associated with scripts are relevant to understanding the infant's organization of knowledge. This is because scripts are temporal and causal sequences of action, within which variable elements may be inserted to provide structure to the experience. The representations formulated during the previewing process resemble such scripts because they depend on causal connections and also incorporate events over time. Exposure to previewing episodes helps the infant experiment with causal connections, predict temporal sequences, and test their consistency over time. Thus, previewing reinforces the infant's developing subjective capacities.

An understanding of the way in which internal working models evolve provides a more profound understanding of how the caregiver represents the dyadic relationship and guides it in the direction of either adaptation or dysfunction. For example, when parents manifest dysfunction during interaction with the infant, this dysfunction often stems from patterns acquired during the parents' own childhood experiences. An examination of parental representations may therefore enable the therapist to predict a rigid and inflexible social interaction. Such parents tend to resist change by adhering to patterns that comply with previously set expectations. In contrast, adaptive caregivers tend to disclose internal representations that are flexible and resilient, enabling them to generate highly adaptive interpersonal behaviors.

George and Solomon (1989) examined the correlation of the internal working models of caregivers with the infant's security of attachment and demonstrated a strong association between them. Children who manifested a relaxed demeanor, coupled with an eagerness to interact with their mother after a period of separation, were inherently secure in their attachment to their caregiver. When interviewed, the mothers of these securely attached children conveyed two significant and distinctive characteristics. First, their responses reflected a realistic consideration of potentially attachment-threatening situations. This finding suggests that mothers with securely attached infants are capable of processing external information relevant to their role as the caregiving figure. Second, such mothers appeared to possess an objective representation of themselves and of their child, and were capable of integrating this knowledge with situation-specific information. These representational capacities permitted them to manifest supportive and effective caregiving behaviors. For example, such mothers described their decision for either withholding or providing support according to the particular situation. Such decisions were based on careful considerations of the child's developmental capabilities and needs. Their comments indicated that both mother and child participated in what has been referred to as a *goal-corrected partnership:* a situation wherein each dyadic member considers and evaluates the needs of his or her partner before engaging in purposeful action.

In contrast to the adaptive mothers, researchers have found that mothers of children with a lower degree of security were incapable of assessing themselves and their children effectively and that they excluded important information from their perceptions of the infant. For example, these mothers described themselves as individuals who were ineffective in meeting the child's needs, because they did not know exactly what the child needed or how the child perceived the environment. Characteristically, such caregivers distorted, ignored, or denied their own perceptions of relevant cues concerning their child's capabilities. For instance, some of these caregivers minimized potential threats to the child, discounted the child's distress, and commented that their support was unnecessary because of the child's precocious independence. Others displayed tendencies to increase potential risks to the child, while overreacting to benign situations. Finally, some mothers were so overwhelmed by threats to the child's security that all they could do was describe their desire to flee from the situation. In each of these cases, the mother's needs dominated and clouded her thinking, such that they overshadowed perceptions of the infant's needs. Moreover, these mothers characteristically failed to describe the relationship with the infant as one involving mutual accommodation. In general, mothers whose infants were insecurely attached seemed less capable of maintaining an objective perception of themselves or of their infants.

The following vignette exemplifies this point.

THERAPIST: What changes in your infant have you noticed in the past few weeks?

CAREGIVER: He sucks his fingers. I hate it when he does that. I don't have any control over it. I feel he has so much control over me. No matter what I tell him, he still puts his fingers in his mouth.

THERAPIST: What do you mean by control?

CAREGIVER: I mean obeying me. He doesn't obey me. The older he gets, the less control I have over him.

THERAPIST: How does his behavior make you feel?

CAREGIVER: I just want him to love me and not resent me. As his autonomy increases, I feel like his affection for me decreases.

Using a different research approach, Zeanah, Benoit, and Barton (1986) asked a group of 37 parents shortly after the birth of their infants to describe their representations of their infants' personalities and behaviors during both general and specific situations. Subsequently, 1 year later when the infants were 12 months old, the parents were interviewed to discuss their responses to their infants' behavior during episodes when the infant manifested distress or was difficult to control. Parents were asked to characterize their overall relationship with the infant, to articulate what pleased and displeased them about the relationship, and, significantly, to express how they expected the relationship with the infant to change over time as the infant became more adept developmentally. The infants' attachment behavior was evaluated using the Strange Situation procedure (Ainsworth & Wittig, 1969). Forty-three percent of the infants were securely attached, 37% were avoidantly attached, and 20% were ambivalently attached.

The researchers' classification of maternal representations was based on the following qualities:

1. *Richness of Perception.* The relative poverty or richness of the parents' description of the infant as an individual and of the parents' relationship to the infant.

2. *Openness to Change.* The parents' flexibility in internalizing new information about the infant.

3. *Flexibility.* The caregivers' receptivity to infant developmental change.

4. *Intensity of Involvement.* The amount of maternal preoccupation with the infant and/or the mother's psychological immersion in the relationship with the infant.

5. *Coherence of Narrative Descriptions.* The overall sense of order contained in the mother's representation of the infant. In particular, coherence in this regard focused on the organization and logical flow of ideas and feelings regarding the infant and the relationship to the infant.

6. *Maternal Sensitivity.* The mother's ability to convey, in descriptions of the infant, both a recognition and valuing of the infant's affective

experience. In particular, sensitivity referred to whether the mother perceived the infant as experiencing a variety of emotional states and biological needs or whether the mother viewed the infant as an individual with unique needs, and whether the infant's needs for dependency and autonomy were accepted in a developmentally appropriate fashion.

Some caregivers manifested estranged representations, indicating a distorted impression of the infant. In these cases, the mother seemed preoccupied or distracted by other concerns, confused or anxiously overwhelmed by the infant, or self-involved and insensitive to the infant as an individual.

Maternal representation of the infants, based on the interview with the mother, disclosed that 46% of mothers had "balanced" perceptions, 30% had "disengaged" perceptions, and 24% had "estranged" perceptions. Furthermore, mothers who demonstrated "balanced" representations, in which infant autonomy was not viewed as a threatening phenomenon, tended to have securely attached infants. This study is noteworthy because it demonstrates the strong correlation between the nature of maternal representations of the infant shortly after birth and subsequent attachment patterns that become evident when the infant is 12 months old. Observations of caregiver ministrations during previewing episodes validate the notion that the evolution of a maternal internal working model is a continual process during which the caregiver devises and experiments with a diversity of current and anticipated responses.

The Infant's Perspective

From Perception to Representation. Although the caregiver, through her representations and subsequent ministrations, introduces the infant to future developmental attainment, considering the infant's representational capacities is also crucial in order to understand how he contributes to the previewing process. For this purpose, it is necessary to examine the infant's emerging representational abilities in the context of the caregiver's interpersonal behaviors.

As has been noted, numerous developmental events consolidate during the first 2 years of life. None, however, is as seminal for understanding the infant's ability to engage in interpersonal communication as is the emergence of the *sense of self*. Although it is not possible to tap the infant's subjective perceptions directly, researchers can ascertain the nature of these perceptions by following the evolution of the infant's ability to recognize himself and others. The sense of self is a developmental milestone that gradually emerges from the constitutional organization inherent in the infant. Understanding how the sense of self emerges provides insight into how the infant coordinates his perceptions of the external world and his unique position in it.

At birth a diversity of developmental skills exist in an inchoate state. These skills allow the infant to perceive and process information about the external world in a rudimentary fashion. Stern (1985) has pointed out that, during the first 2 months of life, affective and cognitive processes cannot readily be separated from one another. Thus, learning and perception appear to be affect-laden. As a result, researchers have been able to interpret cognitive development during this period, as well as during most of infancy, by evaluating the overt emotions manifested by the infant. By 2 months of age, dramatic changes in the infant's behavior become apparent. Specific developmental skills, including eye-to-eye contact and social smiling (which allow for a better engagement with the external world) and tendencies such as the pursuit of sensory stimulation, appear to crystallize (Bruner, 1977; Cohen & Salapalek, 1975; Lamb & Sherrod, 1981; Lipsitt, 1983). Also by this time infants appear to possess distinct preferences with regard to the sensations they seek. Another characteristic evident at this time is that infants appear to have an overall tendency to form and test hypotheses about what is occurring in the world; that is, young infants seem continually to be evaluating and appraising their status and their role with respect to external phenomena (Kagan, Kearsley, & Zelazo, 1978). The infant is perpetually asking such questions as, is this stimulus different from or the same as the previous one? or, how discrepant is this stimulus from the previous one? Thus, it appears that initially the infant is in a state of what has been referred to as "alert activity"; although the infant has not yet begun to interject purpose and intention into his actions, he nevertheless appears to possess mechanisms that motivate him in the direction of experiencing the diverse phenomena of the external world (Stern, 1985).

This organizing tendency leads to the infant's categorization of events in the external world. *Categorization* has been defined as the process whereby perceptually distinctive stimuli that nonetheless share certain qualities are treated equivalently (Berlin, 1978; Medin, 1983). Researchers have suggested that from quite an early age—perhaps as early as 3 months—the infant formulates categories of experiences that are relatively invariant (Resnick & Kagan, 1983). Each new experience the infant encounters in the environment will reinforce or slightly modify the previous categorization. One example of this would be the infant's ability during the first months of life to distinguish between different colors and to categorize them in a manner similar to adults' categories (Bornstein, 1981). In a recent series of experiments Hayne, Rovee-Collier, and Perris (1987) tested 3-month-old infants' acquisition and long-term retention of category-specific information. Infants who were trained with a perceptually different category of stimulus on 3 consecutive days generalized, responding to a novel instance of the original training category, but not to a stimulus from a novel category. These infants were, in other words, able to categorize stimuli. Two weeks later, when infants displayed no evidence of remembering their prior training experience, categorization was reinstated if the investigators used a stimulus from the original training category as the retrieval cue.

These data are among the first to document retention of category-specific information in infants over extended intervals. Thus, 3-month-old infants are able to categorize and can exhibit this skill with similar forms of stimulation even after 24-hour intervals. Moreover, these same infants were also able to engage in categorization after an interval of 2 weeks had elapsed, if provided with cues appropriate to the stimuli. The researchers concluded that categorization may be viewed as the product of repeated retrieval whereby infants differentially exploit their memories of individual stimuli. This study is noteworthy, because it emphasizes that even at a very early age infants begin to form cognitive groupings of their experiences and are able to use these categorizations to respond to the world in a predictable fashion.

For the purpose of mental economy and efficiency, the infant's representational capacities are fueled by his need to *separate* representations, organizing the social interactions to which he has been exposed (Stern, 1989). By formulating an impression about which characteristics belong to which experiences, the infant begins to discover which characteristics of an experience are *invariant* and which features are *variant* (Gibson, 1979). Otherwise, the infant would need to possess a memory capacity that records every interaction with the caregiver and consequently generates a vast array of expectations—a virtually impossible feat. Given the complexity of that task, it is more likely that the infant forms general *categories* of interactions and then, on the basis of such generalizations, formulates expectations about future events.

Another capacity that contributes to the infant's emergent sense of self is the skill of *amodal perception*. Amodal perception refers to the ability to transfer information perceived through one perceptual modality—such as sight—to another perceptual modality—such as touch. This skill explains how individuals come to coordinate and integrate sensory impressions, permitting them to arrive at the conclusion that what is seen, heard, smelled, and touched may in fact originate from a single entity. Another way of phrasing this ability is to say that amodal perception refers to the innate ability to coordinate information that is perceived through different perceptual modalities, but that nevertheless emanates from a single external source. For example, Meltzoff and Borton (1979) conducted an experiment whereby they blindfolded 3-month-old infants and allowed them to suck one of two different pacifiers. The pacifiers differed in the texture of the nipple. After the infant had gained some experience touching the nipples with his mouth, the blindfold was removed. Following rapid visual comparison of both nipples lying side by side, the infants spent significantly more time looking at the nipple they had sucked. This finding suggests that from a very early age infants may be able to form an internal representation of what an object, such as a nipple, feels like, as well as a representation of what the nipple looks like, and may subsequently be able to reconcile the two perceptions.

During this period of the infant's development, caregiver previewing behavior contributes significantly to the infant's emerging amodal perceptual capabilities and to the resulting coalescence of a coherent sense of perception. For example, when the caregiver engages in "baby talk," she does not merely preview speech for the infant, but also incorporates other perceptual communications into her behaviors. Thus, the auditory aspect of speech will be coordinated with rhythmic stroking of the infant and with exaggerated facial expressions that capture the infant's visual attention. When the infant responds positively, the caregiver is motivated to repeat these behaviors, fostering amodal integration of the speech through auditory perception, tactile perception (stroking), and visual perception (facial expression).

What about integration of other perceptual modes and other qualities of perception, such as intensity? Are infants equally gifted in recognizing these qualities amodally? Lewkowicz and Turkewitz (1980), using heart rate as an outcome measure in a habituation paradigm, examined 3-week-old infants with respect to which levels of light intensity (luminescence of white light) corresponded best with certain levels of sound intensity (decibels of white noise). The infants were habituated to one level of sound, and attempts at dishabituation were then made with various levels of light, and vice versa. The results of this observation disclosed that these very young infants were able to correlate certain absolute levels of sound intensity with specific absolute levels of light intensity. Moreover, the matches of intensity level across perceptual modes that the 3-week-olds found to be most correspondent were the same matches selected by adults. As a consequence, the ability to transfer from audio to visual modes and vice versa appears to be established, at least in rudimentary form, by 3 weeks of age.

Finally, of all the perceptual transfers, the most problematic to imagine is how an infant transfers information about shape between the visual and auditory modes. The transfer of shape is more readily imagined across the tactile and visual modes. But speech itself is generally a visual as well as an acoustic phenomenon. Studies have shown that attention to speech rises considerably when the lips are in view; 6-week-old babies tend to look more closely at faces that speak (Haith, 1980). In addition, when the actual sound produced is in conflict with the lip movements observed, the visual information unexpectedly predominates over the auditory. Thus, infants, as well as adults, tend to hear what they see, more than what may actually be said (McGurk & MacDonald, 1976).

Each of these observations reinforces the view that infants appear to experience a world of perceptual unity in which they are capable of perceiving amodal qualities in any modality or form of human expressive behavior, and that they are subsequently able to represent these qualities *abstractly* and transfer them to other modalities. Developmentalists such as Bower (1974), Moore and Meltzoff (1978), and Meltzoff (1988) have hypothesized that from the earliest days of life the infant not only elaborates, but also acts on abstract representations of the various qualities in any given experience. The experiences that the infant represents abstractly are the shapes, intensities, and the temporal qualities of events and experiences that he perceives. Thus, amodal perception plays an important role for integrating potentially diverse experiences of self and other, as well as for coordinating physiological and psychological functions.

Another capacity by which young infants may experience a sense of emergent self is through physiognomic perception. Werner (1948) posited that emotion serves as a common denominator for converting stimulation from one modality to another. This researcher has suggested that physiognomic perception arises from repeated exposure to the human face, with its myriad emotional expressions. The existence of physiognomic perception in young infants is only speculative at this time. Nevertheless, previewing exercises that expose the infant to new didactic skills in an atmosphere of positive emotion are likely to enhance the infant's physiognomic perceptual abilities.

Stern has also described a third quality of experience that the infant is exposed to as a result of interaction with the caregiver. This quality, referred to as *vitality affects,* is defined as the characteristic impression left by an emotion. Some examples of vitality affects include feelings of surging or fading emotions, crescendo or peak emotions that occur after a period of emotional build-up, and bursting emotions. These emotional experiences occur daily to infants, elicited by changes in appetite, motivational state, and tension. Vitality affects often insinuate themselves into interactions between mother and infant. During previewing exercises caregivers rely on various vitality affects to mediate and reinforce their infants' behaviors. By expressing surging joy, waning attention, and other transitional emotions, mothers communicate with their infants in a manner that is accessible to the newborn. Thus, vitality affects represent another aspect of the dyadic communication that is reinforced during previewing exercises, fostering the infant's sense of coherence and organization and thereby hastening the consolidation of a sense of self.

Amodal perception and vitality affects are an analogy to categorization and may be found in the infant's perception of interpersonal stimulation deriving from the caregiver. For example, suppose that the infant is engaging in a particular interaction (e.g., playing) for the first time. No representation of the particular experience that is taking place yet exists. By the time the interaction has taken place, however, the infant begins to identify the invariant aspects of the interactive sequence. After repeated exposure to the experience, the infant identifies the invariant features of the experience and, significantly, creates *prototypes* that represent the particular interactive moment. Gradually, an *internal working model* that embodies the infant's evaluations and expectations about play sequences evolves. During previewing exercises with the caregiver, the infant will begin experimenting with and testing these representations. From the repetitive exposure to such interactions the infant begins to abstract about the new developmental achievements, their precise function(s), and their interpersonal implications. As he begins to recognize that precursory changes represent invariant features of a more global or generalized function (i.e., a particular skill), the categorization of precursory changes into a global function provides the infant with a representational arena for coordinating subfunctions into more evolved skills.

From Representation to Action. By approximately 3 months, skills in the area of amodal perception and categorization have congealed, permitting the infant to formulate abstractions about his responsivity to the world around him. For Stern (1985), this is the period when the *core self* consolidates. The core self consists of four rudimentary characteristics that describe the infant's subjective awareness of both the external world and his own role as a participant in that world.

The first component of the core self is a sense of *self-agency,* which means that the infant possesses a sense of authorship of his own actions and nonauthorship of the actions of others. In other words, the infant believes he has volition and control over self-generated actions and is able to develop expectations about the consequences of his actions. The next component of the core self is *self-coherence,* which signifies that the infant has a sense of being a nonfragmented, physical entity with boundaries and a locus of integrated action, both during activity and at rest. The third component of the core self is *self-affectivity,* which refers to the infant's experience of inner qualities of feeling that are associated with the experience of the self. Finally, by this juncture, the infant possesses a *self-history,* which means that the infant has a sense of enduring, of a continuity with his own past, so that he goes on being and can even change while remaining the same. In essence, the core self results from the integration of these four basic self-experiences, along with a social awareness of the world. Once the core self has consolidated, the infant is able to respond to the stimuli presented by the caregiver, including, most significantly, her previewing manifestations indicative of imminent development.

The caregiver's previewing behavior fuels the infant's understanding of the external world in other ways as well. Specifically, previewing may be understood as a particular kind of language that the caregiver uses to help the infant organize his perceptions of external reality. As has been noted, previewing encompasses the immediate behavioral gestures of the caregiver. If a caregiver previews crawling to the infant by exercising his limbs in a particular way, for example, she communicates the message that crawling consists of that particular combination of neuromuscular alignment and movement. Thus, the caregiver's physical manifestations communicate unique and distinctive messages to the infant. This mode of communication, in which the content of the message and the means used to convey the message are the same, is referred to as the *analogic mode* (Watzlawick, Beavin, & Jacobson, 1967). When the caregiver engages in previewing exercises with the infant, however, she not only is conveying a message about the current activity, but is also orienting the infant toward the interpersonal implications that will arise from imminent developmental achievement. When the caregiver previews the future changes of crawling, for example, she is communicating to the infant the notion, "This is what the sensation of crawling will feel like someday soon when you develop sufficient skill to crawl on your own," while simultaneously conveying to the infant, "This is how you and I will interact when you are able to crawl by yourself." These messages are symbolic, though, in the sense that the simulated crawling behavior serves as a metaphor for the infant's future experience when he successfully negotiates this developmental milestone. The communication of symbolic messages occurs through the *digital mode*. During digital communication, the means used to represent the message is different from the message itself. The most sophisticated type of digital communication is language, whereby objects and concepts can be signified by arbitrary symbols. This is not to suggest that the manifestation of previewing exercises resembles the digital mode of communication in the same fashion that words do. Nonetheless, previewing does signify an effective and unifying form of communication for the infant because it combines elements of both digital and analogic modes of communication. As such, it is a flexible mode of communication that exposes the infant to the direct visceral experience of analogic communication, while at the same time conveying a symbolic or digital component.

Exposure to these two powerful aspects of communication during previewing exercises further aids the infant in consolidating connections between internal and external perceptions. Furthermore, because much of this communication involves the mother's messages about the infant's current and future developmental states, the infant is receiving immediate assistance in his efforts at self-definition and self-consolidation.

As the infant progresses beyond a sense of core self, he also begins to recognize that his perceptual capacities are different from the perceptual capacities of others. This realization, which occurs between 7 and 9 months, is enhanced by the infant's awareness that he can share inner subjective experiences with others. For this subjective sense of self to emerge, Stern postulates that there must be a shared framework of meaning accompanied by a means of communication with the caregiver. Because at this point in their development infants are still preverbal, the subjective experiences that they undergo and seek to share with the caregiver must not require translation into language. Previewing exercises may fill this role and being a mix of both analogic and digital forms of communication, they are likely to be important in the emergence of the subjective self.

As the infant becomes aware that others possess their own separate subjective experience, a quality Trevarthan (1980, 1985) has labeled intersubjectivity, the caregiver's regulation of the infant's subjective experience attains preeminent significance. What is the quantity and quality of the subjective experience to be shared? Once the infant begins experiencing these concerns, he is firmly on the path to a sense of self-agency and self-mastery, and the repeated previewing exercises engaged in by his mother serve the infant as a check on reality and an encouragement to proceed with the task of self-integration.

In achieving a sense of subjective self, the infant also begins a process that Stern describes as "affect attunement." Stern states that the broadest and most clinically important aspect of relatedness between mother and infant is the sharing of affective states. This sharing of emotions is sometimes referred to as *parental mirroring* and other times is called *empathic responsiveness* (Hoffman, 1977).

The final stage of self-development occurs during the 2nd year of life, when language emerges. At this time, infants begin to imagine and represent places, events, and things in a way that involves symbols. By this juncture they are also able to conceive themselves as objective entities. The infant can now entertain a perception of how reality ought to be in contrast to how it actually is. In other words, as Stern points out, the infant can begin to engage in speculative fantasy.

If the infant's needs have been insufficiently met or if a dramatic negative change occurs in his environment, he risks embarking on a self-delusionary path characterized by wishes and withdrawal. Inadequate or faulty previewing can contribute to the infant's risk for psychopathology in several ways. If there is an implied threat communicated to the infant by the caregiver as a consequence of her own feelings of inadequacy, the child may experience insecurity that taints his future mastery efforts. This kind of negative previewing may cause the child to become precocious in his relationship with the caregiver, by engaging in maturational skill without fully appreciating its implications for the dyadic relationship. Without being exposed to previewing exercises, the infant will fail to attribute any particular significance to the achievement of developmental milestones. Lacking a clear understanding of the value of his own achievements, the infant will have difficulty establishing a coherent, meaningful relationship with the external world and with others.

Just as a lack of previewing can expose the infant to future psychopathology, dyadic treatment also can use strategies derived from the previewing process as an interventive technique to prevent this outcome. One reason previewing is such an effective intervention strategy is that it focuses attention on future events. This prospective approach alerts the therapist to the emergence of potential conflict in the caregiver before the conflict is subjected to defensive operations or becomes an entrenched pattern of behavior within the dyadic relationship. Previewing thus focuses on the caregiver's subjective perceptions of the future and allows the therapist to understand the implications of these perceptions on the dyadic relationship. As a preventive technique, previewing allows the caregiver to become attuned to both the infant's and her own perspective, and to integrate adaptive, growth-enhancing behaviors into her interaction with the infant, based on the therapist's guidance.

CONCLUSION

This chapter has introduced the reader to the concept of previewing, a unique phenomenon that occurs within the dyadic relationship and allows the caregiver gradually to introduce the infant to the contours of imminent developmental change, as well as to the implications such change will have for the relationship between mother and infant. The previewing process itself may be divided into several components. First, the caregiver must be able to represent images of the infant's current and prospective development on the stage of active consciousness. Subsequently, the caregiver will convert these representations into previewing exercises during which the infant is specifically introduced to a particular developmental milestone in a supportive fashion. The caregiver will here use various intuitive behaviors, such as visual and vocal cuing, as well as bodily support, to simulate the behaviors characteristic of the upcoming milestone. Finally, the caregiver will be sensitive to the infant's desire to cease the previewing activity and return to his earlier developmental status.

To engage in adaptive previewing, the caregiver must be alert to her own representations of infant development. She must also recognize, however, that the infant too possesses a particular perspective on events. As development proceeds, the infant gradually distinguishes his own sense of self from that of the others around him, particularly the caregiver. The caregiver's sensitivity to the infant's development allows her to devise previewing exercises that are appropriate to his particular level as he begins to differentiate a core sense of self. The caregiver's previewing behaviors during the first 2 years of life are especially important because the infant is striving to forge an adaptive relationship with the caregiver—who serves as his guide to imminent development—while at the same time attempting to assert a sense of self and autonomy. This chapter has sought to describe the process of maturation that the infant undergoes during this period. Only a caregiver who is sensitive to the implications of these events can help the infant achieve an appropriate balance between his reliance on her goal-oriented partnership and the urgings of his own autonomy.

This chapter has also discussed scenarios in which the infant is deprived of exposure to previewing. In such situations, the infant will experience developmental events as arbitrary phenomena and his relationship with the caregiver is likely to be insecure. In these cases dyadic treatment using previewing techniques as a form of intervention may overcome emotional conflict in the dyad. By introducing previewing into the relationship the therapist provides, perhaps for the first time, organization for the rapport between caregiver and infant, enhancing the perceptions of developmental trends, as well as the role of the caregiver in fostering the infant's development. The following chapters explore these themes in greater detail.

Chapter 2

The Role of Parents in Infant Development

INTRODUCTION

Until recently most researchers in the area of early childhood development believed that the primary relationship experienced by the infant during the first several years of life was the relationship with the mother. Indeed, attachment theorists have commented that infants are *monotropically matricentric* in orientation, meaning that the infant tends to focus his proximity-seeking behaviors on one significant other person and that this person is, more often than not, the mother. Moreover, laboratory paradigms that evaluate the level of emotional security inherent in the infant's attachment relationship have relied primarily on evaluating the infant's relationship with the maternal figure, rather than the relationship with the paternal figure. The underlying assumption, then, has traditionally been that the mother generally assumes the predominant caregiving role as a result of both biological and social factors, and as such, it is the mother whose guidance and support results in the infant's ability to establish a primary relationship during infancy.

In the past decade, however, many of these assumptions have been questioned and have come under closer scrutiny. Studies have revealed that infants display a flexible ability to bond closely with virtually any adult figure who interacts with them on a regular and consistent basis and provides them with adequate stimulation. Although some studies suggest that infants may prefer interacting with mothers, preference for fathers has also been demonstrated, especially during play activity that relies more heavily on motor skills. Thus, the infant's preferences do not appear to be grounded in the parent's gender per se. For example, when fathers are trained to introduce the infant to certain behaviors, the infant orients to the father for these kinds of cues just as readily as to the mother. Thus, as a result of intervention, as well as the amount of time the father devotes to interaction with the infant, preferences can be minimized and virtually disappear.

As social mores have changed and as research findings have been reported, professionals have recognized that the father's role in the infant's development is important for many reasons. Where the mother is a victim of a developmental deficit, the infant may have no adult figure, besides the father, who can facilitate maturation and guide the child through the challenges posed by imminent developmental change. It then becomes crucial to determine whether the father possesses the same capacity for nurturance that is generally attributed to the mother. In addition, is the father's sensitivity to maturational trends comparable to the mother's, so that paternal *previewing* behaviors can be used to enhance the infant's exposure to imminent development and reinforce rapport within the dyadic relationship?

Studies of paternal behaviors and attitudes suggest that fathers, in fact, manifest skills comparable to mothers' skills for providing the stimulation necessary to promote adaptive development. Fathers observed with their newborns manifest many of the same behaviors that have been identified in new mothers as being *intuitive,* including gazing, holding patterns, and frequency of vocalization. As a result, fathers may be as competent as mothers in previewing imminent development for their progeny.

This chapter reviews the evidence demonstrating how fathers contribute to the promotion of optimal interpersonal adaptation during the developmental change that ultimately leads the infant toward self-regulation. Following a review of recent studies that have investigated the paternal role in fostering the infant's adaptive development, there is a discussion of how the therapist can interact with fathers to enhance their previewing capacities.

EARLY PREDICTORS OF THE FATHER–INFANT INTERACTION

Paternal Mental Representations

Some fathers become active participants in their child's daily care because of their own father's lack of involvement (Radin, 1985; Russell, 1983). Other fathers who became involved with their infants appear to be conforming to a model of participation established by their own paternal figures (Sagi, 1982). Diverse factors that lead to enhanced paternal participation in child care include the father's attendance at childbirth classes and presence at the actual birth (Russell, 1983).

Paternal *mental representations* either in the form of dreams or fantasies during the wife's pregnancy have demonstrated that childbirth and the arrival of an infant represent significant psychological events for fathers. The content of such dreams and fantasies suggests that fathers, just as mothers, possess a deep psychological need to develop an attachment with the infant and to play a seminal role in the infant's development (Trad, 1990). The most typical paternal fantasies involve concerns about the physical condition of the wife or infant, and about being a good father and having enough money to support the family financially. A typical fantasy is the fear that the wife will give birth to a deformed infant. A second common theme involves the father's positive feelings at the impending birth and his assumption of the role of fatherhood. A third theme focuses on the fear of damage or trauma to the self or spouse unrelated to the pregnancy. Lastly, fathers tend to report dreams concerning preparation for the impending birth and the change in life patterns the birth will bring.

With respect to the studies that have attempted to document the perceptions of expectant fathers, Herzog (1982) reported on the experiences of 103 first-time fathers whose wives had given birth prematurely. Herzog identified two distinct groups. The first group included fathers who were highly cognizant of their feelings and fantasies pertaining to the pregnancy and were labeled the "attuned group"; the second group was "out of touch" with these feelings.

Herzog found that fathers experienced three kinds of fantasies. During the fathering phase, attuned fathers reported fantasies relating to "plumbing, circuitry and other varieties of connecting imagery" (p. 90). During the second trimester, fathers were concerned with the infant's personality and fantasized about playing with the infant. The expectant father began to think of the fetus as a separate individual, with an identity apart from that of the parents. The sex of the child was visualized as well during this period. Fantasies during this stage were often aggressive or intrusive. For example, some fathers expressed a wish to "hurt the baby, as well as welcome it" (p. 90). By the end of the pregnancy such fantasies declined, and reveries turned toward preparations for the arrival of the child in the real world. These fantasies are important not only for ascertaining the psychological status of the expectant father, but also for revealing the similarity of expectations shared by both mothers and fathers.

Sherwen studied primiparous expectant couples with a minimum of a high school education. Subjects came from a similar socioeconomic background, had no medically or psychologically diagnosed illness, and were in the third trimester of the pregnancy. The researcher divided the subjects into three groups and used various instruments including the Imaginal Processes Inventory (the "IPI"), developed by Singer and Antrobus (1972). This scale focuses on such factors as the frequency of the fantasizing, positive reactions, frightened reactions and visual imagery, problem-solving themes, present and future temporal orientations, bizarre fantasies, and fear of failure.

The Bem Sex Inventory (Bem, 1974) was administered to determine the sex role orientation of the prospective mothers and fathers. Bem, who devised the instrument, was persuaded that individuals may display both masculine and feminine qualities (referred to as androgynous sex type) depending on situational demands. Subjects rate themselves and are classified as "masculine," "feminine," or "androgynous." Finally, the researcher administered the Bills Affectional Relationship Questionnaire (Bills, 1980), which measures the father's affectional bond with the infant before and after delivery, as well as the extent of the father's involvement in the pregnancy.

Overall, expectant mothers and fathers were "not significantly different" in their fantasy patterns. Expectant mothers, however, did have a higher degree of night-dreaming fantasy and a higher degree of frightening or anxiety-filled fantasies. With regard to the issue of whether the parents' sexual role orientation affected fantasy patterns, Sherwen found that fathers with a "feminine orientation" had the highest scores on fear of failure in daydreams, bizarre daydreams, and fear reactions to their daydreams, as well as in their daydreaming frequency. On the other hand, fathers with a "masculine orientation" had the highest scores on present-oriented daydreams. An inverse relationship was found between paternal daydreaming frequency and paternal involvement with the infant.

Significantly, these studies demonstrate that fathers and mothers do not appear to have significant differences in the content of their fantasies. In addition, there is evidence supporting the notion that the sex role orientation of the father contributes to the degree of his involvement with the infant. Expectant fathers experience high levels of fantasy comparable to the levels experienced by expectant mothers, and these fantasies tend to involve the same anxieties, fears, and aspirations embedded in the fantasies of pregnant women. As a consequence, fathers most likely undergo deep psychological change and a period of evaluation during their wives' pregnancy. These psychological changes are an appropriate area for inquiry during treatment.

As a result, it is recommended that therapists treating pregnant women should also involve prospective fathers and encourage the fathers to discuss the fantasies they are experiencing, with particular emphasis on fantasies dealing with the fears and anticipations surrounding the infant's birth. Fathers should be invited to participate in the sessions and to express their perceptions and predictions whenever possible. This paternal emphasis may be particularly important because after the birth of the child, attention will undoubtedly focus on the infant first and the mother second, leaving the father to deal with the ramifications of his fantasies himself. To avoid this outcome, the therapist should emphasize the seminal role played by the father and his contribution to infant development.

Therapists treating dyads should explore paternal representations whenever possible, either by involving the father directly in the treatment or by exploring the issue with the mother and encouraging the mother to ask the father to speak about these fantasies. One reason such fantasies need to be investigated and discussed openly is that fathers tend to be excluded from the medical processes during the pregnancy and delivery, at least psychologically. This feeling of exclusion may persist and intensify after the birth when the mother becomes preoccupied with the infant's care. As a result of this exclusion, some fathers may direct their feelings of resentment to the infant, which may then have several ramifications. First, the mother may sense the resentment and, if only to protect the infant, draw closer to the baby in an effort to shield him from exposure to the father's negative emotions. This heightened closeness between mother and infant can only exacerbate the situation, however, creating a division between the parents. Second, the infant will ultimately be deprived of exposure to previewing experiences that the father can provide during the early months of life, and this deprivation may have a detrimental effect on the infant's development.

For example, as cited earlier, fathers may preview a particular kind of motor coordination to infants during play activity. For these reasons, it becomes imperative for the therapist to attempt to ascertain information about the father's fantasies during the pregnancy and to use this information in formulating a strategy for helping the father establish a more intimate and adaptive relationship with the infant that encourages previewing imminent development.

Because the father's fantasies, present as early as the third trimester, are not dissimilar from those of the mother (Sherwen, 1986), these fantasies can be used as imaginative rehearsals to prepare the individual for dealing with outcomes in a situation that has aroused concern (Fletcher & Averill, 1984; Lederman, 1984; Levy & McGee, 1975; Rubin, 1984). When defined in this fashion, fantasies represent an important mechanism for coping with the problems of everyday life (Klinger, 1981). In this regard, the role of fantasy is particularly significant because its relationship to previewing behavior enables both the caregiver and the infant to engage in an imaginative rehearsal of imminent developmental and interpersonal change.

Fantasy can be a vehicle to prepare the individual for the ultimate assumption of a social role, such as parenthood. These definitions apply to the function of fantasy in the life of the expectant parent. For example, expectant fathers may harbor fears and anxieties about the ways that the infant's arrival will alter their relationship with their wives, about how they will cope with the additional burden of supporting the infant financially, and about the as yet undetermined ways in which the new baby will change the lives of all family members. Previewing exercises before the birth during intervention may provide the father with an arena to work through some of these issues. Similarly, fantasy activity for the new father represents a kind of imaginative rehearsal, in that he can preview what he thinks the infant will be like and the nature of the relationship he will share with the infant. Lastly, previewing exercises enable the father to begin accepting the role of fatherhood with its changes in responsibility.

The Role of Self-Esteem

Other factors of the father's psychological makeup have been found to affect the degree of involvement with the child's birth. For example, Coysh (1983a, 1983b) determined that fathers with high levels of self-esteem before the child was born were more likely to participate in daily child-care activities after the birth. In addition, McHale and Huston (1984) found that fathers tend to be more involved when mothers harbor egalitarian attitudes toward childrearing.

Recent investigators have determined that fathers who are active in child-care experience enhanced self-esteem, self-confidence, or satisfaction with the new insights acquired about the caregiving role (Lein, 1979; Russell,

1983). Russell studied parents involved in a nontraditional role-reversal situation and found that the lifestyle had altered their marital relationship. Approximately 45% of fathers indicated that the change had resulted in positive outcomes, including enhanced sensitivity, sharing of emotions, and empathy between the couple. However, another 40% reported negative consequences stemming from the nontraditional arrangement and, in particular, commented on greater conflict and dissatisfaction, irritability, and a diminished amount of intimate time shared between the couple. This finding was particularly evident among families in which the nontraditional childrearing patterns occurred due to financial necessity rather than to choice. Russell also discovered that mothers may have special difficulties in adjusting to the changed balance in affective relationships between the father and child.

THE FATHER AS AN ENHANCER OF DEVELOPMENTAL SKILLS

The Father's Intuitive Skills

Several factors suggest that the father plays a noteworthy role in the infant's early maturation and that his behaviors affect the emergence of developmental competence. Research on parental roles has indicated that the typical American middle-class family has become increasingly child-oriented and that a greater homogeneity of parental roles is taking place. The focus of authority within the family has recently shifted, with fathers yielding more decision-making power outside of the home to mothers, while assuming some of the nurturant functions traditionally associated with the maternal role. This shift should result in a greater sense of psychological intimacy and closeness between father and infant.

Greenberg and Morris (1974) performed one of the earliest studies of father–infant interaction. They found that all of the fathers expressed strong paternal feelings, with 97% of fathers rating themselves from average to very high on these emotions. These observations are similar to those of Parke, O'Leary, and West (1972) who relied on observational sessions of fathers interacting with their infants. Ten-minute observations were made for three consecutive days following the infant's delivery. The presence of holding patterns and posture, gazing at the infant, vocalization, touching, rocking, imitating the infant, participating in feedings, and sharing the infant with the other parent were all noted. The findings of this study demonstrated that the fathers were just as involved with their infants as the mothers and that fathers' manifestations did not differ significantly from mothers' behaviors, particularly with respect to behaviors such as gazing, holding, vocalizing, and feeding. To confirm these findings, Parke and

O'Leary (1976) also studied similar behaviors in a group of fathers of lower socioeconomic status who had neither attended childbirth classes nor been present during delivery, as was the case with the first group of fathers studied. As in the earlier study, this latter group of fathers was found to be extremely interested and active in early interaction with their infants. In fact, in the family triad, the father was more likely to hold and visually attend to the infant than was the mother.

These findings have numerous implications. First, many of the interpersonal behaviors observed in both studies fall into the category referred to earlier as *intuitive behaviors*. These behaviors include visual gazing, vocalization, appropriate holding and feeding behaviors—all of which are designed to provide the infant with a degree of stimulation adequate to promote the experience of contingency. As can be seen from the preceding cited studies, these behaviors do not appear to lie within the exclusive province or skill of mothers. Rather, fathers of newborns often manifest these behavioral manifestations to the same degree as their wives.

Other researchers, most notably Richards, Dunn, and Antonis (1977), have conducted follow-up studies of normal first- or second-born children to examine the long-term participation of fathers in childrearing. Although at both 30 and 60 weeks most fathers played with their children on a regular basis, only a minority routinely undertook caregiving activities. Fathers were more active in participating in the infant's maturation at 60 weeks than at 30 weeks, and this difference was particularly prominent if the infant was a girl. No social class differences emerged from the study.

The observations of the researchers contained records of all adults who interacted with the children. The principal data on father participation came from interviews with the mothers that were carried out when the infants were 30 and 60 weeks of age. For a number of parental activities—such as feeding, playing, bathing, and performing daily chores around the house—the mother was asked if the father performed these chores frequently, occasionally, or seldom. Mothers were also asked to comment generally about their husbands' role in child care and to describe the events of the immediately preceding week. This latter inquiry probed all visits to the home by friends or relatives, as well as the mother's excursions from the home without the child.

The analysis of the reports revealed that half of the fathers were present at the birth. Presence at birth was not significantly related to social class, educational history of the mother, her parity, or to the age of their older children. Most husbands took several days off from work at the time of the birth but thereafter did not play a major role in caring for or performing primary caregiving tasks involving the infant. When analyzing the data based on different caregiving activities, the researchers found that although the majority of fathers engaged in play with their infants regularly, only a minority engaged in caregiving activities on a regular basis. These numbers increased from 30 to 60 weeks, particularly for the category of taking children out of the house without the mother. Almost half of the fathers were performing this task and feeding their children regularly at 60 weeks. At both ages there was a clear hierarchy of paternal activities, with changing diapers and bathing as the activities in which fathers rarely participated and playing as the most frequent behavior fathers engaged in with their infants. No differences in paternal participation were related to the sex of the child after 30 weeks. At 60 weeks, however, more fathers of daughters than fathers of sons were moderately or entirely nonparticipating in caregiving activities. This finding may reflect that as the infant develops, the father identifies more readily with a son.

The researchers summarized the results of the study by noting that only a minority of fathers participate in caring for their children on a regular basis by engaging in regular daily activities such as feedings and diaper-changings. The interview material suggested that a low degree of participation was usually expected from the father, and several fathers who were only minimally involved in infant care were rated as being "very good" in these activities by their wives. This finding was consistent with the view that child care was perceived as women's work. Moreover, the presence of the father at the birth correlated to some degree with the father's later participation in care. It appeared likely that both the presence at the birth and the subsequent degree of interaction were associated with a characteristic attitude about the degree of involvement a father was supposed to have regarding child care.

As noted, evidence of the ability to manifest intuitive behaviors suggests a capacity to represent the infant's future development, particularly in areas such as somatic, socio-affective, cognitive, and motivational skills. In turn, the representational skills associated with intuitive behaviors are a vital component of previewing. Previewing is the ability to represent how imminent developmental change will influence the interpersonal contours of the relationship and to design interactional behaviors that help introduce the infant to these changes, thereby easing the transition to new developmental achievement and changes in the relationship. Because these studies indicate that fathers have a well-developed capacity for manifesting intuitive behaviors, fathers may also possess an inherent ability to preview imminent developmental change for the infant that is comparable to the mother's previewing skills.

Interestingly enough, one area in which fathers appear to possess caregiving skills comparable to those of mothers is feeding behavior. Parke and Sawin (1975), for example, determined that paternal sensitivity to an auditory distress signal in the feeding context—such as a sneeze, spit up, or cough—was as pronounced as the maternal sensitivity to these infant manifestations. These researchers were able to demonstrate that, like mothers, fathers responded to this type of distress cue by modifying their behavior.

As such, fathers would cease feeding momentarily, would look closely to check the infant's status, and would vocalize to verify the infant's breathing functions. This study also determined that infants consumed almost as much milk when they were held by fathers as when they were held by mothers. The findings of this study are significant because feeding has traditionally been viewed as an activity almost exclusively within the province of the mother. The results of the study, then, dispel the myth that feeding is or should be a maternally dominated activity.

DIFFERENCES IN ATTACHMENT BEHAVIOR TOWARD THE PARENTAL FIGURES

Although the father has been viewed as an integral member of the nuclear family, relatively little material has been generated on the role played by the father in the infant's life and on the nature of the father–infant attachment relationship during the first years of life. To explore these themes, Pedersen and Robson (1969) conducted a study investigating the role of paternal involvement in infant care. The study included 45 families and their firstborn infants. The fathers were between 19 and 40 years of age, with a mean age of 27 years, and their educational level ranged from the completion of secondary school to a professional degree. Subjects were recruited during the mother's final trimester of pregnancy.

The investigators made home visits when each infant was 8 months and 9½ months old. At the second visit interview data were secured on father participation in the infant's care. These observations focused on detecting infant developmental differences, particularly in stranger anxiety and separation anxiety. Structured situational tests also took place at certain points in the visit. For example, shortly after entering and explaining the procedures to the mother, one of the researchers approached, picked up, and held the infant in a supportive fashion. The second researcher, who functioned as an observer, then noted the infant's reaction.

Caretaking was rated on a 9-point scale based on the variety and frequency of the father's caretaking activities. Investment was defined as a measure related to caretaking activities performed with the infant. Investment activities included pronounced positive emotional involvement with the infant. Researchers also recorded a measure of the time spent during play activity. Another variable, irritability level, charted the father's threshold of irritation and reactivity to the infant's prolonged fussiness or crying.

The results indicated that the majority of the fathers showed a high degree of emotional involvement with their infants. The researchers noted that infants appeared to be strongly bonded with the paternal figure and that there appeared to be no biological or constitutional impediment to a strong attachment between the father and infant during the first months of life.

Among others, Ban and Lewis (1974) have studied attachment patterns in a sample of 1-year-olds. The main question posed by the investigation was whether the *attachment behaviors* the infant directed toward the mother were significantly different from the attachment behaviors directed toward the father. Infants were observed when they were 1 year of age. Observations of the infants and their parents occurred during two visits to the laboratory, 1 week apart. On the first visit, half of the children were accompanied only by the mother, whereas the other half were accompanied only by the father; this situation was reversed during the second visit. At each visit, infants were placed in a room filled with toys, and parents were instructed to hold their infants on their laps and then to place their infants on the floor when a signal was given. Parents were told to respond to the child's initiation of interaction, but not to initiate interaction with the infant. This sequence lasted for 15 minutes, during which observers watching through one-way mirrors coded for specific types of attachment behaviors. These behaviors included:

1. *Infant Gazing Directly at the Parent.* The amount of time the infant's eyes and head were turned in the parent's direction.
2. *Infant Touching of the Parent.* The amount of time any part of the infant's body made contact with the parent's body.
3. *Infant Proximity to the Parent.* The infant's staying in a delineated space immediately surrounding the parent's chair.
4. *Infant Vocalization Directed to the Parent.* All vocalizations that were not cries, sneezes, or coughs.

The results of the study revealed that for so-called proximal behaviors (including touching and proximity) no differences were apparent when mothers were compared with fathers. However, mothers engaged in almost twice as much touching and proximity behaviors as fathers during episodes when the infant engaged in gazing or vocalizing. Nevertheless, the overall differences in the nature and degree of attachment behaviors the infants manifested to mothers and fathers were minimal and reached significance only for vocalization, but not for gazing behaviors. Interestingly enough, girls looked for an equal length of time at both parents, whereas boys focused their gaze on fathers significantly more than at mothers. The researchers concluded that although infants tend to respond similarly to both mothers and fathers with respect to their proximal behaviors, their gazing behaviors may depend on both the sex of the parent and the sex of the infant.

Ban and Lewis (1974) observed that during a free-play situation, infants generally appear to be more proximally attached to their mothers than to their fathers. Fathers, however, do receive a substantial amount of gazing manifestations during these episodes. When the patterns of attachment behaviors were considered, it appeared that male infants tend to manifest the full repertoire of attachment behaviors during any given sequence. In contrast, female infants exhibit a lower overall behavioral integration. Finally, boys displayed more consistency in the expression of attachment between parents than did girls.

Kotelchuck (1981) also encountered results tending to confirm that the attachment behaviors infants direct to both mother and father are relatively similar. Approximately 300 children were examined, ranging in age from 6 to 24 months. The results of the study indicate that infants and toddlers relate and react to their fathers in a manner comparable to the responses manifested with their mothers. Moreover, it appeared that the infant's behavior could not be used to discriminate the maternal from the paternal figure in terms of the expression of the response or its temporal duration. Thus, the infant appeared to bond as readily with the father as with the mother.

According to Kotelchuck, the extent to which the children were content with either parent and the similarity of response to the departures and arrivals of both mothers and fathers undermines the argument that the mother–infant attachment relationship is somehow different or more pronounced than the father–infant attachment relationship. Nevertheless, Kotelchuck's findings demonstrated that responses to both parents were not identical, and further inquiry as to whether more children favored one parent over the other or whether there was some qualitative difference in response based on gender would be worthwhile. Kotelchuck determined such preferences by examining whether the child's response to the mother or the father was more profuse. For example, by focusing on the duration of proximity to the mother and father in episodes where both parents were present, Kotelchuck found, interestingly enough, that no discernible preference was manifested by the infant before 12 months. After 12 months of age, however, the majority of children displayed a maternal preference. This difference may be attributed to the father not being the parent with primary responsibility for the child on a daily basis.

Predicting Later Development from Early Attachment

How does the infant's attachment relationship with each parent affect other areas of developmental change? Clarke-Stewart (1978) observed 14 infants in unstructured and semistructured play situations at home when the infants were 15, 20, and 30 months of age. The same infants were observed with either their fathers or their mothers. The researcher collected data from 14 children during five different conditions: unstructured natural observations, semistructured probe situations, records kept by mothers, attitude questionnaires completed by both parents, and standardized developmental assessments. The natural observations included observations of the infants as they behaved naturally and spontaneously at home when both mother and father were home and when the mother was the only parent present. Following a natural observation conducted when the children were 15 months old, parents were asked to choose between pairs of activities. The choices were designed to separate social and/or physical activities (e.g., having a pretend tea party, brushing the child's hair), from intellectually stimulating activities (e.g., reading a story) and from other independent activities (e.g., having the child play by himself).

When the infant was 20 months of age, the nature and quality of his attachment to each parent was evaluated. During the attachment assessment, the parent sat at some distance from the child and was instructed to ignore him for 1 minute, followed by 1 minute of gazing, smiling, and vocalization. Thereafter, the parent called to the infant, engaging in play and social interactions. The parent then left the room and subsequently returned. During this time, the investigator assessed infant's responses to the parent's departure and subsequent reunion. Attachment behaviors were assessed with particular emphasis on the following variables:

1. *Negative Reaction to the Parent's Departure.* Manifested by cries and clinging behavior.
2. *Positive Reaction during Reunion with the Parent.* Manifested by smiles, vocalizations and affectionate touches.
3. *Physical Proximity.* Exhibited by touching and staying close.
4. *Social Interaction.* Displayed by smiles, affectionate touches, and efforts to initiate play interactions.

The study revealed that even at 20 months, no single measure of attachment behavior differentiated the infants' reactions to their mother and father. One notable exception emerged, however. The infants were rated as being significantly more responsive to play initiated by the father than to play initiated by the mother. This preference for play with the father was based on the quality of play, not the quantity of the play. Fathers, for example, tended to engage in play that involved more motor coordination and the physical exercising of the limbs. Moreover, when evaluations of the infant's intellectual competence at each of these ages were made, another difference emerged. The infants' intellectual competence was most highly and consistently related to the mother's verbal and emotional stimulation. Though this study suggests that there are no significant differences in the children's attachment behaviors, it does raise questions about other factors (e.g., cognition) affecting the infant's development.

THERAPIST: Your wife has been pregnant for 2 months now. Have you had any thoughts about the sex of your child?

FATHER: I'm hoping for a girl this time since we already have a boy.

THERAPIST: What appeals to you about having a girl? How would the way you relate to a girl be different from the way you relate to a boy?

FATHER: I don't think there will be a difference in the way I relate until the baby is 5 or 6 years old. Before that time, I would relate to the baby in the same way whether it was a boy or a girl. But by the time the child is 5 or 6, I would talk to a girl differently than I would talk to a boy. I think it would be easier to have another boy than to have a girl because I know more about making good boys than about making good girls.

DIFFERENCES IN PATERNAL BEHAVIOR IN OTHER AREAS OF DEVELOPMENT

Most studies that have focused on the characteristics of paternal behavior have found that just because fathers and mothers are attachment figures does not necessarily guarantee that they will exert psychological significance in children's lives. It now seems apparent that mothers and fathers represent *different* sources of interaction and experience for their children. From infancy, fathers engage in physically stimulating and playful interactions, whereas mothers are primarily responsible for daily caregiving activities and engage in more conventional play that is less dependent on physical stimulation.

According to Parsons (1954), the father embodies or personifies for the child the executive *action-oriented* approach and serves as the primary representative linking the family system with the social system beyond the family. In other words, the father serves as a model for *externally oriented behavior.* From this perspective, fathers are responsible for introducing children to the sex role expectations of the wider world, for encouraging the acquisition of competencies necessary for adaptation to the world, and for inculcating in the child the values and mores of the greater society.

The Development of Play Behaviors

Despite similarities between maternal and paternal attachment behavior, several studies have shown that, especially with regard to play behaviors, there are differences in the way fathers and mothers interact with their infants and young children. For the purposes of this discussion, I will define *play* here to encompass those activities engaged in with another that create a pleasurable affective response in the infant while stimulating cognitive capacity and encouraging experimentation with new skills. At least during the first 2 years of life, play will be viewed as an interactive activity that occurs during episodes of exchange between infant and caregiver. Using this definition of play, Kotelchuck (1975) reported that fathers spent a greater percentage of their time with their infants in play (37.5%) than mothers (25.8%). In reviewing play studies, Parke and Tinsley (1981) found that these differences were revealed not only in discrete behaviors, but were also manifested in the patterns of behavior. As Yogman, Dixon, Tronick, Als, and Brazelton (1977) have commented, adult behaviors were often part of an interactive game, consisting of episodes of mutual attention in which the adult repeated behaviors with only minor variations during each episode. Yogman found that these games were more prevalent during sessions with fathers than during sessions with mothers. For example, mothers and infants played games during 75% of their interactive sequences, whereas fathers and infants engaged in this form of game-playing during 87% of their exchange.

Moreover, as Parke and Tinsley (1981) determined from their review, the content of the games that mothers and fathers played differed as well. Indeed, certain games could be characterized as "mother's games," whereas other forms of interactive activity clearly emerged as "father's games." For example, visual games in which the parent displayed distal motor movements observed by the infant while sustaining the infant's attention were commonly categorized as maternal games and comprised 31% of all the games the mothers played. For fathers, such visual games represented only 19% of the games played. These findings were confirmed by Yogman (1981). Among fathers, however, games relying on tactile and limb movement were frequent. These limb-movement games were correlated with heightened infant arousal and, according to Yogman, represented 70% of all father-infant games and only 4% of all mother-infant games. Mothers, therefore, rarely utilized this type of physically arousing game, but instead used more conventional motor games such as pat-a-cake, peekaboo, and waving, as well as games that relied more heavily on vocalizations and visual interaction.

Moreover, these stylistic differences in play did not appear to be limited only to very young infants. Power and Parke (1981), who videotaped both mothers and fathers playing with their 8-month-old firstborn infants, found that fathers were more prone to bounce and lift their infants than mothers. In contrast, mothers engaged in more gazing games in which a toy or other attractive object was presented and moved in a manner to attract the infant's gaze. Lamb (1976) also found that infants of 8 to 13 months responded differently depending on the parent's gender, with more motor responses exhibited by the infant during paternal interaction.

The nuances of how father and mother differ in their play behaviors with their infants was the subject of an investigation by Power (1985). This researcher studied the mothers and fathers of four boys and four girls during play interaction at three separate times—when the infants were 7, 10, and 13 months of age respectively. The researcher focused on the kinds of individual differences in play style that emerged as a result of the sex of the parent or the sex of the child. Play behaviors were placed in categories based on attention, simple motor exploration, complex relational interaction, pretend play, communicative turn-taking play, and play involving the production of visual or auditory effects.

Findings indicated that, at least with regard to the predominant kinds of play, mothers and fathers behave in a remarkably *similar* fashion. Although mothers spent a greater proportion of their time than fathers encouraging pretend behavior, there were no significant mother–father differences in the encouragement of visual exploration, relational play, communicative play, the production of auditory and visual effects, or in the simple manipulation of objects. One possible explanation for these findings is that the infant's behavior toward the toys or the characteristics of the toys may have been more significant determinants of the kinds of parent–infant play exhibited than were the infant's preferences based on the gender of the parent.

Analyses of play style, however, revealed several significant differences between mothers and fathers, particularly with respect to the timing of the parental toy interventions. When attempting to influence the infant's behavior, mothers were more likely to reinforce and continue their infant's natural curiosity by encouraging the infant to choose the object of play, whereas fathers often disregarded the infant's attention-seeking cues and either interfered with the infant's ongoing activity or changed activities abruptly. Whether this finding reflects a difference in sensitivity that results from mothers' greater experience in the toy-play context or reflects mother–father differences in interaction goals (with fathers believing it is their responsibility, not the infant's, to choose the direction for play) is an issue that warrants further examination.

Moreover, Power reported that although mothers and fathers did not differ in the amount of time they spent directing their infant's play, the time factor was related to infant gender. Mothers of girls were more directive than mothers of boys as the infant's age increased. These results are consistent with other studies that show that parents of girls, particularly mothers, spend more time directing their girls' behavior, whereas parents of boys, especially mothers, are less directing, allowing for greater amounts of independent exploration by the male child. Some of this difference may be a residual effect of stereotyped differences perceived to exist between the genders. As such, preconceived notions relating to differences between boys and girls may affect parental behavior.

Development of Cognition

Ninio and Rinott (1988) attempted to discern if there was any correlation between the involvement of fathers in the care of their infants and the kinds of attributions fathers engage in relating to *cognitive* maturation. It was hypothesized that fathers, as a group, would attribute lower degrees of competence to infants than mothers, and that the greater the degree of the father's involvement with the infant, the less difference there would be between his attributions and those of his wife in terms of their infant's cognitive capacities.

The study involved 160 pairs of parents of 9-month-old infants. Both parents were interviewed extensively prior to the study. *Availability* was defined as the average daily amount of time the father was at home when the infant was awake, including time spent outside the house in the company of the infant. *Interaction* was defined as the average daily amount of time the father was engaged in active encounters with the infant in the form of taking care of, playing with, or otherwise being directly engaged with the infant. *Caregiving* was defined as the average daily number of times the father performed the following caregiving activities with the infant without the mother being present: feeding, including a whole meal, not just a snack; dressing or changing diapers; bathing by giving the infant a full bath; and, preparing the infant for bed. Fathers were viewed as having *sole responsibility* for the infant, on the basis of the average daily amount of time spent alone with the infant. Having sole responsibility meant that the father was the only caregiver attending the infant for a minimum of 1 hour. On average, it was determined that fathers were available to their infants for 2.75 hours per weekday, spending approximately 45 minutes of this time interacting with the infants. Fathers tended to perform only one caregiving activity per day and assumed sole responsibility for the infant's daily needs approximately once every 10 days.

The results disclosed a positive correlation between the degree of involvement in an infant's care and the degree of social and cognitive competence the father attributed to the infant. It was found that the more the father was involved in infant care, the more sophisticated and descriptive were his opinions of infant capacities. Such fathers were able to volunteer detailed reports of infant developmental skill. Furthermore, on the average fathers attributed less competence to infants than did mothers. However, this difference between matched pairs of fathers and mothers decreased the more the fathers were involved in infant care. With highly involved fathers, for example, the difference between the attributions of the fathers and mothers was insignificant. Thus, this study indicates that paternal involvement in infant care on a regular basis results in heightened awareness and perception of infant skill. The greater the degree of interaction between parent and child—regardless of whether the parent is the mother or father—the more sophisticated is the parent in discerning and responding to developmental skill.

Development of Locus of Control

Locus of control beliefs refer to the domain, either *external* (i.e., social world) or *internal* (i.e., psychological world), which is perceived to be the prime force motivating outcome (Seligman, 1972). Thus, individuals with an external locus of control believe that outcome occurs by chance or luck and is beyond their control. In sharp contrast, those with an internal locus of control believe that personal skill can master the environment. Infants begin to distinguish between the internal and the external domains of control at approximately 24 months of age (Kopp, 1982).

It has been found that fathers highly involved in their infants' care exhibited more sophisticated activities designed to stimulate the cognitive development of their children. Radin (1982) and Sagi (1982) each investigated the father's influence on the child's social competence skills as well. Children with fathers who actively participated in child care on a daily basis were evaluated for levels of empathy and locus of control orientation, and these evaluations were compared with assessments performed on children whose fathers assumed the more traditional, uninvolved role. Sagi, although not Radin, found that offspring of highly involved fathers were, in fact, more empathic, suggesting a correlation of this emotional quality with fathers who display an increased amount of supportive, nurturing, and sensitive behaviors toward their children. Moreover, both studies concurred in the finding that high levels of paternal participation resulted in higher levels of an internal control orientation in their infants.

FATHER: (Holds infant in his lap) I like having Tammy around. (Infant kicks. Father readjusts her in his lap and gives her a bottle. She drinks quietly.) I wouldn't want to be deprived of the experience of enjoying her growth.

MOTHER: I think Tammy and David have developed a very close relationship. He's wonderful with her, and Tammy responds to him. While I'm doing housework, I can hear them playing and laughing together. (Infant tries to feed bottle to father. Infant laughs when father makes sucking noises.)

CHANGES IN PREVAILING ATTITUDES ABOUT PARENTAL CAREGIVING

Traditionally mothers have been relegated the responsibility for early caregiving, whereas fathers have been viewed as the economic providers who spend much of their time outside of the home ensuring the family's financial stability. Thus, it is not unusual that most major studies of the earliest factors influencing the infant's development have focused on maternal influence (Josselyn, 1956). Nor is it surprising that when parental attitudes or behaviors have been investigated, it is predominantly mothers who have been interviewed or observed.

By the late 1960s, however, dramatic changes began to occur with respect to these attitudes (Lamb, 1981). First, the focus on mother–infant and mother–child relationships became so unbalanced that researchers were forced to ask whether fathers could be deemed virtually irrelevant entities in the socialization of the child. A second reason for the enhanced interest in both fathers and families in general was that the traditional family structure appeared to be undergoing transition and realignment. Within the last few generations the extended family living in one household, the number of children in the average family, and attitudes toward child-care have all changed dramatically. For example, many mothers now work during the years of the child's infancy, leaving the daily care of the child to surrogates. Moreover, it has become increasingly apparent that modern fathers do not want to be peripheral figures in the lives and socialization of their children. Recent surveys have found that the vast majority of young fathers desire a more intimate relationship with their children (Sheehy, 1979). Also, although full-time mothers obviously spend more time with their children than working fathers, there is a tendency to exaggerate the extent of interaction between mothers and young children and to underestimate the fathers' involvement.

Indeed, as Lamb has pointed out, the quality of the interaction and of the adult's behavior is a far more important factor than the quantity of time spent with the child. Thus, a few hours of pleasurable interaction may be more conducive to the formation of secure attachments than hours of cohabitation with a dissatisfied, harassed, depressed, indifferent, or ignoring parent. Such caregivers are not likely to provide their infants with adequate levels of stimulation and the exposure to contingent stimulation necessary to enhance developmental adaptation. With fathers, as with mothers, there is no necessary correlation between the quantity of time spent together and the quality of interaction. Although fathers generally spend relatively little time with their children, they may exert a significant impact on the child's development. This realization, which has become increasingly evident during the last decade, has motivated further investigations of how fathers—the so-called forgotten contributors—influence the child's development.

The Effects of Parental Employment on the Security of Attachment

The *stability* of the attachment relationship was the focus of a study by Owen, Easterbrooks, Chase-Lansdale, and Goldberg (1984). These researchers studied the attachment relationships to both father and mother of firstborn children in families where the mothers were employed full-time, part-time, or not at all for at least 3 months prior to a 12-month assessment. A follow-up investigation occurred at 20 months. Essentially, the researchers found no relationship between employment status and quality of attachment to mother or father at either time period. When the employment status of the mother changed, however, there were changes in the quality of attachment to the father. The direction of this change was from secure to insecure and it was primarily the female infants who experienced this change in attachment status.

Chase-Lansdale and Owen (1987) examined the quality of infant attachment to both mother and father in middle-class families when maternal employment began full-time during the infant's first 6 months of life. The infant was cared for in home settings primarily by the father. The researchers found no relation between insecure attachment and employment status for infants and their mothers. Nonetheless, a significantly higher proportion of insecure attachment patterns was noted between boys and their fathers, leading the researchers to conclude that such attachment behavior was due to lack of predictability between the infant and caregiver. The researchers concluded that the father's early resumption of employment after the birth may represent a risk factor that influences the infant's attachment to him. As in previous research on the effects of maternal employment on infants, boys appeared more at risk in their socioemotional development.

Stuckey, McGhee, and Bell (1982) asserted that fathers of employed mothers did not increase their participation in the daily care of their children. On the other hand, Gold, Andres, and Glorieux (1979), in a French-Canadian sample, credited high rates of paternal involvement with buffering the effects of maternal employment on the child. Cowan and Cowan (1987) and Zaslow, Pedersen, Suwalsky, Rabinovich, and Cain (1986) determined that as hours of maternal employment increased, fathers increased their participation in household tasks.

A series of studies by Pedersen (1975) showed that fathers in single wageearner families played more with their infants than fathers in dual-earner- families. Observations of these families revealed that when both parents returned from work at the end of the day, it was the mother, rather than the father, who engaged in a significantly greater degree of social play and verbal interaction with the infant. These findings are particularly interesting in light of the results of the study by Chase-Lansdale and Owen (1987), which raise concern about the possibility of the infant developing an insecure attachment with the father, particularly if the infant is a male. More research needs to be done to evaluate these hypotheses.

These data indicate that fathers do interact directly with their offspring during infancy and that this interaction has an effect on infant development and on the formation of attachment relationships. Studies have revealed the distinctive benefits fathers provide for their infants as a result of the qualitatively unique nature of the interactions they share with the infant (Schachere, 1990). For example, children with involved fathers have been found to be more competent in numerous areas of developmental acquisition. Moreover, it has been demonstrated that fathers possess the resources to become competent caregivers and that a well-defined attachment relationship can readily develop between infants and their fathers.

Although these studies have raised some ambiguities, certain findings with respect to fathers remain definitive. In particular, infants form attachment relationships as readily with fathers as with mothers, and the majority of fathers express a desire to become actively involved in the infant's care. Thus, the father should be viewed as an additional resource for the infant's development. The therapist should foster intuitive behaviors and representational skills through previewing exercises in the same manner as with the mother in order to encourage the father to use his representational capacities and to engage in previewing with the infant.

A Case Study

One case I treated illustrates how the attachment bond may be fostered between father and infant, and the degree to which paternal involvement can enhance infant development. In this case, the family's decision to reverse traditional roles with respect to the care of the child was due, in part, to the mother's significantly more advanced employment status and potentially more rewarding career. The father in this family was employed as a maintenance mechanic for a large airline corporation, whereas the mother worked as a financial analyst on Wall Street. Almost immediately after the birth of this couple's son, the family decided that the mother, Mrs. G, would take an extended leave of absence after her maternity leave was over and remain at home to care for the infant, Ian. Initially, it was planned that Mrs. G would remain at home until Ian was old enough to attend nursery school.

When the child was 21 months old, however, Mr. G was laid off from work due to a management reorganization. Although he knew that his prospects for obtaining other employment were favorable, Mr. G decided that at least for several months he would remain at home and share some of the responsibilities involved in the care of his son. During this time Mr. G became accustomed to taking Ian to the park playground. In addition, Mr. G also shared with his wife the responsibility of taking his son for pediatric checkups. Despite his participation, however, Mrs. G remained in the role of Ian's primary caregiver. She interacted with her son for a substantially greater percentage of time each day than did her husband, and it was tacitly understood by the couple that if Ian needed care during the night for feedings or illness, Mrs. G would attend to him.

Although this arrangement worked out well, with Ian displaying all the developmental signs of a well-adjusted infant, when the infant was just over 2 years of age his mother decided to return to work, a decision motivated by the rapid depletion of the couple's financial resources. Mrs. G had been contacted about an unusually lucrative employment opportunity, and because it appeared that Mr. G had become adept at caring for Ian over the past few months, the couple decided that Mr. G would continue to stay home and care for the infant, while Mrs. G resumed employment.

Initially, Mr. G was enthusiastic about this course of action. He believed he had developed a strong bond of affection for his son during the preceding 6 months, an affection that was reciprocated during episodes of interaction. Within the first few weeks of Mrs. G's return to work, however, Ian's interpersonal behavior changed dramatically. Every morning just before Mrs. G left for work, Ian would become upset and would sometimes engage in a temper tantrum, flinging his breakfast food on the floor or banging on his high chair tray with his fists. At other times, he would begin to cry uncontrollably when he saw his mother put on her coat and pick up her briefcase to leave for work.

At this time Ian began to manifest other significant changes indicative of a regression to an earlier developmental stage. For example, prior to his mother's return to work he had been able to articulate several words clearly and with each day he seemed to add words to his vocabulary. His motor skills at this time were also impressive: He was an adventurous and curious explorer of his immediate environment, in keeping with his developmental level. A dramatic shift in the manifestation of these skills was noted when Ian's mother returned to work. The child began to regress developmentally almost overnight. Rather than respond with full sentences, he became taciturn and resumed his preverbal grunting and gesturing; at other times he stuttered. He refused to assist in clothing himself and seemed to dislike the exploration behavior he had previously manifested with delight. Beyond these signs of developmental regression, Ian also manifested a new behavior most appropriately labeled "clinging." Whenever his father dressed him for the park, he became sullen, face downcast. Once at the park, Ian would stay only within the immediate vicinity of his father, often touching his father when another child or a stranger approached him. He would also attempt physically to prevent his mother from leaving the house in the morning by pulling at her coat and crying. Moreover, Ian's habit of stuttering increased when he did speak; in addition, he had difficulty sleeping at night, often awakening in the middle of the night from nightmares that only his mother could quell.

As Ian's parents became increasingly more concerned about these changes, they decided to seek counseling. During the initial interview, it was agreed that Ian's father would bring his son for a weekly session and that both parents would be present for family sessions every two weeks. When treatment began, Ian was often reluctant to stay in the treatment room alone with the therapist. As a result, Ian's father joined us during the sessions. The presence of Mr. G appeared to comfort Ian, who generally stayed in close proximity to his father. After several sessions, Ian agreed to draw some pictures and play with the toys scattered around the room, provided the therapist allowed him to arrange them himself and did not interfere with his arrangements without permission.

Shortly thereafter, Ian was able to attend the sessions alone with the therapist while his father waited outside, as long as the door was kept open. Occasionally, he would run out to "check" if his father was still there. Once when Ian went to check on his father, Mr. G was not there. He had gone to get some water. Ian became very distressed and when his father finally returned, Ian, while pulling his father's hand, insisted that they go home.

In the therapist's sessions alone with Ian 3 months later, he would engage in a ritual game. During the ritual, he would lie on the floor on his back with his arms pressed tightly against his sides. He would remain very still and indicate "shh" with his fingers. The therapist sat in a chair and watched. Ian would shut his eyes and stay motionless in this position for several minutes. Periodically, he would open his eyes and gaze furtively in the therapist's direction. If the therapist had turned away or was not concentrating on him, Ian would become upset and indicate that the therapist should pay attention and watch him. Ian told the therapist that during this ritual he was pretending to be "sleeping." In addition, the preschooler was also able to tell the therapist that his mother "would get hurt and cut her fingers at work."

From the revelation of his mental representations along with Ian's behavior, the therapist confirmed that the child may have been experiencing separation anxiety disorder, provoked by his mother's return to work and the daily repetition of her departure from the home. The ritual of "playing sleeping" signified Ian's effort to master the anxiety aroused by the separation from his mother without having to be awakened by his fears. When the therapist explored Ian's concern that his mother would "cut her fingers," it appeared that this fear had two sources. First, Ian was genuinely concerned that his mother would hurt herself and, as a consequence, would not be able to return to care for him. Second, this concern also masked a deep-seated anger at his mother for what Ian most probably perceived as a form of abandonment. Interestingly enough, whenever the child spoke of his mother "cutting her fingers," his recently acquired stutter would surface distinctly. The association of the speech impediment with these strong anxieties concerning his mother suggested that Ian was conflicted emotionally about his mother's return to work. Although it was acceptable for him to express his anger in the form of the fear that his mother "would be hurt," on a more profound level Ian's anger at his mother may have been motivated into a wish to hurt her for abandoning him.

With the active participation of Ian's father in the treatment, the young child eventually worked through these ambivalent feelings during play therapy. At this period, Ian strengthened his attachment to his father, who became his consistent daily companion. Ian and his father worked out a schedule that permitted them to have a sufficient amount of play time together, as well as to share daily chores. Mr. G also assumed primary responsibility for Ian's welfare during this period of time. For example, Mr. G purchased all of Ian's clothing, he arranged for visits with Ian's friends, and he took Ian to the pediatrician. In essence, Mr. G performed virtually all of the tasks generally associated with primary caregiving activity that his wife had previously performed.

During the biweekly family sessions, Ian's efforts centered around engaging both parents in the same activity. Frequently, Ian would pretend to cook for and feed both of his parents; at other times, he would arrange the room so that everyone, including the therapist, pretended to be asleep. During this period, Ian would make crackling noises—he would get up after these noises, come closer to either of his parents and tell them to go back to sleep in a very quiet fashion. Ian also played with the light switches in the room, turning them on and off repetitively.

After approximately 20 weeks of remaining at home, Ian's father was offered a new employment position. Both parents decided that Ian was now old enough to be left in the care of a permanent live-in babysitter. The couple hired a young woman who initially appeared to have an excellent rapport with Ian. Within a week of Mr. G's return to work, however, many of the symptoms Ian had first manifested when his mother returned to work resurfaced. This time the child's distress manifested itself only when his father prepared to leave the house in the morning. Indeed, Ian even expressed the fear that his father would hurt himself with his tools, a concern reminiscent of Ian's previous fear that his mother would "cut her fingers." Once again, these fears were worked through during sessions involving Ian's father. In particular, during one session, at the therapist's suggestion, Ian's father brought some of his tools with him, demonstrated to Ian how they worked, and verbalized all the precautions he took so as not to hurt himself. After several weeks of these sessions, the child's symptomatology abated and he resumed progress at a high level of adaptation.

This case is noteworthy in several respects. First, it is significant that Ian's father was able to assume the role of primary caregiver and competently to provide the skills essential for nurturing his son's development. Second, the recurrence of Ian's symptoms when his father returned to work suggests that young children are capable of and, indeed, prone to develop a strong attachment to the father, which is comparable to the attachment to the mother. The point here is that the gender of the adult who takes primary care of the child is not the significant factor. Rather, it is the nature of the involvement and the quality time spent with the child that tend to determine where the child's attachment loyalties will lie. Second, this case indicates that fathers are as capable as mothers in performing primary caregiving responsibilities and providing the daily level of stimulation and support necessary for an adaptive relationship and for optimal development.

Enhancing the Father's Previewing Abilities

As the studies referred to earlier have demonstrated, fathers are capable of manifesting the same competence in nurturing activities as mothers. Moreover, observations of paternal interaction with infants have revealed that fathers rely on the same intuitive behaviors that mothers manifest—vocal and visual cuing, appropriate holding behaviors—to coax forth developmental capabilities in their infants. These findings indicate that fathers are prime candidates for learning how to preview imminent developmental change to their infants.

Enhancing the father's previewing skills occurs most effectively in the therapeutic setting, although, depending on the circumstances of the case, it may not be necessary for the father to attend sessions on a regular basis. Instead, fathers may be instructed in the basics of previewing techniques in a few sessions. The therapist should begin by asking the father to disclose fantasies and daydreams concerning the infant and his relationship with the infant. The father's knowledge of infant development and his sensitivity to understanding the qualities of the infant's behaviors should also be explored at this time. For example, does the father possess a coherent sense of the normative trends of infant development and can he transfer this knowledge to his own infant to predict imminent maturational change? Moreover, can the father analyze infant response on a somatic, cognitive, affective, and motivational level? To discern the father's skill in this area, it may be necessary to conduct sessions with both the father and infant in attendance. The therapist, while observing the father's skills during interaction, can also evaluate any conflict that may somehow be preventing the father from interacting with the infant in a manner that encourages adaptive development.

Assuming that the father's rudimentary skills are adaptive, the therapist can begin introducing the father to various representational exercises that heighten perception of the infant's imminent developmental trends. During this process, the therapist may also wish to use such techniques as modeling and videotaping further to refine the father's perception of the implications of interaction with the infant. Finally, the father may be encouraged to introduce specific previewing behaviors into the interaction that are designed to acquaint the infant with a particular developmental milestone.

In keeping with the flexibility of the dyadic treatment approach, it may be advantageous to have the mother present during these sessions as well. The mother's presence serves a variety of functions. First, it reinforces for both parents the notion that either mother or father can foster the infant's developmental capacities and that both parents contribute to the infant's growth. Second, such sessions help the parents work through any conflict they may be experiencing as a result of the new triadic relationships that have been introduced into their family. Third, these sessions allow the parents to divide up responsibilities concerning specific previewing behaviors. It may, for example, be advantageous for the mother to focus on previewing speech, whereas the father focuses on previewing motor skills, such as walking. This division of tasks is, of course, left to the individual judgment of the caregivers. Finally, and most significantly, these sessions enable the infant to internalize the notion that each of his caregivers has a unique perspective on his development, although both parents are working toward the unified goal of enhancing overall developmental growth. This exposure helps the infant formulate a sense of self and autonomy in an atmosphere of support and contingency.

CONCLUSION

What are the implications of this research concerning fathers of infants for the therapist who is engaged in the treatment of mother–infant dyads or families? Clearly, the bulk of data indicate that fathers are as competent as mothers in providing care to the infant during the first years of life. That is, fathers are as capable as mothers at providing stimulation and instilling developmental skills.

Aside from specific cases in which the mother is unavailable to the child, however, it is also significant that the father can play an integral role in the infant's development. Studies involving paternal fantasies suggest that even during the pregnancy fathers harbor particular kinds of anticipations about the infant that are similar to the fantasies expressed by their wives. Studies have also demonstrated that the therapist can teach the father particular techniques, such as representational exercises and previewing behaviors, that will serve to heighten the father's involvement in the infant's developmental course. Moreover, just as it is essential that the mother possess knowledge of the infant's developmental capacities, so too it is vital that the father be well versed in every developmental change. The therapist can obtain this information by interviewing the father in the same fashion as the mother, and by asking in particular how the father anticipates the future development of the infant. Such queries help identify the father's propensity for previewing maturational potential to the infant.

There is a further reason for therapists to encourage the involvement of the father in the infant's development and, in particular, to encourage paternal previewing behaviors. As has been noted, previewing offers a means of introducing the infant to developmental milestones that are on the verge of consolidation. If the infant is exposed to previewing from both the mother and father, he will have a better opportunity to contrast the different interactional styles and to understand the changes occurring in his own body and in the world around himself from different perspectives. The more the infant is exposed to adaptive previewing of a milestone by both parents, the more he will be able to sense and perceive the complexity of the developmental process. Moreover, if both parents provide support and guidance through previewing, the infant comes to recognize that developmental progression is premised on a relationship with a significant other who gradually guides the infant in the direction of maturational skill. The strength of this relationship propels development forward, providing the infant with the confidence to master the domains of external and internal reality.

As was noted, mothers tend to engage in particular kinds of behaviors such as attention play, visual stimulation, and vocalization, whereas fathers appear to be oriented toward motor skill activities. In one interesting case I treated, the infant had begun to engage in crawling and walking gestures. When I proposed that the mother might consider previewing walking to the infant, she hesitated and then observed that she believed the child would more appropriately learn walking behavior from his father. Her response came as something of a surprise, because this mother had previously demonstrated competence in previewing other kinds of maturational skills, such as language. This response is probably not all that unusual, and it suggests a further reason for encouraging paternal previewing. In some cases mothers will simply not engage in previewing particular kinds of skills. As a result, it remains the father's responsibility to preview and introduce the infant to the imminent arrival of these developmental capacities. This means that the attributions the parents make to the infant are as important as the objective assessment of the infant's developmental status. Thus, if for whatever reason, one caregiver is reluctant to preview certain kinds of behaviors for the infant, the other caregiver should be able to assume that role. This balanced approach also provides the infant with an opportunity to contrast the responses of two different caregivers, both of whom are oriented in the direction of enhancing development.

A third reason to foster paternal previewing is that in certain cases the mother may be unable to provide the necessary encouragement and reassurance for optimal developmental growth. This form of maternal deficit may stem from several sources. First, the mother may be suffering from a psychological illness that prevents her from engaging the infant in an adaptive relationship during the first few months after the birth. Most commonly, this form of impairment occurs as a result of postpartum depression. Other mothers may have histories of psychiatric disturbance that will also hinder their capacities to be fully responsive to the infant and to behave in a manner that promotes optimal development. Beyond these somewhat obvious cases, however, there will also be occasions when even a highly competent caregiver will find that she has reached an impasse and is somehow unable to minister to the infant in an adaptive fashion designed to enhance optimal development. These situations ordinarily arise when the mother encounters a conflict stemming from her own development. In one such case I was involved with, the mother was unable adaptively to preview walking behavior with her infant because of her own childhood memory associated with being lost in a store. By encouraging her infant to walk on his own, this mother experienced a resurgence of her own anxiety when she had became lost; thus she feared that her infant would wander away from her. Although the mother was able to eventually work through these feelings, during this period of time the infant remained developmentally stagnant. In effect, he was reacting to a maladaptive form of behavior on the part of the mother, rather than enacting his own developmental potential during interaction with her. In such situations, which occur not infrequently, it is advantageous to encourage the father as another source of previewing stimulation. Similarly, the mother can bolster the father when he experiences a developmental conflict. In this fashion, both parents act as partners in the infant's overall development.

PART TWO

Assessment Techniques

Chapter 3

Assessing the Interpersonal Status of the Infant

INTRODUCTION

In many respects dyadic therapy resembles other forms of treatment that involve an individual patient and therapist. For example, during the course of treatment an alliance must be forged between therapist and caregiver and from the strength and resiliency of this alliance, the therapist helps the caregiver predict, recognize, explore, and resolve conflict stemming from early life experience. But in other respects, dyadic treatment is a unique, *sui generis* form of treatment. The unique factor in this therapy is the infant's presence; as a consequence, the therapist can *observe* directly during a session how the caregiver and infant enact interpersonal patterns. In addition, because both members will be undergoing development, the therapist will be able to witness how dyadic members adapt to these myriad changes. Does the caregiver embrace the interpersonal consequences of such change, integrating the infant's acquisitions into her repertoire of interactional behavior, while previewing further imminent advance in skill, or does the caregiver fail to acknowledge such changes during her interaction with the infant? As is apparent from the preceding comments, observation and other interviewing strategies play a pivotal role in the diagnosis during dyadic therapy. It is thus incumbent upon therapists using this treatment to become familiar with the methods of observation and to hone their skills in this area.

This chapter provides guidance on how therapists can become skilled observers. It begins with a brief background reinforcing the role of observation in such treatments as dyadic therapy and next outlines the interpersonal manifestations to which the therapist should be alert. The chapter then moves on to a specific discussion of specific developmental phenomena the therapist should focus on during a sequence of observation. These factors include areas such as the psychomotor, affective, cognitive, and language capacities that indicate the caregiver's effectiveness in helping the infant maximize his potential for adaptive communication. Observational skills also acquaint the therapist with *previewing exercises* designed to introduce the infant to imminent developmental change. Finally, because the technique of observation is best conveyed through description, a clinical case exemplifies how observational skills assist the therapist in promoting a more adaptive dyadic exchange.

OBSERVATION—A TOOL FOR ASSESSING THE INFANT'S MENTAL STATUS

Ethology is the study of behavior in the organism's natural habitat (Charlesworth, 1978). Ethologists chart the evolution of behavior in a particular individual by engaging in specific methodologies. First, they observe and record the behaviors of the subject in his or her natural environment. Second, they analyze behaviors as a consequence of the immediate stimulus conditions. Third, they search for underlying neurophysiological mechanisms regulating these behaviors. Ethologists engage in these tasks to discern the relationship between the organism and the environment—both of which can be observed individually or, as is more typical, during interaction. In observing this dynamic interaction, the ethologist articulates and describes the characteristics of *normal* or *adaptive* human behavior. According to Charlesworth any definition of normal behavior in this context must include at least three criteria:

1. The behavior must be typical for most same-age and same-sex members of the species.
2. The behavior must lead to self-maintenance or preservation.
3. The behavior must result in the production or care of succeeding generations of the species.

In addition to ascertaining these broad norms of behavior, however, ethologists are also attuned to individual variation. Thus, ethologists are acutely aware that there would be no species if there were no variation among the species and no evolution of the species if there were no variation among individuals within a species.

How does ethology contribute to the treatment of caregivers and infants in treatment, and why is this discipline pertinent to this form of therapy? The answer to this question implicates some of the factors that make caregiver–infant therapy unique. As has been noted, dyadic treatment highlights the patterns of interaction between caregiver and infant. Indeed, such interaction becomes the centerpiece of the treatment. The dyadic interaction is primary for several reasons. First, although the caregiver can use language to convey her perceptions and subjective states to the therapist (as in most conventional treatment), the infant—at least during the first 2 years of life prior to the advent of sophisticated language skills—cannot. Moreover, even well into the childhood years, children are not as adept as adults in portraying phenomena from their inner world through words. As a result, the therapist must gain access to different levels of their experience, such as emotional, by observing external manifestations—for example, facial expressions (Kopp, 1990). Therefore, observing the infant's behavior either alone, or more significantly, during interaction with the caregiver, becomes the primary route for attaining insight into the infant's perspective.

Second, the arena of interaction most accurately depicts the trends of development and reveals the methods both caregiver and infant use to adapt to the effects of maturational change. Because one of the therapist's main goals will be to assess and treat the dyad's capacity to integrate developmental changes, observation of the interaction over time and under differing circumstances becomes essential. Finally, behavioral manifestations offer the therapist a vivid and rich embodiment of the inner psychological world of both caregiver and infant, and enable the therapist to detect how the interior landscape contributes to the individual's behavior in establishing a relationship with others. Observation of dyadic interaction, then, is not a substitute for relying on the verbal insights provided by the patient; nor does behavioral observation merely serve to supplement the kinds of information the patient offers the therapist through language. Rather, observation of the dyadic relationship over time, as it evolves and transforms itself during the process of development, gives the therapist a palpable artifact for deriving diagnoses and treatment strategies.

THE SCOPE OF OBSERVATION

The primacy of the interpersonal exchange between caregiver and infant requires that therapists understand the specific kinds of manifestations they should observe and how they can derive interpretations and ultimately treatment strategies from these observations.

Some therapists are reluctant to rely on their observational skill because most training programs emphasize use of the adult patient's verbal communications to formulate a therapeutic relationship. Other clinicians are uncertain what phenomena they should be observing and, as a consequence, avoid careful scrutiny of their patients' behavioral displays. But providing the therapist with some straightforward guidance about the kinds of manifestations that should be observed can overcome both of these reservations.

To assess the status of the dyadic interaction at any given time, the therapist should observe and evaluate essentially five types of manifestations. Each of these five behavioral categories is discussed in this chapter. Moreover, as therapists are observing these phenomena of development, they need to keep in mind that the setting, to a certain extent, will contaminate observation of the dyadic interaction in the therapeutic milieu. Contamination by setting means that the environment in which the caregiver and infant find themselves will determine, in part, the interaction that emerges. For example, some caregivers will initially be hesitant about interacting with the infant in the therapist's presence and will therefore refrain from behaviors they generally express in a more naturalistic setting. Other caregivers will need to "perform" and demonstrate the relationship they share with the infant. Such caregivers may tend to exaggerate manifestations with the infant in the therapist's presence.

As a consequence of contamination, therapists should approach dyads without preconceived notions of the types of behaviors that they may demonstrate. Knowledge of the typical developmental trends manifested by infants at particular chronological ages is essential. However, this knowledge should serve only as a blueprint to guide the therapist's observations in any particular case. Each dyad should be considered individually on its own merits. The more therapists understand the *individual dimensions* observed during dyadic interaction, the greater will be their understanding of the developmental processes within that particular relationship.

Assessing Affective Processing

Researchers have confirmed that within the first few days of life infants possess a repertoire of primary emotional displays that manifest during interaction (Field, Woodson, Greenberg, & Cohen, 1982). Eight primary emotions, each with its own corresponding facial expression, have been identified: *happiness, interest, fear, sadness, soberness, distress, anger,* and *disgust.* Because these affective displays attain full expression at a relatively early point in development and persist in substantially the same form throughout childhood and adulthood, they become key indicators for the therapist. Moreover, research has also indicated that there is an inextricable relationship between external emotional displays and the internal psychological experience of the emotion (Abramson, 1990; Cossette, Pomerleau, Malcuit, & Brault, 1990; Izard, 1978; Rosenstein & Oster, 1988; Termine & Izard, 1988).

Within the caregiver–infant dyad, emotional displays manifested through facial expression have further implications. First, by observing the nature and degree of facial expression, the therapist can evaluate whether dyadic interaction is occurring adaptively. The lack of a full spectrum of affective manifestations and the absence of flexibility or fluidity in regulating the transitions among different feeling states may signify a constitutional deficit or an interactional failure between the caregiver and infant (Trad, 1986, 1987). Spitz and Wolf (1946), who observed institutionalized infants deprived of the consistent nurturing of a caregiving figure, noted, for example, that such infants appeared to lack the capacity to manifest the full emotional spectrum through facial expression. Instead, these infants presented an apathetic face to the world. By observing infant facial expression to detect the spectrum of emotional display, then, the therapist can gain insight into the dyad's degree of developmental adaptability.

Recognizing and discriminating among emotional expressions requires a certain amount of skill. Although facial musculature displays emotional manifestations most prominently, the vocalizations and body posture that the dyad manifests during these episodes are equally important. As such, it is worthwhile to address the correspondence between the facial, vocal, gestural, and postural behaviors articulated in unison during these emotional displays.

1. *Happiness.* Smiling is the most common facial expression depicted during happiness. However, the intensity of the infant's smile may range in degree from ambivalent, intermittent, tentative, or only partial, to a brilliant smile. Thus, to interpret an infant's smile adequately, smile behavior should be distinguished by type and related to context and developmental period (Holt, 1990). Vocalizations that take place during the manifestation of happiness include pleasant squeals and gurgles, as well as laughter. Body gestures can encompass arm flapping and clapping, and the infant often displays a jumping-up-and-down posture. The full constellation of these behaviors is generally present when the infant is experiencing a happy state.

2. *Sadness.* Sadness is manifested with a frowning facial expression that may be characterized as mild, moderate, or marked. Crying may also be present. When the infant is experiencing sadness, a dejected expression, vocalizations in the form of sad whining, or crying with the head down may also be apparent. Often the infant's head and body will droop, giving the appearance that the infant feels crumpled and defeated.

3. *Surprise.* As with adults, the infant manifests surprise by raised eyebrows and wide eyes and often opens his mouth simultaneously. Vocalizations include exclamations, whereas body gestures include sudden movements away from the object or stimulus that has caused the feeling of surprise.

4. *Soberness.* This emotional state is sometimes more difficult to detect, because facial expression and gestures may not be as dramatic as with other emotions. In effect, soberness may be characterized by a sudden shift to an expressionless face. The infant will likely depict a posture of sudden stillness during these interludes.

5. *Disgust.* When displaying disgust, the typical facial expression will include nose wrinkling, lower lip raising, and eye closing. For vocal signs of disgust, the therapist should focus on sounds of expiration. Among the most common body gestures associated with disgust are head aversion and an overall body posture that indicates moving back or away from the stimuli.

6. *Fear.* The infant depicts fear by a hyperviligence and widening of the eyes, ensembling a wary appearance. He turns the lips inward, creating a look of ambivalence around the mouth. The fearful facial expression can range in degree from mild to marked. Vocalizations addressing the degree of fear felt by the infant emerge in the form of gasping or overt crying. Among the typical body gestures that occur during an episode of fear are automanipulations such as the placing of hands over the body as if to protect it or hand-to-hand manipulations. The infant may avert his eyes and head while using the hands to cover his eyes. In addition, the infant's body posture may assume distinctive positions at these times. For example, he may lean away from the fearful stimulus, may actually panic and flee, may reach for the caregiver, or may move away without looking back.

7. *Anger.* The facial expression associated with the feeling of anger includes a frown with tensed eyelids and a stare. Sometimes the infant may display a protruded lower lip and a grimaced expression. Low-to-high vocalizations that tend to convey various levels of tension are also common. Body gestures may include fist-making or arm beating, head thrusts, or tantrums. The infant may also move away from the caregiver and hide his face during these sequences.

8. *Distress.* The facial expression associated with the feeling of distress includes pouting lips coupled with a mild, moderate, or full crying expression. The head and face may tremble in an agitated fashion, or the infant may appear immobile and frozen while manifesting head and hand automanipulation.

Observation of emotional manifestations through facial and body expressions also provides the therapist with information about the adaptive nature of the dyadic communication. It appears, in other words, that an adaptive and attentive caregiver will strive to elicit the full range of emotions from the infant. Indeed, within the first 2 years of life this kind of exchange through emotional displays may represent the primary form of communication between caregiver and infant. Thus, the therapist should observe not only the actual facial expressions manifested by the infant, but also the caregiver's skill in eliciting these emotions from the infant and in using such facial expressions as the foundation of a communicative system.

Finally, the therapist should observe both the adeptness and the appropriateness with which the caregiver elicits facial expressions. By this is meant that a congruence should exist between the facial expression and the message the caregiver is conveying. I have seen mothers who laugh spontaneously when the infant experiences pain. Superficially, this is obviously an inappropriate response, but it is maladaptive on a more profound level as well. By manifesting this kind of discrepancy, the caregiver is, in effect, providing the infant with the wrong message, which will ultimately lead to confusion and bafflement, rather than to meaning and coherence with regard to the myriad stimuli the infant is experiencing.

For all of these reasons, observing the infant's facial expression during sequences of interaction with the caregiver can offer the therapist indispensable insight into the dyad's level of adaptation to developmental trends and the challenges of the environment.

Assessing Cognitive Processing

Cognitive processing involves the ability to comprehend relationships between stimuli, and to encode and communicate inferences, conceptions, abstractions, categorizations, and goals regarding the infant's immediate environment (Bloom, 1979; McCall & McGhee, 1977; Piaget, 1952, 1954;

Stern, Beebe, Jaffe, & Bennett, 1977; Stern & Gibbon, 1978; Watson, 1966, 1972). Because infants are not equipped to communicate through verbal language, the infant's ability to coordinate cognitive skills must be inferred from the infant's affective and psychomotor responses (e.g., the facial expression of interest during play). A wide repertoire of emotions can reflect and even predict the infant's *intentions* and the *goals* that motivate him, as well as the infant's ability to formulate strategies for achieving goals. Such adaptational skill emerges from the infant's capacity to associate two or more stimuli and to perceive a cause–effect relationship between them. This particular ability has been labeled *contingency awareness* (Campos, Barrett, Lamb, & Stenberg, 1983; Fagen & Ohr, 1985; Watson, 1966, 1971, 1972). Indeed, with the introduction of a new stimulus, infants begin to engage in a form of contingency analysis. In one experiment designed to assess contingency, infants were exposed to a mobile. Head-pressing against the pillow caused the mobile to turn, and the incidence of contingency (mobile moved when pillow was pressed) was characterized by a significant increase in the head presses against the pillow, while the infant simulta- neously exhibited a distinctive smiling and cooing behavior (DeCasper & Carstens, 1981). DeCasper and Carstens have also demonstrated that as early as the neonatal stage infants can learn and retain contingency relation- ships for relatively long periods. See Table 3–1.

Another aspect of cognitive maturation that the therapist should evaluate within the context of the dyad is *object permanence*. Object permanence is a form of perceptual constancy signifying the infant's awareness that objects exist independently of the person viewing them and will continue in exis- tence even when the individual is not viewing them. Object permanence also refers to a belief in the continued existence of an object even though it is partially or completely disguised from view. According to Corman and Escalona (1969), object permanence may be defined as the child's capacity to conceive objects as being external, and relatively permanent, and as existing independent of his perceptions and actions in relation to the object. For Piaget (1954), permanence refers to an attribute of constancy whereby objects retain their essential character.

The development of object permanence occurs during the first 2 years of life. Many researchers believe that prior to acquiring representational thought, children cannot conceive external objects as being distinct, func- tioning entities independent of the actions that the child may perform on them or independent of the child's perception. Piaget has referred to this period as the *sensorimotor period,* extending approximately through the end of the 2nd year of life. During this time the infant successfully accomplishes tasks that he is incapable of representing mentally. Initially the infant views the world in an egocentric fashion, through actions rather than representa- tions. Nevertheless, as this period progresses, sensory and motor activities are demarcated, and the infant begins to convert temporary mental

Table 3–1.   *Cognitive Development*

Chronological Age	Object Permanence
4 weeks or less	Reflexive interaction with the environment; no active search behaviors; discrimination of red and green from white; no discernible concept of object permanence (through 1 month)[1]
8 weeks	Haptic mode less developed than visual; primary circular reactions; reflex-based habits; discrimination of red and blue from white; active search behaviors (looking and hearing) (through 4 months)[2]
16 weeks	Knowledge about support relations of objects; secondary circular reactions; habit schemes; adjustments to displacement of object; representation of existence and motion of a hidden object; inference of continued movement on an unobstructed path; discrimination of all chromatic stimuli from white; developing sense of object permanence (through 10 months)[3]
40 weeks	Increased ability to manipulate the environment; active search for completely disappeared objects; mental capability to coordinate separate sets of information (e.g., cognitive and perceptual); attributes of permanence (through 12 months)[4]
48–52 weeks (1 year)	Tertiary circular reactions; ability to follow disappearing moving object; ability to integrate information over time; person permanence[5]
72 weeks (18 months)	Maintenance of a model in the physical absence of model; reconstruction of complex movements; object permanence (through 24 months)[6]

[1] Bower, 1972; Corman and Escalona, 1969; Courage, Adams, and Mercer, 1990; Slater, 1990.
[2] Bower and Patterson, 1973; Courage, Adams, and Mercer, 1990; Gratch, Appel, Evans, LeCompte, and Wright, 1974; Streri, Molina, and Millet, 1990.
[3] Goldberg, 1977; Moore and Meltzoff, 1978; Needham, 1990; Spelke and Breinlinger, 1990.
[4] Bremner, 1978a, 1978b; Butterworth, 1977; Diamond, 1990; Gratch et al., 1974; Lalonde and Werker, 1990.
[5] Arterberry, 1990; Harris, 1975; Ramsay-Douglas and Campos, 1978; Saal, 1975.
[6] Bell, 1970; DeCarie and Simineau, 1979; Wachs, 1987.

representations into stable mental constructs that Piaget has referred to as schema.

The evolution of object permanence may be tracked by carefully observing a change in the infant's psychomotor manifestations in the first 2 years of life. The therapist can assess elementary neuromotor patterns by placing the infant in "activation positions" (Katona, 1990). This developmental period is marked by an increased ability to manipulate objects in the environment and by the active search, through both visual and body manifestations, for completely disappeared objects (Butterworth, 1977). Between 5 and 11 months, infants manifest anticipatory visual attention or vigilance (Ruff, 1990). The looking of an infant between events involves the expectation that the event will reoccur. Other researchers also suggest that infants use visual events to construct future expectations and use their expectations to learn about the environment (Benson, 1990; Haith, 1990). The capacity to follow disappearing moving objects surfaces at approximately 12 months (Ramsay-Douglas & Campos, 1978). By 18 months, the infant demonstrates, through the reconstruction of complex movements, that he can maintain a model in the physical absence of the model (DeCarie & Simineau, 1979).

By observing the infant's manipulation of objects and active search for objects, manifested in both visual scanning and body movements, the therapist can ascertain whether the infant is manifesting a degree of object permanence appropriate for his developmental level. In addition, therapists need to be attuned to the caregiver's responses to these manifestations. A caregiver who stimulates the infant's appetite for manipulation of objects in space through such games as peekaboo will be fostering adaptive cognitive growth in the direction of object permanence. When such caregiver behaviors are lacking, the therapist may wish to use *modeling* or other techniques to encourage the caregiver's promotion of these cognitive manifestations in the infant.

Assessing Fine and Gross Motor Coordination

Infants also communicate their internal states through body gestures. Essentially two types of gestures indicate the adaptability of the dyadic interaction: *fine* and *gross motor behaviors*. The development of these movements over time can be analyzed using videotape. During the first months of life, the infant's gestures are confined primarily to gross motor movements, which involve both sets of limbs; for example, pointing with the arm or kicking to manifest discomfort. Fine motor movement involves gestures that demonstrate a sophisticated degree of coordination and typically involve the hands and fingers. Fist pointing with the fingers and picking up a utensil signify two examples in this category of movement. In observing gesturing phenomena, the therapist should note if the developmental trend from gross to fine movement is evident in the infant. In other words, are gross movements gradually being refined in the direction of more sophisticated fine movements? Is the infant able to combine both gross motor and fine motor movements to accomplish a task?

Beyond the categorization of fine and gross motor manifestations, the therapist should also be aware of other physically communicative behaviors displayed by infants. For example, the behavior labeled *startle* is demonstrated by a sudden movement of the body away from a newly introduced stimulus. The infant manifests *regression* by clinging, sucking a digit or the fist, climbing into the caregiver's lap, or assuming the fetal position. Repetitive rocking motions may also be an indication of regression. *Aggressive behavior* is characterized by pushing, slapping, hitting, shoving, kicking, grabbing, and/or biting. In addition, the infant will often approach the stimulus in a menacing fashion during an episode of aggression. *Negativity* and *oppositional* behavior are manifested by head shaking and purposeful head aversion. The infant may move away from the caregiver and refuse to respond to any external stimulus. The therapist should not only observe and categorize these behaviors, but should also attempt to discern the infant's physical skill when displaying these gestures. Does he display such activity continuously or intermittently in spasms? Significantly, does the infant manifest such behavior to engage the caregiver or to disengage from the interaction?

In addition to alerting the therapist to the infant's chronological development, a detailed observation of motor coordination and gestures also provides insight into the adaptive regulation that permeates dyadic interaction. Several researchers have noted that gestures—referred to as *analogic* forms of communication because the gesture replicates a message being conveyed—provide valuable clues for assessing the nature and degree of communication within the dyad. Not only does the infant manifest gestures to the caregiver, but the caregiver commonly reciprocates these gestures with her own. Therapists should thus observe the gestures of both members of the dyad to ascertain whether these body movements are random and disorganized or whether the caregiver and infant use these signals for conveying messages to one another to achieve a more optimal level of adaptation. See Table 3–2.

Assessing Attachment Behaviors

Attachment behavior is a complicated way of describing what is actually a quite straightforward and direct phenomenon—the degree to which caregiver and infant strive to remain within physical and psychological proximity of one another. In an adaptive dyad, the degree of *proximity* will tend to be high, because physical and psychological closeness result in feelings of intimacy and mastery. This closeness between infants and their caregivers manifested particularly in physical closeness, is due to several factors. First, as several researchers have pointed out, the newborn's visual abilities are not as developed as those of older infants and therefore caregivers tend to remain physically close to the infant's visual field to elicit a response. Second, for most caregivers the newborn represents, on some level, an extension of the physical body, and the intimacy experienced during the pregnancy is reexperienced as the mother holds or nurses the infant. This is the case whether the mother bottle-feeds or breast-feeds. As time goes on, however, the infant's burgeoning developmental skills in the

Table 3–2.   Fine and Gross Motor Development

Chronological Age	Psychomotor Development[1-5]
4 weeks or less	*Gross Motor* Supine: side position head dominates Sit: head predominately sags Prone: head droops, ventral suspension Infants spontaneously modulate muscle activity in response to biomechanical context and impose intention on those dynamics to perform task-related movements[1] *Fine Motor* Supine: both hands fisted
8 weeks	*Gross Motor* Supine: rolls part way to side Pull-to-sit: complete or marked head lag Sit: head predominately bobbingly erect *Fine Motor* Prone: head in midposition Points: no arm extension[2]
12 weeks	*Gross Motor* Supine: midposition head and symmetrical postures Prone: lifts head midposition in sustained fashion *Fine Motor* Supine: hands open or loosely closed
16 weeks	*Gross Motor* Supine: head set forward, bobs Prone: verge of rolling Sit: head steady *Fine Motor* Supine: fingering gestures, scratches, clutches
20 weeks	*Gross Motor* Pull-to-sit: no head lag Sit: head erect, steady Prone: arms extended Ability to compensate for balance disruptions caused by reaching; coordination of active muscle-produced forces and inertial forces *Fine Motor* Prone: scratches tabletop Grip: precarious grasp of cube
24 weeks	*Gross Motor* Supine: lifts legs high in extension Supine: rolls to prone Pull-to-sit: lifts head *Fine Motor* Grip: resecures dropped cube

Table 3–2. *(Continued)*

Chronological Age	Psychomotor Development[1-5]
28 weeks	*Gross Motor*
	Supine: lifts head
	Sit: erect momentarily
	Stand: bounces actively
	Fine Motor
	Grip: radial palmar grasp of cube
32 weeks	*Gross Motor*
	Stand: large fraction of weight
	Sit: briefly, leans forward on hands
	Fine Motor
	Grip: grasps 2nd cube
36 weeks	*Gross Motor*
	Sit: erect 10 minutes plus, steady
	Stand: maintain briefly, hands held
	Fine Motor
	Grip: radial digital grasp of cube
40 weeks	*Gross Motor*
	Prone: pivots, creeps
	Sit: goes to prone
	Stand: pulls to feet at rail
	Fine Motor
	Grip: crude release of cube
44 weeks	*Gross Motor*
	Stand: at rail; lifts and replaces foot
48 weeks	*Gross Motor*
	Sits: pivots
	Stand: cruises at rail
	Walks: needs 2 hands held
52 weeks	*Gross Motor*
	Walks: needs only 1 hand held
	Fine Motor
	Grip: tries tower of cubes, fails
56 weeks	*Gross Motor*
	Stand: momentarily alone
	Fine Motor
	Grip: grasp 2 cubes in 1 hand, pincer grip; instrumental pointing
15 months (60 weeks)	*Gross Motor*
	Walks: few steps, starts, stops
	Creeping discarded
	Stairs: creeps up
	Fine Motor
	Grip: tower of 2 cubes

Table 3–2. *(Continued)*

Chronological Age	Psychomotor Development[1-5]
18 months (1 year, 6 months)	*Gross Motor* Walks: seldom falls Stairs: walks up, 1 hand held Small chair: seats self *Fine Motor* Grip: tower of 3–4 cubes
21 months	*Gross Motor* Walks: squats in play Stairs: walks down, 1 hand held Stairs: walks up, holds rail *Fine Motor* Grip: tower of 5–6 cubes
24 months (2 years)	*Gross Motor* Walks: runs well, no falling Stairs: walks up and down alone *Fine Motor* Grip: tower of 6–7 cubes
30 months (2 years, 6 months)	*Gross Motor* Walks: on tiptoe Stands: tries to stand on 1 foot *Fine Motor* Grip: tower of 8 cubes
36 months (3 years)	*Gross Motor* Stairs: alternate feet going up Rides: tricycle using pedals *Fine Motor* Grip: tower of 9 (10 on 3 tries) cubes
42 months (3 years, 6 months)	*Gross Motor* Stands: on 1 foot, 2 seconds *Fine Motor* Grip: builds bridge from model
48 months (4 years)	*Gross Motor* Stairs: walks down, 1 foot on step Stands: on 1 foot, 4–8 seconds *Fine Motor* Grip: imitates gate
54 months (4 years, 6 months)	*Gross Motor* Hops: on 1 foot *Fine Motor* Grips: makes gate from model
60 months (5 years)	*Gross Motor* Skips: uses feet alternately Stands: on one foot more than 8 seconds *Fine Motor* Grip: builds 2 steps

Table 3–2. *(Continued)*

Chronological Age	Psychomotor Development[1-5]
72 months (6 years)	*Gross Motor* Stands: on each foot alternately, eyes closed *Fine Motor* Grip: builds 3 steps

[1] Thelen, 1990.
[2] Fogel and Hannan, 1985.
[3] Ashmead, 1990.
[4] Piaget, 1954.
[5] Gesell and Amatruda, 1974.

area of motor coordination in particular, coupled with the infant's physical growth, necessitate some degree of separation.

Nevertheless, proximity will tend to be reestablished during episodes of interaction when the caregiver exchanges visual, vocal, and gestural cues with the infant. During these intervals the therapist can observe other aspects of attachment behavior that affect dyadic exchange. For example, when the caregiver initiates interaction, does she establish proximity with the infant and, correspondingly, does the infant move close to the caregiver during these episodes? The therapist should also observe whether the reverse occurs. That is, does the caregiver move closer to the infant when the infant begins emitting cues such as vocalizations and gestures that indicate the desire for interaction? The therapist should also observe the overall nature of proximic behavior within the dyadic interaction. For example, does the infant generally stay within the orbit of the caregiver's immediate presence? Does the infant cling to the caregiver? As development progresses, the therapist should be attuned to general trends governing the infant's degree of proximity.

By the 9th month, for example, the infant will most likely have begun crawling. Campos, Qi, Li, Fleener, and Tu (1990) have documented a number of changes that occur in the dyad as a result of the development of crawling behavior including an increase in the caregiver's expressions of anger toward the infant, an attribution of greater responsibility, a greater sensitivity to maternal departures and reunions, and greater visual checking by the infant of the caregiver's location. Thus, as development progresses, the relationship between the caregiver and infant will be affected by the achievement of each developmental milestone.

The infant engages in visual checking, referred to as *social referencing,* to resolve any discrepancy he perceives in the environment. It is fairly easy to recognize social referencing: The infant will take a few crawling steps and then turn back and gaze in the caregiver's direction for reference. Adaptive caregivers recognize this behavior and will wave or call out to the infant when he manifests this cluster of behaviors. A caregiver who fails to acknowledge the infant in this fashion may be conveying the message that she is not interested by or encouraged to promote the infant's developmental progress.

The therapist can also evaluate attachment behaviors by observing how the infant responds in the presence of a stranger or a new adult. Depending on their age, some infants will gravitate immediately to a stranger. This response may be adaptive in the sense that it indicates the infant is curious and interested in new stimuli, or it may be a sign of maladaptation suggesting that the infant is not receiving sufficient stimulation from the caregiver and is thus indiscriminately seeking out another object with whom to interact. If the infant is frightened or surprised by a stranger, for example, clinging to the caregiver suggests that the infant perceives the caregiver as a secure figure and therefore such clinging may be appropriate. On the other hand, excessive clinging may suggest that the infant has not been encouraged to develop the maturational skills necessary for interacting with new stimuli in the environment. Although it is a broad generalization to say that infants who cautiously interact with others while periodically referencing their caregivers are adaptive, this behavior often does indicate an adaptive level of developmental skill. The attachment bond has implications for the infant's future development. Children with a history of insecure attachment are more shy and manifest more behavioral inhibitions than securely attached children (Aaron, Calkins, & Fox, 1990; Kemple & Hazen, 1990), whereas securely attached children manifest a positive orientation toward other social relationships (Howes & Rodning, 1990). Infants have been shown to manifest undesirable attachment behaviors as a result of maltreatment (Barnett, Ganiban, Martin, Cicchetti, & Carlson, 1990), boundary violations in the family (Fish, 1990), stressful life events (Caldera, 1990; Heim & Mangelsdorf, 1990), a caregiver's negative affect (Isabella, 1990), an overstimulative or intrusive caregiver (Gable & Isabella, 1990), or day care (Lamb, Sternberg, & Prodromidis, 1990). In sum, the therapist should use observations of attachment behaviors in formulating an overall portrait of the status of interaction in any particular dyadic pair. See Table 3–3.

Assessing Language

Language in this context refers not to the specific substance being conveyed so much as it does to the *vocalizations* both caregiver and infant use to communicate and share internal states. Even before the infant is born, he is exposed to language. The voices that an infant hears in utero are muffled and difficult to understand, but prosidic features such as rhythm and intonation remain intact (Busnel, Granier-Deferre, & Lecanuet, 1990). For example, newborns have been observed to orient their heads toward a train of brief sounds (Clarkson, Swain, Clifton, & Cohen, 1990). This suggests

Table 3–3. **Attachment Behaviors**

Chronological Age	Attachment Behaviors
4 weeks or less	Undiscriminating social responsiveness: capacity to orient to salient features of environment Orienting behaviors: visual fixation, visual tracking, listening, rooting, and postural adjustment when held Primitive behaviors: sucking and grasping Special signaling behaviors: smiling, crying, vocalizing; behaviors easily disrupted by competing stimuli (through 3 months)[1] By 1–2 months, proportion of time babies looked, smiled and vocalized, as well as moved arms toward people differed significantly from responses to doll[2]
8 weeks	Enhanced eye-to-eye contact Social smiling[3]
12 weeks	Discriminating social responsiveness: discriminates between and differentially responsive to familiar and strange figures Emergence of differential smiling, vocalization, crying More active and varied, proximity-seeking and contact-maintaining behaviors (through 6 months)[1] Greeting response[4] Matching of emotional expressions[5] Face-to-face games (peekaboo, so-big)
16 weeks	Doll: further attention
20 weeks	Doll: more interested in doll
24 weeks	Consolidation of attachment system (24–48 weeks)[6] Turn-taking in facial expression and visual contact; dialoguelike nonvocal exchanges, e.g., infant turns away as a sign for mother to intervene[7] Infant-initiated play Environmental exploration Ritual games relying on repetition and imitation of verbal sequences; linear increase in instrumental use of caregiver (6–13 months)[8] Manipulation of objects
28 weeks	Active initiative in seeking proximity and contact Locomotion and voluntary movements evident in attachment behavior More active and effective greeting responses (through 36 months)[1] Functional and relational play (through 2 years)[4] Active involvement in play[8]
32 weeks	Stereotypical play[3]
36 weeks	Reflective imitation[9] Simple relational play[10]

Table 3–3. (Continued)

Chronological Age	Attachment Behaviors
44 weeks	Presymbolic schemes: understanding of object use or meaning by brief recognitory gestures[11]
	Differentiates between two basic level natural categories[12]
48–52 weeks (1 year)	Begins to construct internal working model-panorama of self and attachment figures for use in planning, understanding, and guiding behavior vis-à-vis caregiver; accessible attachment figure[13]
	Egocentric empathy (through 2 years)[5]
	Infant-initiated play[14]
	Turn-taking behavior[14]
	Awareness of social or task demands by caregivers (through 18 months)[9]
52 weeks	Representational play[3]
	Accommodative relational play[10]
	Autosymbolic scheme: pretending at self-related activities[1]
18 months (1 year, 6 months)	Decentered acts (through 19 months)[15]
	Single-scheme symbolic play: extends symbolism beyond own actions by including others[11]
21 months	Symbolic play: one pretend scheme is related to several actors or receivers[11]
	Grouping or sequential acts[10]
	Social coordination and joint referencing[16]
24 months (2 years)	Make-believe games
	Role-playing
	Rule structures appear
	Parallel play predominates
	Empathy for another's feelings (through 3 + years)[5]
	Multischeme combinations[15]
	Planned symbolic games[11]
30 months (2 years, 6 months)	Awareness of social rules
36 months (3 years)	Goal-corrected partnership: inference about attachment figure's "set-goals"; attempts to alter caregiver actions and goals; reciprocity of increasing sophistication[1]
42 months (3 years, 6 months)	Associative play replaces parallel play
48 months (4 years)	Cooperates with other children

Table 3–3. *(Continued)*

Chronological Age	Attachment Behaviors
54 months (4 years, 6 months)	Calls attention to self

[1] Ainsworth, 1973, pp. 10–13.
[2] Legerstee, Pomerleau, Malcuit, and Feider, 1987.
[3] Emde, 1984.
[4] Haekel, 1985.
[5] Hoffman, 1975, 1977, 1982b, 1984.
[6] Mahler, 1958; Mahler, Pine, and Bergman, 1975.
[7] Kaye and Fogel, 1980; Papousek and Papousek, 1987.
[8] Mosier and Rogoff, 1990.
[9] Kopp, 1982; Lewis and Brooks, 1978.
[10] Fenson, Kagan, Kearsley, and Zelazo, 1976.
[11] McCune-Nicolich and Carroll, 1981.
[12] Ellis, 1990.
[13] Bowlby, 1980; Bretherton, 1987.
[14] Ross and Kay, 1980.
[15] Fenson and Ramsay, 1980.
[16] Baldwin, 1990.

that the infant, even from a very early age, will *perceive* and *respond* to a caregiver's vocalizations. The infant's own *expressive* language development begins with small throaty noises in the 1st month of life. By 2 months, these vocalizations assume a particular pattern such that the infant verbalizes in response to the caregiver's stimulation. This social response matures by the 3rd month to encompass chuckles, giggles, verbal turn-taking, and repetitive and rhythmic vocal exchanges (Anderson, 1990).

At 4 months of age, the infant laughs out loud in response to specific caregiver cues and expresses a distinct preference for *motherese sounds* (Cooper, 1990; Fernald & Kuhl, 1987). Thereafter, linguistic development is rapid. At some point after 6 months, infants will evince an "m-m-m" sound in the presence of the mother. Single consonant sounds, such as "ba" or "da" follow, along with a phenomenon that has been referred to as *canonical babbling* (DeBoysson, Sagart, & Durand, 1984; Koopmans-van-Deinun & van der Stelt, 1985). During such babbling episodes the infant repeats a sound over and over as if trying to exert control and mastery over the sound. By 10 to 26 months, the single-word utterances of children are similar to those of, and were probably learned from, their caregivers (Ninio, 1990).

As with the other behavioral dimensions, the therapist can use language manifestations to assess the infant's developmental status and the skill of the caregiver in enhancing maturational attainment. Researchers such as Papousek and Papousek (1987) have observed that adaptive dyads are characterized by a high level of *vocal cuing* in which both caregiver and infant verbalize to exchange affective and cognitive messages. In this fashion, an adaptive caregiver will tend to modify the tone, pace, and frequency of her voice to enhance the positive mood during an episode of verbal exchange. A classic kind of vocal cuing is the caregiver's lullaby to the infant: The caregiver is not so much interested in interpreting the specific words of the song for the infant as she is in instilling a rhythmically comforting mood that will help him make the transition from wakefulness to sleep. Mothers often use a similar process when dressing the child by commenting, for example, "Now we will put on your snowsuit before we go out, because it's cold outside." Although the mother may not actually expect the infant fully to understand the message's symbolic meaning, her tone of voice, coupled with other behavioral manifestations, conveys her purposefulness.

Caregivers whose behaviors are generally maladaptive tend to rely far less frequently on language. One caregiver I treated rarely communicated with her infant by name or engaged in the kind of "nonsense" talk that is so prevalent among new mothers. This absence of vocalization represented a form of deprivation, because the infant lacked guidance from an ever-present, supportive vocal flow to guide him in his efforts toward predicting and mastering developmental change. As the caregiver improved and became more attuned to the infant's developmental trends, the frequency of her vocalizations also increased and the infant correspondingly became more responsive. Thus, the nature and degree of vocalization during dyadic exchange become a significant observational dimension that the therapist should evaluate.

What was particularly striking about the preceding case was that the caregiver's lack of vocal exchange with the infant appeared to exert a significantly detrimental effect on various aspects of his development. Indeed, this infant lagged behind others of the same chronological age in a wide variety of developmental skills. The relationship between language and other developmental milestones has been discussed by Cohen (1990) who observed that infants displaying exceptional competence in language development were more likely to have positive self-perceptions in early adolescence. Because language plays a crucial role in other areas of future development, it is important to pay attention to physical factors, such as middle ear disease (which is prevalent in young infants and children), that may cause language delays (Feagans, McGhee, Kipp, & Blood, 1990).

One reason there may be a strong correlation between caregiver vocalization and other infant developmental skills is that vocalizations serve multiple functions. First, vocalization, like visual cuing and gesturing, is a means for communicating with the infant about immediate events. Second, however, exposure to vocalization enables the infant eventually to learn the arbitrary, *digital* signals of language so that he can begin to engage in symbolic thought processes. The caregiver can facilitate the infant's acquisition of these thought processes through *labeling* or *naming*, in which her nonverbal gestures direct the infant's attention to objects in the immediate environment, thus enabling him to discover what specific words mean (Echols, 1990; Schmidt, 1990).

As a consequence, therapists should be particularly alert to both the quality and quantity of the caregiver's vocalizations. Where vocalization is minimal or absent, the caregiver should be encouraged in techniques for directly stimulating the infant through verbal sounds. See Table 3–4.

Table 3–4. **Language Development**

Chronological Age	Language Development
4 weeks or less	Small, throaty noises
8 weeks	Social vocalizations
12 weeks	Social response: chuckles, giggles; verbal turn-taking; repetitive and rhythmic vocal exchanges
16 weeks	Laughs aloud
	Preference for motherese sounds
	Bimodal perception speech—4–5 months: can detect correspondence between auditory and visually perceived speech-vocalization influences;[1] visual fixation, looks longer at face matching sound; visual/auditory connection originating in infant's intermodal representation of speech[2]
20 weeks	Squeals
24 weeks	Spontaneous vocal-social (including toys)
	Bell-ringing: turns head to bell
28 weeks	M-m-m (crying)
32 weeks	Single consonant, da, ba, ka (canonical babbling)
	Gaze alteration
36 weeks	Controlled polysyllabic vowel sounds; grunts, growls; imitates sounds; responds to name
40 weeks	Vocabulary: 1 "word"
	Da-da or equivalent
	Comprehension: bye; patacake
52 weeks	Vocabulary: 2 "words"
(1 year)	Comprehension: gives a toy (by request)
56 weeks	Vocabulary: 3–4 words
	Comprehension: a few objects by name
15 months	Vocabulary: 4–6 words including names; incipient jargon
18 months	Book: looks selectively
(1 year, 6 months)	Vocabulary: 10 words, including names
	Ball: 2 directional commands
21 months	Vocabulary: 20 words
	Ball: 3 directional commands

Table 3–4.   (Continued)

Chronological Age	Language Development
24 months (2 years)	Speech: jargon discarded; 3-word sentences; uses I, me, you
	Picture cards: names 3 or more
	Ball: directional commands
30 months (2 years, 6 months)	Name: gives full name
	Picture cards: names 8
36 months (3 years)	Book: gives action
	Speech: uses plural
	Sex: tells gender
	Prepositions: obeys 2
42 months (3½ years)	Picture cards: names all pictures; enumerates 3
	Prepositions: obeys 3
48 months (4 years)	Color cards: names 1
	Prepositions: obeys 4
54 months (4½ years)	Defines: 4 words in terms of use
60 months (5 years)	Coins: names penny, nickel, dime
	Pictures: descriptive comment with enumeration
72 months (6 years)	Adds and subtracts: within 5
	Differentiates AM from PM[3]

[1] Legerstee and Moore, 1990.
[2] Kuhl and Meltzoff, 1982.
[3] Gesell and Amatruda, 1974.

Assessing the Infant's Subjective Experience

Efforts to recognize the *subjective* elements of dyadic interaction have produced persuasive evidence indicating how these interactions may become maladaptive. The data on mother–infant interaction indicate that the infant needs predictable sequences of interaction with a significant nurturing figure to formulate a mature and stable *self-concept* (Bowlby, 1973, 1982; Kopp, 1982; Ricks, 1985; Trad, 1986). From the infant's birth, the caregiver facilitates this process by attributing meaning to the infant's behaviors (Shields, 1978; Vygotsky, 1962). By responding intuitively to the infant's manifestations, the parent provides a supportive atmosphere for the development of the somatic, socio-affective, cognitive, and motivational dimensions embedded within these intentions. Nurturance of these behaviors supports the infant's efforts to broaden communication channels (Chomsky, 1965). In essence, a nurturing atmosphere invests the infant's behavior with meaning, whereas constitutional disposition enables the infant to coordinate responses to such stimuli. In this manner, the caregiver's responses transform the infant's signals into a meaningful message that the infant can respond to (Piaget, 1952; Spitz, 1959; Wachs, 1987). Examples of other intuitive behaviors that support these transformations include empathy, rhythmicity, and reciprocity.

Empathy is the psychological state through which the caregiver gains awareness of the affective states of the infant. Hoffman (1982b, 1984) defines empathy as an affective response more appropriate to someone else's situation than to one's own. The emergence of empathy on the part of the infant signifies that he has begun to incorporate the perspective of another—generally, the caregiver.

Rhythmicity is a term used to characterize the mood that imbues dyadic interaction. Adaptive caregiver–infant interactions usually occur in rhythmical patterns (Brazelton, Koslowski, & Main, 1974). Periodic cycles take place in which the manifestations of both members of the dyad become synchronized through mutual entrainment (Lester, Hoffman, & Brazelton, 1985). By following the infant's thresholds for attention and withdrawal, the adaptive caregiver produces synchrony in the interaction. Insensitive stimulation of the infant, on the other hand, produces dyssynchronic responses. Systems of classification for synchronous and dyssynchronic nonverbal communication are still being developed (Eisenhart & Hrncir, 1990).

Reciprocity refers to the infant's thresholds of tolerance and concomitant ability to regulate his attentional states in the context of the caregiver's level of stimulation (Brazelton & Als, 1979). For example, when infants withdraw their attention, adaptive caregivers tend to respond in a similar fashion; when infants return their attention so do caregivers. Thus, harmonious interaction produces a consistent pattern of *mutual* attention followed by inattention.

At approximately the time canonical babbling emerges, infants begin to display signs of *intersubjectivity*. This concept involves the infant's capacity to understand that significant others, such as caregivers, have representations that are separate and distinct from his own. Trevarthen (1980, 1985) explains that for infants to share their mental experience with others, they must possess two skills. First, they must exhibit at least the basic components of individual awareness and intentionality. These qualities are referred to by Trevarthen as subjectivity and imply an incipient awareness of a sense of self and of boundary demarcation. Next, to communicate, infants must also adapt their subjectivity to the subjectivity of others. They must, in other words, demonstrate intersubjectivity. Some researchers have referred to intersubjectivity as the capacity to share meaning with another person, so that both individuals experience the same representation of some object, event, or symbol (Trad, 1990). Although this capacity is not yet fully understood, infants begin to display shared meaning by the end of the 1st year of life if an interactive partner has provided a consistent level of adequate stimulation. Once the infant acknowledges the separateness of the caregiver, the child begins to respond to this phenomenon by manifesting particular cues.

For Kaye (1982), the onset of intersubjectivity marks the commencement of the infant's *capacity to symbolize*. Kaye notes that experiencing a shared meaning with another involves two prerequisites. The first is *intentional significance*, the external representation of some class of things or events, or relations among them, using a sign that remains distinguished from the thing signified. This sign or gesture may assume the form of a manual or facial expression, according to Kaye, but may also take the form of words or melodies. Gestures can designate things without actually being equivalent to the thing itself. Thus, the intention of the sign is crucial to whether it is differentiated from what it signifies. The second prerequisite is that the meaning attributed to the thing is by convention only. That is, a signal is a sign for a particular thing only because the members of a group (e.g., speakers of a specific language) have arbitrarily designated that meaning to it. Moreover, gestures are distinctly human; no nonhuman has ever been shown to have produced a sign with the intention of signifying an event that was remote in time or space, so that the sign designates an event without being the equivalent to it. The development of symbolic thought should be regarded as a social process that can emerge only from interaction with others and the developmental attainment of predictive capacities. Although symbols may have a mental process accompanying them, the symbolic process is distinct from the gesture itself, which reflects an interpersonal act. The mind can represent a symbol, just as it can represent nonsignifying objects, and this form of representation heralds the most sophisticated of the infant's acquisitions in the realm of language development (Werner & Kaplan, 1963). Not only is the infant now capable of predicting maternal speech, but he can communicate intentions to the caregiver using his own language.

A fascinating issue related to these studies involves how researchers can deduce that specific developmental events are occurring within the infant during this period. For example, how do investigators surmise the nature of the infant's experience? One answer is that although infancy is a period when *digital* forms of communication (such as language that relies on arbitrary symbols such as words) are not the primary vehicle for conveying information, *analogic* modes of communication are frequent and common. Among the most prevalent forms of analogic communication used by the infant are primitive vocal sounds and body gestures. These behaviors are classic analogic signals because the infant's message is reenacted and predicted as a gesture, the emblem of an analogic message.

Polysyllabic vowel sounds are manifested next, and the infant begins to imitate sounds in response to hearing his name. By 40 weeks of age, most infants are able to pronounce one word and by 1 year of age can pronounce two words. In addition, the infant can associate specific sounds with specific objects by attempting to express a particular word when an object is presented. At this juncture, then, the infant appears to have inculcated the notion that words are symbolic referents that signify specific objects with the real world (Werner & Kaplan, 1963).

Other signs of subjective development follow thereafter in rapid succession. For example, social referencing in situations of affective uncertainty becomes pronounced by 48 weeks, according to Emde (1984); however, it is not used extensively by infants under 9 months (McComas & Field, 1990). There is also a renewed interest in the caregiver's whereabouts at this time, and separation reactions, whereby the infant follows the mother's every move and becomes distressed at her absence, are also prevalent (Mahler et al., 1975). By 30 months, affective expression is appropriate to the social context and internal feeling states are organized (Emde, 1984). Emde has also pinpointed gender identity at 36 months and oedipal identifications at 48 months. See Table 3–5.

Assessing Individual Differences in Self-Regulation

Even the earliest researchers in the area of development noticed that newborn infants manifested individual differences in their mode of *self-regulation* to the environment (Alessandri & Sullivan, 1990; Fries, 1937; Fries & Lewis, 1938; Fries & Woolf, 1953) and the combination of response systems (neurophysiological-biochemical, behavioral-expressive, and subjective-experiential) involved in the infant's self-regulation (Gunnar, Kopp, Tronick, & Rothbart, 1990). Eventually, these individual differences came to be referred to as *temperamental dimensions* that were exhibited in a unique fashion by each infant and that appeared to remain stable over a period of years, thereby exerting a significant effect on early development.

Buss and Plomin (1975) defined temperament as consisting of the specific dimensions of emotionality, activity, sociability, and impulsivity. These researchers indicated that the dimensions of temperament were inheritable, stable, predictive of adult personality, and adaptive in the evolutionary sense. Rothbart and Derryberry (1981) characterized temperament as the constitutional differences in reactivity and self-regulation manifested by the individual, with "constitutional" interpreted to mean the relatively enduring biological endowment of the organism, influenced during development by heredity, maturational trends, and experience. Thomas, Chess, and Birch (1968) focused on the behavioral style of the individual child and articulated nine dimensions of temperament: activity level, rhythmicity (regularity), approach or withdrawal, adaptability, threshold of responsiveness, intensity of reaction, quality of mood, distractibility, and attention span or persistence. Thomas et al. also identified particular clusters of these temperamental dimensions that persisted over time, leading them to for-

Table 3–5.   Subjective Development

Chronological Age	Subjective Development
4 weeks or less	Imitation as an intentional reproduction of a visually perceived model (through 6 months)[1]
	Discrepancy (through 4 months)[2]
	Social referencing: active search for emotional information from another person and subsequent use of that emotion to help appraise uncertain situations. Develops in 4-level sequence:
	Level 1—lack of facial perception, neonates neither recognize facial expression nor perceive whole faces; newborns scan edges, transitions, contours; no tendency to scan entire face; don't scan interior of face, although neonates seem able to discriminate happy, sad, surprised[3]
8 weeks	Subjectivity: motivated, interior cause of action, motive to know world, motive to communicate with others[4]
	Intersubjectivity: holding, feeding, gazing face-to-face, vocalizing, expressing pleasure, reciprocity, avoidance/ withdrawal, developing control[4]
	Coordination of autonomous function into integrative process[5]
	Contingency (2.5–6 months) establishes expectation of control over environment
	At 2.5 months generally does not learn a minimal affective response[6]
	Social referencing: Level 2 (through 5 months)—facial perception without appreciation of affect[3]
12 weeks	Regulation (12–16 weeks)
	Intersubjectivity/contingency (through 6 months)[7]
	Expectancies (12–16 weeks)[8]
	Discrepancy: prior to 3 months, familiar stimulus evokes stronger response than novel stimulus[2]
16 weeks	Emotional spectrum[9]
	Engagement/disengagement[10]
	Contingency (4 months): consistent evidence of learning and emotional response, smiling, less fussing[6]
	Expectancies: can estimate time intervals and develop expectancies of anticipated behavior[8]
	Discrepancy: after 3 months attention to discrepant event begins to predominate fixation, smiling, vocalization, heart rate
	Subjects who rapidly habituate to standard showed heightened fixation to stimulus change in accord with discrepancy hypothesis. Habituation pattern suggestive of internal representation[2]

Table 3–5. *(Continued)*

Chronological Age	Subjective Development
24 weeks	Differentiation/development of body image (20–32 weeks)[11]
	Social referencing: Level 3 (through 7 months). Emotional responsiveness to facial emotion, emerging emotional resonance by 6 months, response to emotional expression/responsivity correlates with visual organization for different regions of face[3]
	Contingency: learning associated with emotional behavior[6] and with place where learning occurs[12]
32 weeks	Interaffectivity[13]
	Independent locomotion: exploratory forays from emotional base (through 1 year)[14]
36 weeks	Established and differentiated emotional experience (through 12 months)[15]
	Secondary intersubjectivity: mother no longer merely source of pleasure, now an interesting agent
	New form of spontaneous play, symbolic representation—peekaboo, lying down for sleep
	Vocalizes interpersonal interaction[4]
	Affective attunement; realization that subjective experience, attention, intentions, and affective states can be shared with another. Subjective intermeshings through interintentionality and interaffectivity; focuses on shared affect—mother matches temporal beat, intensity, contour, duration[16]
	Social referencing: Level 4—facial expression to reference-action consequence; situational reference; inference of emotional feeling states in another; predicting another's behavior as it impacts on oneself; 2-person communication about a third event; mother pointing or gaze understanding target, visual cliff (through 12 months)[17]
40 weeks	Practicing (through 15 months)[18]
48 weeks	Social referencing prominent in situations of affective uncertainty[19]
	Rapprochement (through 21 months): revival of constant concern for mother's whereabouts, separation reactions shadowing mother's every move[14]
21 months	Emotional object constancy; internalization of parental wishes, rules, standards, symbolic play;[14] few differences between self and other knowledge (18 + months)[20]
30 months	Affect expressions "socialized"[19]
(2 years, 6 months)	Internal feeling states organized[19]

Table 3–5. (Continued)

Chronological Age	Subjective Development
36 months (3 years)	Gender identity[19]
48 months (4 years)	Oedipal identifications (through 6 years)[16]

[1] Meltzoff and Moore, 1977.
[2] McCall and Kagan, 1970.
[3] Klinnert, Campos, Sorce, Emde, and Svejda, 1983.
[4] Trevarthen, 1980; 1985.
[5] Hopkins and van Wufften Palthe, 1985; Papousek and Papousek, 1979.
[6] Lewis, Wolan-Sullivan, and Brooks-Gunn, 1985.
[7] Kuhl and Meltzoff, 1982.
[8] Mast, Fagen, Rovee-Collier, and Sullivan, 1980; Stern and Gibbon, 1978.
[9] Emde, Kligman, Reich, and Wade, 1978.
[10] Beebe and Stern, 1977.
[11] Mahler, 1958; Mahler et al., 1975; Mahler and McDevitt, 1968; Spitz, 1965.
[12] Shyi, Schechter, and Shields, 1990.
[13] Stern, 1985.
[14] Mahler et al., 1975.
[15] Lewis and Brooks, 1978; Kopp, 1982.
[16] Bretherton and Bates, 1979; Klinnert et al., 1983; Stern, 1985.
[17] Hoffman, 1975; 1977; 1982b; 1984.
[18] Mahler, 1958; Mahler et al., 1975.
[19] Emde, 1984.
[20] Pipp, Fischer, and Jennings, 1987.

mulate three main temperamental typologies. These included the "easy" temperament, characterized by positiveness in mood, regularity of bodily function, low or moderate intensity of reaction, adaptability, and positive approach, rather than withdrawal from new situations. In contrast, the "difficult" temperament manifested irregularity of bodily function, an intense reaction to stimuli, withdrawal in the face of new stimuli, slow adaptability to environmental change, and a negative mood. Finally, the "slow-to-warm-up" typology displayed a low activity level, mild reactions, and slow adaptability, often manifested a negative mood, and showed a tendency to withdraw from new stimuli.

As with facial expression, the infant's temperamental profile will be manifested relatively early in life, will persist over time, and will provide the therapist with information about the status of the infant's development. Even more pertinent, however, is the way in which temperament contributes to the dyadic interaction. For example, infants who are breast-fed have been found to manifest more irritability than non-breast-fed infants (Worobey & Thomas, 1990). In addition, newborn infants who manifest low irritability but become highly irritable at five months have been found to have mothers who are less satisfied with their marriages and who have less positive personality traits (Fish, 1990). By focusing on such temperamental traits as attention span, persistence, and reactivity level, the therapist will be able to discern how the infant's temperament is either enhancing or impeding the flow of dyadic communication. For example, how long does the infant heed the caregiver's cues before becoming distracted, and does the caregiver persist when the infant has clearly lost interest? Are the infant's responses appropriately reactive, or does the infant react too intensely or too lethargically to derive benefit from the caregiver's communications?

Moreover, the therapist should also focus on the degree to which the caregiver aligns her own temperamental qualities to those of the infant. In some instances, a caregiver with an easy temperament will be unable to adjust to the behaviors manifested by an infant with a difficult or slow-to-warm-up temperament or vice versa. Through observation the therapist can diagnose these incongruities of interaction and eventually develop strategies for modifying behavior in a more adaptive fashion by sensitizing the caregiver to the infant's unique temperamental displays. See Table 3–6.

Assessing Defensive Operations

Researchers have known for quite some time that even very young infants can manifest *defensive operations*. Tronick and Weinberg (1990), for example, have observed that 6-month-old infants can develop stable affective and behavioral patterns of coping with interpersonal stress. Researchers have also known that the extreme exhibition of these defense styles may implicate psychopathology. In particular, researchers such as Fraiberg (1982) have labeled as pathological three defensive operations that are recognizable during infancy. During the assessment process, the therapist should be alert to manifestations of this trio of defensive operations: *avoidance, freezing,* and *fighting.* If the behavior of the infant's parents allows the child no strategy or defense for dealing with the conflict, internally he experiences helplessness (Solomon & George, 1990).

Avoidance occurs when the infant appears to use his full developmental capacity to block out, negate, and simply avoid the mother. In one case cited by Fraiberg, the infant scanned the room, his eyes resting briefly on a stranger and then on an object; during this scanning activity he passed over the mother's face without a sign of registration or recognition. Obviously, this is an extreme example, but a more subtle form of avoidance may occur when the infant fails to evince distress at the caregiver's departure in the Ainsworth Stranger Situation and instead, becomes friendly with a stranger.

Freezing, another defensive operation, is exhibited by complete immobilization, a frozen posture, and lack of motility and articulation. This response may occur when the infant is placed in a strange environment. However, when the response persists even in a nonthreatening situation or

Table 3–6. Individual Differences in Self-Regulation

Chronological Age	Self-Regulation
4 weeks or less	Regulation: Stage 1—achieves homeostatic control over input and output systems, i.e., "shuts out" and reaches for stimuli, achieving control over physiology[1] Neurophysical modulation (through 2–3 months) Responses biologically determined and reflexive; developing distinction between self and other in perceptual clues (through 3 months)[2]
8 weeks	Regulation: Stage 2—uses system of control to attend to and use social cues to prolong states of attention and to accept/incorporate more complex messages Capacity to learn control/feedback loop coupled with environmentally responsive behavior, leading infant to match adult expectation Internal representation of mastery[1] Sense of volition preceding motor act Predictability of consequences that follow the act Self-affectivity: experience of internal patterns of arousal and emotion-specific qualities of feeling (through 3 months)[3]
12 weeks	Regulation: Stage 3—mutually reciprocal feedback loops; infants and parents press limits of infant's capacity to take in and respond to information, and to withdraw to recover homeostasis; games within dyad for amassing affective/cognitive experience (through 4 months)[1] Sensorimotor modulation: intentional motor responses to stimuli Differentiation of self-action from others (through 9 + months)[2]
16 weeks	Self-permanence emerges Differentiation of self-action from others Consolidation of self-other Learns effect on object and social world (through 8 months)[2] Engagement/disengagement involves capacity to modulate stimulation, particularly in light of overstimulation; infant regulation of his own arousal and of environmental stimulation; use of frame by frame, moment by moment stream of events Engagement: visual perception of how mother is oriented to, how mother is reacted to, how infant moves, infant facial expression and affect Visual gazing directly at target, peripheral vision, head orientation 180

Table 3–6. (Continued)

Chronological Age	Self-Regulation
16 weeks (*continued*)	Reactivity: split-second world, contingent sequences 1/2 second
	Responsivity: 3 kinds—inhibition responsivity, unrelated approach/withdrawal, neither
	Emotions: positive, neutral, negative
	Engagement by face looking, side looking, visual checking
	Development of categories of experience with which to structure the interpersonal object[4]
24 weeks	Regulation: Stage 4—begins to demonstrate and incorporate sense of autonomy
	Infant as signal-giver, feelings of competence and voluntary control over environment
	Burgeoning autonomy as infant stops/looks around, and processes environment as mother allows[1]
48 weeks	Control: ability to initiate, maintain, modulate, or cease physical acts; self-initiated inhibition of prohibited behavior
	Self-recognition and categorical self clearly established; beginning of representational behavior (through 24 months)[2]
60 weeks (15 months)	Sense of continuity between time and space (through 20 months)
24 months (2 years)	Self-control: capacity for representational thinking and evocative memory
	Symbolic representation of objects in their absence
	Sense of personal continuity and independence (through 36 months)[2]
36 months (3 years)	Regulation: modulates behavior according to established precepts
	Elaboration of sense of self
	Self-conscious behavior[2]

[1] Brazelton and Yogman, 1986.
[2] Lewis and Brooks, 1978; Kopp, 1982.
[3] Emde, Gaensbauer, and Harmon, 1976; Stern, 1985; Rovee-Collier and Fagan, 1981.
[4] Beebe and Stern, 1977.

when the infant frequently manifests this behavior, it is likely to be pathological.

Finally, fighting behavior occurs when the infant is virtually unmanageable and appears intentionally to stave off any positive response. Such infants will be prone to throw tantrums and to bite, kick, or scream.

According to Fraiberg, all of these defensive operations suggest that a transformation of affect has occurred. Although individual infants cope with conflict in different ways (Hirshberg, Solomon, Buschsbaum, Stern, & Emde, 1990), Hirshberg (1990) has identified four patterns of infant affective response to conflict:

1. *Positive Affect.* Manifested in exploration of a toy.
2. *Negative Affect.* Manifested in retreat to the caregiver for safety.
3. *Ambivalence.* Manifested by alternating affects and behavior and no conflict resolution.
4. *Unresonant-Flat Affect.* Manifested by a lack of overt emotional response and a prolonged flat state coupled with either avoidance or behavioral stilling.

In an adaptive dyad, affective cues are openly and freely exchanged and are designed to promote interaction. However, when the defensive operations referred to earlier persist, it is likely that an adaptive emotional exchange is absent from the dyad. The therapist should therefore be alert to signs of defensive operations during the assessment.

ASSESSING PREVIEWING

In addition to observing specific behavioral manifestations, the therapist should also assess the facility with which the dyad interacts when the *previewing* of imminent developmental and interpersonal change takes place (Trad, 1989; 1990). As has been explained, previewing refers to the caregiver's capacity to represent imminent developmental change that the infant will undergo, to transform these representations of upcoming skill into dyadic exchanges that acquaint the infant with the developmental acquisition, and to gradually return the infant to his previous level of mastery. Previewing can assume a variety of forms. For example, the caregiver speaking about what it will be like to carry on a conversation with her infant is previewing, as is the mother who exercises her infant's limbs to simulate gestures of crawling when she notices that her infant is beginning to manifest these gestures independently.

Another aspect of previewing to which the therapist should be alert during the assessment process is the rehearsal component of this activity. The observation of numerous adaptive dyads during sequences of interaction reveals that previewing exercises themselves are frequently preceded by *rehearsal episodes.* The reiteration of developmental milestones that have already been achieved characterizes these rehearsals. It is almost as if both infant and caregiver are aware that a new developmental milestone is on the horizon, and yet they feel a need to warm up to or ease into the new experience by repeating developmental achievements with which they both are already familiar. Certain behaviors may be precursors to more complex behaviors. Jensen and Thelen (1990), for example, have observed the outlines of a developmental sequence where the simple flexions and extensions of newborns are converted to controlled jumping behavior through the acquisition of stiffness control and muscle strength. Because the development of one milestone may be contingent on previous development, performing these rehearsals is important for the dyad.

Both dyadic members partake in rehearsals prior to the manifestation of full-fledged previewing exercises. For example, a caregiver who senses that her infant is manifesting behaviors precursory to full-fledged crawling will, prior to initiating exercises that acquaint the infant with the experience of crawling, first rehearse such already mastered behaviors as sitting and rolling over. By doing this, the caregiver is, in effect, conveying to the infant that development is an ongoing and progressive process in which each newly acquired skill implicates older skills that have already been mastered. Thus, this form of rehearsing reinforces developmental growth.

Similarly, the infant engages in a form of rehearsal prior to the onset of previewing exercises. Indeed, the infant may sometimes use these rehearsing manifestations to convey to the caregiver that he is ready to experience an imminent developmental event. Rehearsing may also allow the infant cognitively and affectively to experience the mastery that attends already attained developmental achievement and to use these feelings for motivating a caregiver previewing episode that introduces yet another potentially rewarding experience.

Although previewing encompasses specific kinds of behaviors, it is also an overall attitude that imbues dyadic interaction. Viewed in this sense, previewing signifies the caregiver's capacity to envision an ongoing relationship with the infant that becomes increasingly more sophisticated over time because the infant is continually acquiring new developmental skills. As a result, therapists can observe previewing in two ways. First, they can identify whether the caregiver is attuned to the infant's current development and, if so, how the caregiver uses this knowledge to generate exercises that help acquaint the infant with new developmental trends. Second, therapists should observe the kinds of attributions the caregiver generates with respect to the infant. For example, how does the caregiver conceive future interaction with the infant? Does the caregiver ever refer to upcoming developmental milestones such as the infant's ability to crawl, walk, or talk? Does the caregiver ever preview events, such as the infant's attendance at preschool? Moreover, how is the infant's behavior interpreted by the caregiver in general—with optimism and enthusiasm or with negativity and defeat? It is not simply parental knowledge of infant developmental abilities, but also perception of infant behavior that may alter caregiver behavior in the context of the caregiver–infant interaction. Thus it is important that therapists focus as much attention on the caregiver's perception and interpretation of behavior as on the actual behaviors that are observed during dyadic interaction. Essentially, this means that therapists need to listen to caregiver observations and attempt to test and evaluate how caregivers translate their perceptions into interactive sequences with the infant. For example, how does the caregiver describe the infant's temperamental qualities and subsequently how do these perceptions eventually influence the dyadic exchange?

The integration of direct observations of caregiver–infant interaction with systematic measures of caregiver perception and attitudes concerning the infant is highly recommended for the following reasons. First, such information can be a constant source of new hypotheses and insights into both the infant's behavior and the development of the dyadic relationship. Second, this information guides the therapist in identifying potential domains of conflict. For example, if the caregiver repeats extensively that she and her husband initially wanted a son rather than a daughter or mentions that she is excited about having a daughter because she herself only had brothers, the therapist can focus on whether perception of the infant's sexual/gender identity is impeding or fostering the dyadic relationship and the infant's development. Thus, as the caregiver describes her perceptions, the therapist will be better able to understand how belief systems, attitudes, and perceptions have insinuated themselves into the dyadic interaction.

CLINICAL CASE HISTORY ILLUSTRATING A MENTAL STATUS EXAMINATION OF THE INFANT

The use of observation is perhaps best illustrated by examining an actual clinical case in which the therapist integrated these assessment strategies into the treatment. The case involved a 23-year-old primigravida who was first seen for dyadic therapy when her son was 6 weeks old. The caregiver, Melanie G, had a history of manic-depressive disorder that had first been diagnosed during a suicide attempt when she was 15 years old. Since that time, the patient had been in psychotherapy periodically and was maintained on a lithium protocol. However, another attempted suicide had occurred when she was 19.

During the first few treatment sessions, Melanie appeared stiff and wooden; she evinced minimal facial expression and answered the therapist's questions as if by rote. Overall, her affective demeanor was apathetic. She brought her son with her to these sessions. The therapist noted that the caregiver rarely observed the infant directly or gazed in his direction. Nor did she address any vocalizations to him or call him by name. Instead, she kept the infant in a bassinet and only occasionally, when the infant appeared to fuss, did she make an effort to minister to his needs. She did this by reaching down and shifting the infant's position. When asked to describe the infant's development, the caregiver seemed confused and was devoid of insight. She appeared oblivious to incremental developmental acquisitions and was only able to describe broad milestones, such as the infant's changes in sleep patterns. Most compelling, however, was this caregiver's inability to predict or anticipate future changes.

The therapist believed that at least some of the caregiver's reluctance to engage in open and fluid interaction with the infant was due to the contamination of the therapeutic setting. Nevertheless, because the five basic components of interaction—facial expression, temperamental displays, gross and fine motor movement, attachment behaviors, and vocalizations—were conspicuously absent from the dyad exchange, even over a period of several months, the therapist hypothesized that failure to observe these phenomena suggested that the caregiver's ability to forge an adaptive interaction with the infant was impaired.

During the evaluation of this dyad, the therapist also made a particular effort to perform a mental status exam of the infant. The therapist began with an evaluation of the infant's processing capacities as manifested by the eight fundamental emotional displays. Careful observation of interaction within this dyad revealed that the infant was not displaying a full panorama of emotions. For example, even during direct interaction with the caregiver, the infant rarely displayed interest or happiness. Instead, emotional response appeared to be muted. In addition, the infant appeared incapable of manifesting smooth transitions between emotional states. With respect to cognitive functioning, the infant exhibited little awareness of contingency or discrepancy phenomena, even when he was well beyond the developmental stage when these reactions are prevalent. Nor did the infant display the typical interest in manipulating objects that is commonly viewed as the advent of object permanence. Although fine and gross motor development did mature throughout the treatment, this infant failed to demonstrate the expected upsurge in fine motor behaviors that is characteristic of the 2nd half of the 1st year of life.

Significantly, the evolution of an adaptive attachment relationship did not seem to have occurred within this dyad. On repeated occasions, this infant failed to manifest the capacity to use the caregiver as a secure base from which to explore the challenges of the external world or as a social referent to whom he could turn for guidance. Moreover, the infant's development of subjective phenomena was also impaired. Empathy, rhythmicity, and reciprocity were absent during episodes of dyadic interaction, nor did the infant appear motivated to reinvigorate these sequences with affective tone.

As a result of this infant developmental profile, the therapist used a variety of strategies first to bolster and then genuinely to enhance the caregiver's interactional skills. These strategies included encouraging the caregiver to engage in representational exercises with the infant to enhance her capacity for predicting imminent infant development, viewing videotapes with the caregiver and discussing appropriate interactional sequences depicted on the tapes, and asking the caregiver to attend a group session for caregivers and their infants on a once-a-week basis. This latter strategy exposed the caregiver to different infants of varying ages allowing her to observe interactions of these caregivers with their infants. Throughout, the emphasis was on providing the caregiver with a model of adaptive interaction that she could initially imitate and, as her own developmental skills matured, eventually modify to suit the specific developmental challenge the infant was confronting.

After several months of these strategies, a significant change occurred in this patient's behavior. The therapist observed distinct emotional displays on the part of the infant, and the caregiver was able to recognize these displays and respond to them appropriately through verbalizations and gestures. The caregiver also became more adept at identifying the infant's gross and fine motor movements and was able to describe some of the temperamental characteristics she observed in the infant. Most significantly, the caregiver improved in her capacity to preview imminent developmental change and to generate exercises designed to acquaint the infant with this change. This case demonstrates the continual requirement of observation throughout the course of dyadic treatment, for diagnostic as well as therapeutic purposes.

Chapter 4

Assessing the Interpersonal Status of the Dyad

INTRODUCTION

Although the overall success of the caregiver–infant interaction influences developmental outcome more than either the individual caregiver or infant, it is important for the therapist to gain insight into the way the caregiver contributes to the *mental state* of the infant. This is because caregivers who are adaptive and able to represent upcoming developmental change will be more likely to engage in previewing exercises with their infants. In turn, these exercises lead to an enhanced dyadic rapport. As a result, the therapist's task is to conduct a continuous mental status exam, examining the caregiver's capacity to coordinate her somatic, socio-affective, cognitive, and motivational behaviors during interactive sequences. One way of gaining access to the caregiver's mental processes is to observe how the caregiver responds to the infant.

When the caregiver and infant are attuned to one another, for example, it will seem as if both members of the dyad can read each other's signals and predict future interactions. The members of such dyads have learned to coordinate and respond to one another's somatic, socio-affective, cognitive, and motivational cues. When orchestrated rhythmically, these manifestations allow the members of the dyad to share particular mood states. Indeed, the epitome of this form of interaction between infant and caregiver is captured in previewing behavior sequences, when both members of the dyad share their insights about upcoming development. The following example reflects this form of attuned response:

THERAPIST: Could you tell me about your feelings when your baby gets a shot?

CAREGIVER: (Clutching her baby tightly) I have an enormous sense that there's nothing I can do for her, and I become afraid that she's going to have a very bad reaction. Both times that she had a shot I was not able to eat, and I ended up walking around the room with her and she whimpered. It was scary and upsetting.

Nevertheless, some caregivers are incapable of engaging in this type of emotional responsivity, and the responses of these caregivers appear to be out of synchrony with those of the infant because they cannot manifest a developmentally appropriate response. That is, the caregiver's behavioral cues are not coordinated with her internal state. As a consequence, the infant's capacity to represent a consistent relationship with the caregiver and to develop an awareness of contingency relationships may suffer. The infant experiences the caregiver's behaviors as being disruptive and inconsistent. In turn, these disruptions lead to a feeling of loss with accompanying emotional distress that is manifested through crying or excessive fussing. What is characteristic of these dyads is that neither member of the dyad exchanges affect directly. During such intervals it is almost as if the infant is attempting to recapture and sustain the representation of the caregiver. It is vital to minimize such episodes because infants who are repeatedly subjected to these kinds of discrepancies may eventually develop deficits that hamper adaptive development. Such caregivers are not communicating developmental progression adaptively to the infant in the form of previewing; instead, they are providing the infant with a *dissociated* view of the interpersonal changes that will accompany upcoming maturation. As a result, the infant may come to experience both the process of development and dyadic interaction as uncontrollable events that he is incapable of mastering. Moreover, the infant's discomfort during these periods, if unchecked, may *transfer* across to new domains of interaction.

Once the therapist recognizes such a response, two assessment strategies are available. First, the therapist may choose to intervene by raising this issue with the caregiver directly in a supportive fashion. This should be done only if the caregiver has a relatively stable personality. Another alternative may be to use *modeling* as a type of intervention. During modeling the therapist asks to hold the infant whenever the caregiver becomes upset. Providing a firm and steady grasp of the baby in front of the caregiver while she continues to speak with the therapist is often sufficient to continue the assessment. Moreover, edited videotapes of other caregivers performing desirable behaviors can be shown to the caregiver as a method of enhancing self-modeling. In essence, these strategies permit the caregiver to draw a contrast between the objective perceptions of the infant's developmental status and the subjective perceptions she is experiencing. By contrasting the objective and subjective perceptions of the caregiver, the therapist will come to recognize which perspective is being distorted. Even with caregivers who are well adjusted and who display a keen ability to comfort the infant during times of distress, it is helpful to integrate these strategies into the treatment session.

Separation of the caregiver from the infant provides caregivers with an unparalleled opportunity to reflect on the issue of separation per se. Therapists should always remember that each developmental accomplishment that the infant is about to manifest or is manifesting represents subjectively a *miniseparation episode* for the caregiver. In other words, because caregivers can experience separation as a traumatic event—even caregivers who display highly adaptive skills—it is often worthwhile to encourage them to rehearse the experience of separation from the infant. This assessment technique can be performed either by encouraging the caregiver to place the infant on the floor, by having the therapist hold the infant while displaying various behaviors, or by showing videotaped sessions of caregiver–infant interaction. All of these techniques permit the caregiver to view developmental changes in a more objective fashion and to articulate to the therapist the feelings that accompany the recognition of developmental growth and separation.

The development of a *therapeutic alliance* is a significant aid to the caregiver in preparing for the imminent separations that accompany developmental progress. This is because the evolution of an intense therapeutic bond helps the caregiver explore the significance of the infant's developmental achievements, and most importantly, helps the caregiver explore the interpersonal implications of future interaction with the infant. Eventually, through the potency of this alliance, the caregiver comes to represent the infant in a new light that combines an objective awareness of the infant's development with a subjective sense of how she feels about the baby's growth. In essence, the caregiver's relationship with the therapist helps the caregiver to predict, work through, and cushion the trauma that accompanies the realization of developmental separation. Moreover, just as the infant will continue to grow and develop physically, so too will the therapeutic relationship enable the caregiver to replenish nurturing skills and to continue developing psychologically. The therapeutic relationship, then, serves as a developmental paradigm for the caregiver, providing her with an arena for experiments that heighten developmental awareness. The flexibility that imbues the therapeutic exchange also parallels the somatic, socio-affective, cognitive, and motivational maturation of the infant. The infant will now be permitted to explore his environment, while the caregiver's skills in exploring, understanding, and mastering her interior psychological landscape become more sophisticated. When the therapist enables the caregiver to become an explorer in her own right, ministering to the infant and previewing imminent development appropriately become a pleasurable adventure, in which both dyadic members strive toward mastery of developmental challenges and increased intimacy in their relationship.

ASSESSING PRENATAL AND NEONATAL FACTORS

Prenatal Factors

Prenatal variables, including *caregiver stress, social support, substance abuse, diet, nutritional status, health,* and *lifestyle,* have been associated with infant neonatal and developmental outcomes (Hoffman, Bartlett, Hillman, & Orr, 1990; Oyemade, 1990). Although comprehensive prenatal care has been shown to promote fetal growth, it may not prevent prematurity or other complications (McLaughlin, Altemeier, Sherrod, & Christensen, 1990). Occasionally, environmental factors over which pregnant women have little or no control may affect future developmental outcomes as well. Worobey and Thomas (1990), for example, posit a link between intrauterine contaminants, such as heavy metals (e.g., lead), and cognitive deficits. In addition, the infants of schizophrenic patients who are treated with phenothiazine have shown significant hypertonicity, tremors, and irritability (Coles, Platzman, James, & Herbert, 1990). Pregnant women should therefore be alert to aspects of their environments that may affect the future development of their unborn children, and therapists should be aware of the effects of prescription drugs on the subsequent development of the infant.

More recently, however, a prevalent factor in prenatal and neonatal developmental outcomes has been prenatal exposure to nonprescription drugs. Researchers have found that prenatal exposure to drugs influences the infant's capacity to organize his behavior, modulate actions, maintain attention, handle stimulation, direct and control movements with precision, and initiate interaction with people and objects (Poulsen & Ambrose, 1990). More specifically, drugs such as cocaine, crack, and alcohol have been found to have negative effects on growth in general (Coles, Platzman, Smith, & James, 1990; Eisen, 1990). Moreover, prenatal exposure to crack and/or cocaine results in a tendency in the infant to seek higher levels of stimulation (Gardner, Magnano, & Karmel, 1990), whereas prenatal exposure to alcohol results in cry episodes that last longer and contain more turbulence and variability in pitch (Nugent & Greene, 1990). The negative impact of prenatal exposure to teratogens usually extends to poor postnatal caregiver–infant interactions (Chethick, Burns, Burns, & Clark, 1990; O'Connor, Kasari, & Sigman, 1990).

Ambrose and Poulsen (1990) have developed a clinical profile of mothers whose infants were prenatally exposed to drugs. This profile includes the following features: a childhood history of physical and/or sexual abuse, a home environment where alcohol was abused, polysubstance abuse with crack or cocaine as the drug of choice, history of being reported to child protective services, history of substance abuse during previous pregnancies, history of stormy relationships with drug-abusing men, precarious socioeconomic circumstances, history of unplanned pregnancies, lack of prenatal care, and increased risk of premature delivery.

Therapists should be alert for signs of substance abuse during the initial intake interview in order to intervene and attempt to stave off future developmental impairments from a continued prenatal exposure to harmful substances. Moreover, to evaluate the infant's developmental potential accurately, therapists should be aware of the history of the infant's mother regarding substance abuse.

Neonatal Factors

Neonatal factors also play a role in the infant's development and thus in caregiver–infant dyadic interaction. Dyadic interaction has been shown to be affected by whether the infant was born prematurely (Oehler, 1990) or postterm (Beckmann, 1990). A number of other health-related factors, such as *latent anemia* (Al Naquib & Sadek, 1990), *gestational age* (Als, Duffy, & McAnulty, 1990; Beeghly, Vo, Burrows, & Brazelton, 1990; Kennedy-Caldwell & Lipsitt, 1990) and *birth weight* (Barrerra & Kitching, 1990; Chiodo & Maun, 1990) affect various facets of infant development. These factors not only have biological repercussions but also behavioral repercussions. For instance, whereas gestational age impacts the infant's postnatal feeding ability (Kennedy-Caldwell & Lipsitt, 1990), infants who are small for their gestational age may also manifest such behaviors as increased distractibility and hyperactivity, show less cooperation, and may be more difficult to engage in interaction (Beeghly et al., 1990).

How does the caregiver's perceptions of her infant affect dyadic interaction? Stifter (1990) observed that the parents of colicky infants who require many soothing techniques perceive their infants as being more active, more negative, and less positive even after the colic has dissipated. This finding suggests that caregivers may possess unrealistic perceptions of their infants' status that persist and spill over into future interactions. Feldstein, DiGregorio, Crown, and Jasnow (1990), for example, have observed that caregivers who perceive their infants as more difficult and less adaptable manifest lower magnitudes of interpersonal coordination with their infants. As a result, these caregivers may not be able to engage in adaptive previewing with their infants. The therapist's task in these cases involves assessing perceptions in the caregiver and educating her with regard to appropriate development. Individual behaviors and characteristics are important. Maternal responses to infant cues are influenced by diverse factors such as maternal problem-solving skills (Hron-Stewart, Lefever, & Weintraub, 1990), level of illusory control over the infant (Donovan, Leavitt, & Walsh, 1990), competence in social relationships (Beckwith, 1990), depression (Teti, Gelfant, & Pompa, 1990), and perceptions of infant health and temperament (Feldstein et al., 1990). Another factor is whether or not the caregiver is employed. Some infants of employed caregivers are placed in day care, which may be stressful for both members of the dyad (Hertsgaard, Wanner, Jodl, & Mason, 1990). In addition, maternal employment may also affect the quality of the marriage relationship. Owen and Cox (1990) found that the marriages of full-time employed caregivers were significantly lower in the quality and intimacy of communication between husband and wife. The infant may sense tension between his parents and this may affect his development. Moreover, different individuals have different ideas about who should perform certain child-care tasks, and because these ideas may often be based on gender (Welles-Nystrom, 1990), this may also affect the quality of the marital relationship and the caregivers' subsequent interaction with their infant. However, in addition to these individual behaviors and characteristics, environmental factors should also be taken into account when assessing caregiver behaviors. Camli and Wachs (1990), for example, have associated higher levels of crowding and home traffic with less maternal involvement, verbal interaction, and maternal responsiveness. All of these factors play a role in determining the caregiver's ability to engage in adaptive previewing with her infant.

How can the therapist assess the perceptual cues the caregiver is communicating to the infant? One method is direct questioning. Another method that may be helpful is to have the caregiver relate the events of her daily life, particularly as they involve the infant. When caregivers who are asked to tell a story about when they were growing up recount stories with themes of rejection and/or achievement, they tend to be less involved and more intrusive in a free play setting (Fiese, 1990). By asking caregivers to relate an event in their own lives, therapists may gain insight into how the caregiver's representation of her own childhood affects her relationship with her infant.

The therapist should adopt the attitude that the infant's interpersonal behavior during play with a caregiver is less a response to current maternal behavior than a reflection of the relationship history (Houck, Booth, & Barnard, 1990). For example, does the caregiver coordinate her attention to the infant's explorations? Does she facilitate the smoothness of the infant's transition from one play behavior to another? Or are her interactions with the infant overstimulating or intrusive?

Another method that may be helpful in assessing the caregiver's cues to the infant is to have her read a story that contains strong negative emotions. During the recitation the therapist should pay particular attention to the caregiver's interactions with the infant (DeBaryshe, 1990). If the story is sad or frightening, an adaptive caregiver will generally attempt to shield the infant, perhaps by wrapping her arms around the child or cradling him in her arms. During such sequences adaptive caregivers appear *intuitively* to attempt to shelter their infants, as if embracing them in a natural cocoon. Asking the caregiver about infant visits to the pediatrician, particularly when the infant received an immunization, can often trigger a similar response. On numerous occasions I have seen caregivers physically shudder and wrap their arms around the infant when relating such an event. In fact, many caregivers report that they "felt the shot" or "hurt for the baby" when this occurred. This empathic ability to match and experience the affective distress of the infant indicates that the caregiver is attuned to the infant's emotional states and has learned to adopt the perspective of the infant. Moreover, such a response suggests that the caregiver is attuned to the overall developmental status of the infant.

ASSESSING PARENTAL INTUITIVE BEHAVIORS

Just as there are infant modes of adaptive behavior, so too are there parental modes of behavior that indicate the degree to which the caregiver is providing a nurturing environment for the infant's development. During the interviewing process it is essential that the therapist focus on these aspects of caregiver adaptation for two primary reasons. First, if the caregiver is not nurturing the infant's maturational processes, the child will be at risk for a wide variety of developmental disturbances, including most notably, depression (Trad, 1986, 1987). Second, because the therapist can convey messages to the caregiver through both language and through sophisticated therapeutic strategies, it is often the caregiver who is most susceptible to initiating changes in the direction of adaptation.

The four types of intuitive behaviors that therapists should assess in treating mother–infant dyads are (a) visual cuing, (b) holding behavior, (c) vocal communication and degree of playfulness, and (d) meaning attribution.

Visual Cuing

One of the modes of caregiver adaptation that the therapist should be alert to is *visual cuing*, which is the tendency of the caregiver to remain in the middle of the infant's visual field and to attain direct eye-to-eye contact with the infant (Papousek & Papousek, 1987). When this form of contact is achieved, caregivers often display an exaggerated *greeting response*, using rhythmic noises and hand gestures. Adaptive caregivers often initiate face-to-face sequences with the infant. One of the first observations the therapist should make during the interview process is the degree to which the caregiver engages in visual cuing with the infant. Visual cuing begins to occur during the first days of the infant's life and will continue thereafter in virtually all dyads regardless of infant age. The following exchange addresses these observations:

THERAPIST: Can you tell me some of the differences you have noticed in Tammy between the last couple of weeks and this week?

CAREGIVER: (Smiling eagerly) She's learned to crawl. It's slow and steady and she can actually coordinate and balance enough to get her hands and feet moving in the right direction (becoming increasingly excited) and crawling!

THERAPIST: (Prompting) Yes.

CAREGIVER: It's hard to keep her sitting because she's interested . . . (looks at baby directly) Hello there . . . in everything so she'll move to get over to whatever interests her . . . and she's trying to teach herself to sit up by moving to her side and pushing up on one hand.

THERAPIST: It seems she is keeping herself busy by learning new things.

CAREGIVER: Yes, she's very busy. She loves having her bath. The freedom of being able to sit in the water and splash . . . (turns her attention to the baby who is watching another child make gurgling noises) I wonder what Tammy is saying now.

Holding Behavior

When the caregiver holds the infant in the therapist's presence, it allows the therapist to observe yet another behavior that indicates adaptive regulation and interaction, *holding behavior.* The adaptive caregiver tends to hold the infant close to her body, to gently caress and speak with the infant, and to cradle the infant supportively in her arms. This nurturing posture that is evocative of a supportive caregiver is distinctively absent in maladaptive caregivers, whose holding gestures tend to be stiff and awkward.

Holding behavior has been labeled as intuitive by Papousek and Papousek. Appropriate holding gestures appear to convey a variety of messages to the maturing infant, and for this reason therapists should assess whether or not caregivers are sensitive to the location, action, duration, and intensity of their touches (Harrison, 1990). First, the mother's secure embrace reinforces the infant's sense of boundaries. This is especially important during the first few months of the infant's life, when he is just beginning to differentiate between his own body and that of his mother. By holding the infant firmly yet gently, the caregiver ensures that the infant's gradual recognition of his separate physical boundaries is smooth and adaptive. In addition, it is through appropriate holding behaviors that the caregiver communicates her presence as a supportive partner to the infant. Indeed, during the first few months of life physical touch in the form of holding behavior may represent the primary means of communication between mother and infant.

Holding behavior also provides the caregiver with the opportunity to engage in other kinds of behaviors that promote infant development. Soothing behaviors, which may be manifested during holding episodes, have positive effects on infant development (Gunnar, 1990; Rothbart, Halsted, & Posner, 1990). Stroking gestures also enhance infants' weight gain and improve behavioral development (Blass & Smith, 1990). Because caregivers' soothing behaviors have been observed to correspond to developmental changes (Rothbart et al., 1990), it seems reasonable to suggest that these behaviors, like holding behaviors in general, are intuitive. The following dialogue captures the intimate nature of holding behavior:

THERAPIST: You seem to know exactly when she wants to go to sleep.

CAREGIVER: I can almost feel her moods when I hold her. When she snuggles back in my arms, I know she's tired. Then she just drops off to sleep. At other times she leans forward and I know she wants me to play with her.

THERAPIST: You seem to be saying there is a communication that occurs on the basis of touch.

CAREGIVER: Yes, I think that describes it. We communicate in many ways, but the way I hold her definitely conveys a particular message, and the way she positions herself gives me a "reading" on how she is feeling.

Vocal Communication and Degree of Playfulness

Adaptive caregivers will also provide an adequate amount of stimulation for the infant and will demonstrate this stimulation through a specific kind of *vocal communication* and a *degree of playfulness*. The vocal communication referred to here involves two alternating forms of phonetic utterance. The first form relates to the interactional context of the situation and tends to orient the infant. In this regard, the caregiver might say, "You're not alone, Mommy is here." This kind of orienting utterance is followed by the second form of vocal communication, which involves the execution of some non-sense speech interspersed with melodic contours, rhythm, tempo, variations of voice pitch, and quality. Researchers have referred to these special uses of prosody and intonation in mothers' speech to infants, which highlight individual words and partition the speech stream, as *motherese* (Fernald, 1990a). "Yuh, yuh, ho, ho, ho," might represent one such example of motherese.

Caregivers use infant-directed speech to express affection and to label objects for the infant. The infant's siblings, in contrast, have been shown to use it to control the infant's behavior and to express negative and positive affect (Fernald & Dorado, 1990). In addition, a caregiver who interacts verbally with her infant is previewing language to her infant. Not only does the infant learn which objects the words refer to, but he also begins to recognize the *social* aspects of vocalizations beyond their communicative *intent* (Pan & Snow, 1990). Adults attribute intentionality to the infant's use of syllabic sounds, and the positive response of caregivers to these types of infant vocalizations encourages the infant's language development (Beaumont & Bloom, 1990; Bloom, 1990).

Research has suggested that even in infants as young as 2 months, their vocalizations offer significant feedback cues during social interaction (Papousek, 1990). Crying, for example, seems to differ according to its social context (Thoman & Acebo, 1990). In addition, crying not only brings satisfaction of the infant's biological needs, but actually initiates social interaction with the caregiver (Gustafson, Brady, & Hinse, 1990). Both crying and noncrying vocalizations allow the caregiver to respond appropriately to the infant's signals for interaction. The infants of caregivers who tend to engage in fewer verbal interactions vocalize less frequently than infants of caregivers who vocalize more often (Culp, Culp, & Friese, 1990; Stevenson & Roach, 1990). Thus, it is important for caregivers to engage in vocal communications with their infants to foster the infant's acquisition of language. The following example addresses these observations:

THERAPIST: What recent changes have you noticed in Tammy?

CAREGIVER: The latest change has to do with her coordination with a toy. She's able to hold something and spin it, to make the toy perform an action and she knows she's doing it. It's deliberate.

THERAPIST: She couldn't do that before?

CAREGIVER: Not consistently, not all the time (baby smiles and gurgles at therapist). It takes her about 45 minutes but she can wiggle her way backward about 3 feet. She moves around more easily, and she can hold her head up. I think she relates to what's going on around her . . . (to baby) "Right honey?" (Baby smiles at mother.) "Yes, yes, you know you can do so much more now, right?"

Meaning Attribution

Virtually all caregivers engage in a phenomenon that has been labeled *meaning attribution* (Emde, 1980; Papousek & Papousek, 1987; Sosa, Kennell, Klaus, Robertson, & Urrutia, 1980). Meaning attribution occurs when the caregiver attaches meaning to all of the infant's behavior—this is beyond merely a verbal labeling or cataloging of infant action and expression, but is instead a highly personalized interpretation of the child's behavior and the implications of that behavior. The caregiver, in other words, "reads" the infant's state and attributes her own private expectations to these behaviors.

CAREGIVER I: He's curious about the mirror now.

THERAPIST: What does he do when he's in front of the mirror?

CAREGIVER I: (In a monotone) He stares.

THERAPIST: Does he smile?

CAREGIVER I: Yes, he smiles (unenthused). He smiles when he's lying down. I don't think he can hold his head up and smile. He can't do two things at once.

THERAPIST: What is he thinking when he looks in the mirror?

CAREGIVER I: Maybe he doesn't know it's his own face.

(A few moments later)

THERAPIST: Let me hear what you've experienced when you see her on the floor knowing that her movements, no matter what she does, aren't going to do it.

CAREGIVER II: (Smiling and looking at baby) I have thought of that. (Baby gurgles.) She's talking to you (staring at baby). I don't know if it's such a scary perception for her, but I think about it. Her way of communicating at this point is to lift up her feet and bang them down. (Baby makes a loud noise.) She makes that particular noise, the raspberry noise, or she cries. All the things that she does are ways of saying; "I want something else," "I want something different." That's how she communicates with me.

Meaning attribution is an important phenomenon of adaptation if the caregiver uses attributions to create *shared meanings* with the infant. Thus, if the caregiver's attributions are positive and motivating, she may spur the infant on to attain a future developmental milestone. This phenomenon is frequently seen in adaptive caregivers, who are acutely aware of each nuance of infant behavior and who seek to describe that behavior and then to draw conclusions and inferences from it. Maladaptive caregivers may also be prone to engage in meaning attribution, although their attributions tend to be negative, such as "he's slower than his brother was at his age." This form of comparison can lead the caregiver to be disappointed in the infant and to convey negative emotions that will be debilitating to the infant's adaptive development.

The therapist's task during the sessions is to isolate and assess sequences of dyadic interaction, like various snapshots, and to evaluate these sequences in terms of the modes of adaptation the infant is conveying and the intuitive responses the caregiver displays. Ultimately, the therapist must also ask about the emotional repercussions created within the dyad.

ASSESSING THE DEVELOPMENT OF MUTUAL INFLUENCES

Dyadic Regulation

Related to the forms of intuitive responsivity is the dyad's repertoire of *regulatory capacities*. Brazelton and Yogman (1986) have delineated four stages of regulation manifested by the infant within the first 2 months of life. Therapists should be acquainted with these stages, because they serve as guides enabling the therapist to ascertain whether the dyad possesses a developmentally appropriate capacity for regulation.

During the first stage of regulation, which according to Brazelton and Yogman spans the initial weeks of life, the infant's development of regulatory capacities provides a form of *homeostatic control* over input and output. In other words, adequate developmental acclimation to the environment can be demonstrated by the selective capacity to absorb sufficient stimulation, while simultaneously shutting out or obliterating unpleasant or overly complex stimuli. Infants who can comfortably make the transition between states of active stimulation and states of quiescence are actually revealing an incipient ability to exert control over their environment. In addition, such infants are beginning to display the capacity to balance physiological imperatives with the needs of their environment. The therapist can evaluate whether the infant has attained this developmental level of control by observing how the infant negotiates between different states of consciousness, from full alertness to subdued wakefulness to sleep. The following illustration indicates how a responsive infant regulates behavioral responses:

As the session begins, the infant, a 4-week-old female, appears fully alert. She gazes briefly at the door when the therapist enters, smiles, and begins engaging her caregiver with cooing and throaty noises, while gently gesturing with her arms. The infant gazes at objects as they are placed in front of her. As the infant begins to whimper, the caregiver brings a bottle and cradles her child in her arms to feed her, alternating between making eye contact with the infant and the therapist. When the infant indicates she has finished the bottle by turning her head, the caregiver places the child against her chest, stands up, and rocks back and forth while lightly patting the infant's back. At first, the infant appears curious and interested in her surroundings, by raising her head and looking around the room, while making soft noises. As the caregiver gets involved in a discussion with the therapist, she continues to rock the infant back and forth in her arms. Soon after, the caregiver looks at the infant, and notes that she has "one sleeping baby on her hands." After about 15 minutes, the caregiver sits down and lays the baby on her stomach across her lap. The infant continues sleeping quietly for the rest of the session.

If the infant is experiencing difficulty in making these transitions, which may be manifested in the form of excessive fussiness, crying, or other signs of distress, the therapist should note that the infant's capacity for regulation may be impaired and that the caregiver is not helping the infant to regulate between various behavior states. Studies of sleep disorders have confirmed that impairments may be caused by biologically, psychologically, or environmentally based disorders (Minde, Popiel, Leos, & Falkner, 1990; Parker and Popiel, 1990). Because infants with these types of disorders may not present for treatment until they are toddlers or preschoolers, researchers must learn about the developmental precursors of these difficulties to stave off future negative development (Anders, 1990; DeGangi, 1990). The therapist should therefore assess whether the impairment may be due to a constitutional factor inherent to the infant or may derive from the cues being emitted by the caregiver.

THERAPIST: How do you feel when Christian is crying?
CAREGIVER: I'm feeling . . . (in a tense voice) I'm a little nervous.

THERAPIST: What do you think makes you feel this way?

CAREGIVER: (Accusatory) Because he doesn't want to calm down. He's so difficult to handle sometimes.

THERAPIST: (Encouraging) What do you think you should do to communicate your desire to calm him?

CAREGIVER: (Explanatory) I have to walk around with him. He's tired. He's tired and he, uh, can't get the hang of falling asleep right. (She pats the baby on back absently while staring into space; baby continues to cry.)

The second stage of adaptive regulation manifests itself by the end of the first month of life. Now the infant's fundamental skills in attaining control acquire a more sophisticated and refined quality. During this second stage, regulation is evidenced by the infant's ability to attend to and use the social cues of those around him, particularly the signals provided by the caregiver. The infant begins to display *differential responses* to varieties of facial expression, and this developmental capacity is manifested most clearly in two phenomena. First, the infant *displays* a more prolonged attention span and adheres to caregiver cues for a longer period of sustained and uninterrupted interaction. Second, and even more telling, the infant now begins to *match* adult expectations, in the sense that a particular cue evokes a specific response anticipated by both members of the dyad, thus synchronizing the dyad's production and reception of social signals (Naud & Manikouska, 1990). Therapists observing adaptive dyads with infants of this age will note sequences of harmonious interaction that demonstrate the coordination between the infant's and the caregiver's responses. The illustration below demonstrates such observations:

A 10-week-old infant is cradled in her caregiver's arms and is gazing at her. The caregiver makes smacking noises with her lips, and the infant smiles and attempts to reach with her arm in the direction of the caregiver's lips. The infant manages to graze the caregiver's nose. The caregiver places the infant in a standing position while supporting her. The infant inserts her hand in the caregiver's mouth. Now the caregiver and infant are face-to-face approximately 3 inches apart. The caregiver leans her head forward to touch the infant's head, pulls away, and leans forward again. The infant begins to do the same, leaning forward in anticipation of meeting the caregiver's head and leaning back slightly when the caregiver does the same.

As adaptive regulation progresses to the 3rd and 4th month of life, this reciprocal feedback becomes more evident and begins to dominate virtually all of the exchanges between caregiver and infant. Brazelton and Yogman characterize this period as one during which mutually interactive feedback loops enable both the infant and caregiver to begin expanding the infant's thresholds for absorbing and responding to new stimuli. Adaptive interaction now attains a *rhythmic* quality that is analogous to other physiological processes (e.g., regular respiration). These pulsations of responsivity can be observed in waves of attuned interaction during which the caregiver expands the level of stimulation, then gradually tapers off, and finally allows the dyadic exchange to recede to the point where the infant can comfortably withdraw into either quiescence or drowsiness. Therapists observing regulatory responses at this stage will be impressed by two phenomena. First, a range of cognitive and affective cues imbues the dyadic interaction, demonstrating that the infant has attained myriad skills in both of these domains. Second, the dyad's capacity to make smooth transitions between states is present and possesses a quality of fluidity and regularity that suggests that dyadic exchange is occurring *synchronically*. The infant's motor skills are also more developed by this period. The caregiver can place the infant in a sitting position that he will maintain for several minutes with support. This new position facilitates face-to-face interactions. The following illustration demonstrates the emergence of this quality of autonomy:

> (A 4-month-old male infant, Charlie, plays with a stuffed rabbit. Therapist sits on floor next to him. Infant gazes up and gives the therapist a beaming smile. Therapist lifts infant to standing position and turns him to face room. Another mother is lifting her infant out of his seat as well. Charlie watches intently for a minute and then tries to move toward other mother and child.)
>
> THERAPIST: Charlie is clearly very curious at this point in his development.
> CAREGIVER: Yes, he has been very curious recently. (The therapist lifts the infant up again and takes him to the mirror. Fascinated, the infant reaches out and touches his reflection, while gurgling happily.)

By the 5th or 6th month of life, when the infant progresses to the fourth stage of adaptive regulation, a new form of autonomous functioning emerges. Now the infant begins to assume the role of interactional *initiator*, as he signals a wide variety of cues to the caregiver. Adaptive caregivers will demonstrate a facility in translating and responding to such cues in an appropriate fashion during this period. As a result of this burgeoning autonomy, the infant will display such developmental capacities as a heightened sense of awareness, coupled with curiosity about environmental stimuli and enthusiastic reliance on the caregiver's guidance in exploring the diverse stimuli of the environment (Landry, Richardson, & Garner, 1990). Motor skills become even more refined, as the infant is able to sit alone for several seconds and to roll from his back to his stomach.

Needless to say, many of these regulatory capacities may be absent in infants who are brought into therapy by their caregivers. In addition, infants who are temperamentally difficult may not demonstrate these capacities and may cause the caregiver to experience stress and decreased marital satisfaction (Portales, Porqes, & Greenspan, 1990). Thus, the infant's ability to self-regulate, which has been considered a component of the infant's temperament, influences the quality of the dyadic exchange. It is vital for therapists to gain familiarity with the expectable levels of adaptation to evaluate each particular dyad diagnostically and to administer the most efficacious treatment. If the caregiver appears oblivious to infant cues, for example, it will be virtually impossible for her to initiate regulatory interaction characterized by the harmonious exchange discussed earlier. Nor will a caregiver who fails to distinguish between infant states of arousal and quiescence be adequately equipped to guide the infant during sequences of transition between states.

The following excerpt is from a case history of another infant of 6 months who failed to demonstrate these regulatory capacities:

THERAPIST: (Noticing baby in carriage next to mother.) I see that Charlie is stirring as if he is about to wake up.

CAREGIVER: (Leans forward to look in carriage, responds in a lackadaisical tone.) Yeah (waves hand as if to say, don't worry about him) he ate before we came here.

THERAPIST: Oh, he ate before you arrived? (Waits for explanation of the relevance of this comment) What did he have?

CAREGIVER: (Laughs nervously) A bottle of milk (stares into space).

During the entire therapeutic process the therapist should attempt to discern the level of the infant's adaptive regulation to the environment and to identify the caregiver's response to these capacities, as well as to pinpoint areas of weakness that will be most susceptible to treatment techniques.

Regulation of Autonomous Functions

The caregiver plays a vital role in the infant's development of autonomy. Research suggests that the development of autonomy depends on the emotional support and assistance the infant receives during positive interactions with the caregiver (Berlin & Cassidy, 1990; Heinicke, 1990; Ward, Brinckerhoff, et al., 1990; Ward, Carlson, et al., 1990), and the caregiver's conception of her role as a mother (New, Richman, & Welles-Nystrom, 1990). Based on the normal trends of developmental adaptation, an infant of approximately 2 months of age will begin to display manifestations that underscore an incipient capacity to coordinate autonomous functioning and to integrate disparate skills of responsiveness. Typically neonates display sharp, almost acute, *transitions* between states. During periods of alertness, a newborn will evince heightened motility, heart rate, respiration, and visual/vocal signals in the form of knitted brows, frowning, clenched fists, body stiffness, and fierce crying. Interestingly enough, such infants appear capable of reverting almost immediately to a sleep state. This distinctive abruptness in the neonate's developmental ability in negotiating between states of consciousness indicates early *autonomous functioning*, which is largely a physiological response unfiltered by cognitive and affective developmental skills.

The tendency to make abrupt transitions between states gradually subsides by the 2nd month of life, however, as the infant begins integrating responses in a smoother and more coordinated fashion. In contrast to the first weeks of life, for example, by the 2nd month the infant no longer cries uncontrollably nor does his body become contorted with displeasure when presented with distressful stimuli. The earlier reaction that was predominantly physiological is now superseded by highly sophisticated responses implicating cognitive and affective skills that enable the dyad to communicate in a more subtle fashion.

In the following example, the caregiver had been holding her 2½-month-old son on her lap while she talked. The baby had been playing with a stuffed bear. After several minutes, the caregiver looked directly at the infant's face.

CAREGIVER: You probably feel tired . . . don't you? You don't want to play with the bear any more? (The caregiver waited for several seconds and then began stroking the baby's cheek.)

THERAPIST: How did you know he was tired?

CAREGIVER: He is not moving as much. He always becomes less active and quieter when he wants to nap. I can sense this from his movements.

THERAPIST: Do you think you can predict his needs most of the time?

CAREGIVER: Yes, it's not that hard to do now. I have become accustomed to his rhythms. (Caregiver gently places baby in carriage on his stomach and continues to rock him.)

Infant Engagement/Disengagement

This mode of adaptation involves the infant's capacity to modulate the degree of stimulation filtering in from the environment (Beebe & Stern, 1977). The therapist can best assess *engagement/disengagement* when the infant is exposed to overstimulation. During periods of engagement the infant will generally orient to the caregiver by gazing at her directly and scanning her face. Disengagement occurs when the infant breaks this interactive sequence to approach another stimulus, by averting gaze, or to convert to another behavioral state, such as sleep. What the therapist should be looking for when observing these sequences is the infant's ability to transfer between behavioral states smoothly and nondisruptively. The caregiver meanwhile should be guiding these transitions by demonstrating sensitivity to the infant's various affects and moods. Maternal sensitivity for guiding the infant's transitions does not appear to be related to factors such as the caregiver's age, the behaviors used to assist the infant, or the caregiver's emotional and verbal responsivity (Moran, Pederson, Petit, & Krupka, 1990; Vyt, 1990). Depressed caregivers may not exhibit the necessary emotional responsivity and as a result appear less sensitive (Teti & Gelfand, 1990; Trad, 1987). In addition, substance abusers have been shown to be less sensitive to their children's cues and dysfunctional in virtually all maternal interactive behaviors (Hans, Bernstein, & Henson, 1990). During the initial assessment interviews when the caregiver is playing with the infant, the therapist might ask the caregiver to comment on what she thinks the infant is thinking and feeling. Caregivers who are reluctant to engage in this exercise may actually be conveying to the therapist their difficulties in representing the infant's affective and motivational status.

If this is the case, the infant's developmental status may be at risk. Unless the caregiver possesses the capacity to represent the infant, she will be unable to convey this perception back to the infant, and he, in turn, will be unable to establish coherent internal representations and perceptions about imminent developmental events and situations. In essence, the infant's predictive capacities will be stifled. The following vignette exemplifies these observations:

THERAPIST: One question that we always ask mothers is "What do you think Tammy is thinking?" This helps us understand whether the mother is picking up on the infant's cues.

CAREGIVER: I don't think she thinks that much.

THERAPIST: What do you think causes her to stop interacting with you and begin interacting with something else?

CAREGIVER: I think it's like the expression, "out of sight, out of mind." What she doesn't see, she doesn't remember, because she doesn't understand language yet and she can only remember when she sees me.

Imitation

Paralleling the ability to coordinate responses is the infant's tendency to engage in *imitation.* The proclivity to duplicate the caregiver's reactions is referred to as imitation and occurs as early as the neonatal stage. Imitation is a crucial developmental achievement because its presence suggests that the infant is beginning to forge sophisticated mental representations of his interactions with the caregiver. When engaging in this activity, the infant is gradually attempting, through a series of purposeful behaviors, to capture the caregiver's attention and elicit a response. The developmental capacity to imitate also suggests that the infant is beginning to comprehend contingency responses. By imitating the caregiver's responses, the infant is, in essence, conveying his wish to elicit a particular response in the caregiver—a response that the caregiver elicited in the infant when she first displayed that particular gesture, expression, or behavior. For example, Jones, Raag, Collins, and Hong (1990) found that although infants produce equal numbers of "closed lip," "bared teeth," or "open mouth" smiles to toys and inattentive mothers, they produce mostly "bared teeth" smiles to attentive mothers. It is important to recognize the interactive nature of infant's imitation and its implications for future interpersonal development. Imitation may be construed as a form of interpersonal exchange that regulates ongoing interaction and promotes communication. Not only do infants imitate their caregivers, but caregivers also engage in imitation with their infants. For example, caregivers imitate infant speech to confirm the infant's utterance and highlight a new occurrence in the child's speech (Uzgiris, 1990). However, there are individual differences between the caregiver and infant in some imitative behaviors (Nwokah, Hsu, & Fogel, 1990), not a surprising finding given the unique personalities of the caregiver and infant. Infants who appear unmotivated to imitate their caregiver's behavior may be indicating that the relationship within the dyad is impaired and the channels of communication and responsivity have not been established. The following example involving a 3-month-old female infant illustrates this developmental capacity:

> (Caregiver enters room holding infant facing away from her. Therapist comes into room and baby looks up, curious and surprised. Each time therapist smiles at baby, she smiles back. Each time therapist protrudes his tongue, so does baby.)
>
> THERAPIST: Look at her, Christine's imitation skills are so good. Do you see how she follows me with her eyes and imitates my gestures? How old is she now?
>
> CAREGIVER: (Looking down at baby proudly) She's almost 3 months.
>
> THERAPIST: (Smiles broadly at infant, as infant maintains eye contact and returns a smile, gurgling and waving her arms as if in response to each of therapist's queries.)

Attachment Behaviors

Although the consolidation of the *attachment* system becomes evident during the second half of the first year of life, its precursory manifestations—*proximity* and *interaction-seeking*, which are infant behaviors that are directed to the caregiver—emerge as early as the neonatal stage. In fact, the infant appears motivated to seek out emotional and cognitive exchange with a particular figure who serves as a haven for the infant during periods of distress, while simultaneously providing a *secure base* during periods of venturing forth and exploration.

The therapist can best assess the presence of the attachment system when observing interaction between mother and infant. The therapist should ascertain whether a dynamic interplay between proximity seeking and caregiver responsiveness takes place during sequences of interaction and whether such sequences take place in a reciprocal fashion. Special attention should be given to contingent maternal reactions to infant responses (e.g., protests, cries) upon which the attachment is based (Gewirtz & Peláez-Nogueras, 1990). These reactions include touching, talking, comforting, picking up, and reassuring. Are vocalizations comprehensible to both members of the dyad? Blicharski and Feider (1990) suggest that the quality of attachment in the dyad is related to the comprehensibility of vocal communication. Furthermore, therapists should particularly observe the emotional reactions of the dyadic members during separation and reunion sequences. Infants in day care, in the absence of their mothers, have been observed to manifest a significant drop in cognitive performance due to sadness and distress (Harsman, 1990). Although the lack of an attachment figure may impede the infant's development, however, so may the opposite kind of parental arrangement—an overly enmeshed relationship with the caregiver. The following illustration highlights these points:

A 12-month-old infant is standing, holding onto a chair with both hands. He begins to interact with the therapist, smiling at him. The therapist reaches out to the infant and the infant lets go of chair as if to move toward the therapist, but grabs onto his mother instead. The infant maintains physical contact with his mother (holding her hand), while reaching with his other hand for the therapist. The therapist lifts the infant into his or her arms, and the infant visually tracks his mother as she walks across the room. The mother returns with different toys for the infant to play with and positions him on the floor among them. The infant looks at his mother, attempts to catch her eye prior to picking up a toy, and then begins walking toward her.

Greeting Responses

During the first 3 to 4 months of life several other developmental phenomena also emerge that provide the therapist with insights into the dyad's degree of adaptation. Among these phenomena are the *greeting responses,* which are manifested following an appropriate visual cue by the caregiver or in reaction to other forms of stimulation. This social response becomes evident during episodes of interaction with the caregiver. The specific and characteristic greeting response emerges at approximately 3 months of age (Haekel, 1985). Once again the therapist's task during the therapeutic process involves observing whether a full emotional spectrum is being displayed and, if so, the degree to which the infant coordinates these emotions with the caregiver's cues.

> (Billy, an 11-month-old infant, is sitting with therapist playing with pots and pans, banging them together and vocalizing.)

THERAPIST: Billy, are you a member of an orchestra?

> (Billy turns to the therapist and makes a questioning sound similar to "Eh?" He smiles briefly at the therapist prior to returning to his toys. The therapist reaches out to Billy, who extends his arms to grab those of the therapist and stands up. The therapist lifts up the child, and another therapist brings over a bright red play mat. Billy looks at the mat and excitedly waves his arms. Billy's mother places him on the mat. Billy falls forward onto his stomach and begins to whine, seemingly frustrated because he cannot sit up and spin a toy in front of him. The mother places the toy closer to him. Billy laughs with delight and then resumes his own playing activities.)

Duetting

Observers have reported that the exchange between the infant and caregiver is especially compelling because of its degree of intimacy. Kaye and Fogel (1980) refer to this type of rhythmic unity as *duetting*. In essence, duetting represents a kind of turn-taking between the infant and caregiver that involves facial expressions and visual contact. During the first few months of life, the infant's facial expressions and gestures are often displayed at random. With the advent of duetting at approximately 6 months, however, the infant gains the capacity to engage in dialoguelike nonvocal sequences of exchange with the caregiver. Therapists should attempt to discern the quality of such exchanges. For example, some caregivers are often overly talkative and inattentive to the infant's signals. As a consequence, communication actually represents more of a maternal monologue than a sequence of genuine turn-taking. Infants exposed to such interactive sequences generally display one of two responses. Either the infant will become distressed at being subjected to overstimulation and will manifest this distress by fussing or crying or, in some instances, the infant will withdraw into a state of apathy, as if to shield himself from exposure to the barrage of uncontrolled stimulation.

As with many of the other forms of adaptive development being discussed here, duetting can be observed during interactive sequences within the dyad; to assess the phenomenon, the therapist should make every effort to encourage the caregiver to interact with the infant during the sessions.

(Therapist holds and talks to the baby, turns her toward the mirror)

CAREGIVER: (Standing off to one side catches baby's eye and begins to clap her hands. Baby breaks into a wide grin. Mother forms two fists and waves her arms up and down while whispering "Bye-bye, bye-bye, bye-bye, bye." Baby observes behavior, catches on quickly, and imitates mother). (Mother is thrilled.) Yes, yes, bye-bye. (Baby, turning to face mirror, waves her arms, kicks her legs, and laughs gleefully.)

Expectancies, Contingencies, and Discrepancies

At some point between 3 and 6 months, infants who are developing normally will begin to display signs that they are aware of *expectancies, contingencies,* and *discrepancies* in their environment. Expectancies have been described as the capacity to develop and maintain anticipations about the future (Mast et al., 1980). These researchers pretrained 3-month-olds to move crib mobiles with 6 to 10 objects by foot kicking. Subsequently, the infants were exposed to crib mobiles containing 2 objects. When these infants were compared with a control group of infants, the infants in the experimental group had higher kick rates, their visual attention decreased, and their negative vocalizations increased. Moreover, this cluster of responses lasted for 24 hours, leading the researchers to conclude that the experimental infants had developed an internal representation of a reward-expectation sequence that was maintained on the stage of active consciousness. Similarly, McDonough and Mandler (1990) observed that a group of 23-month-old infants previously engaged in a particular action, performed this action significantly more often than infants who had not previously engaged in the action.

Stern and Gibbon (1978) have highlighted other qualities associated with the infant's development of expectancies. These researchers note that only if the infant can estimate time intervals will he be able to anticipate particular responses. Expectancies emerge from the mother's repetition of patterns of behavior that are slightly varied over time. Each time an adaptive caregiver varies her response, she waits for the infant to become habituated to the new response and then provides a reciprocal cue. As a result of this rhythmic stimulus–response interplay, the infant comes to expect that particular stimuli will lead to particular responses and becomes upset if the expected response is not forthcoming. One way that therapists can assess whether the infant has attained an awareness of expectancies is to observe interactive sequences between caregiver and infant. If, when the caregiver emits a particular response, the infant scans her face and then exhibits a corresponding response and, subsequently, the caregiver smiles and the infant imitates this smile, it would appear that a sequence embodying an expectancy has occurred. The following vignette with a 3-month-old exemplifies this phenomenon:

THERAPIST: Billy seems to really enjoy it when you watch him so closely, imitate his expressions, and smile at him. It's very interesting. Before he used to make buzzing noises and now he makes these happy faces and gets you to respond. Do you think that he makes those faces purposely? Or do you think it's just a matter of chance?

CAREGIVER: I think he expects something.

THERAPIST: I agree with you. How do you explain the emergence of his reactions? What do you think he expects?

CAREGIVER: Well, I think he has discovered that I respond to his cues, so he knows that smiling makes me happy also. He smiles and then he feels happy too.

THERAPIST: When do you think he was able to make this connection? When did he develop this capacity?

CAREGIVER: (Smiling) I guess he learned that when he makes that face, I respond with a smile. I think he began to make that connection by himself.

THERAPIST: Do you ever play with him by making faces at him and imitating his faces?

CAREGIVER: Yes.

THERAPIST: Why do you think he likes that?

CAREGIVER: Because he gets the response he expected. It must be like getting a reward.

THERAPIST: Has your husband noticed the same smile that you've been telling us about?

CAREGIVER: (Smiling) Yes. He does it with him also.

THERAPIST: How does your husband describe it?

CAREGIVER: (Laughing a bit, amused) The same way I do, as the "Funny Face." He makes the face back at him and they play.

Contingency awareness is related to the developmental phenomenon of expectancy awareness. Contingency awareness refers to the infant's ability to associate a specific stimulus with a specific response. For example as Lewis et al. (1985) demonstrated, an arm movement may be contingent upon a specific audiovisual response. The achievement of this developmental milestone is crucial, because it assists the infant in attaining a sense of mastery and control over his environment.

A third form of adaptation, referred to by researchers as *discrepancy awareness,* also represents a seminal aspect of the infant's cognitive development. Discrepancy awareness, as described and investigated by McCall and Kagan (1970) among others, refers to the infant's heightened sense of attention, which is manifested by increased heart rate and visual fixation, at stimuli that are somewhat divergent from anticipated stimuli. The infant will attend to such a discrepant stimulus with fascination and concentration that suggest he recognizes the difference between the stimulus and another stimulus to which he has already become habituated. Although the emergence of discrepancy awareness can occur earlier, in most infants of 4 months this type of response will be readily apparent. Therapists should test the infant's ability to respond to discrepant stimuli by presenting the infant with a variety of different toys in well-paced succession. After the introduction of one toy, the therapist should wait for the infant to habituate to the stimulus and then should introduce a stimulus that is slightly discrepant. The infant's responses to the toys should be monitored closely. When a different response is observed, the therapist should note the response and assess whether it indicates an awareness of the discrepant feature of the toy. Another way of ascertaining whether the infant has attained the ability to distinguish discrepant stimuli is to ask the caregiver to describe the range of the infant's reactions to different objects or different caregiver responses. Such questions as "Do you think he knows the difference between your moods? Can he recognize the different facial expressions you exhibit? If so, how do you know?" are helpful in eliciting information about the infant's ability to distinguish discrepancies. "Does the baby recognize differences among toys and other objects?" is often a sufficient inquiry to elicit discussion about such phenomena as discrepancy awareness, contingency awareness, and expectancy awareness.

These developmental phenomena are significant additions to the infant's spectrum of hierarchial adaptation for a variety of reasons. First, discrepancy, contingency, and expectancy awareness all represent cognitive modes of development, although evidence of the attainment of these milestones is generally assessed by observing the infant's emotional response—for example, the infant may cry when he experiences a disrupted contingency or expectancy or may respond to a slightly discrepant stimulus with curiosity. But although the therapist assesses these milestones by evaluating the infant's emotional status, asking the caregiver about the infant's responses and watching for evidence of these phenomena represent the primary means of checking the infant's cognitive development, at least until his acquisition of language. Second, the caregiver plays an active role in stimulating the infant's achievements of these cognitive milestones. Thus, if an infant of 4 months appears oblivious to discrepancies or does not seem to have gained an awareness of contingency situations, the deficit may lie with the caregiver, who is failing to adequately stimulate and motivate the infant's development. In such cases, the therapist can model appropriate forms of interaction with the infant and request that the caregiver imitate these behaviors.

Core Self

Researchers such as Emde et al. (1976), Rovee-Collier and Fagan (1981), and Stern (1985) have suggested that by 2 to 3 months of age infants begin to exhibit the indicia of a *core self*. This core self is a precursor to the sense of self that begins to consolidate by the end of the infant's 2nd year of life. The core self is manifested by such developmental phenomena as sustained eye contact with the caregiver, a flexible and easy ability to smile and coo, and sustained periods of visual scanning that are followed by an appropriate response to a particular behavioral cue. Such outwardly manifested indicia of development have corresponding internal representational equivalents, such as a memory of motor acts and schema involving patterns of arousal. As evidence of this developmental achievement, researchers point out that within adaptive dyads an infant of approximately 3 months of age will demonstrate specific intentions and will manifest certain behaviors to initiate a particular interaction. By the time the infant has attained this developmental level, behavioral responses are no longer diffuse. Instead, they are far more economical, as the infant strives to imbue each gesture with a particular meaning and to conserve the expenditure of unfettered energy. Therapists treating dyads, therefore, should use the therapeutic process to observe whether the infant's behavior indicates the development of a core sense of self. The following excerpt illustrates these observations:

> (Infant Christine is lying on her stomach in the middle of a group of other infants. Caregivers are discussing the feelings of a mother when she sees her baby in a helpless situation. Christine interrupts by gurgling loudly.)
>
> CAREGIVER: (Excited) She's talking to you!
>
> THERAPIST: I think she is trying to communicate something to us. She's trying to engage us through vocal and visual signals. These are two of many skills she has for engaging people.

Affect Attunement

Affective expression has been shown to play a crucial role in early caregiver–infant interactions; mothers consider it to be the primary communicative system during the child's first two years (Reilly, 1990). *Affect attunement* has been defined as the pattern of reciprocal behaviors, as well as the emotional harmony that permeates a dyad in which the infant is achieving the full benefits of adaptive development (Stern, 1985). Perhaps the best way to describe affect attunement is to say that the infant and caregiver are sharing and validating affect in the sense that the caregiver matches the temporal beat, intensity, contour, and duration of the infant's responses. Affect attunement refers to a quality that encompasses far more than the earlier imitation sequences engaged in by the caregiver and the infant at 6 months. Instead, during attuned interactions, responses are gradually modified and refined, and the entire interactive sequence appears to adhere to a rhythm of sustained regularity. It is as if both caregiver and infant can *predict* the signals of one another. Research has suggested that because infants respond selectively and appropriately to affective vocal expressions at an age when they do not discriminate affective facial expression consistently, infants initially rely on vocal rather than facial cues in responding to emotional expressions (Fernald, 1990b). In fact, vocal communication has been claimed to be the most informative channel for emotional expression (Reilly, 1990).

For therapists treating dyads in which the infant is between the ages of 8 months and 1 year, it is crucial to look for the indicia of affect attunement during the assessment process. If even a minimal level of such attuned, reciprocal interaction exists, the therapist's task in promoting adaptive interaction will be far easier during treatment. Sometimes, however, the caregiver has not managed to forge this type of reciprocal interaction with the infant. This may result because the caregiver is emotionally unavailable to the infant (Osofsky et al., 1990) or has an unsupportive relationship with a significant other (e.g., the husband) (Levitt & Coffman, 1990). In these cases, intervention for the purposes of restructuring the dyadic relationship becomes a priority because affect attunement, perhaps more than any other developmental phenomenon, catalyzes adaptive interaction. The following illustration captures the quality of attuned interaction:

> (Infant in session begins to cry. Another mother turns to her child, who seems to be content in therapist's arms, looks at him with a worried frown. At that moment, baby begins to whimper. Therapist attempts to distract him by placing him in the midst of some toys right near his mother, but not facing her. Baby refuses to sit and turns expectantly toward his mother, who is taking out a bottle of juice. Baby reaches out for the juice.)

CAREGIVER: Here, would you like some juice?

THERAPIST: It looks like that's exactly what he expected.

CAREGIVER: (Smiles knowingly)

THERAPIST: Do you think it's the juice or you that made him stop crying?

CAREGIVER: Probably both, my knowing that he wanted the juice and my offering him the juice.

> (Mother cradles infant in her arms to feed him. He begins to turn to face her body. At the same time, mother begins to lift her arm to bring baby closer to her. As both mother and child shift positions it seems as if they are engaged in a well-practiced, orchestrated series of synchronized movements.)

Intersubjectivity

The infant's developmental capacities in the area of *intersubjectivity* are further acquisitions to explore during the assessment process. Intersubjectivity and subjectivity refer to the infant's capacity to maintain an innate representation of the caregiver's face, as well as his own face, on the internal domain of consciousness and to use these representations for motivating and initiating responses in the environment (Trevarthen, 1980, 1985). Trevarthen inferred the achievement of subjectivity and intersubjectivity from infant manifestations such as facial expression, vocalization, knit brows, coos, lip movement, hand movements in response to holding, sustained eye contact, smiling in response to the caregiver's face, and displays of imitation. The ability for early imitation can be documented through such mannerisms as tongue protrusion, mouth-opening gestures (Meltzoff & Moore, 1977, 1983) and exaggerated emotive gestures that are evidenced by very young infants (Field et al., 1982).

By the end of the 2nd month, the presence of these responses reveals that the infant is reacting to the stimulus represented by the face of the caregiver. To exhibit this sophisticated array of responses, *representations* must develop internally in the infant's consciousness. These behavioral manifestations suggest that development is moving in an adaptive fashion and also indicate that the infant is becoming increasingly motivated to achieve familiarity with the external world and with others.

Therapists treating infants should, therefore, look for these hallmarks of developmental progression, which are most prominently exhibited during sequences of interaction with the caregiver. If these responses are absent, the therapist should explore further the infant's ability to form mental representations of either the caregiver or the external world and should rule out whether these capacities may be impaired. The implications of such a developmental deficit may be dramatic, particularly with respect to the infant's later ability to achieve a coherent sense of self. Unless the infant achieves the developmental skill of representation within the first months of life, he will be unable to coordinate his responses to the vast number of stimuli impinging from the environment. Nor will such infants be able to perceive these stimuli as emanating from the figure of the caregiver, who serves as a guide and regulator to external phenomena, continually introducing the infant to new stimuli. The following comments from a caregiver in treatment suggest an infant who has achieved specific internal representations of each parent:

THERAPIST: Have you perceived any differences in the way Charlie responds to various forms of stimulation?

CAREGIVER: Yes, there are very big differences in the way that he relates to my husband and me. (Emphatic) Oh, there you are! When we are sitting at the dinner table, and he is babbling and looking at my husband there are certain noises that he make, sort of like an "eh, eh" noise, and this has happened more than once or twice. With me, though, he says "mm, mm, mm." He uses different noises and different strategies. I am certain that this is his way of telling us he knows the difference between us.

Social Referencing

A developmental characteristic described as *social referencing* (Klinnert et al., 1983) represents another mode of dyadic regulation. Social referencing generally refers to the infant's active search for emotional information from the caregiver and the subsequent use of that information to assist him in appraising situations that are either novel or rife with uncertainty. The dyad uses social referencing to communicate attitudes toward particular stimuli (Baxter, Knieps, & Walden, 1990). For social referencing to occur, *joint referencing* must be established. That is, both the caregiver and infant must focus on the referent of the message to understand its meaning (Walden & Johnson, 1990).

The outward indicia of social referencing may be broken down into four components, depending on the developmental status of the infant. During Level 1, which spans the time from birth through the 2nd month, the infant lacks the capacity either to recognize facial expression or to perceive whole faces. Instead, neonates characteristically scan the edges and contours of surfaces (Haith, Bergman, & Moore, 1977). Nevertheless, despite their relatively undeveloped ability to respond to facial expression, neonates do display an ability to discriminate among extreme displays of emotion, such as happy, sad, and surprised faces (Kestenbaum & Nelson, 1990).

A discernible progression in social referencing begins to surface during Level 2, from the 2nd to 5th months of life, when the infant's ability to differentiate among various facial expressions becomes more pronounced. At 6 months, when the infant attains the Level 3 of social referencing, even more dramatic changes are apparent. During this period, the infant displays the developmental capacity to scan the center areas of faces and exhibits a corresponding emotional responsiveness to a wide range of caregiver expressions. In fact, the caregiver's face begins to attain the status of a true referencing or orienting point, as the infant uses his heightened visual capacity to scan and interpret caregiver expression prior to demonstrating a particular response. This capacity consolidates by 36 weeks of age, when the infant moves to Level 4, the most complicated level of social referencing. At this juncture the infant is developmentally capable of relying on the caregiver's expression to infer a particular emotional state and to formulate a response based on this inference.

As Klinnert et al. demonstrated in their research involving a visual cliff, developmentally adaptive infants of this age will use the caregiver's emotional status to coordinate their actions. If the caregiver expresses danger through facial expression, the infant will not move toward the visual cliff; however, if the caregiver expresses a confident facial expression, the infant will readily negotiate the visual cliff without hesitation.

Therapists treating dyads should be attuned to the nuances of social referencing. In particular, in infants of up to 1 year of age it is important to observe the degree to which the infant relies on the caregiver as a guide to behavior. If the infant does not refer to the caregiver's face prior to initiating action, this may signify some form of discord within the dyad. One phenomenon that is generally evident in infants with clinically depressed caregivers, for example, is a tendency to develop precociously to stave off the emotional repercussions of being repeatedly exposed to the caregiver's negative affect. Such infants will often display a readiness and almost overeagerness to interact with the strange figure of the therapist, while exhibiting a corresponding lack of interest or apathy toward the caregiver. This extreme response signifies that the infant has not become accustomed to using the caregiver as a social referencing figure. As a result, the infant may experience subsequent difficulty in representing and eventually predicting upcoming developmental changes.

THERAPIST: Could you explain why it is that when Christine sees you display an angry facial expression, she gets angry?

CAREGIVER: (Softly, as baby is sleeping on her shoulder) I guess that I make her nervous or make her feel a little insecure.

THERAPIST: Insecure because she's not sure what's happening to you?

CAREGIVER: (Thinking) She's not sure what's happening with me, but maybe she's picking up on my sense of intolerance. I think she's aware of that. As a matter of fact, I can remember one day being very frustrated. I don't remember exactly what made me angry. I can remember she was sound asleep in her swing and I told my husband, "I'd better get rid of this mood before she wakes up." I didn't want her to know I was upset.

THERAPIST: So what happened? Do you think she was able to understand some of your emotions?

CAREGIVER: After she woke up, she remained very subdued.

Awareness of Autonomy

Signs of *awareness of autonomy* on the part of the infant and an awareness on the part of the caregiver to the process of boundary consolidation are further evidence that the infant is developing along adaptive channels.

This mode of interpersonal awareness suggests that the dyad is gaining an awareness of differentiated function and physical boundaries. No longer is the caregiver perceived as an integral part of the infant's own functionality; instead, the recognition of autonomy has begun to emerge, and with this realization comes a new tendency to explore the environment and practice this perception. Infants of approximately 7 months who fail to demonstrate a tendency to explore their environment enthusiastically may be revealing a developmental deficit and the therapist should look for these signs during the intake interview.

> (An 8-month-old infant is sitting on the caregiver's lap and playing with a toy. He begins to whine and whimper. She places him on the floor away from her. Baby continues to cry.)

THERAPIST: (Carrying baby to his mother) I think he needs to be with Mommy.

CAREGIVER: (Smiling and reaching out to child) Come here. I know you like to be with me. (The infant gropes for his mother's arms and, once settled on her lap, reaches up and grabs fistfuls of her hair, touches her chin, and buries his head in her shoulder, mouthing her blouse.)

Stranger Reactions

A form of behavioral adaptation the therapist should be familiar with is the degree and sophistication with which the caregiver is attuned to the infant's responsivity to stimuli. One aspect of infant responsivity that is best assessed during the first months of life involves the infant's reaction to strangers.

Kurzweil (1990) observed that under several types of circumstances infants recognize their mothers within a few days after birth. By approximately 1 to 3 months of age, the infant should begin to display an identifiable level of differential responsiveness upon being exposed to various figures. As a corollary of this phenomena, the infant's response to the caregiving figure can be compared with the infant's reactivity to a stranger (e.g., the therapist). Legerstee et al. (1987) followed eight infants biweekly from 3 to 25 weeks of age. These researchers observed that by the age of 1 to 2 months infants were capable of discerning differences among the caregiver figure, a stranger figure, and a doll. These infants manifested signs of recognition through such behaviors as increased gazing, smiling, vocalization, and bodily gesturing. Moreover, these indicia of recognition were more pronounced when the caregiver, as opposed to the stranger, served as the stimulus. Thus, the therapist may ask the caregiver to compare the infant's response to him or her with the infant's response to the caregiver. In addition, the caregiver should be asked if she knows how the infant manages to recognize her and to differentiate among her behaviors, expressions, and moods.

The pathway of adaptive development indicates, then, that the infant recognizes the caregiver, as evidenced from outwardly observable responses, by the 3rd month of life. The therapist encountering an infant who does not exhibit these signs, should question the infant's developmental status. A rapid method of assessing infant responsivity involves comparing the infant's response to the therapist (who represents a stranger), with that to the caregiver. From such observations, the therapist can form a preliminary assessment of infant responsivity. Initially, the therapist should rule out neurophysiological deficits as a cause of the infant's failure to distinguish between various stimuli or as an etiology of the infant's failure to exhibit more pronounced signs of recognition when exposed to the caregiver's face. Once neurological deficits have been ruled out, the therapist should investigate whether the caregiver is failing to provide the infant with sufficient stimulation to elicit a differential response. In addition to asking the caregiver directly about perceptions of infant responsivity, it is helpful to formulate an impression of the caregiver's contributions to the infant's behavior. For example, does the caregiver appear outwardly depressed, with flat or muted affect such that the infant is exposed to a minimal adaptive response? Does the caregiver spontaneously engage the infant in playful exchanges of the type that would foster the infant's perceptual capacities, or is the caregiver dysfunctional and apathetic when providing stimulation for the infant? Does the baby smile when the caregiver approaches? After a distressing event, does the baby stretch out his arms to the caregiver seeking comfort? Does the baby play the same game with the caregiver that he refused to play with the stranger? If the caregiver's behavior conforms to the diagnosis of a psychopathological condition (e.g., depression), the therapist should assess specifically how her interactions affect the infant's responsivity at any given point.

During an initial session with the caregiver and her 4-month-old son, the therapist encouraged the mother to describe the infant's level of responsivity. In particular, the caregiver was asked to identify differences in the infant's responsivity to her, as opposed to the therapist.

THERAPIST: Do you notice any differences that allow you to assess Charlie's awareness of me? (Therapist smiles and leans toward baby)

CAREGIVER: He seems very . . . weary and subdued. He's not that way with me.

THERAPIST: How is he different with you?

CAREGIVER: Well, he gurgles a lot and smiles at me, sometimes he tries to reach for my hand.

THERAPIST: What about his response to me?

CAREGIVER: I guess he knows you're someone new, different, not familiar. So, I think he's sort of sizing you up, because he doesn't know what to expect from you yet.

Self-Recognition and Object Permanence

During the 2nd year of life, the infant evinces signs of *self-recognition* and *object permanence*. Self-recognition evolves gradually through a series of stages. Bertenthal and Fischer (1978) tested for the presence of self-recognition by placing a rouge mark on the infant's nose and then placing him in front of a mirror. Alternatively, a toy hat was lowered onto the infant's head while he gazed at the mirror image of himself. Throughout these sequences, the caregiver was instructed to ask, "Who is that?" If the infant's response demonstrated recognition, it was inferred that the child had achieved a sense of self-identity. Often by this age, the child's facility with language is such that he can use pronouns to refer to himself and others. During the intake process it is important for therapists to speak to infants of this age to ascertain the level of self-awareness. This milestone represents the consolidation of numerous earlier developmental achievements, and if the child has not attained a sense of self that can be communicated by 2 years of age, the therapist's task during treatment may involve reconstructing the entire dyadic relationship.

(Mother is holding baby in front of the mirror.)

THERAPIST: Of all the developments that you've noticed during the past 6 months what was the least expected change?

CAREGIVER: He knew his name right away (looking in mirror and touching her face).

THERAPIST: Can you tell me at what age he first rolled over?

CAREGIVER: (Still staring in mirror, continues touching face; does not make eye contact with infant) He just started that last month.

THERAPIST: So now he'll turn around when you call his name?

CAREGIVER: (Watching mirror) Yes—try it.

CONCLUSION

This chapter has attempted to provide the therapist with a convenient blueprint for evaluating the interpersonal status of the dyad during the initial intake process. As has been emphasized, in addition to assessing both caregiver and infant independently, it is crucial for the therapist to attain a sense of how the dyad functions as a unit. To this end, discerning the mode of communication used by the dyadic members and ascertaining how the caregiver promotes the adaptive development of the infant represent two of the therapist's primary goals.

Beyond articulating these broad principles, however, this chapter has sought to specify the manifestations to which the therapist must be alert from the outset of treatment. One section was devoted to caregiver intuitive behaviors. These various manifestations have been identified among researchers as hallmarks of an adaptive parental response that promotes the infant's development. Among these behaviors are visual cuing, whereby caregiver and infant maintain eye contact for sustained periods and eventually use this behavior to communicate various messages; holding behavior, which provides the infant with a secure sense of boundary differentiation and ultimately fosters the capacity to perceive an independent sense of self; and vocal communication, whereby the caregiver develops a full-fledged mechanism for exchanging information with the infant. In addition, vocalization also promotes the infant's skills in progressing to symbolic thought through the use of language. Finally, the therapist was alerted to the significance of playfulness and meaning attribution in the infant's development. Through playfulness, the caregiver provides the infant with a requisite degree of stimulation necessary for optimal growth. Meaning attribution functions as a double-edged sword. Caregivers who attribute positive meanings to their infant's manifestations are more likely to be sensitive to precursory manifestations of developmental skill and to promote such skill through previewing. On the other hand, caregivers who ascribe negative attributions to their infant's behavior are likely to have a pessimistic view of development that will eventually be represented by the infant.

The chapter then discussed the infant's developmental acquisitions during dyadic interaction. Included in this discussion were such phenomena as dyadic regulation, regulation of autonomous functions, infant engagement/ disengagement, attachment behaviors, imitation, greeting responses, duetting, expectancy, contingency, and discrepancy awareness. These manifestations implicate both cognitive and affective development. Nevertheless, evidence indicates that their manifestation is, to a large extent, contingent on the caregiver's ability to evoke particular responses in the infant and to foster various patterns of interaction. Other phenomena strongly influenced by the caregiver include the development of the core self, affect attunement, intersubjectivity, social referencing, and awareness of autonomy. Stranger reactions and the cognizance of self-recognition end the therapist's checklist of developmental events for investigation during the intake process.

Chapter 5

Assessing Unconscious Defense Operations Affecting Dyadic Interaction

INTRODUCTION

The efficacy of dyadic therapy has been praised in recent years by research-ers who now advocate early intervention for the resolution of conflict within the mother–infant relationship, as well as for behavior modification toward more adaptive interaction. Theorists have attributed the potent effects of dyadic treatment to a complex process, which begins when the caregiver and therapist establish an alliance. As a result of this alliance, the caregiver who harbors unresolved conflict can project it into the domain of exchange with the therapist, whereas the unconflicted caregiver relies on the relation-ship with the therapist to derive model behaviors conducive to adaptation. Subsequently, caregivers can use the insights obtained from interacting with the therapist to enhance perceptions and behaviors manifested during the relationship with the infant. For this process to occur, however, the caregiver must develop sufficient *trust* in the person of the therapist. Only by trusting the opinions and attitudes of the therapist will the caregiver be able to relinquish any inappropriate attributions relating to her subjective perceptions of the infant's behavior.

Therapists should be cognizant that the evocation of trust within the caregiver can trigger two different reactions, depending on the mental status of the caregiver. A well-adjusted caregiver's feelings of trust toward the therapist are likely to be reminiscent of the trusting relationship the caregiver experienced early in life. Resurrection of this positive memory will activate in the caregiver a repository of interpersonal skills fostered during her own childhood that she can now transfer to her relationship with the infant. Thus, a therapeutic alliance results in access to two sources of nurturing capabilities: the therapist's objective viewpoint and the previ-ously submerged memories of adaptive caregiving that emanate from the caregiver's past. In contrast, maladaptive caregivers may initially experi-ence the therapeutic relationship with somewhat less sanguine conse-quences. For these caregivers, the memories of childhood that are awakened may be distressing and may lead to the emergence of interactions that thwart an adaptive exchange. When treating such caregivers, therapists should be aware that at the point when progress appears imminent, the caregiver may become frozen in a debilitating cycle of maladaptive behav-ioral patterns. To counter this phenomenon, the therapist must attempt to instill adaptive modes of interaction by sharing the insights gained from the assessment.

This description suggests that the process of effecting change within the dyadic relationship is straightforward. Nothing could be further from the case, however. Indeed, the therapist will discover that as with any other patient, caregivers are subject to *unconscious defense processes* that insinuate themselves into the relationship with the therapist and/or infant. The therapist's task involves analyzing these psychological mechanisms and their effect on the individual caregiver's personality and interpersonal patterns. Moreover, it has become increasingly apparent that even infants, whose psychological capacities are still forming, are already capable of manifesting defenses which, although they are relatively rudimentary replicas of adult skills, can still influence interpersonal exchange. Those engaged in dyadic treatment have often had the frustrating experience of experiencing how these defenses cast a shadow on dyadic exchange, thwarting what should be a spontaneous, growth-enhancing experience for both mother and infant.

This chapter is devoted to exploring the defensive operations in both caregiver and infant. Unless the therapist approaches dyadic treatment equipped to analyze and, when necessary, help the caregiver overcome the often defeating intrusion of these defenses, the optimal goals of this form of intervention may not be achieved.

THE RELATIONSHIP OF INTERNAL WORKING MODELS TO DEFENSE OPERATIONS

Bowlby (1969) was among the earliest theorist to propose that even very young infants develop *organized internal perceptions* or *schemas* incorporating the preeminent features of their relationships with their caregivers. Bowlby hypothesized that as a result of interacting with significant others in the external world, the infant constructs *internal working models* that incorporate and preserve in memory key aspects of relationships. As a result, the infant begins to perceive the future and even engages in predictions about future behavioral sequences. To fulfill its fundamental purpose, the structure of the working model should be relatively congruous with the reality it represents.

It is important to understand that the infant's working model of the world contains models correlating to the self and the principal caregiving figures. A key component of the working model of the self is a perception of how acceptable the self is to the attachment figure (Bowlby, 1973). In other words, Bowlby believed that relatively early in life the infant inculcated the caregiver's attitude toward him. Conversely, a crucial feature of the infant's working model of the caregiver is the caregiver's accessibility, emotional availability, and supportiveness. Under Bowlby's theory, the internal working models of the self and attachment figures evolve almost simultaneously because both are derived from actual interpersonal transactions the infant experiences with the caregiver. As explained by Bretherton (1987, 1990), a child who experiences, and thus internally perceives, attachment figures as being primarily rejecting may form an internal working model that depicts the self as being worthless. In a similar manner, a child who experiences the parental figure as being emotionally available and supportive will most likely construct a working model of the self that incorporates elements of competence and affection.

Theorists posit that the construction of complementary internal working models corresponding to the self and attachment figures is a seminal part of the developmental process. As the child matures, Bretherton explains, attachment relationships also undergo change. The child becomes more competent physiologically and begins to manifest more sophisticated cognitive and emotional capabilities. In turn, these developmental events lead to modifications in the caregiver's responses to the child. Such modifications in caregiver behavior are incorporated into both the child's and the parent's internal working models. Bretherton adds that the affective quality of the dyadic relationship may also change because of external influences on the child and caregiver. For example, the attachment figure may gain or lose social support or may experience increases or decreases in life stress, which in turn cause changes in the caregiver's attitude toward the infant. Nevertheless, although the internal working model inevitably undergoes change, Bowlby comments that it would be incorrect to view internal working models of the self and the caregiving figures as being in a state of continuous flux. Instead, behaviors and thought patterns that are initially under deliberate control tend to become more ingrained and less accessible to the infant's awareness as they become more habitual (Bowlby, 1980). Eventually, the content of the internal working models becomes fixed, resulting in a relatively stable view that affects how the infant interprets his interpersonal world.

Bowlby's theory of internal working models has several implications for the therapist conducting dyadic therapy. First, the therapist should be sensitive to the fact that during the first years of life the infant is constructing internal working models and will therefore be acutely attuned to the caregiver's behaviors. Second, because the infant's internal working models are in the process of construction, they are likely to be more malleable and susceptible to change than will be the case at a later date. Thus, infancy becomes a crucial developmental period for shaping the individual's internal perceptions of self and others. Third, the caregiver as an adult, is likely to possess internal working models that are more fixed and resistant to change, unless discrepancies between objective events and subjective perceptions become unmanageable. The therapist's task in modifying the caregiver's attitude toward the infant, then, can be arduous because the caregiver's internal working models are already consolidated, and the therapist may need to share his insights actively and assertively to modify interpersonal behavior.

As will be discussed later in the chapter, in many circumstances, defensive operations may also hinder the development of internal working models that incorporate adaptive perceptions of the self and others. Bowlby (1980) has emphasized that defense operations can be viewed as processes that exclude information from the content of the working models. Defensive exclusion is believed to occur in response to conflict. Until recently, it was difficult to envision how an individual could either selectively or defensively exclude aspects of external or internal reality from further appraisal without first becoming conscious of these phenomena (Freud, 1966). Substantial evidence now suggests, however, that the material contained in an individual's internal working models undergoes many stages of selective processing before it reaches awareness, with opportunities for exclusion at each level (Trad, 1990).

Because internal working models guide the ability of the individual to function, some form of selectivity or screening of incoming information in the service of adaptation is normal and unavoidable. Defensive exclusion, however, represents a process whereby the exclusion of information interferes with the development of internal working models. As an illustration, an excessively harsh or neglectful caregiver may habitually ridicule the child's security-seeking behaviors, rejecting the child or otherwise disavowing or denying the child's feelings toward attachment figures. Mahler et al. (1975) note that such an infant would then develop a model of the mother that segregates the mother's "good" (adaptive and contingent) responses from her "bad" (noncontingent) responses. Mahler et al. also point out that for a parent to provide an appropriate amount of autonomy and emotional support at different phases of development, the parent must develop along with the child. Under these circumstances, it is common for a child defensively to exclude from awareness the perception of the bad, unloving parent, and to retain conscious access only to the loving model of the good parent. Because an internal working model of an unconditionally loving and supportive parent does not correspond to the reality the child is experiencing, this idealized but inaccurate model is maladaptive and inherently distorted. Although defensive processes may provide relief because they keep the child from experiencing the mental pain, confusion, or conflict associated with a rejecting caregiver, they are also likely to cause further distortions in the child's internal working model, which will lead to discrepancies between subjective perceptions and external experience. Inaccurate working models, in turn, interfere with the development of effective coping skills and other capacities designed for optimal adaptation.

Bowlby also suggests that an individual's internal working models of the self and of the parents play a decisive role in the intergenerational transmission of attachment patterns (Bowlby, 1973). Individuals who attain adulthood with relatively stable and self-reliant personalities, he notes, normally have had parents who were supportive and responsive to their needs when they were infants but who also permitted and encouraged autonomy. When questioned by therapists, such parents tend to be relatively candid concerning their own working models of self, of their children and of others, and also indicate flexibility about possible revisions and modifications in their working models.

MOTHER: I wonder if the baby will have my personality traits. I wonder if he will try to analyze everything the way I do. If he does, he will go insane.

THERAPIST: (To father) Have you thought of the effect of your wife's emotional makeup on the baby?

FATHER: I don't feel that she is so ill that it's noticeable. I don't worry about her giving this condition to the baby. I don't think it will affect his growth even when he realizes she has an illness. He will see that she is just like everybody else—caring and concerned.

As these researchers suggest, then, the dependency of infants in early life does not imply that they are merely passive recipients of their mother's ministrations (Behrends & Blatt, 1985). Indeed, all available data suggest that the neonate is a highly organized entity, with perceptual and memory systems that contain the capacity for processing information learned about the external environment. For example, DeCasper (1979) demonstrated that infants 24 to 36 hours old could repeat a pattern associated with the sound of the mother's voice, which they were able to distinguish from the voices of other people. According to Behrends and Blatt, the establishment of mother-infant unity, and the internal working models that the infant develops as a result of this relationship, provide a foundation for the developmental sequences leading to self-regulatory capacities throughout the life cycle.

Nevertheless, a familiarity with the concept of internal working models is not sufficient if the therapist wishes to assist the caregiver in promoting developmental change. It is necessary, as a next step, to examine how the infant processes experiences from the external world and transforms them into internal working models that modulate his relationship to himself and his caregiver. These processes include internalization and identification and will be explored in the next section.

MECHANISMS THAT MODULATE THE PERCEPTION OF EXTERNAL REALITY

The therapist conducting dyadic therapy must understand how the infant and caregiver come to develop internal working models and subsequently use these representations to predict and motivate interpersonal exchange.

These processes involve fundamental skills that explain how individuals perceive external phenomena and transform these phenomena into a rich internal tapestry of experience that is reflected back to the external environment. The focus here is on the mental abilities that enable individuals to categorize and represent their perceptions of external reality in order to influence the relationships that play a seminal role in their lives.

Internalization

The concept of *internalization* has undergone refinement since it was first introduced. Freud (1938), who first proposed the concept, noted that internalization occurs when the individual selects certain events from the external world and integrates these experiences into his internal world. Thus, internalization enables the individual to replicate and retain events in the external world by generating internal representations of these events. In other words, in Freud's view, once an external phenomenon is fully internalized, it becomes a permanent fixture of the individual's interior landscape. Hartmann (1939), who expanded Freud's notions, stated that internalization refers to all those cognitive and affective processes by which the individual transforms real or imagined interactions and characteristics of his environment into a structure that allows for internal regulation. By 1962, Hartmann and Lowenstein had further elaborated on the process of internalization, noting that prior to internalization the individual engages in the process of transformation, whereby external phenomena are converted into *internal analogues*. This latter definition explains the process of internalization and provides insight for understanding how the caregiver's previewing exercises of imminent developmental events lead the infant to develop predictions about these events. Hartmann and Lowenstein have emphasized that it is the relationship with the caregiver that becomes internalized, suggesting that the individual absorbs the nuances and subtleties that make up dyadic exchange between mother and infant. This definition suggests that internalization involves the presence of at least certain infant regulatory capacities that intentionally select aspects of external experience and convert these perceptions into internal images.

For Schafer (1981), the primary relationship between caregiver and infant is also the matrix that fuels internalization. The concept of regulation is key to Schafer's (1968) definition. Schafer observes that two individuals are involved in the dyadic relationship—mother and infant—and each may be said to be regulating the other. In Schafer's view, internalization emerges from the mother–infant relationship; mother and infant regulate each other, using their perceptions to shape the characteristics of their relationship. By observing this dyadic interaction, the therapist will thus be able to infer information about the infant's regulatory capacities. Most importantly, the therapist should ascertain whether there is a rapport within the dyad during sequences of behavior and whether the infant exhibits behavioral manifestations that are appropriately responsive to those of the caregiver. The infant's ability to imitate, which can be observed as early as the neonatal stage (Field et al., 1982), serves as an indication of the further acquisition of internalizing capacities, because imitation discloses a means whereby information is being memorized and internalized.

Moreover, through repetitive interactions with the environment, the infant develops expectations relating to how particular events will evolve. Because of this repetition of experiences, these expectations congeal and are most likely to become internalized by 3 months of age (Fagen, Morrongiello, Rovee-Collier, & Gekoski, 1984; Watson & Ramey, 1972). Evidence of the infant's ability to harbor internalized expectancies has been demonstrated by studies showing that the infant becomes upset when an expected or anticipated interactive sequence is violated. In one such study, a 3-month-old is seated facing the mother who is actively engaging the infant. Upon a signal, the mother freezes and ceases her interaction, although she continues to gaze at the infant. Three-month old infants become mildly upset by this maternal response, indicating that an expectation of continued maternal responsivity was violated (Tronick, Als, Adamson, Wise, & Brazelton, 1978). Thus, the infant's reaction to violated expectations provides evidence that he has *internalized* various components of the dyadic relationship.

> (Caregiver has come to a mother–infant session for the first time. Her baby is on the floor lying on his stomach. As the caregiver talks to the therapist, the baby begins to whimper. She looks at him quickly and continues talking to the therapist.)
>
> THERAPIST: Why is your baby making those noises? (Baby starts to cry loudly and flap his arms.)
>
> CAREGIVER: He wants me to roll him over. Whenever he starts to whimper like that, he signals that he is tired of being on his stomach. (Infant continues to cry and flap his arms.) I roll him over as soon as he starts whimpering.
>
> THERAPIST: (Picks up infant and places him on his back. Infant stops crying.) He looks much happier now.
>
> CAREGIVER: Yes. I always roll him over like that at home before he starts crying. He is used to me responding right away.
>
> THERAPIST: It is okay for you to take care of him while you are talking to me.

The emergence of regulatory capacities in the infant relate to the negotiation between external experience, so-called *objective reality*, and internal experience, or what has been referred to as *subjective reality*. Schafer has noted that internal regulations coexist with external regulations. As an example, the infant may rely on external support, such as caregiver holding behavior, to supplement efforts at self-control. The status of an individual's regulatory capacities depends on circumstances such as his state at a given time and the strength of established internalizations. Moreover, internal regulations can be projected back into the environment without losing their function as an internalized experience. The overall process of internalization, then, refers to all those phenomena whereby the individual transforms both the interactions with and characteristics of his environment into an internal regulatory system.

Caregiver previewing promotes the infant's abilities to internalize and self-regulate. During previewing exercises, the caregiver must coordinate her own and the infant's external perceptions to generate coherence for the current experience, while simultaneously motivating predictions about imminent interpersonal experiences. As a result, the infant internalizes the previewing episode and uses it to derive predictions and expectancies about future interaction.

Another concept—*identification*—is also important for understanding how the infant comes to adjust internal perceptions to external reality. This concept refers to processes that transform external material into internal reality.

Identification

The term *identification* refers to the modification of the individual's behavior and thus, the individual's own sense of self, to increase resemblance to an object (e.g., caregiver) that has been internalized as a model. Identification implies a relationship with the object in its most evolved form (Fuchs, 1937; Greenson, 1954; Knight, 1943).

During the initial stages of development, boundaries between the self and object are still in the process of formation, allowing identification to take place directly (Jacobson, 1954, 1964). According to Schafer (1968), not all internalized objects are converted into identifications. Identifications are constructed from objects and they may decompose into the original objects during states of regression.

An awareness of these processes is vital for understanding how individuals begin to generate representations concerning the external world. The most powerful of these processes is internalization, the means by which the infant incorporates phenomena perceived from the external world into an internal system of self-regulation. For internalization to take place, the infant must be encouraged to develop skills of self-regulation. Self-regulation involves the ability to coordinate the demands of the external and the internal worlds simultaneously. Identification is one form of internalization and provides insight into how individuals incorporate key interpersonal events that they experience in the external world. The internalization of the caregiver–infant relationship serves as the prototype that fosters self-regulation.

The process of internalization should alert the therapist conducting dyadic therapy to the complexity of the interaction between mother and infant during the first 2 years of life. From the outset of treatment, the therapist should be attuned to the infant's developmental status and the nature of his behaviors. By observing these behaviors, the therapist acquires information about types of phenomena the infant is internalizing. In addition, the caregiver's behaviors will alert the therapist to how the caregiver is responding to the infant and how she is helping the infant develop an adaptive internal working model. For example, does the caregiver attend to the infant's manifestations and respond appropriately, while simultaneously providing the infant with sufficient opportunities for exercising skills in the area of autonomy and independence? What is the infant's response to episodes of caregiver absence, and how does the infant greet the caregiver during reunion episodes? How does the infant interact with strangers? Does he prefer them to the caregiver, or does the infant show an appropriate curiosity toward strangers, while still referencing with the caregiver? Most significantly, do the infant's behaviors suggest an ability to anticipate the caregiver's behaviors, and is the caregiver adept at predicting infant responses? The answers to these questions will offer insight into the status of the infant's relationship with the caregiver and the way in which the infant is internalizing this relationship and evolving internal working models of the self and caregiver.

THERAPIST: Are there any milestones that your baby will develop that you feel might threaten your bond with him?

CAREGIVER: I'm afraid he might be smarter than me and try to control me.

THERAPIST: How are you going to feel when he starts exploring on his own?

CAREGIVER: Terrific! When he comes back, I'll ask him what he learned.

THERAPIST: As he grows, you may experience less control over him. How does this make you feel?

CAREGIVER: I just want him to love me. I don't want him to resent me. I am afraid that once he starts to get more control over his body, he might have less affection for me. He'll feel as if he won't need me anymore.

MECHANISMS THAT MODULATE THE PERCEPTION OF INTERNAL REALITY

To infer the subjective experiences of both caregiver and infant, the therapist using dyadic therapy must observe the external behaviors manifested by caregiver and infant. In this regard, dyadic therapy challenges the therapist to design sophisticated strategies to evaluate the interpersonal patterns between infant and caregiver. In particular, the therapist should attempt to understand how the caregiver conveys *meaning attribution* to the infant. During the initial phases of treatment, therapists will recognize that some caregivers are biased when they are asked to discriminate between the meaning they attribute to infant behavior and the actual behavior the infant manifests. The caregiver's ability to make attributions in an objective fashion benefits the dyadic relationship and enhances the infant's development. For example, a caregiver who engages in positive attributions is most likely encouraging the infant's adaptive development. One caregiver I treated, for example, was eager to attribute developmental achievement to the infant's manifestations. This mother interpreted the infant's early vocalizations as precursory forms of language. This attributional style made it easier for the caregiver to engage in previewing behaviors with the infant, because she was eager to view his behaviors as evidence of maturational attainment. On the other hand, the inflexibility with which some caregivers cling to their attributions can hamper adaptive development. For instance, occasionally caregivers will make statements such as, "Since Billy is a boy, I expect him to talk late," or "I know Sharon cries because she is just a colicky baby. In my family all the babies are colicky. So I am not surprised she is that way, too."

These statements are similar in that the caregiver has introduced into the dyadic exchange *preconceived* interpretations of the behaviors the infant will display. Such comments are reminiscent of the findings of Fraiberg (1982), who observed that parental attributions stemming from their own past experiences tainted the interaction with the infant. As treatment progresses, however, the therapist will often note changes in such caregivers' perception of the infant. This change in the caregiver's attributions reflects the viability of the therapeutic relationship. Unlike the caregiver, the therapist is able to view the infant from a fresh and objective perspective. Each gesture, each episode of the interaction, and each attempt to elicit a response on the part of the infant can be perceived and interpreted not only as a discrete signal that reflects the infant's developmental status, but also as an independent representation of the infant's unique personality. The therapist, then, comes to view the infant in a relatively objective fashion that is uncontaminated by inappropriate attributions. Moreover, the therapist manifests a fresh perspective to the caregiver who, in turn, internalizes this more objective view of the infant. Therapists should also become adept at interpreting the precise nature of the caregiver's attributions to infant behaviors. Thus, from the onset of treatment, the therapist serves as an independent observer who can distinguish between the infant's objective behaviors and the caregiver's subjective attributions to these behaviors. The caregiver should be encouraged to use the therapist's objective perspective to evolve a new perspective of the infant. As the treatment progresses and the potency of the therapeutic relationship heightens, caregivers also *contrast* their interventions with the therapist's interventions to incorporate a more objective point of view. Finally, by the conclusion of treatment, caregivers will have internalized and identified with the therapist's viewpoint to the extent that they can interpret the infant's behavior objectively.

CAREGIVER: (After placing baby on the floor) If I am taking care of her, but I start fantasizing about something else, will she perceive that?

THERAPIST: She is not going to perceive exactly the same thoughts that you are having in your mind. She may, however, be able to perceive the mood connected with your thoughts.

CAREGIVER: The mood . . . ? You mean she will pick up on my mood? Hm . . .

THERAPIST: Yes, infants can sense mood, which is essentially an external manifestation of how you are feeling with regard to what is going on at that moment.

CAREGIVER: (Disbelieving and skeptical) But that can be so subtle. It's amazing anybody can pick up those cues.

THERAPIST: Think about how many skills and capacities babies have for relating to the external world. One way they are going to engage your attention is by picking up on your moods. So they depend on that ability to read, to feel, and to represent the interaction they are having with you.

One of the prime goals of dyadic treatment is to *predict* the caregiver's future attributions and to explore with her how preconceived attributions affect the dyadic relationship, so that she can achieve and communicate to the infant a more objective interpretation of his behavior. Ultimately, caregivers must resolve any ambivalent feelings they experience from the continuous process of development. These ambivalent feelings distort not only their perceptions, but their interactions as well. Ambivalence is aroused because as the baby develops, he gains independence and autonomy from the caregiver. Some caregivers experience this autonomy as a threat to their already established rapport with the infant and seek to stifle development to maintain the intimacy of the relationship. Caregivers should leave treatment with a *model* for interpreting dyadic interaction that will permit them to respond adaptively without being threatened by the burgeoning independence that comes with development.

CAREGIVER: (Holding her 7-month-old infant) I've noticed that she cries when she's with certain people, and I'm wondering if I'm just reading into it or if it's her mood. I have one brother she won't tolerate. Even if she's only in his arms for a minute, she starts to cry. She's done it with other people, and I began thinking that maybe these people all shared a particular characteristic. Were they all smokers as opposed to non-smokers? Maybe she's smelling something? Are their hands cold? Do they feel nervous and she's picking up on that? I can't put my finger on any one quality that these people have in common.

THERAPIST: Could you describe the relationship between you and your brother?

CAREGIVER: We didn't speak for many years, but when I was pregnant he approached and said "It's time to heal old wounds. Let's not go over the past, but let's start fresh" We're getting along very well now, just beautifully . . . we actually like one another (surprised), which is nice, because for a while we couldn't tolerate one another and . . . he . . . everybody loves this guy. It has been a slow start, but it's been good except (looks at baby as if for confirmation) the baby doesn't like him—she cries.

THERAPIST: How do you explain that?

CAREGIVER: I have no explanation for it. The last time he held her and she cried he was wearing heavy cologne, so I think she may be responding to something external.

THERAPIST: You had mentioned other possibilities besides the external features.

CAREGIVER: (Looking away) Yeah—I don't think my brother is nervous because he's very comfortable with his own kids.

THERAPIST: Do you think he may be nervous about your baby in particular?

CAREGIVER: That's the most obvious explanation (becoming flustered) . . . I don't know.

THERAPIST: This is an important question. It really helps us to distinguish something. When the parents begin to attribute ways of relating to the world to the baby, this is a good example of whether this is a pure attributional style on your part or whether in fact she is responding to external factors. You have come to realize that she is responding selectively to a particular individual.

CAREGIVER: Can a response be that intense, with someone this young?

Externalization and Projection

Externalization and *projection* are two potent defense processes that can be reflected in the individual's characteristic style of interaction. It is not unusual for either or both of these phenomena to emerge during intervention. Projection in this context refers to a process whereby a thought or feeling is subjectively experienced as unsettling and is subsequently attributed to a specific person. Apprey (1987) explains that individuals use projection to rid the ego of anxiety associated with unacceptable or incompatible instinctual wishes. The individual then exteriorizes these wishes or relocates them in an object. During true projection, the exteriorized wish that has been attributed to an object in the external world "boomerangs" back to the individual, who now perceives the projection as a threat apparently originating outside the individual's self. This description of projection captures the almost persecutory quality associated with the concept. Externalization, on the other hand, is a more diffuse process and refers to the individual's tendency to project moods, thoughts, wishes and conflicts into the external world. Externalization is similar to projection in kind, but somewhat different in degree. It is an internal process whereby the individual seeks to avoid blame and attack on self-esteem or seeks to counter fear. During episodes of externalization, the individual manages to stave off fear, but does not experience the boomerang effect associated with projection.

To understand the implications projection and externalization have for a caregiver with an infant, it is necessary to examine how these psychological capacities develop. Among the major challenges confronting the developing child is the task of gradually differentiating his sense of self from the external world (Novick & Kelly, 1970). Whether motivated by action-oriented processes (Piaget, 1937) or a pleasure principle process (Freud, 1915), the transition to a coherent sense of self takes place during the first 2 years of life (Stern, 1985). According to Freud, those experiences that cause displeasure are projected outward.

The differentiation of the self from the external world, and especially from significant objects such as the caregiver, is partially determined by what the infant comes to know and feel about himself. Because the infant becomes aware of himself primarily through the interaction with the caregiver, the capacity for using caregiver behaviors to derive generalized principles about the outer world emerges. According to Freud, *generalization* is a natural mode of thought whereby the individual attributes certain universal truths to the external world. During the long period when the child is dependent on the ministrations of the caregiver, the child attributes to his parent his thoughts, feelings, and actions. Moreover, generalization may also be used as a defense to stave off painful emotions that arise during interpersonal experiences. Gradually, the child becomes aware of his capacity to execute his own wishes in the form of actions and thus his ability to alter both internal and external conditions. However, as development progresses, the child internalizes responsibility for his own actions and thoughts (Freud, 1965).

As unconscious derivatives emerge in action or thought, the child may say, "You made me do that" or "You put that thought into my head." In this regard, *projection* serves a defensive function, enabling the child to attribute his own internal perceptions to another. Externalization, on the other hand, refers to those defensive processes that attribute subjective phenomena to the outer world in a more general way. Externalization is more closely associated with an impairment in differentiating capacity, implicating the child's initial inability to distinguish between himself and the external world. Externalization may also function as a defense to avoid the painful emotions caused by accepting devalued aspects of the self. In contrast, projection develops after boundary differentiation has occurred.

According to Novick and Kelly (1970), considerable psychological development must take place before the child can employ projection. Such development primarily occurs as a result of internalization, which is the process that the infant uses to create an internal representation of external experience—often referred to as the "inner world" (Hartmann, 1939). By this definition, internalization is a regulatory process whereby the infant enhances his opportunity for autonomy by formulating internal representations that assist him in modulating and responding to the stimuli of the external world. Internalization enables the infant to heighten his adaptive functioning and develop resources for dealing with the challenges posed by environmental stress (Meissner, 1971). This occurs because internalization allows the child to incorporate perceptions of the external world into the fabric of self-regulation. Exposing the infant to previewing exercises enhances his ability to internalize phenomena.

A parent who projects indiscriminately may hinder the processes of adaptive development. For example, infants who become the main objects of parental projection are narcissistically injured. This disturbance is rooted in the incorporation of the projected devalued aspects of the parent's sense of self and the infant's incapacity to integrate his own positive aspects of the self. That is, the parent provides no means for distinguishing between acceptable and unacceptable behavior, and the infant—child-to-be—consequently fails to internalize rules governing appropriate conduct. Children who are subjected to their parent's projections may also experience intense anxiety and guilt in expressing their impulses. In these cases, parental projections continually reinforce impulses, hindering the development of an adaptive and autonomous defensive system to regulate behavior. The extensive use of externalization can also lead to a pathological imbalance within the family unit, creating a closed system in which members of the family become alienated or isolated from one another (Brodey, 1968). Projection, in contrast, promotes an intense fusion or bonding between mother and child that stifles adaptive development and precludes relationships with others. Caregivers who rely on these forms of behavior may be creating deficits in their infants' functioning that will be difficult to eradicate at a later stage because the infant is evolving a coherent sense of self and the caregiver's unregulated responses intrude on his development. Such intrusion may permanently impair the infant's ability for representing adaptive behavior.

From this discussion it becomes apparent that for the therapist treating mother–infant dyads the task at hand is a thorough exploration of the interpersonal behaviors manifested by the caregiver to determine whether projection and/or externalization are insinuating themselves into the dyadic exchange. Ideally, therapeutic explorations should begin during the pregnancy period. Projections tend to emerge during pregnancy, when the mother may, as one example, fantasize that the unborn infant is going to "devour" or "kill her." If the therapist is treating the caregiver while she is still pregnant, such material should be explored in depth through inquiry and techniques designed to encourage the expression of such representations. Nevertheless, even if treatment does not commence until after the birth, the therapist can, by asking the caregiver to describe her perceptions during the pregnancy, explore these fantasies and evaluate whether representations of this type were present prior to the birth. It should be remembered that virtually all new mothers, particularly first-time mothers, harbor fantasies about the infant. Nevertheless, projections are distinctive both in their aggressive content and in the exaggerated affect that fuels them. Such expectant mothers are, in effect, aggressively projecting negative feelings, thoughts, and persecutory fantasies onto the fetus.

THERAPIST: Have you had any dreams about your pregnancy?

CAREGIVER: I dreamt that my girlfriend had a baby. I also had a baby. I can't remember if it was a boy or a girl. We were both breastfeeding our babies. I felt that my baby did not want my breast. I said, "Oh my goodness! I don't have any milk!" I thought that I could buy some and put sugar in it like a formula. The baby was angry because I hadn't fed him for a long time. I put my nipple in the baby's mouth and he pushed it away. I was scared because I didn't know what to do. I had to think fast because the baby was very hungry.

Therapists conducting dyadic treatment must remember that, at least until the infant is able to communicate through language, the infant's subjective impressions will be communicated primarily through the caregiver. That is, the caregiver will express to the therapist what she perceives to be the infant's emotional needs. This process can become cumbersome because the therapist may experience difficulty in distinguishing whether the caregiver's elaborations are based on accurate intuitive perceptions or distorted projections. Observations of the dyadic interaction, however, can also provide access to the infant's direct experience. This more objective guide requires that the therapist evaluate the infant's developmental status and the caregiver's response to that developmental status.

CAREGIVER: He can't talk yet, but he's aware of everything. He just can't verbalize it.

THERAPIST: How do you think he's processing all of this in his mind?

CAREGIVER: I think he's conditioning himself to solve new problems, being his own person, being an individual, and I think since we are going through a battle of our own, I think he is trying to resolve it as a person as best he can. I know he does not want to hurt me.

The process of imitation should also be mentioned in this context. Kagan (1958) refers to imitative learning as the "initiation and practice of certain responses (gestures, attitudes, speech patterns) which result from copying the behavioral patterns of a model" (p. 296). Although imitation occurs when one person copies another person's manifestations, the presence of imitation does not necessarily provide insight into the relational or affective bond between the mother and infant. When the person being imitated is one with whom the imitator identifies, however, the acquisition of particular behavior patterns is most likely.

Within the context of the caregiver–infant relationship, imitation can lead to identification which, in turn, stimulates further imitative behaviors. For example, the infant increases his repertoire of behaviors by imitating the caregiver. This interpersonal behavior helps the infant to learn and eventually internalize appropriate emotional responses. As a consequence, infantile patterns of imitative behavior awaken the identification processes that promote the ego's early development (Hendrick, 1951). When behavioral patterns are acquired in this fashion, they become ingrained and, as a result of subsequent identifications, provide motivation for the evolution of even more elaborate structures and, eventually, the emergence of a coherent personality. If, however, the caregiver is projecting undesirable wishes onto the infant to relieve her own distress, the infant is likely to have two responses. First, he may internalize the caregiver's attitudes and incorporate them into his evolving working models of the self and other. Residues of persecutory feelings will thus become entrenched in the infant's perception of both himself and his mother, leading to feelings of both worthlessness and devaluation. Second, the infant is likely to reflect these behaviors back to the caregiver. Thus, a caregiver who projects negative emotions onto the infant may well have these projections confirmed as the infant begins to behave in a rejecting and disdainful manner toward the caregiver.

CAREGIVER: He cries all the time and I can't figure out what he wants. I get so frustrated with him. (Baby fusses in caregiver's lap). Do you want your bottle? (Baby whimpers. Caregiver angrily throws bottle into bag. Baby begins to cry loudly and swings fists at caregiver.) If he doesn't stop crying I'm going to throw him against the wall.

Because therapists should be acquainted with normal, adaptive developmental events, they will be able to evaluate whether adaptive interaction is proceeding within the dyad. If the caregiver has either projected or externalized unresolved unconscious material to the infant, the therapist should intervene to preclude the caregiver from further interfering with the infant's emerging representational capacities. Focusing on the enhancement of the caregiver's sense of self, through the use of the previewing exercises described in an earlier chapter, is generally an effective strategy in these cases.

CAREGIVER: (Infant cries and therapist takes him to look out the window while speaking to the infant in soothing tones. Mother sits and shakes her head. Therapist tries to interest the infant by pointing at certain things.) I don't think you can get him to do anything right now. That's the way he behaves at home sometimes.

THERAPIST: Do you think he may want you to soothe him?

CAREGIVER: (Nods) I don't know. When he gets in this mood, he doesn't want anything. He doesn't want to do anything. It's strange.

THERAPIST: Your descriptions of your baby remind me of the descriptions you have made about yourself when you have a problem. How do you feel right now?

CAREGIVER: (Caregiver tries to put bottle in infant's mouth. Infant rejects it and she slams it back into her bag. She gets up and walks with him more.) I feel very frustrated with him. Taking care of him is sometimes like being imprisoned.

Projective Identification

Projective identification is a concept first introduced by Klein (1952). This theorist postulated that projective identification differs substantially from projection because it exists only during interaction between two or more individuals. In contrast, projection is preeminently an intrapsychic phenomenon that may or may not take place during interpersonal exchange. Although projective identification has intrapsychic characteristics, it generally occurs between individuals when the projector strives unconsciously to elicit within another individual particular thoughts, emotions, and experiences that are in some fashion connected to the projector's own inner perceptions. During the process of projective identification, the projector may activate in the individual an experiential state that corresponds with either the projector's self-representation or alternatively, the projector's object representations drawn from the projector's internalized object relations.

Apprey (1987) has defined projective identification as "an unconscious defensive process which exteriorizes an incompatible aspect of one's self organization into a representation of an object in ways which permit an unburdening of an unacceptable attribute or a preservation of an aspect of one's self away from hostile primary process presences. In the process of actualizing the delegated self-organization, one maintains a fantasized picture of control and oneness with the object. The result is that there is a change in the subject's own self representation as well as a change in the perception of the object" (p. 5). In this sense, projective identification suggests an impairment in the recognition of boundaries. Grotstein (1985) has explained that if projective identification is used as a defense, then the self, through translocation, can *split off* unwanted aspects that have been previously internalized. The individual may also maintain the fantasy that he can actively control the object or passively fuse with the object to evade painful emotions of helplessness.

There are, however, some positive variations of projective identification and these include *vicarious introspection, empathy,* and *intersubjectivity,* which represent adaptive strategies for relating to a significant other. According to Hoffman (1977), empathy refers to a vicarious affective response experienced by an individual that is more appropriate to someone else's situation than to one's own. Other notions of empathy include Schafer's (1959) definition that the phenomenon represents the experience of sharing and comprehending the momentary psychological state of another person. Kohut (1959) has referred to empathy as vicarious introspection, whereas Greenson (1960) uses the phrase "emotional knowing." For Racker (1957), empathy refers to a complementary identification whereby the momentary self-representation of one individual closely matches the internalized object representation of another individual at that particular moment.

Related to the notion of empathy is the notion of intersubjectivity, a developmental milestone that first emerges at approximately 9 months of age and implicates the infant's ability for self-regulation. In general, intersubjectivity describes the emergence of the self from its state of undifferentiation. Both Stern (1985) and Trevarthen and Hubley (1978) have noted that this developmental event correlates with the infant's perception that others possess an internal reality that is separate and distinct from the infant's own internal reality. At this juncture, the infant begins to display an awareness of the caregiver's intentions, perceptions, and affects. The awareness of a shared internal reality, which includes both awareness of an internal self and awareness of the internal reality of others, is a prime prerequisite of intersubjectivity. Initially, a more rudimentary form of this skill becomes apparent at 40 weeks of age, when the infant begins to perceive the caregiver as a partner in interactional sequences. By 2 months, the infant has progressed to a form of reciprocal mirroring and by 9 months, full-fledged intersubjectivity may be inferred from the infant's manipulation of objects and efforts to capture the caregiver's attention through pointing and looking gestures.

These manifestations indicate that the infant has perceived he is separate from the caregiver, even though the caregiver may be engaged in meaningful interaction to elicit particular behaviors and responses. Intersubjectivity represents a significant developmental milestone that influences the internal and external perceptual capacities of the infant. As noted, internal perception changes to the extent that the infant recognizes the distinction between himself and his caregiver. External perception is altered in a more subtle manner. When the caregiver realizes the infant's new maturational skills, she spontaneously enlarges her repertoire of manifestations and begins interacting with the infant in a more sophisticated manner.

To fully understand how projective identification influences dyadic interaction, it is necessary to consider how this defense manifests itself. Kernberg (1984) has described the following components of projective identification. First, the individual projects an unacceptable part of the self onto an object. Second, there is generally an empathy between the self and the recipient of the projection. At the same time, however, the individual experiences a desire to control the object. Finally, there is an unconscious wish to induce in the object the content that is being projected. According to Kernberg, empathy is present between the self and object in projective identification because the projector of the fantasy has internalized and identified with the object. This form of empathy is lacking in pure projection. Moreover, in projective identification, parts of the self that are perceived as being "good" can be delegated to the object, thereby impoverishing the self and causing idealization of the object. As a defense process, projective identification can have an overwhelming impact on the caregiver's relationship with the infant and thus on the infant's development. Such is the case when the infant comes to mirror the caregiver's tendency to fuse with the object, impairing not only the development of an autonomous sense of self, but also the ability to distinguish his perspective from that of the caregiver.

For example, if a mother has delegated unacceptable parts of her sense of self onto the infant, she might express such opinions as "The baby is mean" or "The baby is angry." The controlling aspects of projective identification would emerge in such remarks as "I feel rejected when she bites my nipple," or "I can't bear for her to be away from me." Finally, the mother may use the infant to induce the quality that will be projected. This phenomenon is revealed in comments such as "I am afraid her temper will be like mine and will come between us." As a result of projecting into the infant the anger, spite, and aggression that is actually part of her own self-organization, the caregiver's internal working model of the self undergoes alteration. Moreover, the infant's working model of the self also changes. These alterations eclipse the objective profile of infant development and replace it with distortions.

Several conditions are associated with projective identification. For example, fantasies of control or of being controlled by objects appear to be common among caregivers with a proclivity toward projective identification. Grotstein has commented that individuals who manifest projective identification engage in relationships characterized by coercion, manipulation, seduction, intimidation, ridicule, and such histrionic behavior as martyrdom. Caregivers who display a tendency to engage in projective identification often report that they feel as if they are sleepwalking or that they are "possessed," and their outward demeanor may be robotlike and mechanical. Essentially, caregivers who manifest projective identification experience the sense of self as being somehow inadequate or insufficiently equipped to maintain a sense of coherent identity. As a result, myriad maladaptive responses may emerge in an effort to disguise underlying psychological deficits.

Grotstein (1985) has identified some of these responses, including responses that involve external projections onto an object:

1. The return to an undifferentiated state of fused oneness with the nurturing object that blurs the distinction between self and object.
2. The scanning of the environment for objects that contain qualities reminiscent of the self.
3. The externalization of aspects of the self, in order to recognize objects as being familiar and to identify with them.

The following responses involve a transformation of the self and the object:

4. The invasion of an object to control it or be controlled by it, thereby eliminating feelings of helplessness.
5. The communication with other aspects of the self, as well as with external objects.
6. The disavowal of aspects of the self onto an object to further the aims of splitting.

During projective identification, both the self and the object are transformed so that the self may experience episodes of confusion, emptiness, and vulnerability to being controlled by the object.

For the process of projective identification to emerge, there must be an available object. In other words, there must be a significant other (e.g., infant) with whom the caregiver has developed an intimate relationship. If such a relationship exists, the caregiver can project perceptions about the experiences she is undergoing. This process fosters identification.

In contrast, if the caregiver treats the infant as an object upon which to project because of unresolved conflict, a detrimental outcome will follow. That is, the caregiver is developing an internal working model of the infant that is *not* based on the objective evidence of development, but is instead based on her own subjective distortions. The caregiver perceives that the infant has accepted the projection and identifies with her projection. Identification is here experienced as a transforming agent that changes the infant into the caregiver's victim and ultimately into her persecutor.

From the above discussion, it is apparent why an understanding of projective identification processes is vital for the therapist working with parent–infant dyads. As a preliminary matter, it is essential that such therapists attempt to discern the nature of the exchange between infant and caregiver. Evidence concerning the dyadic relationship may be derived from the caregiver's reports, from direct and open-ended inquiries, and from observations of how the caregiver interacts with the infant. A classic example of this dynamic was provided to me by one caregiver who, upon being asked why she had selected a particular name for her child said, "[W]e named him after his uncle and it's funny because even now he always reminds me of this uncle . . . He always seems to want to have his own way and control things." This vignette illustrates how projective identification can be used to transform the infant by endowing him with a particular personality that derives from the caregiver's own representations of past experiences with other objects. The therapist then should determine whether the caregiver is projecting traits onto the object or whether the infant objectively displays the particular behavioral patterns that the caregiver is addressing.

Of equal significance is the way that the caregiver projects feelings and attributes to the therapist. Here, the therapist should keep in mind the role of parallel processes, whereby characteristics of the caregiver's relationship with the infant are reenacted during the caregiver's relationship with the therapist. The therapist will also be called upon to analyze the transference relationship that is evolving during therapeutic encounters. By assessing the transference relationship and the countertransference feelings experienced, the therapist can discern the emotions being projected within the caregiver–infant dyad and within the caregiver–therapist dyad. The key factor is that, at some point, the dyadic interaction will be replicated during interaction with the therapist.

Thus, projective identification may become manifested in three distinct ways. First, the individual receiving the projection (e.g., therapist) would identify his self-representation with the object representation of the projector (e.g., caregiver). Second, there may be a complementary identification, whereby the therapist temporarily identifies with one aspect of the caregiver's internalized self and object representations, while the caregiver, at least temporarily, experiences the counterpart identification. The complementarity in this interaction is reflected by the complementarity in the patient's self and object representations. A third way that projective identification manifests itself is customarily associated with the individual's empathic capacities. In this scenario, the caregiver arouses within the therapist what has been referred to by Racker (1954, 1957) as a concordant identification such that the immediate self-experiences of both individuals are temporarily similar in nature.

> (Caregiver has expressed feeling jealous of her husband because he can go out to work while she has to stay home and take care of their baby.)

THERAPIST: Have you noticed any changes in the way you feel about your baby since you began feeling jealous of your husband?

CAREGIVER: I feel more care and affection for the baby. I also feel more relaxed with him. I just feel special with him. I feel as if he's always going to be there for his Mommy—much more than his Daddy.

THERAPIST: Are you concerned that your special relationship with your baby may change?

CAREGIVER: The only thing that may change it is if my baby becomes smarter than me. (Caregiver holds infant close to her face and speaks in low tones.) If he is smarter than me, he might be able to control me.

THERAPIST: How might he control you?

CAREGIVER: (Still speaking softly, as if to the infant) By saying or doing certain things that I didn't teach him, or things that make me wonder where he got his ideas from—ideas that I didn't teach him.

THERAPIST: Could you give me an example of the kinds of ideas he could have or behaviors he could manifest to make you feel as if he controls you?

CAREGIVER: He could say, "Mommy, you don't understand" or "You need to do this." I can't just rely on my instincts when I'm caring for him because they are not always accurate.

THERAPIST: Could you give me an example of a time when your instincts weren't accurate?

CAREGIVER: I think there are certain things he might want to do while knowing that I don't want him to do them. He behaves that way sometimes. He knows that I don't want him to throw all of his toys out of his crib, but he wants his own way and I have to do whatever he wants.

If therapists determine that a projective identification is operating within the dyadic exchange, they should attempt to analyze the "fit" between what each participant is experiencing. That is, are the experiences of caregiver and infant complementary to one another? Tansey and Burke (1985) have identified three categories of interactional fit when projective identification is involved. In the first category, the individual projects his own self-representation onto a recipient, resulting in a concordant identification. The second category occurs when the individual projects an internalized object representation to the recipient individual, resulting in a complementary identification. Finally, projective identifications may be both complementary and concordant.

During dyadic interaction, projective identification can signify a maladaptive response on the part of the caregiver. The infant is sensitive to the nuances of caregiver manifestations and is likely to be attuned to the projections. Such tendencies are maladaptive because they represent instances in which the caregiver is not responding to objective dimensions of infant maturation, but is rather grafting preconceived notions and attributions onto the interaction.

The therapeutic relationship can reverse this debilitating trend of projections and projective identifications in both the infant and caregiver. Intervention is efficacious because it offers strategies whereby patients externalize their imaginative inner realities onto a neutral and objective observer (the therapist) for assessment and interpretation. As intervention progresses, a therapeutic relationship develops, enabling the therapist to become identified with the patient's inner world and to serve as a model for adaptive interaction. This relationship may be split between an "idealized" and an "objective" relationship. The caregiver will inevitably strive to involve the therapist in such issues. One way of resolving the effects of projection is by discerning which aspects of the internal object the caregiver projects onto the external world. These tendencies need to be evaluated, and the conflict that underlies them needs to be resolved within the therapeutic relationship. Thus, the therapist should assess the experiences of the caregiver's daily life because they dominate her emotions and the internal representations. Through the exploration of these relationships, signifying aspects of primitive experiences, the caregiver can integrate the split-off and projected feelings from her past.

Finally, projection needs to be understood as a phenomenon that implicates both a subject and an object—whether the object is internal or external. The adaptive caregiver is attuned to the infant's complaints and is eager to engage in ameliorative behavior to help the infant undergo or dispel painful affect. In contrast, however, if the caregiver is maladaptive and engages in projections, the infant will experience and internalize the maternal object as continuously undergoing frightening transformations. Thereafter, the object becomes contaminated with subsequent projections and is further infused with negativity and contempt.

The goal of dyadic intervention is to prevent the emergence of debilitating patterns of projective identification and, in cases where such patterns of maladaptive interaction have been established, to replace these patterns with more adaptive behaviors that will generate qualities of contingency, reciprocity, and attunement. To do this, the therapist must first observe and then engage the dyad directly in previewing exercises that promote adaptation.

The overwhelming thrust of this research indicates that these early patterns of interaction between infant and caregiver create and perpetuate enduring personality structures. The therapist engaging in dyadic treatment needs to recognize that one member of the dyad—the caregiver—will bring these patterns into treatment for evaluation and analysis by the therapist.

INFANT DEFENSIVE FUNCTIONING

Just as caregivers manifest various defenses—such as externalization and projection—that can intrude into the domain of interaction with the infant, so too have researchers determined that even very young infants are capable of displaying defensive phenomena that can interfere with an adaptive relationship with the caregiver.

Fraiberg (1982) has identified a group of pathological defenses in infants between 3 and 18 months of age who have experienced danger and deprivation. The infant defenses observed by Fraiberg include *avoidance, freezing,* and *fighting,* which are summoned from a biological repertoire based on the model of "flight or fight." Fraiberg explains that a defense operating during infancy is not a full-fledged "defense mechanism." When considering the presence of defense mechanisms in infancy, Fraiberg notes that it is helpful to adhere to the views of Wallerstein (1976), who distinguished between "defense mechanisms as a construct" and defenses as "actual phenomena." A behavior that serves defensive purposes can be observed, Fraiberg notes, whereas Wallerstein points out that a defense mechanism is a theoretical denomination. The therapist may, for example, observe exaggerated sympathy in a patient as a behavior, but the unconscious process whereby a cruel impulse is converted into its intellectual opposite cannot be observed. In this regard, therapists may observe behaviors that serve a defensive purpose at any point in development; in the case of the infant, if the child is capable of registering a danger or threat to his functioning, he will react to the danger with a behavior that serves as a defense.

Using the manifestation of an objective behavioral response as evidence of an infant defense, Fraiberg reports on three manifestations—avoidance, freezing, and fighting—that can be observed in young infants subjected to maternally depriving experiences. In some of these children, an avoidance response was manifested by the infant's scanning behavior as he briefly looked at his mother's face without a sign of recognition. There was no pause in scanning or a flicker on the infant's face that would reveal an awareness of or a sensitivity to the caregiver's presence. The freezing defense consists of almost complete immobilization, a freezing of posture, motility, and articulation. Finally, while manifesting the fighting response, infants can display irritability and distress when in situations in which their responses are frustrated or overtly ignored by caregivers.

Fraiberg's work is valuable because it suggests that even very young infants who have been exposed to adverse circumstances will manifest defensive behaviors. The objective manifestation of these behaviors indicates that the subjective capacities of the infant are highly sensitive and will function to protect or shield the infant from exposure to negative or noncontingent situations. Therapists conducting dyadic therapy should, therefore, be alert to such infant defense manifestations and should view them as a sign that interaction between infant and caregiver has gone awry and necessitates intervention.

CAREGIVER: (Holds baby in her lap and shakes a rattle right in front of her baby's face. Infant starts to cry and wave her arms. Caregiver continues to shake the rattle. She says to her infant) Listen to the rattle! You like that, don't you?

THERAPIST: She can't focus on the rattle when you hold it too close to her face. She doesn't understand where the noise is coming from.

CAREGIVER: (Moves rattle away from the baby's face and allows her to focus on it. Baby starts to smile and laugh.) I knew you liked rattles! (Caregiver again shakes the rattle close to the baby's face. Baby buries her head in the caregiver's stomach.)

THERAPIST: How do you think she feels right now?

CAREGIVER: (Stops shaking rattle.) She must be tired of it.

A variety of factors that emerge from the caregiver–infant relationship may function to affect the degree to which the infant manifests defensive functions. These factors include the infant's temperament and the nature of the attachment relationship that has evolved between mother and child.

With respect to temperament, the infant's disposition will likely exert an effect on how the caregiver responds to him. For example, a temperamentally demanding infant may require a greater degree of attention from the caregiver. In turn, these increased demands may cause the caregiver to grow resentful toward the infant and to manifest such resentment through her behavior. The infant may thus be subjected to rejecting and other negative behaviors that cause him to engage in the defense of avoidance to escape from the debilitating emotions the caregiver arouses in him. In a similar fashion, a slow-to-warm-up infant, who appears to manifest an apathetic response, will often initiate fewer interactions with the caregiver, who fails to understand that this more muted style of response merely reflects the infant's constitutional endowment. As a result of this misinterpretation, the caregiver in these circumstances may also adopt a resentful attitude toward the infant, and as with the infant whose disposition is too active, the defensive response of avoidance emerges. To prevent these forms of dysfunctional interaction, the therapist, from the outset of dyadic treatment, must ascertain the infant's temperament, explain temperamental classifications to the caregiver, and work to ensure that an appropriate match exists between the temperaments of the dyadic members.

Equally as devastating to the functioning of dyadic interaction as a temperamental mismatch is attachment deprivation. Attachment deprivation occurs when the infant experiences a prolonged separation from or deprivation of the caregiving figure. Attachment deprivation may occur as a result of physical separation from the mother or because of the mother's own inability to offer the infant a sense of emotional security. Robertson and Bowlby (1952) have identified three phases in an infant's response to separation: protest, despair and detachment. Protest can begin immediately after separation from the caregiver and is manifested by infant crying and other signs of obvious distress. During the succeeding phase, despair, the infant continues to exhibit a preoccupation with the missing parent, but the behavior also suggests an increasing hopelessness. Physical movement diminishes and the infant becomes withdrawn and inactive, ceasing to make demands. As detachment occurs, the infant becomes increasingly more withdrawn and at this point will manifest an avoidance reaction to the caregiver.

As a result, the therapist conducting dyadic treatment needs to evaluate the status of the attachment relationship between caregiver and infant. Is the relationship secure, in the sense that the infant responds to the caregiver, is distressed by her absence, and is enthusiastic about her return, or is the relationship insecure in the sense that the infant uses the defense of avoidance to extricate himself from interaction with the caregiver? These responses need evaluation, and if an avoidance response is present, the therapist must devise treatment strategies that prevent the infant from relying on these mechanisms of defense to deal with external experiences and the relationship with the caregiver.

CONCLUSION

This chapter has sought to pierce the veil that shields many of the subjective processes modulating dyadic interaction. As was discussed, the caregiver–infant interaction is governed by the internal working models of both members. In particular, however, the infant's internal working model is in the process of development and will be strongly influenced by the behaviors and attributions of the caregiver.

Such processes as internalization and identification help to explain how the infant comes to inculcate content that he will use to construct his internal working models. The caregiver's use of externalization, projection, and projective identification will contribute to the way in which the infant comes to perceive the world. Some of these psychological processes may thwart adaptive development because they preclude the dyadic members from perceiving developmental change as an objectively verifiable phenomenon whose repercussions will affect the dyadic rapport. Other processes, such as empathy, enlarge the caregiver's view of the infant and promote an adaptive relationship.

The therapist engaging in dyadic therapy needs to explore how these subjective processes become manifest and, above all, must observe the interaction between infant and caregiver. Subsequently, the therapist should engage in inquiry with the caregiver to discern the degree to which she is weaving subjective processes into the relationship without conscious recognition of their origin, purpose, or effect on the dyadic exchange.

Chapter 6

Assessing the Role of the Infant in the Development of Family Relationships

INTRODUCTION

It is not sufficient for the therapist to view the infant as a developing individual or as merely a member of the intimate dyad he shares with the caregiver. Rather, virtually all infants are born into families that are already formed and that carry generations of a psychological legacy of interaction with the world. When the infant is viewed in this light, it becomes apparent that he inherits not merely a sophisticated constitutional and genetic endowment, but a social and environmental one as well.

This chapter elucidates the vast ramifications of the infant's role as a family member and helps the therapist understand the infant's perceptions of either marital harmony or discord and emotional alliance or turbulence. It is important for the therapist to know how the father has perceived the pregnancy and birth in respect to his relationship with his wife, whether sibling rivalry threatens to disrupt the relationship between parents and infant, and whether the parents are using the infant as a scapegoat for their own emotional conflict. But in addition to probing these general issues, it is crucial for the therapist to understand the perspective of the infant who may be caught in the throes of such dysfunction.

As researchers have concentrated more efforts on the role of the infant, a paradoxical finding has emerged; although the infant may be a focal point of presenting symptomatology or a kind of magnet for psychopathology that attracts attention initially, case studies reveal that often the entire family structure is experiencing malfunction. That is, by studying infant behaviors and perceptions, researchers have become more attuned to the convergence of infant and family psychology, and to the significance of viewing the infant's role from the global perspective of the family dynamic. This concept, of course, is not new. From the seminal studies of Spitz onward therapists have recognized that the infant does not develop in isolation. Rather, the caregiving environment and the bidirectional response provided by caregiver interaction significantly shape the infant's personality and emerging sense of self. Nonetheless, researchers are now recognizing more clearly that beyond the dyadic relationship between caregiver and infant lies the domain of family interaction encompassing the marital relationship, the relationship among siblings, and triadic interactions of various permutations, all of which exert a definitive impact on the infant and affect his development.

As will be explained, it is only after achieving an understanding of the infant's position in the family that the therapist can surmount maladaptive patterns. Moreover, by assuming the infant's position, the therapist can better understand the degree to which adaptive previewing is or is not occurring. In turn, such perceptions will permit the therapist to devise effective treatment strategies for creating equilibrium within the family unit and asserting adaptive strategies.

FAMILY STRESS AND THE LIFE CYCLE

In its most familiar definition, the family is a group of persons united by relational bonds who undergo and share a series of common experiences. But the family may also be viewed as an entity, a kind of symbolic individual, that experiences its own unique life cycle. At some point during the life cycle of the family—whether the family is highly adaptive or dysfunctional—it encounters a period of stress (Boss, 1983). These challenges to the family's capacity for adaptation not only come from external forces but also arise from the normal developmental processes experienced throughout life. The therapist engaged in dyadic treatment must explore how these *stressful life events* influence development in the family and, in particular, development of the infant. Terkelsen (1980) distinguishes two kinds of important life changes that occur in families—*first order developments*, which involve no substantive alteration in identity or self-concept, and *second order developments*, which involve transformation of meaning and status as a result of stress. Marriage and the birth of a child are second order developments because the individuals undergoing the experience change their concepts of "self" and "family." One of the tasks in therapy is to identify the processes that help families acclimate to stress and evolve more cohesive relationships as well as the processes that prevent other families from coping effectively, so that a downward spiral toward maladaptive behavior patterns and dysfunction emerges. For example, a family that is likely to overcome stress with adaptive strategies is one in which both caregivers successfully departed from their own families and established separate adult identities without trauma. When stressful events arise in these families, they are likely to employ adaptive forms of interaction to surmount the event and evolve more cohesive bonds of unity.

Because stress can exert such a potent effect on family dynamics, how are parental attitudes conveyed to newborns at these times? During the first 30 months of life the infant inculcates messages about the external world and about himself primarily as a consequence of parental interaction. Initially, for example, the infant craves physical comfort, so that the dramatic shift from the soothing prenatal atmosphere of the womb to the external environment is as nondisruptive as possible. Over time, the infant becomes sensitized to the stimuli and cues of the external world, learning how to influence and predict the responses of others, including most significantly, the caregiver's responses. Infant response occurs most commonly in behavioral cues addressed to the primary caregiver. The infant also becomes adept at imitating behaviors during this period, as he begins to engage in patterns that evoke particular types of caregiver reactions, helping him convert the world into a contingent and predictable domain (Trad, 1990). Some typical examples include crying, which will motivate the mother to provide warmth and body contact, or the emission of particular vocalizations that the mother recognizes as a signal to initiate play behavior. As the infant experiments with his repertoire of responses, he comes to realize that he can master the universe for the purposes of fulfilling various needs—provided that the caregiver is receptive to his manifestations. Eventually, the capacity to interact with the environment acquires an emotional dimension for the infant, and his feelings of mastery are essentially converted into affective responses referred to as *esteem*. Adaptation occurs when the caregiver validates these feelings of competence and independence through such techniques as developmental previewing. Encouragement of the infant's efforts through previewing exercises introduces the infant to the interpersonal and emotional consequences of the developmental processes. In particular, previewing behaviors acquaint the infant with upcoming developmental milestones and with the effect the acquisition of these milestones will have on his relationship with the caregiver. For example, from the period of infancy to toddlerhood, the child will develop skills for feeding himself, anticipating and avoiding dangerous objects and situations, and managing the functions of his own body in relation to the environment. Through adaptive previewing, the infant will be supported toward balancing his needs with those of others, a requirement for family coexistence.

The therapist can enhance diagnosis of the family's status by discerning connections between caregiver–infant maladaptive behavior and the dynamics within the family unit. Crowther (1985) has determined that measures of clinical depression in one parent are often correlated with maladaptation within the marital unit as a whole. Thus, impaired interaction with the infant may correspond to marital distress and dysfunction. A major implication of this research is that assessment and therapeutic evaluations concerning the emotional status of a parent should consider the status of the marital relationship and should examine how any conflict between husband and wife may impact on the infant. If, for example, the mother reports depression, but the husband reports marital adjustment, the husband needs to be incorporated into the dyadic treatment to explore whether the marital relationship is in fact adaptive or whether one marital partner is disguising or evading the presence of conflict. Conversely, if psychopathology occurs concurrently with marital conflict and maladjustment, concurrent marital therapy may be recommended at the same time that the mother and infant are being seen for treatment.

THERAPIST: Has Judy been spending more time playing by herself?
CAREGIVER: She doesn't come to us to play as much as she used to. She's becoming much more independent and playing by herself very often.
THERAPIST: What factors do you think account for this change?

CAREGIVER: The problems I have with my husband. It is very traumatic to Judy. She knows everything that is going on between us. We seem to be fighting all the time and the baby just avoids us. It's as if she can sense when a fight is about to begin.

To validate the infant's growing mastery over the environment, both caregivers must be competent not only in recognizing when developmental achievements have occurred but also in previewing the interpersonal implications of future developmental achievements. For validation of perceptual messages through previewing to operate as a developmentally enhancing phenomenon, it should be appropriate to the needs, developmental abilities, and readiness of the child. Such validation must be rendered in a clear, direct, and specific fashion, designed to motivate the child toward further maturational achievement. If the caregivers are fighting between themselves, their perceptual insight into the infant's experiences will become far less acute. Morever, as is suggested by the preceding vignette, the infant often can sense this change in the status of the marital relationship and withdraws from the controversy surrounding him.

In addition, caregivers may be incapable of sharing their feelings openly with the infant because they harbor developmental deficits emanating from their own family of origin. As Gaffney (1986) has pointed out, during the course of the pregnancy some expectant mothers and fathers may undergo a form of regression to an earlier developmental state that impairs self-confidence. This regression may stem from the uncertainties aroused by the prospect of parenthood and a desire to return to previous levels of development with which the parent(s) felt more secure. This lack of self-confidence may, in turn, cause the caregiver to feel depressed and helpless, resulting in the conversion of these debilitating feelings into anger that is displaced onto the infant. Thus, unresolved conflicts from the caregivers' own pasts can suddenly surface with the advent of a new baby, threatening the relationships within the family. In a related study, Condon and Dunn (1988) found that when caregivers have an indifferent or negative first impression of their infant at birth, this reaction can exert a potentially enduring detrimental effect on patterns of caregiver–infant attachment. In such situations the infant often becomes the parental *scapegoat,* meaning that some conflict harbored by the parent is foisted or displaced onto the child. Unless the caregiver, with the therapist's assistance, explores and resolves the source of this anger, the infant may become a scapegoat bearing the brunt of the caregiver's anger and frustration, while the underlying emotional conflict is continually thwarted. Although relatively few caregivers experience these feelings, it is vital for the therapist to explore whether such emotions existed at the birth in order to trace familial maladaptation and to institute treatment that will rectify this pattern and prevent further scapegoating.

In evaluating the role of the infant in the family, the therapist should also consider the role of *developmental dyssynchrony* on the life span of the family. As explained by Budman and Gurman (1988), developmental dys- synchrony refers to a conflict that has arisen because an individual or family is experiencing a pivotal period of life transition during which a sense of identity is lost. Budman and Gurman highlight several key times when such a pivotal period may occur. First, during late adolescence or young adult- hood the individual may experience difficulty in separating from the par- ents and establishing an independent identity. Failure to establish a signifi- cant romantic relationship in young adulthood is another such pivotal time, as is the period when a woman appears to be approaching the end of her childbearing years without being able to have a child. A similar crisis may occur when an adult experiences the death of a spouse or when a serious illness is diagnosed in the individual or in another family member. Another instance of developmental dyssynchrony occurs when a man or woman in midlife experiences dissatisfaction in the marital relationship or when a child is still dependent on family members when he has reached middle age.

Any of these situations may motivate individuals to seek treatment. Ac- cording to Budman and Gurman (1988), the therapist's line of inquiry in seeing such patients should include specifying and describing the develop- mental dyssynchrony in question as well as clarifying the individuals' per- sonal narratives and perspectives on the situation. In addition, the therapist should help patients toward actively achieving their developmental goals by reasserting and if necessary reformulating a position within their families. In other situations the therapist may need to assist individuals in accepting that they may not be able to fully resolve the developmental crisis. More- over, treating a developmental dyssynchrony frequently occurs in an inter- personal context where the participation of other family members is advan- tageous.

The theory of developmental dyssynchrony is particularly useful within the context of dyadic treatment because it encourages the therapist to view the family from a developmental perspective. Indeed, numerous research- ers have suggested that the advent of a new infant into the family repre- sents, in and of itself, a developmental crisis. If the infant is the first child, the parents will be forced to alter their marital relationship to accommodate the infant's needs. If, on the other hand, the family already has at least one child, the birth will require the other family members, including the infant's sibling, to realign themselves into new patterns of interaction.

The arrival of a new infant may further trigger conflict within the family because the husband and wife may for the first time be adopting the responsibility of parenthood. The onset of these roles may provoke a period of developmental dyssynchrony because the new parents will be reeval- uating their status in their families of origin as well as attempting to replicate effective patterns of nurturing derived from their own childhood experiences. These events will often cause confusion and a period during which the prospective parents feel that they are losing their old identities, whereas their new identities as parents are just beginning to surface.

As a result, the therapist treating a dyad should use thorough inquiry techniques to determine whether the motivation for seeking therapy is the parents' feelings of developmental dyssynchrony. Moreover, developmental dyssynchrony represents an upheaval in the individual's identity, so it is likely to disturb the representational process. There may be an absence of previewing behaviors within the dyad because the caregiver must first maintain a lucid perception of imminent developmental change before she can eventually exhibit it to the infant in the form of previewing exercises. Thus, an absence of previewing may indicate developmental dyssynchrony on the part of the caregiver, and the therapist should elucidate this crisis by relying on the inquiries described earlier.

THE EFFECT OF THE NEWBORN ON THE MARRIAGE

Almost immediately after the conception of an infant, both caregivers will begin noticing alterations in their own relationship and patterns of interaction. Caregivers with whom I have discussed this process have observed that despite recent sociological changes in attitudes concerning the mother's role in childrearing, it is still expected that the mother will maintain emotional equilibrium within the marriage and balance the multigenerational dimensions of the relationship she establishes simultaneously with the infant and her husband. The following dialogue is from a case that illustrates how the arrival of a newborn affects the sense of equilibrium and modes of interaction between the parents:

THERAPIST: In what ways do you feel that your relationship changed after you learned about your pregnancy?

CAREGIVER: That's one of the things that surprised me about our marriage. We've known each other a long time, almost 12 years, and we've been married for seven years . . . (drifts off, puts baby on floor) and yet when I became pregnant . . . I felt that my husband and I grew closer.

THERAPIST: Has the baby's birth affected the relationship with your husband?

CAREGIVER: Not on a deep level . . . but sometimes I feel it's safer to love the baby.

THERAPIST: Can you explain what you mean by that?

CAREGIVER: Ian's birth really changed our marriage. I don't know what it is (resigned, shrugs shoulders). Sometimes I think it's me.

THERAPIST: (Focusing) Can you be more specific about the changes you've noticed?

CAREGIVER: I used to feel as if I had everything I needed to be satisfied (embarrassed). I had a good job, a good home, and a good husband. I kind of stopped taking care of my husband and he's been telling me this for years. I just said, "Well, I'm sorry, I'm really busy." I guess that my attitude has really taken its toll on the marriage. I just never noticed. The quality is not there anymore.

THERAPIST: Do you feel the change is only within you or between you and your husband? What has changed?

CAREGIVER: I feel exhausted! Friday night I always make a special dinner and set the table and do all the outward chores and we'll sit down to have a wonderful meal . . . I enjoy doing that, preparing a meal like that, I don't find it tedious or burdensome. But now the television goes on, my husband is exhausted . . . it's like pulling teeth to get a conversation going. That's the difficult part. We really have to put extra effort into it— it feels very strenuous. We don't communicate the way we used to. Maybe it's because of the baby who distracts us.

THERAPIST: (Confirming) So is it the exhaustion that changes the quality of the relationship with your husband (prodding), or have you sensed there might be other things?

CAREGIVER: It's all the responsibility . . . taking care of an infant, changes in work status. For me, I went from being a working adult spending all my time with other adults to interacting with the baby all day and being at home. Your world and perspective shrinks tremendously. Many times I feel left out of the adult world. I know I devote my energies to the baby, sometimes at my husband's expense, but I can't seem to help it.

THERAPIST: What would be the best balance for you?

CAREGIVER: I think both of us should spend a little more energy working out a balance in the marriage relationship and in our attitudes toward the baby.

One of the issues the therapist should explore during dyadic treatment is how the marriage and other family relations have changed since the conception of the infant. As exemplified in the preceding dialogue, some of the changes may be dramatic, whereas others may be more subtle. Many mothers with whom I have discussed this issue have noted that they are expected to bear the emotional burden of the infant's birth and arrival. In general, it is the mother who shoulders a disproportionate amount of the responsibility for nurturing the infant, and this added responsibility can occasionally lead to feelings of resentment that affect the mother's attitude toward the infant and her husband. Also, in many modern marriages both caregivers work full-time prior to the birth of the infant. Nonetheless, it is usually the mother who is expected to leave her job and become a full-time homemaker after the birth of the infant, a transition that may cause lingering regrets and create conflict for the mother. If this conflict is not worked out within the context of the marriage, it may ultimately be enacted in the relationship with the infant.

The advent of an infant in the household significantly alters interactional patterns between the caregivers themselves and between the caregivers and their offspring. The therapist's task is not only to probe these issues but also to assist the parents in expressing and resolving conflict, so that the infant's presence will enrich, rather than disrupt, the relationship between the caregivers. As may be seen from this analysis, included in the concept of "family" is the notion of numerous dyadic, as well as triadic relationships, each of which must be synthesized harmoniously to solidify the adaptive alliance within the family structure.

A thorough perspective on the life span of families has been provided by McGoldrick and Carter (1982). These researchers note that the family life cycle perspective views symptoms and dysfunction in relation to normal functioning over time. This perspective locates problems along the spectrum the family has traversed in the past, the goals it is currently attempting to master, and the future events and experiences toward which it is moving. To understand the family life cycle, McGoldrick and Carter recommend that the family be viewed as consisting of more than the sum of its parts and that the family life cycle be considered the major context for the development of family members. The authors comment that the family represents a basic unit within which emotional development springs forth.

One point emphasized by McGoldrick and Carter is that the emotional system of the family should be considered for at least three generations. In addition, the therapist should analyze the family in both its horizontal and vertical configurations. The vertical flow in the family system includes patterns of relating and functioning that are transmitted down the generations in the family tree, primarily through the mechanism of emotional triangulation (Bowen, 1978). This vertical flow incorporates all the family attitudes, taboos, expectations, labels, and emotionally charged issues to which individuals are subjected as they are growing up. The horizontal flow in the family life cycle is generated by anxiety from the stresses on the family as it moves through time. These stresses would include normally expected developmental events, such as the departure of an adolescent child from the household, as well as developmental crises, such as the death of a family member.

McGoldrick and Carter articulate essentially three generations that the therapist should analyze—the grandparents, parents, and children—as well as six stages of the family life cycle. These six stages include the period when individuals are young unattached adults seeking to establish their own identities while still maintaining ties to their families. This stage is followed by the period during which individuals find a partner and enter marriage. Next comes the stage of a family with young children. The family then matures to the phase in which the children reach the adolescent years. Eventually, these children mature to the point where they are prepared to leave the confines of the nuclear family. The final stage involves the family in later life, at which time the parents gradually assume the role of grandparents.

A key to understanding the family life cycle portrayed by McGoldrick and Carter is an understanding of the transitional periods between different stages of development. During these periods individuals tend to reassess their identities and reevaluate their role within the family. Indeed, it is almost a cliché that at such periods of transition individuals are prone to seek treatment. As has been noted previously, one of these seminal transition periods occurs with the birth of an infant. If a caregiver with a new infant enters the treatment setting it is more likely than not that she or another member of her immediate family is experiencing the transition to parenthood as a kind of crisis situation.

It is therefore advisable to utilize some of McGoldrick and Carter's strategies. For example, the therapist should ascertain the full history of three family generations whenever possible. In addition, it is important to review how the parents have negotiated various periods of transition during their own life cycles and how they are adjusting to the birth of the infant.

Elderkin (1975) advocates a similar kind of evaluation of the family unit during the process of psychotherapy. For Elderkin, the family should be viewed as a total unit within which the child is a functioning member. Disturbances in interaction manifested by the child should be viewed as a response to the family as a whole, rather than as merely an individual response. For example, parental pressure, inefficiency, and indifference may in fact be causing the maladaptive behavior that has caused the parents to seek treatment. Behavioral disorder may also be viewed as an effort on the part of the infant to disrupt a rigid system within the family and to revise entrenched patterns of dysfunction. Elderkin also suggests that the child's disturbing behavior may represent an effort to restore adaptive patterns that have been disrupted. The infant or child is, in other words, striving to regain a stable or homeostatic balance in the interrelationships among family members. In fact, much of the literature concerning the family as a unit highlights the breakdown of family homeostasis as a cause of behavioral disorder and the restoration of a homeostatic balance as an objective of therapeutic efforts (Satir, 1967).

When a caregiver or family presents for treatment, the adults in the family frequently characterize the infant or child as the presenting problem. Although in certain cases factors relating to the infant's constitutional endowment may indeed have upset the family's equilibrium, more often than not the problem affects the entire family and has its etiology in the interactional patterns among family members.

Researchers have thus advised that therapists treating infants and young children attempt to discern the sequences of interaction within the family, the coordinated practices of the family, and, in particular, the intersection between the child's development and the family's development. It is vital to consider each of these factors when formulating a treatment plan. Moreover, therapists should focus particularly on times of developmental *transition* within the family. By developmental transition is meant a stage during which some new milestone is consolidating within a child, or some event of dramatic significance is occurring within the family. The birth of an infant and his integration into the family structure is one such milestone, as is a career change on the part of a caregiver. The reason developmental transitions are so significant is that researchers have determined that these are times when family members tend to "get stuck" in resurrecting and repeating old patterns of dysfunctional behavior. This tendency occurs because a period of developmental transition is one of upheaval: The individual becomes anxious about prospective challenges and, to buffer this anxiety, relies on old dysfunctional patterns of interaction. In addition, because periods of developmental transition are times of stress, unresolved conflict tends to be resurrected.

As a result, families are most vulnerable to dysfunctional behavior during periods of developmental transition. Therapists should be aware of this phenomenon and should recognize the value of using previewing exercises during this time. Through previewing, family members can represent and then enact prospective developmental events. By focusing on upcoming transitions in development, the therapist is able to explore unresolved areas of conflict with family members. Previewing also facilitates an understanding of parental expectations concerning the child and of the internal working models of family members. For all of these reasons, a thorough examination of the familial environment is recommended for therapists conducting dyadic therapy. Moreover, previewing represents a valuable treatment tool that therapists can use to diagnose and intervene during periods of developmental transition and, significantly, before such transitions have caused upheaval and conflict in the family unit.

Therapists conducting dyadic treatment should thus examine on a profound level the motivations of the caregiver who seeks treatment. In particular it is important to determine whether the child's problematic behavior reflects misalliances and emotional conflict that actually emanate from the parents. Until they rectify this situation, the family will be unlikely to look toward future developmental change with optimism or to engage in previewing behavior that could acclimate the infant to those future events.

DYADIC AND TRIADIC RELATIONSHIPS WITHIN THE FAMILY

Each family creates its own structure from which the therapist can derive an understanding of the fundamental interpersonal patterns that govern human development among those individuals (Brazelton, Als, Tronick, & Lester, 1979). From birth onward, the human infant manifests predictable behavior patterns when interacting with specific adults in the environment. These predictable patterns generate differentiated behaviors, as do more sophisticated regulatory systems of communication that enable the infant to build a model of his relationship with each caregiver and with the family as a whole. Only if the caregivers themselves manifest predictability toward the infant, however, will the infant be able to achieve his full developmental potential.

The family structure serves as a vehicle that stimulates and reinforces previewing behavior. Previewing behavior by both caregivers signifies an attempt to *predict* and *guide* the direction of the infant's future development so that he can begin to define his own consistent perspective on interpersonal relationships. If the infant experiences predictable patterns of response even from birth, such patterns will encourage him to interact further to elicit a greater number and variety of predictable interpersonal responses. The infant experiences predictability as being pleasurable and feels a sense of mastery and competence when caregiver actions fulfill his expectations. Moreover, the caregivers are likely to share and validate their insights about infant response with one another. Eventually, the caregiver's capacity to commune in a significant fashion will influence the infant's representational models of interaction, allowing him to incorporate the implications of new developmental acquisitions within the interpersonal arena. In turn, evidence of the infant's development motivates caregivers to continue predicting future developmental acquisitions in a more complex fashion. Indeed, parents typically share their aspirations about the infant's development with one another and jointly devise previewing exercises to acquaint the infant with future development. Although dyadic interaction between the infant and one caregiver is vital to development, optimal development occurs when other relationships within the context of the family, such as the relationship between both caregivers, complement the dyadic context.

THERAPIST: Which developmental change has provided you with the best indication of your baby's progress?

CAREGIVER: His language skills. I take care of him. I feed him. I change his diapers, and I let him listen to the music. I feel soft music is helpful to him because he can develop better speech patterns on his own. In other words, I'm trying to teach him to be independent. But certain things I know I have to help him do. As far as helping him to talk, I know it's just going to be a natural thing for him. He is only five months old and he is already saying, "Mama, Dada. . ."

THERAPIST: How old was he when he first started pronouncing "Mama and Dada"?

CAREGIVER: About four and a half months.

THERAPIST: What changes have you noticed in his speech since then?

CAREGIVER: I've noticed that he's been talking more frequently. For the last month or so he hasn't said "Mama." He's been saying "Dada." And I've noticed that he hasn't been saying anything new lately, so I might have to start teaching him new words and concepts. I think he wants me to teach him new words.

THERAPIST: What do you think he wants you to teach him?

CAREGIVER: I think he probably wants me to teach him some basic words so he can communicate with us more effectively. I would like to teach him words like "society," "man," "boy," "God."

THERAPIST: Why do you want to teach him these particular words?

CAREGIVER: Because I would like him to learn more about how other people think and about abstract concepts. I want to teach him that, and I want him to know that whatever he's involved in, he will have to consider what is around him, whether it refers to people, to himself, or even to God. Ultimately, all of these things will teach him who he is in life. I think language will help him have a sense of identity.

Considering the complexity of the family structure is important for several reasons. First, interaction with two individuals who vary in physical appearance, style of behavior, and personality provides the infant with confidence during diverse developmental challenges by instilling the concept that he can maintain positive interaction with different individuals. Thus, he learns that there may be a variety of methods for handling a situation effectively. The presence of various interactive partners also prevents the infant from becoming mired in the patterns of a single partner and helps to diffuse the intensity of the dyadic interaction. For example, on those occasions when the mother may not be in the mood to interact with the infant, another family member (e.g., the father or a sibling) can assume a prominent role. At times when the father is not available, a sibling or a member of the extended family can step in. These diverse interactional styles ultimately help the infant coordinate and differentiate function, increasing his flexibility with the styles of exchange manifested by different family members. This exposure benefits the infant as he strives to formulate his own unique sense of identity while balancing his responses to various individuals.

These principles are illustrated by the visual object fixation of a 3-week-old infant. Such fixation is characterized by periods of rapt attention, folowed by abrupt and brief turning-away episodes that seem to function as recovery periods, enabling the infant to retreat from his investment in the object. During the periods of attention, the infant's face, arms, legs, toes, and fingers move in a jerky fashion; however, when the infant averts gaze, these movements cease. But the infant's behavior in the presence of an adult is distinctively different. With adults, the infant acts in *affective synchrony* and modifies his behavior in response to the feedback messages he receives during episodes of *reciprocal interaction* (Brazelton et al., 1979). In essence, by fostering the development of self-regulatory behaviors, a nurturing figure shapes the development of the infant. Exposure to several adaptive styles of different adults will therefore enhance the infant's repertoire of responsivity.

During observations of the infant manifesting this form of affective synchrony, it becomes apparent that an exchange of information is occurring. According to Brazelton et al., the parent becomes sensitive to the limits on the infant's attention span and the necessary phase of recovery that balances the child's emotional investment in behavior. In turn, the infant learns about himself as he achieves physiological and interpersonal homeostasis within this environment. This awareness replenishes the infant during subsequent previewing episodes when he communicates to the caregiver that he has experienced sufficient exposure to an imminent developmental change. A sensitive caregiver will adjust the cues emitted and will work synchronously to transmit meaningful messages within the limits set by the infant. As the infant develops his capacity to attend to external phenomena, he learns how to achieve an optimal state of attention for both objects and people, and how to articulate control over them.

Thus, a *triadic system* that encompasses both caregivers and the infant may be more suitable for optimizing his development than a dyadic exchange between only one caregiver and the infant. As a consequence, the earliest model for learning about the interpersonal implications of development should occur within the family and should include both caregivers. Although the infant can experience reciprocity within a dyad, the enhancement of available organization and richness in a well-balanced triad allows for a readjustment by any two members when there is a violation or disruption within the relationship. Each member becomes sensitive to necessary readjustments and is able to achieve the homeostasis essential for maintaining communication within a regulatory feedback system.

Parenthood itself should be viewed as a distinct developmental phase for both mother and father. The frequent alterations of parental attitudes that occur contemporaneously with the child's rapid development suggest that it is not merely the child who undergoes maturational change during the family life cycle. Schecter and Corman (1979) have noted that the specific parental task at a given stage of the child's development is shaped to a degree by the parents' unique social and family group as well as by the individual personality of each parent—including expectations and idealizations.

THERAPIST: How does the infant's development affect you on an individual level?

CAREGIVER: Now he can climb on chairs by himself. But I don't want him to learn to stand up on them. He goes from the chair to the table, and sometimes I'm afraid he will fall and hurt himself.

THERAPIST: So it goes both ways now: He's more independent, but he also has more dangers to confront.

CAREGIVER: Yes. I'm happy that he's starting to explore more, but he's learning how to do more things every day. Sometimes I am afraid for him and wish he would slow down a little—not be so curious.

In addition, the actual developmental experiences of the child directly affect parental and familial attitudes. Parenthood is a developmental phase that transforms the parents and involves marked shifts in the family's equilibrium. Parental expectations—often idealized—of the parent–child relationship play a potent role in shaping developmental processes. For example, as determined by Brackbill, White, Wilson, and Kitch (1990), the family's basic dynamic for establishing relationships can be used as a predictor of the infant's temperament at 8 months. These researchers relied on dimensions of healthy family functioning (Barnhill, 1979) and grouped these dimensions into four themes: identity processes, adaptability to change, information processing, and role structuring. Parents who received high scores during the prenatal interview in areas such as individuation, cogent communication, flexibility, and role reciprocity tended to have infants with "easy" temperaments at 8 months of age. In contrast, parents who manifested enmeshment, disorganization, and rigidity tended to have infants with "difficult" temperaments. In addition, the infant's behavior and development may modify parental attitudes and behaviors significantly. If the marital relationship is harmonious, the differences in the parents' styles of behavior will tend to complement one another, so that the infant is exposed to two varied, but adaptive, kinds of supportive relationships. If emotional conflict troubles or strains the marital relationship, however, the parents' diverse styles of interaction may lead to noncontingency and distress. In effect, the parents will be asking the infant to "choose sides" between them and express a preference for one parent over the other.

These findings intensify the significance of early intervention in families with new infants to prevent the entrenchment of maladaptive behavior patterns. In particular, therapists working with new families must examine and analyze the representational skills of both parents, their ability to preview adaptive patterns of behavior, their conceptions of the infant's development, their ability to share intimacy between themselves and to convey this intimacy to the infant, the degree of dyadic and triadic rapport, and finally the capacity of the family to withstand the effects of triangulation. According to Kerr and Bowen (1988a, 1988b, 1988c), triangulation may be defined as a dynamic equilibrium established by a three-person relationship that constitutes one of the basic emotional components of the family system. Triangulation is "emotional" because these interactional configurations exist largely as a result of the anxiety that fuels them. When the level of anxiety is low, the relationship between two individuals remains comfortable. Because emotional and environmental forces can easily disturb relationships, however, they usually do not remain in a state of complete equilibrium for long periods. Inevitably, when anxiety levels rise, a third person becomes involved to defuse the anxiety between the twosome and dissipate it into a three-person relationship. The capacity of a triangle to disperse anxiety and contain it at reasonable levels makes it a particularly flexible relationship. Triadic rapport may be examined by observing all three family members simultaneously; when this is not possible, the therapist may gain valuable insights by listening to the comments of one caregiver about the other caregiver or by posing inquiries that explore how the marital relationship has changed since the birth and the arrival of the infant in the household.

The importance of understanding the role played by the infant from the perspective of the family is significant for a variety of other reasons as well. For example, if the family is functioning as an adaptive and integrated unit, the infant will most likely have the opportunity to observe interaction between the mother and father that will serve as a model for deriving further predictions about the nature and scope of adaptive interaction. In essence, then, parents who expose the infant to such interaction are engaging in a kind of previewing, whereby they portray the nature of meaningful exchange between two individuals. As a result, the infant does not become locked into or fixated on a single style of interaction. By observing both mother and father, the infant will also formulate a perception of how the mother relates to the father and how the father reciprocates phenomena to the mother in a supportive fashion. This exposure further expands the infant's universe of perception and stimulates him to engage in predictions about what will occur during development. In other words, if the relationship between the caregivers is adaptive, the infant will be motivated to participate in a similar form of interactional rapport. As such, the infant will come to rely on these perceptions of mother–father interaction to validate his own perceptions.

Obviously, the preceding scenario most likely occurs when interaction between the mother and father is adaptive. In certain instances, however, interaction between the parents will be maladaptive and the conflict embedded in the marital relationship will emerge during interaction between the parents. The infant exposed to this form of conflict repeatedly will become sensitive to it and will begin to predict that virtually all interaction occurs in this fashion. As a result, he may come to generalize the notion that interactions are situations of conflict and turmoil. Because this conflict cannot be resolved, it will generate negative emotion. In turn, negative emotion causes feelings of helplessness that can become magnified into feelings of depression and hopelessness. This cycle of debilitating emotions would most likely prevent the infant from developing self-regulatory capacities and would undermine his motivation to interact with the caregivers.

If the infant perceives a conflicted relationship between the caregivers, two outcomes are likely to ensue. First, he may withdraw from interaction to shield himself from the debilitating affect that accompanies negative or conflicted exchange. One detrimental effect of withdrawing from the caregiver is that the infant will begin to deprive himself of the stimulation and exposure to interpersonal situations that are essential for formulating predictions about imminent developmental change. Lacking the ability to predict, the infant becomes further mired in the overwhelming effects of development that he experiences as being uncontrollable and may come to experience the emotions of hopelessness associated with depression. Alternatively, the infant may have precisely the opposite response to parental conflict. Rather than withdrawing, he may instead seek to escape from the conflicted ambience through precocious development. In such cases, the infant's predictive abilities will also become impaired, because he will strive to practice skills prior to the advent of full maturational potential and as a result of the absence of a supportive caregiver.

To avoid either infant withdrawal or precocious development, the therapist's first task is to explore the conflicted relationship between the parents and to enlighten them regarding the effect such conflict has on the infant's development. Once this has been accomplished, the therapist should encourage both parents to focus on representational exercises that enable them to understand the nature and scope of infant development in a more neutral fashion.

Optimal caregiving, to a substantial extent, depends on the parent's ability to interpret the infant's behavior accurately so that parental manifestations can meld with those of the infant (Parke & Tinsley, 1987). One method of measuring competence is to assess the degree to which caregivers adjust their behavior in response to infant cues. Concentrating on this criterion, Parke and Sawin (1975) found that paternal sensitivity to an auditory distress signal in the feeding context—such as sneezing or coughing—was just as pronounced as the maternal reaction to a similar cue and that fathers responded to infants in a highly adaptive manner that was comparable to a maternal response. Moreover, infants being fed by mothers and fathers consumed the same amount of milk.

Nevertheless, researchers have documented some differences in father-versus-mother responsivity to the infant. For example, Yogman et al. (1977) determined that mothers and fathers engage the infant in different types of play behavior. Mothers, for instance, were more prone to visual games, in which a motor movement is shown to the infant and the infant's eye movements display heightened attention and gazing behavior. In contrast, fathers rely more on tactile and movement games involving motor skills. Studies have also shown that the infant receives the most enriching stimulation when play occurs in the presence of both caregivers. For example, Parke, Grossman, and Tinsley (1981) found that parents conveyed more positive affect in the form of smiling toward the infant and demonstrated a higher level of exploratory behavior while in the presence of the other spouse. Parke and Tinsley suggest that this phenomenon may be because parents who interact together verbally stimulate one another by focusing the partner's attention on aspects of the infant's behavior. This behavior, in turn, evokes affectionate or exploratory behavior in the parent, which is exhibited to the infant. This enhanced form of stimulation may also be attributed to an optimal marital relationship and to the tendency of such episodes to strengthen the nuclear family's sense of security as an integrated unit. Pedersen (1975), for example, commented that a "good baby" and a "good marriage" go together, and Belsky (1984) found that the father's general level of involvement with the infant was reliably and positively related to the overall level of marital adaptability.

Feldman, Nash, and Aschenbrenner (1983) have investigated the effect of the marital relationship on the infant's developmental status by studying mothers in the third trimester of pregnancy and repeating the assessment again 6 months postpartum. These researchers found substantial support for the influence of the marital relationship on understanding the dyadic relationship between mother and child; the overall quality of the marital relationship also predicted the father's involvement in caregiving, playfulness with the infant, and overall satisfaction with fatherhood.

EXCLUSION OF THE FATHER

Discussions of caregivers and infants often assume that the primary caregiver is the mother, rather than the father. This is not so unusual because the mother not only carries the baby within her body and nurtures it from her own milk, but also traditionally has been relegated to the role of primary caregiver. With the advent of the neonate, the couple is suddenly transformed into a threesome, creating, for the first time, a permanent system of interaction called a "family." The transition to parenthood generates a general decrease in marital satisfaction, a reversion to more traditional sexual roles—even in those families with dual-career couples—and an overall diminishment of self-esteem for the wife and mother (Cowan & Cowan, 1984). The woman may feel this particularly because of discrepancies between social expectations and the reality of motherhood. The change to parenthood also tends to provoke most couples in the direction of more traditional gender roles. Indeed, relatively few couples share household and child-care responsibility equally after the birth of the child. These phenomena occur although most modern couples have a more equitable distribution of responsibilities in the early phases of their relationship and marriage. Furthermore, modern couples confront a variety of challenges not faced by older generations (Bradt, 1988). For example, the egalitarian marriage and dual-career families have come to predominate during the past few decades notions of gender equality, according to this researcher. Nevertheless, reality has a habit of clashing with innovative cultural mores, and despite modern ideas, many new parents find that after the child is born, the mother is expected to serve as the primary nurturer. If this occurs in a family seeking treatment, the therapist may wish to explore whether the return to more traditional nurturing patterns has aroused feelings of resentment in either parent.

THERAPIST: In what ways does your baby remind you of traditional parental roles?

CAREGIVER: I have the baby all day. I give him to my husband when he comes home from work, and all of a sudden the baby goes to sleep in my husband's arms. Sometimes it feels as though the baby knows how to do different things with each of us. But sometimes I resent this because I have the burden of taking care of the baby all day.

One way of eliminating disparities between parental roles may be to have husbands attend childbirth classes with their wives and participate in the delivery. In addition, fathers should be encouraged to demonstrate skills of intimacy with their young children. These skills are often ignored, making the father feel even more isolated from the attachment bond forged between infant and mother. Therapists involved in dyadic treatment should, therefore, be sensitive to the father's role in the household and should strive to include him in either regular or intermittent therapy sessions.

Gurwitt (1976) has recommended strategies for helping fathers acknowledge their feelings of insecurity or resentment at being excluded from the mother–infant rapport. These strategies to deal with uncertainty stemming from the infant's birth encourage fathers to voice feelings of rejection and envy at their wives for giving birth to and breastfeeding the infant—two physiological functions from which fathers frequently feel emotionally excluded. To help fathers overcome envy and resentment, Gurwitt has suggested two basic strategies. First, fathers should be encouraged to voice fears and anxieties concerning the impending birth. Second, the father should become more involved with his wife, by participating in classes for prospective parents and by accompanying the expectant mother to the obstetrician on routine visits.

It is vital that therapists treating mother–infant dyads attempt to include the father so he can resolve these negative feelings and become fully integrated into the family unit. Unless the father feels that he is an integral figure in the infant's development whose influence is as significant as that of the mother, he may harbor resentment toward both his wife and infant. Such resentment may be directed toward the infant, or if directed toward the mother, she in turn may transfer the resentment to the infant (Abelin, 1975). Equally as damaging, the mother may become enmeshed with the infant in a suffocating relationship that excludes the father and hinders normal development. If this occurs, the infant will be deprived of previewing experiences with the father. The birth must therefore be treated as a developmental transition that requires realignment of the original alliances between husband and wife.

A study conducted by Belsky (1985) suggested one way of reinforcing adaptive interaction that includes mothers and fathers. Families were randomly assigned to one of four treatment groups, and infants in all groups were compared at 1, 3, and 9 months to examine the effects of a basic neonatal intervention. In half the families, both caregivers were the target of the intervention, whereas in the remaining families, the mother was the sole target. The intervention itself consisted of passive or active exposure to the Brazelton Neonatal Behavioral Assessment. This assessment exposes the parent to a variety of neuromuscular and other skills that the infant manifests even from birth. An advantage of this assessment is that parents see the magnitude of the infant's constitutional endowment and developmental potential. During the Assessment, the caregivers were informed about the developmental capacities manifested in the evaluation. Half the parents in each group then actively elicited responses from their newborns under a therapist's direction, and the remaining parents listened to a detailed description of the infant's performance. Following this exposure, the researcher observed that the caregivers who had been engaged in more active participation with their infants subsequently displayed an increased number of episodes of adaptive interaction, suggesting that early intervention enhances interaction between the caregiver and infant.

SIBLING RIVALRY

When there is already one child in the household, the advent of a new infant can arouse feelings of insecurity and inadequacy in the older child. In effect, the older child may feel left out and excluded. Although it may sound like a cliché, it is especially important that the parents do not ignore or alienate the older child during this period immediately after the birth of the second child. In particular, children should be reassured that the new infant will not usurp their position in the household. Siblings who feel isolated may turn to their fathers—who may also feel alienated because of the intimacy between the mother and newborn. Such alliances, which can breed resentment and erupt in dysfunctional behavior at a subsequent date, should be avoided. In addition, the arrival of a new baby creates a form of stress that may lead the family to form certain triangular relationships. The therapist's task is to detect and neutralize these triangles before they threaten the infant's development. To deter these maladaptive patterns, the therapist should explore how each family member feels about the newborn and resolve any negative feelings in an adaptive fashion.

THE INFANT AS SCAPEGOAT

Parental stress can affect the infant and toddler in insidious ways by causing him to become a *scapegoat* for the parents' own conflicts. If the parents are in conflict, they will be in conflict with the infant as well and will seek to entangle the infant in their dysfunctional relationship (Bell & Vogel, 1968; Lask, 1982). Whitaker (1976) has described a phenomenon of simultaneous *alliance* and *distance*, whereby the union of two family members functions to exclude and ostracize a third family member. Conflict that cannot be expressed overtly is in effect foisted on this family member. While estranged from one another, both parents may feel a unique and special closeness with the infant, who will receive contradictory messages as to how he should feel and/or act with each parent and will implicitly be coerced into taking sides in the parents' battle. During this process, the infant is alternately disparaged by one parent while being validated by the other. As a consequence, the parents inculcate a series of discrepant responses that gradually erode the child's capacity to develop an autonomous and coherent sense of self.

Using the infant as a scapegoat is common in maladaptive families because the infant's developmental immaturity makes him susceptible to parental attributions of blame and dysfunction. That is, it becomes easier to blame the infant than to confront the problem. The child performs an indispensable function by becoming the focus of the parents' submerged conflict (Bell & Vogel, 1968), thereby diverting attention from the real conflict, which remains in eclipse. Once the conflict is displaced onto the infant, the family can maintain a precarious sense of unity. In this fashion, the infant's function comes to resemble the function of a neurotic symptom, representing a compromise mechanism that allows the individual to deal with the underlying conflict. In this sense, the symptom must perpetually recur whenever the underlying conflict threatens to erupt. Repetition of the symptom achieves two goals: First, the seemingly unresolvable conflict is staved off along with its attending anxiety; second, because the symptom contains residues of the core conflict, a feeling of gratification emerges with each repetition. Foisting conflict on the scapegoated infant accomplishes similar dysfunctional goals: It enables the caregivers to avoid dealing with their real conflict, and by displacing it onto the infant, the caregivers avoid the possibility of severing their own relationship, which would likely trigger even greater anxiety. Moreover, the caregivers derive a distorted form of gratification from channeling the conflict onto the infant. Where one infant in the family has become the subject of such hostile emotions, it is often best to begin treating this infant within the context of the family. The primary therapeutic goal in such a situation is to create a *transition* or moderate alteration in the distorted patterns of alignment, so that the focus is diverted from the infant, who has served as the repository of unresolved conflict, and in the direction of the suppressed problem. Beginning treatment in this fashion liberates the infant from the scapegoating processes and allows him to explore his own sense of identity, which has previously been obliterated by dysfunctional family patterns. Nevertheless, no matter how ameliorative this treatment is for the scapegoated infant, the therapy will be palliative only if the entire family eventually receives counseling to determine the dynamics of a particular infant's selection as the repository of the family's negative emotions as well as to determine the nature of the conflict the family has displaced onto the infant. In addition, if the therapist detects that the infant is a potential scapegoating target, it is imperative to evaluate the psychopathology that has insinuated itself within the family's dynamics.

Precisely how does one infant become the family's scapegoat? At some point during the marital union the parents recognize that they require a channel for dissipating their tensions (Bell & Vogel, 1968). The latent hostilities between them prevent the direct expression of their problems, however, because there is always the danger that one partner may become too angry, leading to a permanent severing of the relationship. A number of variables make an infant the most vulnerable target for scapegoating and a vehicle whereby the family can concentrate and discharge tensions. First, infants and young children are relatively powerless to challenge their parents. Moreover, infants and young children are ill-equipped to counter their parents' more developed adaptational skills. Although the parental defenses may be relatively maladaptive compared with those of adaptive parents, such defenses are still far more sophisticated than those of their infant children.

The infant is also an especially susceptible focus for the parents' unresolved conflicts because an infant's identity is as yet unformed. According to Bell and Vogel, infants and young children can be readily molded to adopt the particular role that the family assigns to them. When the infant assumes many of the characteristics the parents dislike in themselves, he becomes an especially fitting object upon which to focus parental anxieties and frustrations. Furthermore, the "cost" of a dysfunctional infant in the family is relatively low in comparison with the parents' "gains" from creating an object for displacement of their own conflicts. Nevertheless, the therapist cannot ignore the insidious implications of scapegoating on the infant's development. Just as the infant is likely to become a scapegoat because of his psychological vulnerability, so too scapegoating can result in permanent damage because the infant internalizes distorting perceptions into his working model of interaction.

Because scapegoating is so common and yet so often ignored, it is important to emphasize that therapists working with infants and young children should examine the precise role and effect the infant has on the overall dynamics of the family. Has a particular infant been chosen as a scapegoat because of his or her sex or because of birth order within the family? What does the family gain through scapegoating? The answer to this question often lies in the psychiatric history of the parents during their infancy relationships with their own parents. A mother who is experiencing problems with a son or a father who distances himself from his daughter may be reenacting the scenario of his or her own childhood and inadvertently forcing the infant to participate in a drama beyond the child's adaptational skills. Overall, the therapist should always evaluate the family as a cross-generational unit to discern how deviant nurturing patterns replicate themselves across generations and are unwittingly thrust on a newborn infant.

Psychotherapy basically promotes individuation from the parental model and encourages the concomitant assertion of autonomy. When a dyad is referred for treatment, the therapist should evaluate and engage every family member to assess whether the process of individuation is being thwarted (Whitaker, 1976). This intervention prevents feelings of disloyalty from emerging among family members in treatment. When parents are actively engaged in the therapeutic process, it helps family members to feel less disloyal about moving in a direction that may be antagonistic to the parental model and that may challenge parental authority. A vignette from a case history follows:

(During this session, parents are arguing about money. Husband ignores wife's interpretation of her argument by playing with infant. Finally, husband states that he is angry at his wife for wanting to buy a coat for $3000. Wife tries to explain.)

MOTHER: I want a coat for Christmas so I've kind of been looking around. I know we're not going to buy an expensive coat because it is way out of line with our budget. So I said to Martin (father), I just want to look at the coats for 10 minutes . . . (Infant plays by herself on the floor.)

FATHER: (Interrupts) You're really not telling the whole story. You have no qualms about me getting you a coat. An expensive coat! You buy very expensive things all the time . . .

MOTHER: I would never buy a coat that costs $3000. (Begins to explain how saleswoman asked her to try it on) First I said, "No, why bother to try it on." Then I said, "Well, since my husband's around, maybe I'll try it on." (Husband goes to interact with infant who has been playing by herself across the room.) I tried it on, and it really looked gorgeous. It also felt good. I haven't felt good in a long time. I've been working very hard with the baby. I'm really angry about all of this. I felt good. I asked him to please look at me, and he would barely look at it on me. (Imitates husband's voice) "I've got to watch the baby, I've got to watch the baby." I said, "I'll watch the baby. Would you just look at this? Doesn't it look nice?" He gave me one criticism after another about it.

FATHER: We can't afford an expensive coat right now . . . (Infant goes to mother.)

MOTHER: He's been yelling at me because I said I'd do the books. I said, "How can I do the books if I have no access to your account?" (Infant tries to interact with mother, who holds her hand.) I'm very upset about the way we fight in front of Natalie. In fact, people at the store said, "That poor child."

(The husband explains his solution to the problem: using cash instead of writing checks so account won't be overdrawn.)

MOTHER: I don't think that's the answer. When I ask him how he feels about babies, he says he can get along with zero children. Give me a break! (To husband) Natalie gives you a lot. Natalie really gives you a lot. (To therapist) She's very attached to him, and I don't want her to keep giving to him because he's such a schmuck.

THERAPIST: (To father) What do you think about your wife's observation? (The infant isn't responding to father's attempts to play with her.)

FATHER: It's just my wife holding my daughter hostage against me . . . what's new? She always does it!

MOTHER: I had a dream last night that Natalie was drowning and I couldn't save her. I'm very frustrated. I'm really . . . really frustrated. That's probably why I'm exploding. It seems like he doesn't want to be in this relationship. He has this "special" relationship with Natalie. But . . . (Husband is ignoring her, trying to play with infant. Infant is not responding to him.) What about me? Where do I fit in?

PARENTAL DIVORCE AND REMARRIAGE

Two potent events may evolve from stress in the family: divorce and remarriage. These pivotal events result in a realignment of the family structure. A longitudinal study by Hetherington (1989) analyzed the effects of divorce and remarriage on children's adjustment. The study found that individual characteristics—the child's temperamental disposition; a supportive family milieu; and extrafamilial factors such as social support systems, their availability, and how children made use of them—played important roles in either exacerbating or shielding the children from the negative consequences associated with their parent's marital disturbances.

The original sample included 144 well-educated, middle-class white parents and their children (Hetherington, Cox, & Cox, 1982). Half the children were from divorced families in which the mother had been granted custody, the other half were from nondivorced families. Within each group, half the children were boys and the other half were girls. At the time of the 6-year follow-up, the sample included 124 subjects of the original 144 families who were available for study. A new group of demographically matched families was added at this time to include 30 sons and 30 daughters in each of three groups: a remarried mother–stepfather family configuration, a nonremarried mother-custody family configuration, and a nondivorced family configuration.

The researchers reported that the first 2 years following the divorce were relatively troublesome for the families in the sense that conflict tended to disrupt the relationship between the child and the parent with whom the child was living. During this interval, most of the children and many of the parents underwent emotional distress, accompanied by somatic and behavior problems, disruptions in normal family functioning, and significantly, difficulties in adjusting to new roles and relationships associated with the family's altered status. This finding suggests that the realignment of family relationships precipitated by divorce exerts a traumatic effect on virtually all adults and children who undergo the experience. Nevertheless, in keeping with the findings of other studies of divorced children, the researchers also found that after the 2-year crisis period, the majority of parents and children appeared to be coping in a reasonably adaptive manner and displayed improvement in psychological profile. Superficial conflict had at least diminished. Beyond this superficial improvement, however, the investigator found that a trio of factors—the individual child's temperament, familial influence of the parent, and social support outside of the family—helped to determine the success of the child's adjustment.

Hetherington focused on temperament because this factor has been found to affect the child's capacity to adapt to change, as well as the child's vulnerability to adversity (Garmezy, 1983; Rutter, 1983). For example, temperamentally "difficult" children have been found to be less resilient to change than temperamentally "easy" children. The caregiver's capacity to adapt to the infant's temperament so that a "good fit" is created also assuages the effects of a difficult temperament. Although individual differences in temperament may be biologically based, Rutter (1987) has commented that the heightened risk of the temperamentally difficult child is, at least in part, due to interactional patterns initiated by the parent. In this regard, Rutter has suggested that the difficult child is more likely to be both the elicitor and the target of the parent's aversive responses. In contrast, during stressful events the temperamentally easy child is less apt to receive criticism and displaced anger, which provides him with better developmental skills for coping with stress and adversity. In addition, Hetherington found that temperamentally difficult children were less adept than temperamentally easy children in coping with abusive and other maladaptive behavior from parents. In fact, increased stress was correlated with diminished capacity for adaptability in these children. With temperamentally easy children under supportive conditions, however, stress at low or moderate levels actually enhanced levels of adaptation. Regarding the familial aspects of these findings, Hetherington noted that high levels of stress and personality problems on the part of the mother increased the probability that she would engage in negative or punitive behavior toward the child. This synergistic effect occurred most often with temperamentally difficult children.

The second factor, intrafamily relationships, also affected the children's capacity to adapt to the divorce. Divorced mothers differed from their nondivorced counterparts in the degree of punishment and control they exerted over their children, as well as in the degree of discipline they imposed. For example, divorced mothers tended to be ineffectual in their control efforts and gave numerous instructions with minimal follow-through behaviors. These mothers complained more often and were frequently involved in disputes with their children, particularly their sons. Moreover, once these negative exchanges between divorced mother and son had occurred, they were likely to persist, perpetuating a pattern of dysfunctional behavior. Parental supervision was also diminished in the divorced families, as contrasted with the nondivorced families.

The third factor isolated in the Hetherington et al. study was the child's social support network. Even during the preschool years, the social and cognitive development of young children from divorced homes was heightened if they attended nursery schools with explicitly defined schedules and rules consistent with discipline and the expectation of mature behavior. This study indicates that the repercussions of divorce may be long-lasting. Therapists who treat children from divorced homes need to examine all of Hetherington's factors in diagnosing such children and in developing treatment strategies that enhance adaptive functioning in the family unit.

CONCLUSION

This chapter has sought to place the infant within the context of the family unit. In doing so, the family has been portrayed as a total system within which the infant develops. As a consequence, the reception the infant receives on joining the family has been evaluated from the point of view of the parents, as well as other family members. In particular, this chapter has examined such phenomena as the arrival of the infant in the family from the perspective of the parents; the feelings of exclusion the father may experience both during the pregnancy and after the birth; the feelings of sibling rivalry that the infant may engender among other family members; the tendency of parents to submerge their own emotional conflict by foisting it on the infant who, in turn, becomes a scapegoat for the marital conflict; and the effect of divorce and remarriage on the family unit and particularly on the infants and young children in the family.

One reason it is necessary to devote a chapter to the infant's position within the family is that the infant—among all family members—remains in a developmentally fragile and vulnerable position. Although adults will suffer emotional consequences if they experience conflict, their identities are in large part intact, and as a consequence, they are better equipped with a psychological mechanism to overcome or at least manage developmental crises. In contrast, the infant, although possessing a relatively sophisticated constitutional endowment, lacks a fully formed internal representation of working models of the external world, of significant others in his environment, and of himself. Because of this psychological inchoateness, the infant may attract—much like a lightning rod—the emotional conflict around him. This outcome may be especially insidious because representations of such emotional turmoil may become entrenched in the infant's internal subjective perceptions of self and other.

As this chapter has emphasized, the therapist must therefore seek to adopt the perspective of the infant as a member of the particular family into which he has been born. Only in this way can the therapist fully appreciate how the infant is perceiving reality, formulating internal working models, and gaining a sense of what future developmental events will bring for his own autonomy and rapport within the family unit.

Chapter 7

Assessing Parallel Processes

The Caregiver–Therapist Relationship as a Reflection of the Caregiver–Infant Relationship

INTRODUCTION

The unique qualities associated with dyadic treatment involving a caregiver and infant have been discussed in earlier chapters. However, an additional feature of dyadic treatment distinguishes it from other forms of intervention. This feature has been referred to as *parallel process*. The phrase parallel process was originally coined to describe a fascinating phenomenon that occurs when therapists in training receive supervision from senior practitioners. As will be seen, the parallel process can be applied as a model for discerning common or duplicative patterns between the caregiver–infant and caregiver–therapist relationships.

During the supervisory experience that most therapists undergo as part of their training, the demeanor, manifestations, and, most significantly, the affective tone of the therapist under supervision frequently replicates the mental state of the patient being treated by the therapist. After reviewing numerous cases, researchers recognized that this process of psychological *replication* was not coincidental; rather, the theorists who initially described the phenomenon were persuaded that the interactional patterns of the patient are somehow absorbed or incorporated by the therapist. During treatment the patient acts as an *evoker* of these manifestations while the therapist assumes the posture of the *recipient*. When the therapist undergoes supervision, however, these roles are reversed: Now the therapist becomes the evoker and the senior supervisor adopts the recipient role. As a result, the therapist in training manifests a process of interaction that parallels the interactional atmosphere with the patient that predominates during treatment. One of the advantages of assessing parallel process phenomena is that the therapist gradually gains insight into the subjective perceptions of the patient. When these subjective perceptions are contrasted with the therapist's objective assessment of the case, a more profound understanding of the patient's conflict becomes evident. Parallel process phenomena also offers guidance for devising effective treatment techniques when assisting the patient in overcoming conflict.

Interestingly enough, dyadic therapy incorporates many features of the parallel process encountered among the therapists undergoing supervision. The parallel process occurs during dyadic therapy because the caregiver and infant represent an interactional unit with the potential for or actual enactment of conflict. In this interactional unit, one member (the infant) functions as the evoker and the other member (the caregiver) acts as the recipient. These interactional patterns are then paralleled during the therapeutic relationship between caregiver and therapist, in which the caregiver evokes a particular emotional tone in the therapist, who serves as the recipient. As a result, the therapist attains insight into the subjective perceptions exchanged between caregiver and infant, as well as the affective tone that infuses this relationship. This chapter addresses the full implications of the parallel process as it emerges during dyadic therapy. The premise is that the transference bond between caregiver and therapist will disclose the nature of the conflict between caregiver and infant because the caregiver usually replicates key aspects of her or his general style of interaction when forging a transference relationship with the therapist. From the contours of this relationship, then, the therapist will be able to discern behaviors that are or will be enacted with the infant.

DEFINING THE PARALLEL PROCESS IN DYADIC INTERVENTION

The techniques for training a therapist have long involved a system within which the therapist meets with the patient on a regular basis and subsequently meets with a supervisor to review the content of these sessions. These supervisory meetings not only monitor the course of the treatment and the techniques used by the therapist, but also act as an arena for exploring the therapist's subjective experiences. That is, the therapist establishes a relationship with the supervisor that facilitates *reenacting* unresolved conflict in a manner similar to the one used by the patient during sessions. This duplication is highly advantageous because it provides the therapist and supervisor with insights for resolving the patient's conflict and for instituting techniques that promote adaptive behavior.

Researchers have referred to this phenomenon, whereby the therapeutic relationship that characterizes a particular case is replicated when the therapist himself or herself subjects the case to scrutiny or supervision, as the parallel process (Arlow, 1963; Caligor, 1981; Gross-Doehrman, 1976; Langs, 1989).

Significantly, the parallel process is also evident when therapists engage in dyadic therapy. In dyadic treatment, however, the parallel process has a further dimension that offers more profound insight into the conflict disturbing the dyad. Specifically, the subjective perceptions and emotional tone experienced by the therapist can be used for further exploration of the caregiver's psychological status and behavior patterns. The parallel process allows the therapist to experience what both the caregiver and infant are experiencing during their interaction. This is an especially valuable bonus in dyadic treatment, because the infant's inability to speak and express his own views can be a potential barrier to understanding his perspective. The parallel process, however, overcomes this barrier, and the therapist is able to obtain insight into the infant's subjective perceptions.

Researchers such as Searles (1955) have described this mirror-imaging of the initial therapeutic relationship that is reenacted during supervision. Searles observes that the emotions experienced by supervisors, including even their subjective perceptions about the therapist, often lead to valuable clarifications of processes that characterize the ongoing relationship between the therapist and patient. Applying this model to dyadic treatment, the processes at work in the relationship between caregiver and therapist are often reflected in the relationship between caregiver and the infant, because the therapist assumes the role of the infant during these sessions. In other words, during dyadic therapy the caregiver oscillates between experiencing and reporting, whereas the therapist oscillates between identifying with the caregiver and/or infant and observing the caregiver and/or infant (Arlow, 1963). In the context of dyadic therapy, the therapist has an opportunity to share with the caregiver transient identification with various aspects of the infant's mental functioning. This occurs because the caregiver begins to reveal how she borrows defenses from the infant to fend off her own anxiety associated with the material which the patient presents.

Theorists such as Meerloo (1952), Blitzsten and Fleming (1953), and Ackerman (1953) have described the supervisor as having a considerable degree of emotional involvement in the therapeutic situation. The supervisor often finds that the arousal of emotions within himself signifies a reflection of the relationship between therapist and patient. Adapting this model to the dyadic framework between caregiver and infant, when therapists find themselves experiencing potent emotions during the session, they should be alert to two possibilities. The first is that the source of this emotion may lie chiefly in the therapist's own repressed past. This would cause the therapist to perceive the caregiver and infant as being strikingly similar in their mode of operation. The second possibility is that the source of this emotion may lie in the caregiver–infant relationship, primarily with the infant. If this is the case, the therapist should reflect on the interpersonal phenomena that have been occurring in the caregiver–infant relationship and, ultimately, on the responses of the infant.

Searles (1955) has noted that both negative elements, such as anxiety-laden processes, and positive elements, such as pleasure derived from a collaborative effort, are carried over from the patient–therapist relationship to the therapist–supervisor relationship. For example, in dyadic therapy, if a therapist experiences a special fondness for the caregiver during a particular phase of the treatment, this may be in part because the caregiver and infant are very fond of one another.

During dyadic therapy, the caregiver projects replicative emotions to both therapist and infant. This will cause the caregiver to behave in a similar fashion toward both therapist and infant, allowing the therapist to perceive similarities between the caregiver's mode of functioning in the therapeutic relationship and the caregiver's mode of functioning in the dyadic relationship with the infant. The caregiver may also demonstrate negative attitudes toward both the infant and the therapist. Another possibility that therapists should be alert to is that the caregiver may utilize the infant's conflicts as defenses in the therapeutic relationship to prevent further exploration. Such behavior also leads the therapist to perceive major parallels when comparing the therapeutic relationship with the mother–infant relationship.

One reason the parallel process is such a compelling phenomenon in dyadic treatment is that the therapist can enter into both the caregiver and the infant's subjective interpersonal experience, just as the caregiver is able to experience the infant's subjective interpersonal experience, as well as the more neutral attitude of the therapist. As the caregiver becomes more attuned to participating in the dyadic process, she begins to experience emotional learning and communication evoked by the infant, a parallel process contoured by the infant's interpersonal integration needs. This process is initiated by, evoked by, and centered in the infant's self. The caregiver, as an observer, experiences herself as engaging in cognitive and affective processes, responding with a delayed reaction, autonomous and centered in the infant's own need system. In effect, then, the parallel process becomes a kind of reciprocal process. Reciprocal process in this context refers to the interpersonal response evoked in the recipient during the parallel process. Thus, the parallel processes are in the realm of field theory. That is, all mothers, who are unique, are responding in a similar nonunique way to the conscious and preconscious cues of the infant or therapist as evoker.

The perspective on mother–infant treatment under discussion here views the parallel process experience as continually unfolding and evolving. As the effect of the parallel process becomes intensified, the therapist brings into the realm of conscious experience and knowledge unconscious meanings and functions of which the caregiver was previously unaware. In most instances, an adept therapist will be able to translate the infant's perceptions of the caregiver into direct language. This is particularly the case with sources of anxiety and depression, although positive aspects that contribute to the caregiver's growth will also become apparent. In this fashion, the therapist will be taking the infant's disguised and displaced images (constituted as unconscious perceptions and reactions to such perceptions) and reintroducing them into the therapeutic interaction, by revealing their direct meaning and significance. These perceptions are based on the real and actual implications of the caregiver's behaviors toward the infant, as selectively perceived by the infant in terms of his or her therapeutic needs. In essence then, the therapist is presenting the caregiver with objective perceptions of the caregiver's implied messages, many of which may indicate implicit or actual conflict in the relationship between caregiver and infant. Such material will often contain unconscious interpretations to the therapist and a derivative working through many of the ramifications and sources of the caregiver's subjective perceptions.

It is important to recognize, then, that much of the information processed during the parallel process originates outside of conscious awareness and only enters awareness as the process continues. Messages that can be tolerated in awareness are sent directly without modification to the conscious system where they are stored in the superficial unconscious subsystem. In contrast, incoming information that provokes anxiety or depression is transferred to a deep unconscious system for silent processing. This information is subjected to primitive processes, although it may subsequently be processed with considerable logic and wisdom. All such information, however, departs from the deep unconscious system in altered form; it is accessible to the conscious mind only through displacement and disguise. This realization suggests a powerful unconscious influence without availability to conscious adaptive resourcefulness. Thus, the therapist should be mindful that the parallel process phenomenon can awaken a good deal of material that had previously been processed unconsciously. As a result, the therapist should be cautious about interpreting this possibly potent information. Of help in this regard is that presumably the accumulation of knowledge combined with the caregiver's positive identification with the therapist may permit a new technique for managing the conflict of both caregiver and infant. The parallel process serves as a powerful therapeutic tool whereby the therapist can awaken the caregiver's perceptions to certain of her own behaviors, as well as certain of the infant's behaviors that she had previously misconstrued or ignored. In effect, the parallel process enables the caregiver to obtain new perspectives on the subjective perceptions of both herself and the infant in a supportive and nurturing atmosphere.

In dyadic therapy the therapeutic situation always involves a *triangular relationship* among therapist, caregiver, and infant. This triangular relationship may encourage the development of rivalries between the caregiver and infant with regard to gaining the therapist's attention or between caregiver and therapist with regard to gaining the infant's attention. Rivalry occurs because the conflicts in one relationship affect and are reflected in the other relationship so that a two-way process exists—a parallel process in which the caregiver's problems with the infant are related to the caregiver's relationship with the therapist, and vice versa.

As a result of the parallel process, when therapists reflect on the session, they should be alert to the possibility that the source of aroused emotions may lie in the caregiver–infant relationship, primarily in the caregiver herself. It may be said, therefore, that the therapist's experience reflects the dynamics between caregiver and infant. Exploring this reflection is a vital component of the therapeutic process because it offers insights into any conflict or potential conflict that may trouble the caregiver–infant relationship. The value of the parallel process as a therapeutic tool is reinforced in numerous circumstances. At a minimum, the therapist gains insight from parallel process into the *complexity, subtlety,* and *depth* of human relationships. After recognizing the nature of this complexity, the therapist becomes sensitive to the complexities that must infuse the caregiver's other relationships.

The following case illustrates how the parallel process works in dyadic therapy. The caregiver, who had entered treatment with her infant, appeared evasive with the therapist. She manifested this demeanor by distancing, avoiding contact, claiming not to hear the therapist; indeed, the caregiver foiled the therapist's every attempt to reach her. Subsequently, the therapist experienced a feeling of depletion during a session. Attempts to engage the caregiver in discussion met with evasive responses that generated further emotional depletion in the therapist. Significantly, the caregiver's relationship with the infant paralleled these behaviors and emotional manifestations. For example, the caregiver tended to distance herself physically and emotionally from the infant. Frequently, she avoided both physical and emotional contact, despite the infant's efforts to establish contact. When the caregiver described what was transpiring with the infant, her tone of voice sounded defeated, or she was often silent, appeared morose, and was not clearly focused. Thus, the emotional tone the caregiver manifested to the therapist mirrored the lethargy and stupor in the caregiver's descriptions of her infant.

There are two predominant trends in mother–infant therapy designed to identify and explore different levels of meaning. First, there is a filtering out of those unconscious caregiver perceptions of the infant that are most threatening. Second, acute disturbances in the mother–infant relationship tend to surface, at times jeopardizing the continuity of the treatment when the therapist interprets in areas intolerable to the caregiver's capacity to function effectively (e.g., you might hurt your baby). When this occurs, the caregiver no longer experiences the treatment as an arena for learning. In general, therapists should view caregiver–infant intervention as a process of ever-increasing insights in which the meanings and behaviors the caregiver was previously unaware of are brought by the therapist into the realm of conscious experience. Cognizance of the parallel process assists the therapist in achieving these goals.

PARALLEL EVOLUTION OF THE TWO RELATIONSHIPS

No event is as pivotal to progress in treatment as the development of a *therapeutic relationship* between the therapist and the patient. In the treatment of a caregiver–infant dyad, the forging of a therapeutic bond that can endure the rigors of intervention is often a complex matter because in most instances the caregiver has already established a relationship with the infant prior to entering therapy. One of the therapist's first tasks involves deciphering the nature of that relationship. In accomplishing this task, the therapist will become familiar with how this particular caregiver relates to significant others in her life, and in particular, how she communicates with the infant in a manner that either enhances or impairs developmental acquisition and adaptation. Moreover, the therapist will also be challenged to establish a therapeutic relationship with the caregiver. Above all, the therapist's relationship with the caregiver should not compete with or impede the caregiver's ongoing relationship with the infant—a relationship that must continue and endure well after therapy has ended.

The therapeutic relationship between the caregiver and therapist will, in some ways, resemble other therapeutic relationships. Such similarities emerge as a result of the caregiver's proclivity to project conflict or the potential for conflict onto the person of the therapist. At the same time, however, the caregiver–therapist alliance is distinctive in dyadic therapy because of the infant's presence. With individual treatment, the patient generally discloses information about interaction with significant others in his or her life. From this narrative, the therapist infers the subjective dimensions of these other relationships that occur beyond the therapeutic setting. But in dyadic therapy, the presence of the infant affects the significance of the caregiver's narrative. Not only does the therapist hear the caregiver describe events that have occurred outside the therapeutic milieu, but during sessions the therapist also is an eyewitness to the relationship between caregiver and infant. As a result, dyadic therapy involves the *parallel evolution* of two relationships. In addition, the therapist should establish a rapport with the infant through play and other modes of physical interaction that rely on gestures and behavioral cues. By establishing such a rapport, the therapist can begin to experience the infant's perceptions of the relationship with the caregiver, just as the rapport between caregiver and therapist provides the therapist with insight about the caregiver's perspective on the infant's interactions.

As noted earlier, the *parallel process* refers to those interpersonal patterns individuals manifest in one relationship (e.g., caregiver–infant) that are reenacted and reflected in a relationship with a different person (e.g., caregiver–therapist). The parallel process assumes a qualitatively unique dimension when both caregiver and infant are in treatment. While the caregiver is continually exploring her relationship with the infant during sessions, she must simultaneously negotiate strategies for traversing from the relationship with the infant to the relationship with the therapist. Thus, dyadic treatment allows the therapist to examine the caregiver–therapist relationship while directly exploring the vicissitudes of the caregiver's subjective perceptions of her relationship with the infant. Dyadic therapy therefore offers the therapist a unique opportunity for contrasting the dimensions of the caregiver–infant relationship with the parallel manifestations that emerge in the caregiver–therapist relationship.

An understanding of the dynamics of the parallel process is of overriding importance for the therapist conducting dyadic therapy because, unlike individual treatment, it allows the therapist to observe how the caregiver manages multiple relationships simultaneously. Dyadic therapy explores and contrasts three kinds of relationships within the treatment setting:

1. The effect of the caregiver's past relationships on the caregiver's relationships with the infant and the therapist.
2. The effect of the relationship of the caregiver–infant relationship on the caregiver–therapist relationship.
3. The effect of the caregiver–therapist relationship on the caregiver–infant relationship.

The multiplicity of relationships embodied in the structure of dyadic treatment yields benefits for therapists in terms of diagnosing conflicts that threaten to impede adaptive interaction and in terms of devising effective treatment strategies for resolving conflict. For example, dyadic therapy allows therapists to observe interpersonal patterns carefully and to explore caregiver comments in evaluating whether they represent the caregiver's genuine attitude toward the infant. When the caregiver then interacts with the infant overtly, therapists can focus on aspects of the caregiver's behavioral style and can verify whether initial impressions regarding the caregiver's interactional skills were accurate. Moreover, as therapists observe interaction between caregiver and infant, they can contrast these observations with the subjective impressions the caregiver has provided through narrative reports.

The parallel process also introduces flexibility into the therapeutic milieu. For example, if the caregiver is hesitant about interacting directly with the infant in the therapist's presence, the therapist can attempt to engage the infant. By doing this, the therapist will be able not only to experience the degree to which the infant effectively communicates through behavior cues, but also to use these interactions with the infant as a catalyst for motivating the caregiver to externalize and explore her subjective perceptions about the infant. During such exchanges with the infant, the therapist should be cognizant of the infant's developmental status. As an example, does the infant exhibit *stranger anxiety* —withdrawing in distress—when the therapist makes overtures of interaction? Such a reaction may be adaptive and indicate that the infant has, in fact, established an attachment to the caregiver. Adaptability may also be inferred from the way in which infant and caregiver refer to each other during interaction. *Social referencing* —turning to the mother while observing her emotional reactions—helps the infant resolve uncertainties or dangers posed by the environment while promoting exploration. If the therapist approaches the infant, and the caregiver encourages this interaction by reflecting positive affect back to the infant, then this response implies the caregiver's approval and should evoke minimal distress in the infant. The therapist should also be sensitive to an infant who relates too readily with a stranger figure while manifesting indifference to the caregiver's social referencing. Such infants may be displaying a developmental precocity that suggests a need to evade a nonresponsive or rejecting caregiver. Keeping these emblematic responses in mind, the therapist should make every effort to interact with the infant, because this form of therapist–infant interaction is vital for understanding the relationship between caregiver and infant. In addition, the caregiver may reveal how she transfers strategies from her interaction with the infant to stave off anxieties associated with the material she is exploring with the therapist.

Beyond its use as a diagnostic tool, the parallel process is also valuable for treating maladaptation within the dyad. After determining the particular aspects of the caregiver–infant interaction that are maladaptive, the therapist can begin interacting with either the caregiver or the infant in a manner that more effectively uses positive developmental skills. Thus, the therapist may model an appropriate style of interaction with the infant, the caregiver can observe the interactions, and the therapist can then encourage her to enact an appropriate interaction with the infant. As the treatment progresses, the caregiver will replicate the adaptive aspects of her relationship with the therapist during her interactions with the infant.

Finally, the therapist's emotional responses to both the dyad as an entity and the mother and infant individually are significant. These subjective impressions may further clarify the caregiver–infant relationship and isolate interactional failures. Just as in individual treatment, the therapist treating a mother and infant will experience some form of countertransference response. The presence of the infant and the caregiver's interaction with the infant, however, do enable the therapist to understand and work through this countertransference response because the ongoing relationship between caregiver and infant during the therapeutic sessions provide objective behaviors through which to analyze subjective impressions.

During the initial phases of dyadic treatment the most effective means of assessing the caregiver–infant relationship are *direct observation* and *inquiry*. In this regard, it is important to observe whether the caregiver appropriately diverts attention from the infant to interact with the therapist. In some instances the caregiver's perceptions may be so intermeshed with the manifestations of the infant that she is unable to interact with another individual. In other cases the caregiver may appear overly eager to interact with the therapist and may seem virtually oblivious to the infant's presence. This latter attitude is manifested by the caregiver's neglect of the infant and apparent urgency to establish an exclusive rapport with the therapist. Either tendency suggests that the caregiver may have difficulty in modulating and differentiating between relationships. These extreme responses suggest the presence of an underlying psychological conflict that impedes adaptive interaction.

From work with numerous caregivers in dyadic therapy, it appears that they adopt essentially three attitudes toward their newborn infants. The first attitude is conveyed by caregivers who manifest *adaptive maternal attitudes* concerning their roles and who have established a mutually fulfilling rapport with their infants. These caregivers possess coherent subjective representations of their relationship with their infants that emerge vividly when they describe the relationship. Such caregivers do not have to "see" the baby continuously to remain attuned to his needs. In these cases, caregivers appear to have developed a bond that connects them with the infant even when the child is absent. This bond enables the dyadic members to preview one another's responses. Evidence of this bond is displayed in such anecdotes as the familiar, "I know her cries . . . there is a cry when she wants to be put to sleep in her crib, there is another type of cry when she wants to have her diaper changed" or "I woke up because I knew she was feeling thirsty."

In contrast, therapists will also encounter caregivers who are at virtually the opposite end of the spectrum. Such caregivers appear to harbor ambivalent subjective representations of their relationship with their infants. This emotional ambivalence may cause them either to monitor the infant almost continuously to discern his needs or to relinquish unnecessary contact with the infant because of their own sense of failure. In effect, these caregivers cannot sustain their representations of the infant because these representations trigger a psychological conflict. When observing caregivers in this category, it becomes apparent that they have difficulty relating to others (e.g., the therapist) while simultaneously ministering to the infant's needs. Attending to one individual (e.g., the therapist) becomes an all-consuming affair, precluding meaningful interaction with others (e.g., the infant). This interactional style may be referred to as an *enmeshed maternal attitude*. In one such case I treated, the caregiver was unable to respond to my inquiries or even to relate a coherent history of her relationship with the infant. Each time I addressed the caregiver, the infant became noticeably irritable and fussy. What was so striking about these episodes was that the caregiver seemed to lack the fundamental interpersonal skills—such as appropriate eye contact, vocalization, holding behaviors, adaptive stimulation, and previewing—that normally guide the interaction of adaptive caregivers and their infants. In fact, despite this caregiver's ostensible zeal to comfort the infant, the more irritable the infant became, the more frenetic and disorganized was her response. As a consequence, whenever the infant cued or signaled the caregiver to initiate interaction, the caregiver devoted her energies to determining how to respond to the baby. Virtually all her efforts, however, stifled the baby's response. In these cases latent psychological conflict impedes the flow of intuitive skills that usually emerges spontaneously in adaptive caregivers, enabling them to minister to the infant in a nurturing fashion.

Another type of caregiver whose interpersonal skills seem deficient may appear oblivious to the infant's cues, ignoring even the most fundamental signals emitted by the baby. Such caregivers have an *avoidant maternal attitude*. This type of caregiver possesses impaired intuitive behaviors and appears incapable of establishing a stable relationship with the infant. In these instances the mother almost always ignores infant signals. It should be emphasized that not only are both of these latter types of caregivers responding inappropriately to the infant, but their interpersonal deficits also interfere with other relationships in their lives. In particular, such deficits may hinder the caregiver from establishing a therapeutic alliance with the therapist.

When caregivers become either overly enmeshed with the infant or avoid infant cues, a debilitating series of emotional responses interferes with the adaptive care of the infant. The caregiver's interactional deficits infiltrate and undermine the capacity to respond intuitively to the infant. As a result, the caregiver becomes overly preoccupied with the infant and fails to establish an appropriate rapport with the baby or, conversely, ignores the infant, thereby exposing him to emotional indifference and apathy. The caregiver's inability to relate to others reinforces her feelings of overpreoccupation or hopeless indifference, leaving the infant to experience further interpersonal stress while failing to establish a meaningful relationship with the caregiver. In either case the caregiver is also ill-equipped to establish a therapeutic alliance with the therapist. The following clinical vignette examines these issues:

THERAPIST: Can you share your thoughts about what it means to be a baby? What does it mean to have ongoing needs that require nurturance?

CAREGIVER: Um . . . (long silence).

THERAPIST: (Encouraging) What thoughts come to mind when you think of your baby?

CAREGIVER: (Glances repeatedly at baby) I . . . I don't know (laughs nervously while moving the baby away from her sight).

THERAPIST: (After a long silence) Could you share your feelings about raising your baby?

CAREGIVER: It's very difficult to take care of an infant.

THERAPIST: Could you describe some of the difficulty?

CAREGIVER: Well . . . she's so completely dependent on me. During the pregnancy—the fear that I was going to have a deformed baby—even though I had amniocentesis and they said everything would be all right—was overwhelming. Now, I have other fantasies . . . sometimes when I see her asleep and I don't hear her breathing. I'm terrified that she is . . . (looks away, embarrassed) . . . that she may have stopped breathing. With my older daughter I got scared so I put mirrors in front of her nose, to see if she could fog a mirror.

THERAPIST: Have you felt sometimes that Karen may stop breathing?

CAREGIVER: No, I haven't felt that (in an adamant, defensive tone) . . . I'm not scared that I could drop her either.

THERAPIST: Have you thought you could drop her?

CAREGIVER: Not drop her, but sometimes I accidentally brush her head against the wall or something . . . (smiles self-consciously). I'm used to where my body ends, but then sometimes I kind of forget how delicate and fragile the baby is.

THERAPIST: Are you suggesting that sometimes you are not aware of the boundaries of the baby's body?

CAREGIVER: Yeah, even when I was pregnant . . . I'd forget where my stomach ended and I would brush against people or into them . . . and sometimes I was reckless . . .

The therapist's initial efforts, then, should be devoted to establishing therapeutic relationships with both the caregiver and infant, and to observing the parallel relationship between the caregiver and infant. Where the caregiver is adaptive, establishing such a rapport becomes a relatively straightforward task and will likely evolve after the first few sessions. Where conflict precludes adaptive exchanges, however, forging this kind of relationship and creating an atmosphere to evaluate conflict candidly become more problematic. In such instances, the therapist should observe the caregiver's behaviors closely—especially with the infant—and gradually raise key issues empathically through inquiry. As an example of the emergence of the caregiver's interpersonal deficits while relating to the infant, in the preceding dialogue the caregiver referred to her "reckless" behavior during her pregnancy. This recklessness may indicate a latent motivation to hurt either the baby or herself. The therapist should be alert to such nuances and implications in the caregiver's remarks and should attempt to find evidence validating these comments while observing the parallel process of interaction.

THE EFFECT OF TRANSFERENCE PHENOMENA ON THE PARALLEL PROCESS

The concept of a unique relationship that evolves between patient and therapist during treatment was first proposed by Freud (1933), who coined the term *transference* to describe this phenomenon. For Freud, the transference was a significant component of the psychoanalytic experience in which the therapist was a figure with whom the patient reenacted unresolved conflict stemming from early periods of development. Subsequent theorists have expanded the concept and applied the notion of the *transference relationship* to other forms of treatment, such as psychotherapy, family therapy, and group therapy. Thus, the concept has been applied to various formats within the patient–therapist relationship. With the exception of a few commentaries (e.g., Fraiberg, 1980), however, the transference relationship has not been fully explored in the context of caregiver–infant intervention. Because this form of treatment presents a unique opportunity for the therapist to explore the caregiver's interpersonal skills, it warrants a discussion of how transferential issues emerge during caregiver–infant therapy.

When discussing caregiver–infant intervention, several factors should be remembered. First, as in other forms of treatment, the caregiver is likely to develop a relationship with the therapist imbued with transferential overtones. Second, through observing the dyadic exchange between mother and infant, the therapist will witness how the caregiver reenacts aspects of other relationships in her interactions with the infant. In effect, the caregiver will be "transferring" (displacing) behaviors to the context of her exchange with the infant although, strictly speaking, the term transference generally applies only to the patient–therapist relationship. Because the infant will exhibit numerous manifestations, this form of transference is likely to change as the infant undergoes developmental transformation. The therapist will be able to monitor the changes in the caregiver's attitude to the infant as a consequence of these developmental changes. In a parallel fashion, the caregiver's attitude toward the therapist is also likely to change as the infant develops. The therapist should be particularly sensitive to changes in the caregiver's attitude toward the treatment during periods when the consolidation of a developmental milestone is imminent. Thus, a distinctive situation is created during caregiver–infant treatment, because two observing adults—therapist and caregiver—can *consensually validate* their perceptions about the infant. In this fashion, the infant's developmental changes enable the therapist to establish objective criteria for exploring the caregiver's transference. This process contributes to the accurate monitoring of progress during the treatment.

Essentially, then, caregiver–infant therapy allows therapists to test hypotheses about both the transference between therapist and caregiver and the transference between caregiver and infant. During treatment, the infant's objective behavioral manifestations serve as *independent* variables. Because therapists know a good deal about the processes of development, they can use observations of infant development as barometers for determining whether the caregiver is exhibiting a *flexible* response that will promote adaptive development or is causing the emergence of *inflexible* patterns. By carefully observing the responses of the infant, therapists can perceive whether the caregiver is relating to the infant as an individual with unique constitutional and interpersonal qualities or is using the infant to reenact earlier, unresolved intrapsychic and/or interpersonal conflicts. Comparing the caregiver's relationships with both therapist and infant provides therapists with further insight for testing the caregiver's tendency to transfer residual conflict onto others. Therapists should keep in mind that not all the caregiver's manifestations are the result of the transference onto the infant. Indeed, one of the prime challenges confronting therapists involved in dyadic therapy is to differentiate between caregiver behavior that is maladaptive because of an inherent deficit in one or both of the dyadic members (e.g., a "mismatch" of temperaments between caregiver and infant), and behaviors that are maladaptive due to the caregiver's unresolved conflict from an earlier developmental period (e.g., a wish to control the baby by inducing him to behave in certain fashions).

What are transference phenomena and how can the therapist recognize them? According to Freud (1893, 1894, 1895a, 1895b, 1895c, 1933), transference reactions are new editions or facsimiles of the fantasies aroused during the progress of the treatment. Freud also noted that transferences have the peculiarity of *replacing* an earlier person in the patient's life with the person of the therapist. For Wolstein (1964), the transference is a complex mode of interpersonal relatedness that occurs during the relationships of everyday life as well as during therapy. The transference phenomenon loses its conceptual utility when applied to everyday life, however, because the individual does not ordinarily understand it and such comprehension does not ordinarily lead to insights and changes in personality. In therapy, though, a distortion motivated by transferential issues becomes a vivid and telling experience that can help the caregiver explore unresolved conflicts.

Moore and Fine (1967) have defined transference as the *displacement of feelings and behaviors,* originally experienced with the significant figures of one's childhood, onto individuals in current relationships. These researchers add that the transference process promotes the *repetition* of unconsciously perceived attitudes and emotions. In this sense, the individual establishes a *false connection* between the phenomena experienced in the past and the phenomena being experienced in the present (Stolorow,

Brandchaft, & Atwood, 1987). Among the primary properties of the transference that have been emphasized by Blanck and Blanck (1986) are the
following:

1. The transference involves patterns of organization that include memory, affect, and behavior.
2. Such patterns underscore early life experiences that have not only
   persisted throughout the patient's life, but have also influenced the
   patient's personal relations.
3. The persistence of such patterns is responsible for displacement from
   the past onto the present. This final factor, in fact, represents a deficit
   in reality testing and thus a distortion of reality—the ingredient that
   lies at the core of the transference experience. When such a distortion
   occurs, there is confusion not only between past and present but also
   between the patient's representations of significant relationships and
   the patient's real experiences with such individuals.

The Blancks have suggested that the mode of transference is regulated by
the level of the patient's development. In other words, the individual
repeats in the present earlier experiences with the primary object (e.g.,
caregiver) because such earlier experiences were either overly gratifying or,
in contrast, because the individual experienced deprivation during such
interactions. Thus, the transference emerges as a consequence of a *developmental deficit.*

For these reasons caregivers are likely to replicate past experiences
during their interactions with the infant or the therapist. For example, a
depressed mother whose conflict is rooted in the apathetic care she herself
received from her caregiver may transfer this flat, apathetic attitude to her
infant, thereby inducing these same feelings in the infant. In essence, the
caregiver has effectively transferred to her infant emotions derived from
her past. The interpersonal accentuation that the caregiver can manifest is
crucial, because it reveals how significant the transference relationship is in
the context of the caregiver–infant relationship.

An important point should be made about the therapist's role in the
transference during dyadic treatment. Traditionally, the therapist was
viewed as a neutral figure who reflected back to the patient only the content
of what the patient had enacted in the session. Waelder (1956) and Wolstein
(1964), among others, have noted that under this theory the therapist was
assigned the role of a kind of depersonalized observer. Over time, however,
the concept of the therapist's role has changed dramatically. Just as formats
of psychological treatment that differ from psychoanalysis have emerged,
so too the role of the therapist has been significantly reevaluated. In particular, the active participation of the therapist in the therapeutic process casts
a different complexion on the therapeutic relationship. Transference dis-

tortions are interpreted within the *interpersonal* arena in which the therapist—both as participant and observer (Sullivan, 1953)—ostensibly discloses his skills to the scrutiny of the patient who is at once the individual being observed and the participant. Distortions are transferred into the interpersonal situation as a response provoked by the therapist's inquiry. In this regard *inquiry* activates defensive operations when it activates memories involving dynamically guarded experiences. The activation of the transference creates a pressure within the interpersonal field that corresponds to the content being elaborated by the patient. Such a scenario permits the patient and the therapist to enact the material being discussed (Levenson, 1972). The prevailing view of transference phenomena is that the therapist's interventions (e.g., inquiry) stimulate the emergence of both real or distorted beliefs on the part of the patient. Whether the patient addresses the therapist's personality objectively or in a distorted fashion can determine the extent to which the patient will be able to respond to the treatment.

The therapist's role as an active participant is especially evident during treatment formats such as caregiver–infant intervention. The therapist must not only actively encourage the caregiver to explore and interpret her subjective perceptions about the infant, but should also foster the caregiver's interventions by interacting directly with the infant. This approach enhances the therapist's ability to assess and diagnose dysfunction. Moreover, the therapist's more active role is not an impediment to treatment; rather, theorists have actually postulated that the therapist may stimulate the emergence of a transference relationship by assuming this more active posture (Sullivan, 1954; Tauber, 1954; Trad, 1987).

How does the therapist recognize that a transference relationship is emerging in the patient? Numerous signs point to its presence. Two such signs are the caregiver's willingness to engage in free association and eagerness to report dreams during sessions. A catalogue of responses indicating the emergence of a transference relationship follow, with comments describing what is likely to occur during caregiver–infant psychotherapy.

First, the caregiver may verbalize an unreasonable or irrational dislike of the infant or the therapist. In these situations, the therapist may comment or ask questions designed to gather more information about these feelings. If this reaction is actually a transference reaction, the caregiver will tend to ignore the question or the main issue being probed or, instead, will provide an evasive answer. The caregiver may, in this context, also accuse the therapist of being overly intrusive. Some caregivers rely on this strategy because they are threatened at the prospect of exploration. Occasionally, negative feelings may be redirected to the infant who lacks the developmental capacity to challenge the caregiver.

A second indication of the emergence of a transference occurs when the caregiver becomes overly involved with some personal characteristic of the therapist that is irrelevant to the therapist's ability to work with the dyad. The caregiver may express an excessive liking for the therapist, may feel that the therapist is the "only person able to solve the problem," and may affirm that no one else in the world could successfully treat the caregiver. This phenomenon is an example of what has been referred to as an *idealizing transference,* whereby the patient displaces emotions of an exaggerated and grandiose nature onto the therapist. The caregiver here becomes preoccupied with the therapist to an unusual degree in the intervals between sessions and may find herself conducting imaginary conversations with the therapist, which she usually reports to the therapist. The caregiver may also disclose that she has dreamed about the therapist or about the infant. An example of the opposite response, an extreme *devaluing transference,* is encountered with a caregiver who complains that she dreads the hours she spends in treatment and is consistently uncomfortable throughout the session.

Other telltale indicia of a transference reaction include the caregiver's difficulty or even impossibility in focusing on any aspect of her progress or on problems during sessions. In these circumstances, the caregiver may unnecessarily digress or may use the infant's presence as a diversion to avoid discussing certain issues. Some caregivers will make unusual comments or will include notable omissions in their narratives—both of which indicate that some information is intentionally being withheld (resisted) from the therapist. Some caregivers will be vague about the source of any problem with the infant or will discuss problems as if consulting the therapist as yet one more of many professionals in their lives. The inability to be punctual for appointments or the display of other disturbances concerning time arrangements, such as leaving before the session is ended, are further clues that a transference may be developing. Other patients may habitually run over at the end of the hour and at that point suddenly raise key issues for discussion or they may indicate that they don't want to leave. Disturbances about any aspect of the arrangements of sessions, once these arrangements have been previously agreed upon, also fall into this category.

The evolution of a transference is also apparent if the caregiver continually argues, seeks affection and approval inappropriately, remains uninvolved or indifferent about problems in her life, or continually interacts in a mechanical way without demonstrating emotional investment. On the other hand, the caregiver may become highly defensive or exhibit extreme vulnerability to the therapist's observations or interpretations. For example, the caregiver may express disagreement or resentment at the therapist's views regarding the infant's development. Or, the caregiver may consistently misunderstand or persistently demand reassurance. In other cases, the caregiver will seek to elicit a particular emotional response from the therapist by engaging in provocative and dramatic remarks or by asking double-edged questions. A transference is also indicated when the caregiver selectively asks leading or argumentative questions of the therapist, rephrases the therapist's inquiries in the form of declarative statements, and uses them as an opportunity to digress.

When monitoring the transference the therapist should observe the caregiver's facial expression, voice pitch, and emotional tone, particularly uncontrolled fits of laughter or affective displays that are inappropriate to the content of the narrative being disclosed. The caregiver may also alter body position in characteristic ways, for example, with uncontrolled or nervous movements of the legs, or by the crossing and uncrossing of the arms and legs. The transference can also cause regressive behavior that may confuse the infant who is in the throes of a developmental impasse due to the lack of adaptive interaction. In fact, the caregiver may disguise her own regression while interacting with the infant. Finally, the caregiver may report transitory somatic complaints during treatment, although there appears to be no somatic basis for the symptomatology. Each of these phenomena indicates that on some level the caregiver may be using the therapist as an object upon whom to displace various emotions stemming from earlier development. The therapist should help the caregiver work through these manifestations so that she becomes more receptive to exploring unresolved conflict before it is displaced further onto either the relationship with the therapist or the relationship with the infant.

While noting these signs, the therapist should also attend to dream material. When evaluating a dream, the therapist should not forget that the primary objective of dyadic treatment is to assess the nature of the interaction between caregiver and infant. In so doing, the therapist will evaluate hypotheses regarding the caregiver and infant and attempt to test the validity of these hypotheses. The caregiver's dreams act as a kind of barometer for contrasting perceptions as they emerge in the dream with the fantasies of daily life, as well as for contrasting the observations of the interaction between caregiver and infant being recorded by the therapist.

As the transference intensifies, mechanisms of projection may come to predominate the caregiver's responses. Projection is a defensive process in which an aspect of the self is expiated from consciousness by being attributed to an external object to quell anxiety and alleviate conflict (Stolorow, Brandschaft, Atwood, & Lachmann, 1987). Once a transference reaction has occurred, projection may or may not emerge depending on the extent to which the caregiver uses this process as a defense against subjective dangers. If signs of projection are encountered in the caregiver, the therapist should closely direct the caregiver's attention to the infant's response. Has the infant begun to manifest irritable or apathetic affect? In these instances, the therapist, while exploring the issue with the caregiver, should assume the role of a neutral figure and engage the infant in an adaptive fashion to defuse the negative affect the caregiver is discharging into the interactional milieu.

The transference may therefore be said to be an attempt on the part of the caregiver to revive and reenact, in the therapeutic situation and in the relationship with the infant or the therapist, a developmental deficit stemming from her own childhood. As the transference is worked through, the caregiver will be able to expose areas of conflict, to recognize the conflict, and to develop alternative strategies for overcoming it. As she becomes more involved in the treatment, the relationship with the therapist becomes cast in images from earlier experiences of the caregiver's world of object relations. Here again, the therapist must attend to the infant's reactions to discern the effect of the caregiver's transferential phenomena and to neutralize their impact on the infant's development.

Two other significant concepts are important in this regard because they facilitate understanding of how the parallel process phenomenon can be rebuilt in an enhanced form of communication between caregiver and infant during dyadic treatment. These two concepts are intersubjectivity and *projective identification*. Both of these concepts attempt to describe and explain how the subjective perceptions of one individual are communicated to another individual without the use of language.

The term *intersubjectivity* (Trevarthen & Hubley, 1978) refers to a developmental milestone in the evolution of self-regulation that occurs when the infant is approximately 9 months old. By this time, the infant has begun to emerge from a state of undifferentiation and has come to recognize the presence of others who are separate from himself, both physically and psychologically. As noted by Stern (1985) and Trevarthen and Hubley (1978), with this realization comes the recognition that others possess a separate internal reality. The infant's attainment of intersubjectivity is manifested through evidence of an awareness of the caregiver's intentions, perceptions, and affects. A recognition of the possibility of a shared internal reality, which includes both awareness of an internal self and an awareness of an internal reality in others, is a prerequisite for intersubjectivity. As intersubjectivity achieves full fruition, both separation/individuation and new forms of experiencing union with others begin to emerge.

It is important to recognize that it is not just the infant who achieves intersubjectivity and uses this capacity for understanding the caregiver's motives and internal state. The caregiver also must rely on intersubjective skills to comprehend the infant's perceptions and motivations. In this sense, intersubjectivity, much like previewing, serves as a substitute kind of language for better grasping the full implications of the infant's inner experience.

Related to the quality of intersubjectivity is *projective identification*, phenomenon initially introduced by Klein in 1952 and subsequently elaborated on by that researcher. Projective identification differs substantially from general projection, in that it occurs only in the context of interaction between two or more individuals. In contrast, projection is predominantly intrapsychic and may or may not evolve in an actual interpersonal relationship. Projective identification, although it has intrapsychic characteristics, primarily derives from direct human interaction in which one individual unconsciously attempts to elicit thoughts, feelings, and experiences within another individual that in some way resemble his own. Projective identification is, therefore, only successful to the extent that the recipient identifies with and receives the material being projected. During the process of projective identification, the individual who is projecting may awaken within the therapist an experiential state that matches, to some degree, either the projector's self-representation or, alternatively, the projector's object representation from any of a multitude of the projector's internalized objects (Tansey & Burke, 1985).

In dyadic therapy, projective identification assumes an added dimension because of the presence of not only the infant but of the therapist as well. If we assume that the caregiver will be engaging in projective identification, then we may assume that both the therapist and the infant will be the recipients of the caregiver's unconscious thoughts, feelings, and experiences. As a result, the therapist will gain more profound insight into the kinds of unconscious material the caregiver is projecting to the infant. Moreover, the infant's responses will provide insight into how the infant has come to understand and interpret the phenomena being projected by the caregiver. In addition, projective identification helps the therapist understand how the residue of unconscious conflict is transmitted to the infant and significantly, how the infant perceives this conflict. As a consequence, the therapist can diagnose conflict and identify its source far more readily than in other forms of treatment.

It is worthwhile to explain how projective identification manifests itself in the context of the therapeutic encounter. According to Tansey and Burke (1985), the patient may evoke within the therapist an impulse to attack and criticize. As a result, the therapist begins to identify his own immediate self-representation with the sadistic object representation of the patient. In other cases, a predominantly masochistic patient may assume a sadistic role as his or her immediate self-representation and begin attacking or criticizing the therapist, who begins to feel like a victim. Both of these scenarios encompass what Racker (1957) describes as complementary identifications in which the therapist temporarily identifies with an aspect of the patient's internalized representations of self and object, while the patient, at least temporarily, experiences the representations of the "other" that is opposite from his own. The interaction signifies the complementarity of the patient's internalized self and object representations. In a third kind of projective identification, the patient arouses within the therapist a concordant identification such that the immediate self-experiences of both individuals are temporarily similar (Racker, 1957).

The primary advantage gained from projective identification is that therapists acquire insight into the emotional awareness of the patient and his or her internal world. This occurs when therapists attempt to determine the nature of the patient's feelings or subjective experience as well as the nature of their own feelings. Therapists attempt to ascertain, in other words, the extent to which the two experiences either match or complement one another. Three configurations are possible: First, the patient has projected his or her own self-representation into the therapist, resulting in a concordant identification in the therapist (Racker, 1957); second, the patient has projected an internalized object representation into the therapist causing a complementary identification in the therapist (Tansey & Burke, 1985); third, a projective identification may contain both complementary and concordant elements.

The benefits from projective identification increase in the dyadic treatment setting primarily because both the caregiver and infant are present. As a result, the caregiver may engage in projective identification with the infant and vice versa, providing the therapist with an opportunity to observe in a neutral fashion how members of the dyad transfer emotional perceptions. Subsequently, the caregiver will engage in projective identification with the therapist, as will the infant during episodes when the therapist enters into direct interaction with the child. These diverse interactions enable the therapist to gain a more profound understanding of how the caregiver and infant each represent "self" and "other" and of the process used to project these representations during interaction. Diagnosis and treatment are thus facilitated because any deficits in these fundamental internal working models of the caregiver and infant are readily exposed early in the treatment.

THE EFFECT OF THE THERAPIST'S REACTIONS TO THE PARALLEL PROCESS

It is also important for therapists to monitor their changes in attitude during treatment. In the opening phases of the treatment, for example, it is not unusual for the therapist to experience negative feelings, such as frustration, toward the caregiver. A caregiver who seems to possess encyclopedic knowledge about the development of the infant and who insists on correcting the therapist may easily evoke negative feelings. At the beginning of the treatment it is not unusual to find that the greater the caregiver's ability to master the interaction with the infant, the less receptive the caregiver may be to the therapist's interventions. Under these circumstances the therapist absorbs and responds to the unacceptable, unconscious, or preconscious aspects of the caregiver without conscious awareness. Referred to as toxic-affective-uncritical merging by Caligor (1981), this experience is subjectively induced and takes over the therapist. For example, the therapist may experience profound feelings of anxiety, rage, or confusion. To deny these unacceptable and disassociated responses, the therapist often winds up responding to the caregiver as the caregiver has responded to the infant. It is vital to recognize that the parallel process enables the therapist, caregiver, and infant to reverse roles and alternate between both evoking and receiving emotion. Also significant is that the parallel process may activate intrapsychic conflict, of which the therapist may be unaware. As the treatment progresses, however, the therapist will be able to reflect upon and channel these powerful emotions more effectively. Therapists should also focus on their emotional response to the caregiver's adaptive skills.

Moreover, therapists should observe when they are identifying with the caregiver, particularly with respect to using a common methodology for warding off anxiety. This occurs because the therapist shares with the caregiver transient identifications with various aspects of the infant's mental functioning. Many of these phenomena, however, do not stem from the therapist's childhood. Rather, these emotions may emanate from the therapist's observations of the caregiver's or infant's own manifestations (Schlessinger, 1966).

Therapists who have analyzed their own emotional response to the dyadic interaction will be able to offer a model of adaptation that caregivers can eventually replicate to enhance their relationship with the infant. An anecdote from a case history will provide a vivid illustration of the impact that the therapist's feelings may have on the treatment. The caregiver reported a dream to me during the 8th month of treatment, when our work together was drawing to an end, as we had previously agreed. This caregiver was extremely well educated and prior to motherhood had been employed in a professional capacity. During the initial weeks of treatment, she had displayed the kind of assertiveness and authority over the infant's development that is typical of the first stage of dyadic treatment. If anything, this caregiver was somewhat obsessional in her responses to the infant. Although this attitude sometimes aroused a countertransference reaction of resentment, I remained neutral. As therapy progressed, however, the caregiver became less inhibited and more emotive. This change in attitude was coupled with a greater receptivity to my observations and to the manifestations I displayed during modeling episodes with the infant. At approximately this time, the caregiver reported that her relationship with her husband was also improving and that for the first time since the infant's birth they were sharing the joys, as well as the fears and anxieties, that accompany parenthood. The caregiver also told me that she had previously had a strained relationship with her own mother and that one of her greatest fears during pregnancy had been that she would replicate this cold, unempathic relationship with her own infant. She noted that she believed therapy had helped her to overcome this fear, so that she could now relate to the infant competently in a more spontaneous and reciprocal fashion. Several weeks prior to a planned summer vacation that would interrupt the treatment schedule for more than 5 weeks, the caregiver reported the following dream:

CAREGIVER: I was sitting in a pleasantly lit room with two other women. We had all recently given birth and were waiting to see our babies. However, first we were being given some instructions about how to take care of them. At first, I resented that we had to learn this information before we could see our babies, but then I felt it was all right and better this way. The lady who was giving us the instructions was older, about 60. She was kind and knew what she was talking about. She was very well-educated, and I sensed that she had had many children herself. Suddenly, you were also in the room; I was glad you were there. The lady continued the instructions for several minutes. I felt I was learning a great deal. Then she said, "It is time to nurse the babies." We opened our blouses and we were all wearing nursing bras that open on one side. I didn't realize I was wearing one, but I was glad I was prepared. All of a sudden I felt scared, and the thought crossed my mind that I wouldn't have enough milk for the baby. I tried to look at the other women. When I saw them, I realized I would be all right, and that I would have enough milk for my baby. We were now getting ready to nurse and we were all exposed on the left side. But we all put our hands over our nipples, so you wouldn't see. It is as if all of us—all three mothers—felt the same thing. We wanted you to leave now, because we were going to nurse the babies. It was something that we could do by ourselves. It was just that nursing is something private, something each of us wanted to share only with our babies.

I interpreted this dream as meaning that the caregiver was summarizing her experience in treatment and the stages of the treatment she had undergone. Initially, the caregiver felt confident in her role as a new mother and vaguely resented that the older woman in the dream was instructing her. This attitude corresponds to the first stage of treatment when the caregiver exhibits assertiveness and self-competence, or what can be referred to as "encyclopedic knowledge." The caregiver eventually came to accept the interventions of the older woman—an aspect of the therapist— representing the second phase or working through of the treatment, when the caregiver begins to experience the therapy as being more intimate and is able to work through her conflicts. At this time she forges intense feelings with the therapist and is most susceptible to change. Finally, by the end of the dream, the caregiver wished to nurse the infant alone, out of my presence, because it is a "private" experience. This realization correlates with the resolution of conflict concerning her ability to serve as an adaptive mother. Now the caregiver realizes that she is ready to nurture the infant on her own. This dream represented the emergence of the third stage in the therapeutic relationship. The caregiver had identified with the therapist's perspective, explored her conflict, and acquired a more objective view of the reciprocal contributions that both mother and infant bring to the relationship. She was now able to fulfill her caregiving role with a genuine sense of competence and mastery, unlike the pseudocompetence she had manifested when she first entered treatment.

In contrast, the following excerpt from a trainee conducting an intake interview demonstrates the type of attitude that is not conducive to forging a working alliance with the caregiver:

THERAPIST: I understand that the fetus was in the breech position before delivery.

CAREGIVER: Yes, if you mean it wasn't positioned correctly during labor.

THERAPIST: So a Caesarean was performed?

CAREGIVER: Yes.

THERAPIST: And the fetus was premature? How many weeks gestation?

CAREGIVER: I'm not sure . . . I think . . .

THERAPIST: What month were you in?

CAREGIVER: Oh . . . the eighth.

THERAPIST: I see . . . were there postnatal complications?

CAREGIVER: The baby was placed in an incubator . . .

THERAPIST: How old is the infant now?

CAREGIVER: Twelve weeks.

THERAPIST: What has the pediatrician told you?

CAREGIVER: She says the baby is developing very well.

Several obvious flaws in this dialogue suggest the therapist is pressing for information in a way that impedes the emergence of a comfortable exchange with the caregiver. First, the therapist's questions contain an abundance of medical jargon. It is not recommended that the therapist rattle off a litany of questions about prematurity, caesarean birth, physical complications, and infant temperament. Instead, open-ended questions, such as "Could you share with me what happened when the baby was born," usually elicit more spontaneous and unrehearsed information that will not cause the caregiver to become overly self-conscious. Therapists should encourage a natural disclosure so that the caregiver provides insight into feelings and behaviors concerning the infant's development. Second, the exchange lacks spontaneity because the therapist's timing is rigid and mechanical. Rather than giving the caregiver enough time to consider the questions, this therapist's goal seems to be to obtain information for its own sake, without following the caregiver's cues. This is a particularly inappropriate message to convey at the inception of dyadic therapy because it suggests that interaction is one-sided and controlled by a dominant partner—a model that should certainly be avoided with the infant. A more appropriate posture for the therapist to adopt is that of a *participant observer* (Sullivan, 1954) who will be receptive to the patient's own pace, not to the preconceived timing that the therapist believes is appropriate. A third prominent feature of the preceding dialogue is that it lacks an appropriate affective rhythm and tone. Although it is essential to obtain a thorough case history during the initial weeks of treatment, another significant aspect of a caregiver's history is her ongoing emotional state, along with her capacity to share a full range of affects with the therapist. *Affective modulation* by the therapist is vital because it is almost certain that the caregiver's experiences with the therapist will be replicated with the baby. As such, one of the therapist's initial tasks is to support the emergence of the caregiver's emotions in a free and unfettered manner. The therapist can only accomplish this by creating an atmosphere of nonauthoritative negotiated equality and conveying the message that he or she can deal with emotions candidly and respectfully.

As a final comment, the therapist in the preceding example questioned the caregiver about the infant as if the baby did not contribute to the caregiver's dilemma. The therapist at no time referred to the infant by name and repeatedly made references to physiological functions relating to the birth and nurturing processes—the caesarean birth, the caregiver's postpartum complications, breastfeeding, and the infant's schedule— rather than to the emotional experience of giving birth and caring for a young human being. In other words, the therapist here *mechanized* the interpersonal experience for the caregiver. Although obtaining an objective perspective of the caregiver–infant relationship is certainly one goal of the intake process, this approach should not assume priority over allowing the caregiver to express freely the *subjective experiences* she is undergoing with the infant, because it is from these subjective perceptions that the unique relationship between each caregiver and infant emerges.

In sum, then, therapists should avoid the pitfalls of mechanical inquiry during therapeutic interactions by maintaining the flow of the communications in a direct and conversational mode, rather than by introducing clinical jargon. It is important to pace the questions in harmony with the caregiver's verbal rhythms, allowing for listening time and a full disclosure of concerns before raising another inquiry. Nor should the therapist adhere to a rigid script. If the caregiver provides a digression that may yield insight into her subjective experience with the infant, the therapist should be adept at pursuing this unexpected, but possibly productive, line of inquiry. Moreover, from the beginning of the treatment, empathic interactions with the caregiver provide an atmosphere in which the caregiver will feel comfortable about voicing emotional concerns. Only if the therapist displays empathy will the caregiver be comfortable about manifesting these responses. From the beginning of treatment, the therapist should refer to the infant by name and, when the therapist senses that the caregiver will be receptive, should interact directly with the infant. Later in treatment, as the caregiver gradually engages in interaction in front of the therapist, other kinds of interventions can take place. From the outset, however, therapists must convey to the caregiver through their interactions that the infant is a reciprocal partner in the dyadic relationship.

ASSESSING THE PARALLEL PROCESS IN THE DYADIC TREATMENT

The therapist should assess the interpersonal capacities of the caregiver—whether they be adaptive or maladaptive, or lie at some point on the spectrum between these polarities—as early as possible in the treatment in order to begin predicting the future course of dyadic interaction and devising optimal therapeutic strategies. Assessment occurs not only by observing the caregiver's interactions with the infant and analyzing the discrepancies between the caregiver's comments and her actions with the infant, but also by evaluating the therapeutic alliance. A useful strategy to elucidate the caregiver's relationship with the infant is conducting a number of sessions alone with the caregiver, or having several individual interviews with each of the caregivers to observe not only how they relate individually to the infant but also how each interprets developmental phenomena. The therapist may discover different interpersonal processes that become apparent when the caregiver speaks about the infant outside of his physical presence. This form of one-to-one discussion between therapist and caregiver(s) will provide further insight into the caregiver's subjective perceptions and her ability to perceive the infant as an individual with a distinctive personality.

During the assessment phase, therapists are constantly shifting roles. Occasionally therapists are predominantly observers; at other times, they become active participants in the patient's emotional experience. It is possible to characterize the enactment of the caregiver's behavior during therapy sessions as a form of communication. When the caregiver experiences failure in the recognition, recall, or verbalization of a problem, she may express such conflict through acting out during her interactions with the infant or therapist. In other words, just as the caregiver oscillates between identifying with and observing the infant, the therapist may oscillate between exploring and modeling what the caregiver fails to enact with the infant.

The therapist should first consider the infant as an *evoker* of emotion. Examples of the infant's behavior that the therapist should be alert to include avoidance, resistance to interaction, withdrawal, irritability and fussiness, and short attention span. The therapist should observe the experience of the caregiver as a *recipient* of such interpersonal manifestations. In such cases, therapists should look for signs such as stupor, depressed affect, a taciturn attitude, lack of critical thinking, suppressed rage, and withdrawal. When considering the caregiver as an *evoker* figure, the therapist should be alert to the caregiver's resistant-evasive or rejecting behavior. During such episodes it is not uncommon for the caregiver to manifest a "swirl of words," scattered thinking, and anxiety. As the *recipient* of these emotions, the infant's response is likely to be one of stupor, depression, withdrawal, suppressed rage, and confused thinking.

It is particularly important to bear in mind that the caregiver, the infant, and the therapist can switch roles and any of the three can play evoker or recipient. For example, the caregiver may be the recipient with the infant and the evoker with the therapist. The parallel process captured by these descriptions suggests that the dynamics manifested in the caregiver–infant relationship may represent the way the caregiver establishes relationships in life. Such patterns are analogous to ripples of *concentric circles* growing more remote with each periphery, from caregiver to infant and caregiver to therapist.

The clinical implications of the parallel process phenomenon are diverse. The parallel process occurs continually in the caregiver–infant dyad, and unless therapists become alert to its dynamics, they may remain oblivious to its implications. The invariant variable therefore becomes the therapist's reactions. For the parallel process to be a viable therapeutic tool, therapists must be aware of what they are experiencing in their relationship with both caregiver and infant. If therapists do not actively participate in *self-exploration* they may be unable to prevent themselves from acting out personal emotions. Significantly, the parallel process is exhibited most dramatically in situations where the therapist, caregiver, and infant have reached a crisis or conflict, with the resultant heightened disjunctive anxiety and decline into apathy.

Using the parallel process as a therapeutic tool is effective for several reasons. By analyzing the overlap of two relationships, the therapist gains insight into dyadic conflict. The emergence of insight allows the therapist to respond and to devise strategies for overcoming the conflict with its debilitating cycle of negative emotions. When the therapist does not recognize the parallel process, however, the caregiver–therapist relationship may reach an impasse, just as the caregiver–infant relationship may begin to stagnate. If this occurs, the therapist will be fostering the debilitating patterns that the caregiver is experiencing and reflecting in her relationship with the infant.

To prevent this negative outcome, the therapist engaging in dyadic therapy must recognize and decipher the infant's perceptions and the subjective perceptions of the caregiver in a way that enables alerting the caregiver to the source of maladaptation and to its remedy. The therapist must develop a strong sensitivity, tact, and repertoire of appropriate responses for encouraging the caregiver to explore her motivations and to respond to the infant's motivations. In this sense, the mother–infant relationship may be viewed as the perpetual disclosure of a series of new meanings fraught with powerful motivational implications. These goals may be accomplished once the therapist recognizes that the caregiver will be receptive to exploring these meanings and to modifying them consciously before enacting them with the infant.

The therapist also needs to observe carefully the contours of the dyadic interaction between caregiver and infant. Adaptive caregivers will tend to *reciprocate* the infant's manifestations, matching their behaviors to the infant's interpersonal rhythms. It is especially important to diagnose how the caregiver communicates affect to the infant while describing the infant's emotional responses. During such times, the therapist should evaluate whether the caregiver is able to distinguish her mood from the mood she perceives in the infant. For example, one caregiver told me of a new toy she had bought for her infant and commented that the baby seemed fascinated by the face painted on the toy. At precisely that point in her description, the caregiver turned toward her infant and engaged her in a face-to-face sequence of interaction during which the caregiver began to vocalize softly to the infant. I was impressed by the caregiver's intuitive capacity to match the content of her disclosures with appropriate interpersonal cues and to share these behaviors with the infant in a sequence of harmonious exchange. I was also impressed by this caregiver's ability to communicate effectively with me, while simultaneously being alert to the signals emitted by her infant. She was able to forge parallel relationships without becoming confused or overwhelmed, allowing her to divide her attention appropriately between infant and me.

In contrast, another caregiver in treatment appeared impervious and unresponsive to the infant's cues. The attachment between this pair seemed devoid of positive affect and the caregiver attended to the infant only sporadically, using mechanical gestures. Even when the infant attempted to look directly at the caregiver by turning his head in her direction, the caregiver continued to be oblivious to the infant's painstaking efforts to initiate interaction. This caregiver also had difficulty sustaining simultaneous interactions with the therapist and with the infant.

Evaluating the caregiver's developmental adaptability with the infant by assessing her relationship with the therapist is particularly important. For example, if a caregiver is questioned about the infant, it is not unusual for an adaptive caregiver to gaze at or interact with the baby before, during, or after answering, as if to validate consensually with the infant her own perceptions, impressions, and attributions. For such caregivers, interaction with the infant is a continually shared and reciprocated experience. The adaptive caregiver communicates descriptions that provide insight into the infant's perspective. Moreover, adaptive caregivers will also manifest a similar response to the therapist and will be open about sharing perceptions with the therapist in a candid and flexible fashion.

Caregivers whose interactions are organized around conflict, on the other hand, exhibit an entirely different pattern of response. In these cases, the caregiver does not consider or even acknowledge the infant's cues when she is formulating a response. Such caregivers generally don't look at the infant to assess the cues being emitted. Instead, these caregivers gaze into space or at the therapist or plead that they cannot describe or remember the infant's reaction to a particular situation. Interaction in these instances does not represent a reciprocal exchange of information between two individuals. Furthermore, these caregivers appear impaired in their ability to provide insight into the infant's perceptions, thought processes, or motivational perspective.

Therapists should also be cautious when caregivers provide them with *mechanical descriptions* of their babies. For example, does the caregiver attribute mechanical qualities to the infant or describe the infant only in physiological terms without describing the infant's affective, cognitive, or motivational state? Such descriptions characteristically are devoid of any affective tone, the description of transitions between different interactions is blurred or nonexistent, and the meaning attributed to the infant's behavior fails to consider the infant's perspective. Significantly, these caregivers may also exhibit difficulty during the interaction with the therapist. For example, the caregiver may be overly anxious, may resist, or may withdraw from the therapist's inquiries. As a result, the relationship with the therapist will be characterized by a coercive quality, as if the therapist is trying to force information from the caregiver. In effect, the relationship the caregiver is forging with the therapist may be paralleling her relationship with the infant. The therapist should, of course, also keep in mind that the caregiver's inability to express herself may be due to some other precipitating factor, such as the therapeutic setting or the infant's condition on that particular day. Therefore, the therapist should attempt to identify patterns of resistance to interaction that are consistently displayed session after session.

It is also important to focus on the infant's interpersonal behaviors during these observations and to diagnose the patterns that appear to have become entrenched within the dyadic exchange. Unlike older patients, who have developed sophisticated mechanisms of defense that can mask internal states, infant affect is generally spontaneous and unrehearsed, with the exception of recalcitrant patterns. Some caregivers, for example, fail to understand that infants cannot simply abate their cries upon command. In fact, the inability to comprehend the spontaneous quality of the infant's interpersonal capacities is a key indication of maladaptation. One caregiver commented to me that she was convinced the infant cried to "spite her" or to "get back at" her for not paying attention to him all the time. This is a prime example of an attribution organized around conflict, suggesting a failure to understand the infant's developmental capacities. Through interpretation and modeling, I was able to persuade this caregiver that the infant was incapabe of harbong this kind of complex intentionality and that, rather, his cries were more likely a sign of physical discomfort.

Pointing out the similarities and dissimilarities of the patterns manifested over time by the infant will help the caregiver become better attuned to the infant's motivational state. For most adaptive caregivers these observations will not seem incomprehensible because adaptive caregivers generally can adopt the infant's perspective and perceive the underlying motivation. In fact, by sharing perceptions about the infant's behavior, the adaptive caregiver conveys that she is aware of the similarities or differences and is prepared to assist the infant with experiencing change when necessary. For maladaptive caregivers, however, a coherent understanding of the infant's developmental status is either deficient or lacking. Nor are such caregivers able to adopt the infant's perspective and to make appropriate attributions to infant behavior. Some caregivers who manifest these deficits behave as if the infant is a mechanical object whose communication abilities are flawed. As a result, the caregiver tends to abandon her efforts to establish an adaptive system of communication with the infant. By failing to support the infant's skills and to use their own capacities to enhance dyadic communication, such caregivers thwart infant development.

(Baby is lying on his back, on the floor)

THERAPIST: Could you try to put yourself in your baby's position, and see the room from his perspective. Pay attention to the feeling of not being able to move away and yet still perceiving all the things happening around you.

CAREGIVER: If I put myself in his place, it would be pretty scary.

THERAPIST: What scares you: not being able to move or not being able to control the environment?

CAREGIVER: When I think of how much he depends on me it scares me. (Soon after, she turns to watch the baby; he babbles loudly.)

THERAPIST: In some way his behavior conveys the point that I'm trying to make. I believe he is trying to engage us through vocal, facial, and visual cues. These are his ways of engaging people. (Baby again makes babbling sounds.)

The therapist must function as a surrogate caregiver during those periods when the caregiver conveys inappropriate cues or misreads the infant's signals. In effect, the therapist should establish an adaptive relationship with both the caregiver and infant that can later be paralleled by the caregiver in her own relationship with the infant. The therapist in this respect is caring for the infant through modeling behavior, while exploring that aspect of the mother needing nurturance. As a result of this nurturing stance, the caregiver becomes better able to cope with the infant's demands, and she attends to her infant's needs in a more reciprocal fashion.

THE EFFECT OF THE CAREGIVER–THERAPIST RELATIONSHIP ON THE CAREGIVER–INFANT RELATIONSHIP

Just as the caregiver's relationship with the therapist undergoes dramatic transition during treatment, so too her pattern of response to the infant changes significantly as treatment progresses. This transformation occurs, in part, because conflict has been brought to consciousness and resolved during the therapy. For example, because caregivers are attuned to changes in their infant's behavior from the first hours of life onward, they have a tendency to act as the main "journalists" charting the infant's development. Of course, such a disposition is, in large part, adaptive, because it reinforces the caregiver's primary role with the infant as a nurturer. After all, the goal of adaptive caregiving is to achieve a *negotiated equilibrium* that recognizes and fulfills the needs of both members of the dyad in a satisfactory manner.

As treatment progresses, caregivers begin to adopt a more flexible stance that enables them to further enhance their reciprocal behaviors with the infant. The caregiver is now eager to *learn* more from the infant and about the infant and to contrast and interpret the infant's signals from various perspectives. This is because the caregiver has come to perceive the infant increasingly as a unique individual with whom she has forged a communicative network promoting reciprocal fulfillment. The caregiver's change in perception is due to many factors, not the least of which is her increasing exposure to the neutral and objective attitude inculcated by the therapist. The parallel process has also enabled the caregiver to understand the infant's perspective in a more objective fashion.

Presumably, the acquisition of knowledge, coupled with a positive identification with the therapist's approach, may permit a new technique for handling a caregiver's problem when the same problem may be unresolved for the caregiver. The function of the therapist is to help the caregiver become aware of and express her "will not to learn," or those factors that inhibit her "will to learn and change." During the participating aspect of the parallel process, the caregiver comes to experience directly the infant's subjective interpersonal field. The attuned caregiver as participant continually experiences emotional learning and communication evoked by the infant, a parallel process molded by the infant's interpersonal integration requirements. This process is initiated by, evoked by, and centered in the infant's self.

In most situations, an effective therapist translates the infant's perceptions into direct, decoded language with particular emphasis on sources that generate depressed affect or anxiety. Thus, the therapist absorbs the infant's perceptions and reactions and relates them back to the interaction for the purpose of unmasking their meaning. These perceptions are based on the real and actual behaviors of the caregiver and allow for a "working through" of the caregiver's conflict.

Previewing exercises provide a significant additional technique for helping the caregiver negotiate equilibrium with the infant. As was noted earlier, previewing enables both the caregiver and infant to obtain a more comprehensive perspective on the interpersonal implications of the infant's development. In addition, because previewing hones the caregiver's interpersonal skills in anticipating or predicting the future course of the infant's development, these exercises may also enhance the caregiver's sense of mastery in confronting the perpetual changes that attend the infant's maturation. Through previewing, the caregiver can master her role as a facilitator of the infant's developmental trends. Similarly, the infant's responses to these interpersonal behaviors provide the caregiver with the impetus essential for sustaining and enhancing further interactions. The greater the number of these interactions, the more the caregiver comes to recognize the integral role she plays in the infant's life and the integral role the infant plays in maintaining a sense that the two of them are functioning as a developmental unit.

CAREGIVER: My husband and I have been having a difficult time lately. It's been a little strained between the two of us. When I walk away from him with bad feelings, the baby picks up on it immediately.

THERAPIST: Could you describe to me what you have observed? How does your baby respond to these changes?

CAREGIVER: Just the look in his eyes is asking me . . . are you mad at me? Did I do something? Are you going to take care of me now?

THERAPIST: Do you think that he is trying to predict how you will interact with him?

CAREGIVER: Yes. A lot of times he responds to my husband's or my mood changes. The mood is very negative, and he's lying on the floor not talking to us. I hadn't thought of it in terms of trying to draw us back.

THERAPIST: Do you think that he may want to test out that if he tries to interact with you that you will reciprocate?

CAREGIVER: Yes.

THERAPIST: How can you tell that this is the case?

CAREGIVER: Because when I don't reciprocate or meet his expectations, he becomes distressed and fussy for a long time.

CONCLUSION

This chapter has elucidated how the phenomenon of the parallel process, first encountered during the supervisory experience of therapists in training, also emerges in dyadic treatment involving a caregiver and infant. As has been explained, dyadic therapy combines two interactional relationships in one format. The caregiver's relationship with the infant is thus exposed to scrutiny during dyadic treatment, enabling the therapist to understand how the infant functions as an evoker and recipient of emotional response while the caregiver functions as a recipient or evoker. In addition, a concurrent interaction between caregiver and therapist is transpiring that provides a paradigm for understanding the dynamics of a relationship in which the caregiver functions as an evoker of emotional material while the therapist assumes the role of the infant as a recipient.

The presence of the parallel process during dyadic treatment facilitates both diagnosis and treatment strategies. For example, by analyzing the nature of the parallel processes, the therapist can better understand how transference phenomena modify both the caregiver's and infant's responses and how conflict may insinuate itself into the dyadic exchange. The parallel process also helps clarify the therapist's reactions because in dyadic therapy the parallel process exposes the therapist to both the objective and the subjective impressions of these interactions. The juxtaposition of the subjective and the objective experiences results in a more profound understanding of any individual conflict.

PART THREE

Intervention Techniques

Chapter 8

Observation and Other Intervention Strategies

INTRODUCTION

The arrival of a new infant in a family dramatically alters the way both caregivers relate to one another and to their other children. Beyond the all-pervasive changes that will result from the infant's arrival in the home, the newborn will also disrupt the family's mundane patterns of living. For example, feeding and sleeping patterns will be radically changed, and often the couple's sexual relationship will be significantly modified as well. When I first began conducting therapy sessions with new mothers and their infants, I encountered yet another fascinating phenomenon relating to the arrival of a new infant. By approximately the fourth session, most caregivers began to speak spontaneously about their lives both *before* the birth of the baby and *after* his entrance into the household. It was as if the demarcation between their lives pre- and post-baby arrival was clear and distinct. Moreover, each caregiver seemed acutely aware that her identity had assumed new dimensions with the infant's arrival. The infant's entrance into the household, then, represented a new beginning for these parents, who were also cognizant that the baby's birth would alter the lives of the other family members. This chapter provides therapists with an overview of the primary techniques for helping caregivers accommodate to the dramatic transformation that occurs in their daily lives with the advent of an infant.

Once the therapist has diagnosed the degree of adaptation from the case history and from observation of the interactional patterns within the dyad, he or she is challenged to begin devising strategies for modifying behaviors so that parent and infant can forge a more positive dyadic relationship. To accomplish this, the therapist should verbalize observations in a neutral fashion and ask questions that at least initially do not arouse deep-seated conflict. For example, the therapist might ask the caregiver to share her observations concerning when the baby becomes irritable. During the early stages of the treatment the therapist needs to break down dyadic behavior into *discrete units,* so that the caregiver becomes accustomed not only to recognizing the qualities of each infant response but also to categorizing each response into a *pattern.* The degree of eye contact, different facial expressions, and vocalizations are examples of discrete units of infant response. The therapist might then explore at what times the infant coordinates a discrete unit or pattern of responses. These observations should be contrasted with the caregiver's perceptions of the infant's mood. By describing in detail the somatic, socioaffective, cognitive, and motivational components of these behavioral displays, the therapist helps the caregiver to perceive differences among the infant's reactions, so that she can see that each dimension of behavior signifies a separate manifestation. Moreover, by focusing on these discrete manifestations, caregivers will ultimately be able to recognize how their behavior and motivations contribute to the infant's response. This approach will also help caregivers to represent or predict and then preview the infant's imminent developmental and inter-personal changes. This chapter addresses the different techniques for accomplishing these tasks.

OBSERVATION—THE ROLE OF OBSERVATION IN DYADIC THERAPY

A primary goal of dyadic therapy is to diagnose the level of adaptation within a particular dyad and to devise strategies for enhancing that dyad's interactional exchange. One way of achieving this goal is through *observation* of all forms of behavior manifested by the dyadic members. Such observation encompasses behavior that is (a) interpersonal, in the sense that it engages both caregiver and infant in a mutual exchange; (b) noninterpersonal, such as the infant's play with an inanimate object; and, (c) noninteractional, such as the manifestation of sleeping states or withdrawal from others. By observing each of these behaviors, therapists can detect how the dyad functions and, in general terms, how dyadic members communicate with one another.

Infant researchers adopt systematic observational techniques with a clear methodology so that behavior among dyads can be appropriately quantified (Bakeman & Gottman, 1987). Such research techniques may also be applied to the study of an individual dyad. Thus appropriate techniques should be developed to arrive at accurate clinical observations. Among the qualities of dyadic interaction researchers have focused on are the differences between momentary events (i.e., *frequency* of behaviors) and behavioral states (i.e., *duration* of events). A frequency behavior includes such momentary events as the infant's pointing to an object or briefly gazing at the caregiver. A duration event, on the other hand, lasts for a greater length of time and might include an episode of infant play. The differentiation between these two types of events becomes significant once the observer (e.g., therapist) determines what he or she is attempting to observe (Altman, 1974; Sackett, 1978).

For therapists working with mothers and infants it is important to be alert to both frequency and duration events. Moreover, at least initially, therapists should evaluate events (e.g., interactions) using a scale with three *gradations*—low intensity, medium intensity, and high intensity. By relying on this scale, therapists can evaluate virtually any form of behavior within the dyad. Moreover, with experience and exposure to numerous dyads, therapists learn to grade events automatically. That is, as therapists become familiar with individual dyads, they will come to recognize differences in modes of interaction. Therapists can then observe and assess the particular behavior in question, and can evaluate whether the level of intensity is appropriate.

First and foremost, therapists should possess a broad knowledge of the developmental events occurring during the first 2 years of life so that they can contrast their observations with model behaviors indicative of adaptive development. Therapists can compare the maturational trends they observe with what is known to be normal and adaptive. Beyond these models, therapists should also attain a comprehensive history of the infant's and caregiver's development through careful inquiry during the initial phases of treatment. This information provides a method for measuring and validating observations of behavior between the caregiver and the infant. Thus, therapists will be comparing three phenomena. First, they should use the models of adaptive behavior that define normal maturational trends as a background for understanding the particular kinds of phenomena encountered in the dyad; second, they should use both the narrative descriptions and observations of the caregiver to evaluate the level of adaptation within the dyad; finally, they must directly observe the behavioral manifestations of the dyad. From the combination of these strategies therapists can formulate a diagnosis and treatment regimen that has relevance for an individual dyad.

During these observations therapists must assess the role of *individual differences*. Individual differences refer to the unique temperament and style of reacting that distinguishes the dyad from all other dyads. Early on it is necessary to isolate and scrutinize these individual differences and to understand how they are contributing to the infant's development and the relationship evolving between parent and infant.

In addition to isolating both the frequency and duration of significant events, therapists should also be aware of *behavioral states*. Behavioral states encompass those episodes that reflect at any given moment the underlying "organization" of an infant or dyad (Bakeman & Gottman, 1987). The arousal states usually associated with young infants, such as alert, quiet, fussy states, are a well-known example of these conditions (Wolff, 1966). The particular developmental task being observed may require definition of other behavioral states. For instance, Bakeman and Adamson (1984) wanted to determine whether infants deployed attention only to objects, only to people, or to the two jointly. It was therefore logical and efficient for the researchers to code observations pertaining to the phenomenon they were interested in, rather than to code all observations without discrimination. These researchers defined a series of such attentional states, including unengaged, onlooking, solitary object play, person play, supported joint engagement, and coordinated joint engagement. Behavioral states should be labeled and segmented by the observer, whose task it is to isolate the behavioral manifestations into discrete dimensions that are occurring at a given time.

Observing behavioral states can be an extraordinarily helpful diagnostic tool for several reasons. First, focusing on these dimensions protects the therapist from becoming lost in myriad observational detail. Second, behavioral states may qualify the meaning of other acts. Korner (1972) noted, for example, that the infant's state of arousal affected the meaning of many of his acts. For example, when infants are engaged jointly with their mothers, they are more likely to show affective expressions than when they are playing alone with objects (Adamson & Bakeman, 1985). The point here is that once a behavioral state has been evaluated, other behaviors can be analyzed relative to the state during which they occur. As a descriptive strategy this approach is very useful.

· To further distinguish the kinds of behaviors displayed by the infant or caregiver, therapists can classify behavior as being *physically* or *socially* based. Physically based behavior originates with the organism's physiology. A familiar example for coding physically based behavior is Ekman and Friesen's (1978) Facial Action Coding System (FACS). The FACS scores facial movement in terms of visible changes in the face brought on by the movement of discrete muscle groups. This system codes the various facial configurations. In contrast, a socially based approach would code such items as "sadness." Overall, socially based coding schemes require a greater degree of inference on the part of the observer. Thus, when observing the infant's affective manifestations, therapists should observe the degree to which the child displays a full spectrum of emotions and the ability of both caregiver and infant to modify emotional states flexibly. It is also useful to ascertain the extent to which the caregiver helps the infant coordinate his skills in achieving greater mastery over the interactions. Socially and physically based approaches provide descriptions on different levels. Physically based schemes, such as the FACS, can be time-consuming to learn and difficult to apply when observing a particular dyad. As a practical matter, socially based behaviors may provide a more available alternative during observation episodes.

In addition to the basic distinctions among behaviors, it is vital that therapists know how to classify their observations, that is, how to describe any given behavioral unit, either of a *particular event* or a *particular time interval*. The coding of intervals may be summarized as follows: An infant or a mother–infant dyad is observed for a period of time; the period is divided into relatively brief intervals (e.g., 10 to 15 seconds); the observer then categorizes each successive interval or notes which codable events, if any, occurred during each successive interval. Another method of recording is by addressing the *percentage of time* spent in each of the engagement states. This approach includes calculating the onset and offset time of a particular manifestation. Bakeman and Adamson (1984) provided some examples of this technique. Using videotapes, observers recorded onset times for, among other things, the six engagement states defined earlier, as well as affective expressions. From this record they were able to determine that 15-month-old infants and their mothers spent 23% of their observations in supportive joint behavior. This example reveals an important strength of creating a record that includes exact onset times for the various events defined in the coding approach. In this fashion the nature of the events observed (e.g., facial expressions, engagement states) can be related to each other.

In addition, therapists should strive to ascertain the intrapsychic results that are available from individual patients. For example, the therapist must address the complex task of the infant's *subjectivity*. How does the infant process what he feels? To understand the infant's subjective experience, the therapist must rely on observation.

As time goes by, the therapist will learn to predict the infant's behavior and, by observing dyadic interaction, will discern that child's typical patterns of response. Eventually, the therapist will be able to anticipate or predict the infant's response or the behavior that he will try to initiate in his partner. Predicting the infant's behavior taps into the child's subjective experience. Because the infant cannot speak and verbally communicate his subjective experience through language, the therapist must use observational skills to understand these internal perceptions. This kind of observation not only provides insight into such perceptions, but also yields an understanding of the dyadic relationship.

Initially, observation focuses on distinguishing between frequency events and duration events, on ascertaining whether interaction is physiologically or socially motivated, and on determining the intensity of response by a comparison of the developmental phenomena of one dyad with the developmental phenomena in other dyads. From these observations the therapist not only can extrapolate typical patterns of interaction and reaction in a particular dyad, but can also predict the infant's response. When these predictions appear accurate, in the sense that the infant manifests the anticipated behavior, it is likely that the therapist has achieved an understanding of the child's internal perceptions.

Another aspect of dyadic behavior that should be incorporated onto the therapist's observations involves what may be referred to as the *mechanisms of interaction*. Here the therapist should ask such questions as the following: Who initiated the interaction—the infant or the caregiver? Who terminated the interaction and how? Was the transition between behavioral states smooth or abrupt? Moreover, did the initiated behavior exercise the infant's newly acquired emerging developmental skills, or did the behavior appear to hinder the coordination of skills and emerging development? Can a pattern be identified within the interaction observed in that particular dyad? In other words, does the caregiver continually initiate exercises and interactions that assist the infant in articulating imminent developmental acquisitions, or conversely do the caregiver's behaviors appear to limit the infant's scope of development? By addressing these questions during observational episodes, the therapist can obtain a better understanding of how the caregiver and infant are forging their relationship. The therapist should be patient and, above all, should keep detailed records of observations until answers are forthcoming that clarify an understanding of the dyadic exchanges.

After each session, the therapist should write down key observations and reflect on them. Videotaping is also a helpful approach. The caregiver who agrees to permit videotaping during the session can provide the therapist with an invaluable tool for comparing direct observations with the impressions detected by the camera. In addition, many behavioral exchanges that are vital to a successful dyadic exchange occur on a micromomentary level that may be imperceptible to the human eye during normal observation, but that will be available during videotape analysis. Through observing videotapes, the therapist can determine the degree to which the caregiver has incorporated these developmentally enhancing behaviors into her repertoire of response. The videotape may also serve as a teaching tool for demonstrating to the caregiver how she can improve her ministrations with the infant.

Because observation is a key element in the diagnostic and treatment armamentarium for dyads, the therapist should essentially become immersed in observing the dyad's scope of interaction. Initially, it may take several weeks or months to note *discernible patterns* of interaction. Nevertheless, observations will eventually yield insight into the performance of each particular dyad. To this end, the therapist should be alert to the intensity of response, to the dyadic member who imitates interaction, and to the delineation of affective as well as cognitive skills. There should also be an attempt to predict infant response, because the capacity to anticipate the infant's reactions suggests that the therapist has attained an understanding of the infant's subjectivity.

INQUIRY

Beyond direct observation, the therapist's most potent tool for ascertaining information from the caregiver and for directing the course of the treatment is *inquiry*. Posing questions that elicit information makes the caregiver feel that every developmental phenomenon that the infant is experiencing or will experience can be interpreted in a fashion that enhances his developmental skills and the dyadic relationship. Thus, inquiry provides a way to ascertain that the caregiver understands the meaning of these phenomena. Inquiry allows the caregiver to enhance her competence during interactions with the infant by encouraging her to anticipate and predict the behavioral exchange in its broadest sense, and then to devise previewing behaviors that acquaint the infant with upcoming developmental skills.

To understand how inquiry can be used in caregiver–infant therapy, it is necessary to recognize that the therapist is imparting both substantive and procedural skills to the caregiver through this technique. Inquiry involves communicating, through a series of organized questions, all the diverse information the therapist strives to understand and share with the caregiver. Each question focuses attention on a specific capacity of the infant and the caregiver's ability to understand these infant capacities. On one occasion, for instance, the therapist may be seeking to familiarize the caregiver with the infant's perceptual and subjective experience. To accomplish this, the therapist would pose a series of questions that inquire about the infant's visual, hearing, smelling, and tactile responses when exposed to a particular stimulus. Each inquiry would coax the caregiver to a deeper level of analyzing the experience from the infant's point of view until an overlap occurs, enabling the caregiver to perceive and thus experience the stimulus almost entirely from the infant's perspective.

This process is used repeatedly during any given session to awaken or arouse the caregiver's perceptions from a cross-modal perspective. The cross-modal perspective refers to the infant's capacity to integrate perceptions in several sensory domains, such as sight, hearing, and smell. The point here is to convey to the caregiver that each activity she engages in with the infant or each new stimulus to which he is exposed sets in motion diverse sensory responses that affect his somatic, socio-affective, cognitive, and motivational status. Only when the infant's perceptions are understood in this integrated fashion will the caregiver be able to predict the course of future development and use her predictions to engage in previewing exchanges. When used in this fashion, inquiry reinforces awareness of the complexity and potential diversity of infant response. Inquiry also has a procedural aspect that enhances the caregiver's ability to predict or anticipate developmental change and to prevent conflict from interfering with the experience.

When viewed as a process, then, inquiry promotes the caregiver's capacities to match her perceptions of the infant with the representations being posited by the therapist. This exercise facilitates the matching of representations: The caregiver is stimulated to draw on her own intuitive powers and her own observational experiences to provide sophisticated predictions. Inquiry helps the caregiver understand that the infant is continually evolving and that she can anticipate and guide his future development in the direction of adaptation.

Inquiry here embraces the therapist's *questions, clarifications,* and *pauses* that elicit material necessary to carry the treatment forward, including all attempts to resolve ambiguities and uncertainties in the patient's verbal communications (Langs, 1973). Questions also aid in investigating relevant omissions that come to the therapist's attention and encourage the emergence of further fantasy and dream material. Moreover, questions help the patient to elaborate on perceptions, thereby offering the therapist a richer and more comprehensive view of the caregiver's interior life. Learning when and how to use questions during a treatment session is an art. In general, questions should not interrupt the patient's discourse. Such interruptions disrupt the patient's spontaneous thought processes and may convey that the therapist is more interested in obtaining data than in learning about the patient's internal struggles.

As a result, questions should be interposed when the patient reaches a pause and when major themes are being discussed. Another strategy to avoid is asking a series of questions in rapid succession. This form of excessive questioning breaks the patient's chain of thought and forces her to focus on surface material without probing more deeply into unconscious and more profound issues. Finally, it is important to remember that there are many occasions in therapy when silence is more appropriate than inquiry. Indeed, one of the most significant messages that the caregiver derives from treatment is that the therapeutic milieu is one in which she will be listened to; it is a safe haven within which unconscious and otherwise forbidden fantasies may be expressed and explored honestly, without threat or judgment. The therapist creates this atmosphere through the types of questions asked and the flexibility offered the caregiver to elaborate on issues. Particularly in the context of caregiver–infant therapy, it is important for the caregiver to feel she is entering an atmosphere where her innermost emotions about her infant will not be challenged, criticized, or judged.

Clarifications allow the therapist to restate the patient's communication back to her as she made it, or with some minimal alterations (Langs, 1973). For example, the therapist may add an emphasis not used by the patient to cue her to particular thoughts, fantasies, emotions, or conflicts. This form of cuing invites a further exploration of the meaning and implications of issues and thus leads to further insight. Langs has also identified another type of clarification, whereby the therapist explains or elaborates on his or her own remarks either in response to a patient's questions or because of realizing that the comments contain ambiguities.

Clarification may also provide a subtle interpretation. When used in this manner, clarification may be particularly effective because it engages patients in the actual process of interpretation. In addition, when the therapist asks for clarification, he or she may be exercising a form of confirmation. Used in this manner, clarification alerts patients that they have not provided enough insight or probed an issue with sufficient depth to offer insight.

On those occasions when the patient requests the therapist to clarify an inquiry, Langs offers the following advice. First, the therapist should not hesitate to clarify an ambiguity. Second, if the patient expresses confusion over an interpretation, the therapist should clarify it but should attempt to determine the source of the confusion. Finally, when patients seek clarification about an earlier session, Langs recommends that the therapist re-explore why the patient made the request, rather than immediately offering a clarification.

THERAPIST: Can you tell me about how you felt when you first brought the baby home?

CAREGIVER: Fine. We all loved having a baby in the house . . . my husband and my mother, who was always visiting and offering to help.

THERAPIST: So you were happy when the baby first arrived?

CAREGIVER: Yes, very . . . It wasn't until later that I got sad . . . (Pause) It happened suddenly when we were in the park . . . (Patient falls into a brooding silence.)

THERAPIST: (Waits to see if patient will continue, then) What happened in the park?

CAREGIVER: I just . . . I was just overcome with the strangest feeling . . . like I didn't want to see the baby any more . . . (Long pause) It was almost like I was disgusted by the baby . . . (Pause) I never actually said that before, but that's how I felt and I guess I'm glad I finally said it out loud.

Questions and clarifications are an important therapeutic tool for intervention and should be used from the onset of treatment. They convey to the caregiver that the therapist is interested in obtaining comprehensive insight into her relationship with the infant to identify any conflicts that might intrude on the relationship and to obtain consensually validated information.

The techniques of observation and inquiry described hasten the therapist's ability to detect areas of adaptation as well as maladaptation, during dyadic interaction. Thus, these techniques are vital to formulating a diagnostic profile for each dyad. Moreover, such techniques enable the therapist to detect the caregiver's capacity to preview upcoming development adaptively to the infant. After performing these techniques in several sessions, the therapist will likely be ready to institute specific exercises designed to treat dysfunction within the dyad. The caregiver, however, may not be ready to embark on these exercises, and as a consequence, it is often necessary to allow the caregiver a strategic period of evaluation—which I refer to as the *therapeutic pause*—to reassess her relationship with the infant.

During the pause, the caregiver will generally convey to the therapist an appropriate course to pursue in the treatment. Caregivers may express three basic responses during the period of the therapeutic pause. First, some caregivers will express a desire to return to the stage of elaborate description that characterized the therapist's initial observation and inquiry.

They will comment, for example, that they are still uncertain about portraying the infant's emotional or cognitive perceptions and wish to have the therapist continue to guide them in previewing behaviors for the infant. It will be necessary to continue the exercises in observation and inquiry until such caregivers feel comfortable and enthusiastic about probing more deeply into the relationship with the infant. Other caregivers will be relatively silent during this period, without either initiating questions or volunteering insights. In such cases, it is often wise for the therapist to present a brief summary of what he or she has observed during dyadic interaction and to offer an opinion of the type of relationship shared by caregiver and infant. This summary should emphasize the objective status of the infant's development. The summary will often stimulate the caregiver to communicate her perceptions more candidly with the therapist. Finally, a third group of caregivers will be eager to proceed with the therapy and will display this eagerness by raising issues that pertain to a direct conflict with the infant.

The pause is significant for the therapist as well, because it demarcates the diagnostic and treatment phases of the therapy. Although some aspects of the observational and inquiry exercises include a treatment dimension—as when the caregiver is asked to describe her observations of the infant or is asked to predict the future course of his development—until this point in the therapeutic encounter the therapist has primarily devoted energy to formulating a diagnosis. It is now necessary for the therapist to finalize this diagnosis, in the sense that particular areas of discord within the dyadic interaction have been identified and the factors impeding adaptive interaction have been exposed, and to begin devising strategies that will assist the caregiver in exploring and resolving these conflicts.

PERSPECTIVE TAKING

During the next phase of treatment the therapist will engage in the technique of perspective taking. The goal of *perspective taking* is to help the caregiver develop a perception of the infant's point of view and of the infant as a complex and sophisticated entity, who can manifest a unique perspective in the relationship. The caregiver must be attuned to this perspective before she can effectively recognize, nurture, and minister to the infant's needs during adaptive interaction. Once the caregiver begins to display skill at intuitively deciphering infant responses, the therapist's next goal is to guide the caregiver in perspective taking by asking her to interpret and attribute meaning to the infant's various manifestations. Eventually, the caregiver will realize that she not only can sense the infant's mood but, in fact, can also modify mood by engaging in particular forms of behavior.

THERAPIST: That's the first time I heard her make that noise. Is that a new noise?

CAREGIVER: She's been doing it for a couple of weeks.

THERAPIST: That was a very deliberate sound. What does it mean to you?

CAREGIVER: As I was saying earlier, by the time you figure one thing out, the meaning has changed. So, um . . . now (looks at baby and smiles) it could either mean "Gee, I really like this" or "Okay, that's enough, I want to do something else." It's very hard to figure it out, but it helps when I try to understand these changes from her point of view.

Thus, insight into the caregiver's ability to take the perspective of the infant yields information about the relationship that the caregiver is forging with the infant and alerts the caregiver to the infant's separateness and autonomy. Negotiating this delicate balance means that caregivers are able to sustain an internal representation of the infant's somatic and psychological state while perceiving objectively how they are responding to the infant.

Caregivers who engage in perspective taking will therefore not become too engrossed or overwhelmed by the infant's needs, such that an inappropriate response predominates. Nor will they ignore the infant's genuine cues for nurturance. In addition, such caregivers will be able to guide their mates in the nuances of perspective taking, thereby fostering balanced triadic interactions. Thus, caregivers who respond intuitively to the infant and engage in perspective taking will use the infant's presence to reinforce their perceptual abilities about the baby as well as their perceptual abilities between themselves and the therapist. Over time such caregivers will also become more adept at predicting future interactions with the infant.

Caregivers who have deficits in perspective taking (e.g. overpreoccupation with the infant) will likely exert a damaging effect on the family dynamics. The therapeutic task here is to function as a third member of the triangle by helping the caregiver compare her perceptions with the perceptions of the therapist.

To encourage the caregiver's intuitive skills it is necessary to direct the caregiver's attention to the behavior the infant is displaying as well as her own reactions. Similarly, in helping the caregiver develop skills for understanding the perspective of the infant, the therapist must urge the caregiver to focus on her own feelings and to share these emotions with a greater sense of freedom. When the caregiver shares her emotions about the infant's development, the therapist should convey to the caregiver not only that she is an individual with unique feelings but also that it is possible to articulate several interpretations about what is perceived.

An anecdote will help illustrate this point. A young mother I was treating had previously noted that her baby was beginning to intrude on her relationship with her husband. "I don't have the energy to do anything anymore," she complained. "At the end of the day, all I can do is sleep." I commented that it sounded as if the baby was making demands on her and asked her how this made her feel. She paused and concentrated deeply for awhile and then looked at her infant son, smiled nervously, and said, "Sometimes I don't know who's the baby . . . me or him." I conveyed to this caregiver my observation that these were precisely the sort of ambivalent feelings that she needed to share and explore so that she could contrast her perceptions with the perceptions of others.

The steps necessary to developing a therapeutic bond with caregivers who are having emotional difficulties with the infant are multifold. First, the therapist must accentuate and describe infant affective-behavioral displays, so that the caregiver can begin to understand how she is responding to the infant. Once intuitive responses emerge, the therapist should foster skills of perspective-taking, encouraging the caregiver to describe the somatic, socio-affective, cognitive, and motivational point of view of the infant. By adopting the infant's perspective, the caregiver will become more attuned to her own point of view. This realization will fuel her ability to represent the infant. Ultimately, the caregiver should become adept at integrating other interpretations of her own and the infant's behavior. The therapeutic relationship allows the caregiver to integrate the objective and subjective components of the relationship, which reinforces adaptive skills.

CONTRASTING THE PAST WITH THE PRESENT

A unique facet of interviewing caregivers and infants is that the therapist can understand both past and current interactions almost simultaneously, and can observe how the relationship between past and present modulates the infant's development. This statement may seem puzzling, but it is a relatively familiar phenomenon for therapists who engage in therapy with caregivers and infants. Essentially, one of the therapist's main tools during dyadic therapy is *observation*. By observing the interaction between the caregiver and infant, the therapist can help the caregiver distinguish which interactive patterns are based solely on the immediate experience with the infant, which responses derive from previous experiences, and which responses are being grafted onto the relationship. Caregivers should be alerted to how the infant can evoke memories and responses from the past. Thus, the therapist should urge caregivers to represent and contrast past and present and to extrapolate how factors such as infant development can evoke specific modes of interaction.

THERAPIST: Have you ever noticed that sometimes when your baby needs
    something she checks your face more or looks at you directly, eye to

eye? Or, on some days, when you're not feeling very well, that she's picking up on your emotional state?

CAREGIVER: Oh sure. Especially when I am not feeling well physically and I want to rest a little bit. I think at those times she is glad that I put her down. I sensed that she didn't want to sit by herself or even just in the same room with me for any amount of time.

THERAPIST: Does it take her long to realize what you are going through?

CAREGIVER: It's been changing. Now it's almost to a point where it's instantaneous.

THERAPIST: How have you learned about these changes?

CAREGIVER: It happened gradually, over time. I remember how it was when I first brought her home and how alert I am to her cues now. It's a process of comparison.

RECONSTRUCTION

During mother–infant intervention, therapists will often find the technique of *reconstruction* helpful. When used appropriately, reconstruction can lead to a dramatic lifting of repressive barriers and the consequent working through of conflict that is so crucial to progress in treatment.

In general terms, a reconstruction is an effort, based on what is both present in and missing from patient material, to fill in an apparently important gap in a recollection of a pivotal event in the patient's life. Reconstruction also attempts to discern the inner and outer implications of the event for the patient (Langs, 1973). The therapist must account for the gaps in the patient's memory to achieve a full understanding of a particular symptom and the anxieties, conflicts, and fantasies related to it. In sum, then, a reconstruction represents the therapist's effort to help the patient remember missing material that has been so effectively repressed that it remains inaccessible to direct awareness.

Reconstruction challenges the therapist's interpretive skills and when used appropriately can result in substantial progress for the patient. The need for reconstruction arises when the therapist intuitively senses that an explanatory event or fantasy is lacking from the patient's narrative (Langs, 1973). This occurs when the patient discloses material about a particular event but the conscious memories and fantasies appear to lack some pivotal event that could account for her current behaviors and fantasies.

Moreover, unless these lapses are eventually filled in it will be virtually impossible for the therapist to determine the source of the patient's unresolved conflict.

THERAPIST: You speak about a feeling of "resentment" toward the baby and this often comes up during conversations regarding your mother. Do you think there could be some connection?

CAREGIVER: I don't think so. My mother is very pleased with the baby and is always praising the baby. Of course, now that you mention it she does sometimes seem to overcompliment.

THERAPIST: What do you mean by overcompliment?

CAREGIVER: Well, it reminds me of the way my mother treated my sister.

THERAPIST: How is that?

CAREGIVER: My sister was always preferred and I was always criticized. Maybe I've transferred some of the resentment I felt toward my sister onto the baby.

INTERPRETATION

Interpretation may be viewed as the therapist's primary tool for effecting change in the patient on both intra- and interpersonal patterns. In the context of caregiver–infant therapy, interpretations implicate a change in meaning attribution (i.e., intrapsychic) and in the patterns of exchange (i.e., intrapersonal) between caregiver and infant. Thus, not only will the therapist be able to ascertain the effect of the interpretation from the caregiver's reports, but the therapist will also receive direct insight into how the patient applies or fails to apply the interpretation.

Interpretations can be defined as the verbal interventions through which the therapist makes material that was previously inaccessible to the patient's conscious available to the patient in a meaningful manner (Langs, 1973). The derivatives expressed in various verbal and nonverbal communications from the patient form the substrate for interpretations. According to Langs, the primary goal of an interpretation is to make conscious *latent motives* from which disturbed thoughts, fantasies, and interactions germinate. To render meaningful interpretations and to effect change, the therapist must discern the patient's latent content accurately. Thus, interpretation makes the previously latent material available to the patient's conscious, placing the caregiver in a position to reconsider the conflict and her adaptation to it, to assess the illogical and unrealistic nature of her thinking and fantasizing, and to contrast current motives and behaviors in light of these insights.

The goal of interpretation is to enlighten the caregiver's awareness of developmental processes and to provide her with a more objective perspective for interpreting aspects of the infant's current and future development such as how she is interacting with the infant, how she is predicting and enacting her predictions, how the infant is responding to her, and finally, how her predictions are shaping their current relationship. In this sense, interpretation enables the caregiver to step back and view herself as an active participant. At the same time, interpretations should enable caregivers to better understand how conflict stemming from another relationship is or may be potentially transferred onto the relationship with the infant. Overall, then, interpretations should provide insight into the caregiver's primary relationships and the way that they affect the present caregiver–infant relationship.

Langs distinguishes *specific* and *general* interpretations. Specific interpretations relate to specific unconscious derivatives, whereas general interpretations are more superficial and less defined. Therapists should use general interpretations, which are less threatening, in a preparatory manner that encourages the caregiver to focus on material related to latent or manifest conflict. Subsequently, specific interpretations allude to highly individual, well-disguised but evocative, fantasies that provide further insight into the nature of the conflict.

Therapists should keep in mind that the therapeutic alliance facilitates their passport to interpretation. In caregiver–infant therapy two processes continually influence each other: the relationship evolving between caregiver and therapist, and the relationship emerging between the caregiver and infant. In addition, the therapist needs to consider the role of development, which steadily influences each of these processes. Thus, the therapist must use the trends of development as objective parameters to ascertain how conflict is or may be intruding in future interactions to prevent adaptive trends of maturation from emerging.

By contrasting the dynamics inherent in both relationships (caregiver–infant and caregiver–therapist) and the developmental process that unfolds during these exchanges, the therapist can begin rendering interpretations. In this regard, questions pertaining to the infant's development and the caregiver's feelings about such development can assist the caregiver in revealing unconscious thought processes. In addition, by asking the caregiver to predict future interpersonal outcome with the infant—which is essentially what previewing strives to accomplish—the therapist can access the caregiver's unresolved conflict and can use interpretation to modify current or future behaviors.

THERAPIST: You were talking about how you think you will feel when Jessica begins talking.

CAREGIVER: I'm a little disappointed at her (looks at infant and shakes finger to simulate a scolding gesture). . . .

THERAPIST: Can you explain what you mean by disappointed?

CAREGIVER: Well, shouldn't she have started talking by now? I mean she's nearly 12 months, and she only says "Mama" or "Dada."

THERAPIST: Each infant develops differently. From what I've observed, Jessica is a happy baby who is developing at a normal pace.

CAREGIVER: Yes, but . . . I mean, my mother keeps asking when she will talk and I really have no explanation; I can't answer her. After all, my mother always said I spoke early, so I guess I expect Jessica to be the same.

THERAPIST: It's interesting you said you had "no explanation" to share with your mother. Maybe this is one time when you are disappointing your mother, not Jessica.

CAREGIVER: (Thinks about therapist's interpretation) That's interesting . . . I guess . . . I know I've always tried to please my mother and sometimes I sort of resent her meddling . . . but I didn't realize how much I let my mother's comments affect the way I feel about Jessica until you asked me this.

COUNTERPROJECTION

Counterprojection, another effective technique in dyadic therapy, represents a variation on the preceding method of interpretation. The common goal of both techniques is to promote adaptive developmental patterns within the dyad and to provide direct enhancement of caregiver intuition. Although interpretation aims at eventually solving the conflict by exploring the past, counterprojective techniques guide the caregiver's attention to the immediate implications of interactive sequences with the infant. By directing her attention to the interaction itself, the caregiver can begin to understand which behaviors or misperceptions evoke a response from the infant that fuels further discordant or disturbed responses in the relationship.

Counterprojection requires observing sequences of interaction while carefully appreciating the caregiver's narrative. During this monitoring period, the therapist will be particularly alert to the particular flow of information being exchanged between caregiver and infant, and to the signals that thwart adaptive exchange. For example, what are the caregiver's interpretations for not engaging in a sufficient amount of gazing behavior or appropriate holding behavior? If these or other intuitive responses are absent, the therapist should attempt to determine the dynamics involved. Once the therapist has some idea why adaptive behaviors are not in evidence during the interaction with the infant, he or she can begin using counterprojection to overcome these deficits and guide a more attuned perception of the interaction.

Counterprojection may require the therapist to isolate instances where the caregiver is either overidentifying with the infant or projecting aspects of herself onto the baby. For example, if the therapist senses that the caregiver is avoiding the infant and, as a consequence, that the infant is experiencing distress, the therapist may comment on the baby's discomfort. Having assumed the perspective of the infant, the therapist can then reflect back to the caregiver how the infant may be perceiving her behaviors in order for the caregiver to contrast her projections against what the infant is truly experiencing.

THERAPIST: Many caregivers entertain fantasies about their babies (turns to mother for reaction). Do you have any fantasies or wishes about your baby?

CAREGIVER: (Acutely uncomfortable) I don't want to discuss it!

THERAPIST: (Confronting) It will be better to verbalize your thoughts. You may think that by saying what you wish you're confirming it, but it's just the opposite. Usually, when you state your fantasy, it's almost as if you are relinquishing it.

CONFRONTATION

Often in treatment the patient is not yet ready for a full-fledged interpretation that will offer insight and lead to interpersonal change. The therapist will know that interpretation is not warranted because certain unconscious material (e.g., dreams, fantasies) will have been provided by the patient. Instead, the patient will display a series of common defenses, such as denial, avoidance, and rationalization. In these situations, *confrontation* represents one of the therapist's most reliable tools. Confrontation is critical in helping the patient modify and correct interpersonal dysfunctions such as the potential to act out impairments in reality testing or object relationships (e.g., abuse) that prevent the caregiver from dealing adaptively with the conflict (Langs, 1973).

Essentially, confrontations focus the patient's attention on various aspects of behavior and provide the patient with the realistic choices in a given situation. Confrontation is particularly effective in helping the patient to examine resistances. In short, confrontations are interventions in which the therapist directs the patient's attention to a particular behavior and says, in effect, "Consider what you are doing."

THERAPIST: You were telling me about how hectic it gets when your husband comes home.

CAREGIVER: Yes, sometimes it just gets crazy. Billy acts up so much. He gets so excited when he sees my husband. And my husband loves to see this. But then my husband starts playing with Billy and Billy messes up the floor or spills something. It's hard for me to calm him down. I even yell at him, but that doesn't seem to help either (interrupts herself, looks at her son who is playing with a toy truck)—Billy, stop it. Try to sit still!

THERAPIST: It sounds to me as if you have an infant who likes to play.

CAREGIVER: But he gets so excited and my husband just encourages it. I think we have a hyperactive kid.

THERAPIST: Have you ever asked your husband to try to refrain from exciting Billy?

CAREGIVER: Well . . . I guess . . . I guess not. I hadn't looked at it that way.

INTERVENTIONS DURING THE DIFFERENT STAGES

Caregivers often display a distinctive attitude of *autonomy* toward the therapist during the first few sessions and may appear to be in complete control of their infants. They answer all queries as if they are the repositories of knowledge about the infant and, in general, convey a stance of absolute competence. Nevertheless, the therapist who probes this ostensible posture of encyclopedic knowledge will often find that the descriptions of some caregivers are peculiarly mechanistic and inflexible. The infant's growth and development are viewed as linear, impersonal events that are independent of the emotional presence of the caregiver, and the infant himself is viewed much like an object, devoid of subjective experience or of an individual personality. During this phase techniques such as observation, inquiry, clarification, and perspective-taking are particularly useful.

As therapy progresses, however, the caregiver gradually relinquishes this attitude of almost rigid control and autonomy and replaces it with a new perspective that begins to incorporate the more objective attitude of the therapist. By the time this change occurs, the caregiver has become increasingly more receptive to the observations, inquiries, and interpretations of the therapist. During this middle period of treatment, it is as if the caregiver is attempting to gain a new perspective on the relationship with the infant by contrasting the therapist's point of view with her own. This phase is marked by an increased receptivity on the part of the caregiver, whose eagerness to avail herself of the therapist's guidance and insight paves the way for the development of a therapeutic alliance.

This transition of the caregiver from an attitude of encyclopedic knowledge about the infant and her role as the sole, autonomous interpreter of infant behavior, to one of receptivity to the therapist is best illustrated by an example culled from a case history. One mother had been in treatment with her 4-month-old infant daughter for 2 months. Throughout this period she had been thoroughly cooperative, rarely missing a session, arriving on time and dutifully reporting progress she had noticed with the infant during the previous weeks. Although this caregiver was intellectually receptive to my comments, she appeared reluctant to accept my interpretations and continually implied that she thoroughly understood each new manifestation the baby displayed. One week, however, I shared with her that the infant appeared particularly alert and was turning her gaze on others in a way I had not noticed before. The caregiver did not respond to this comment, other than with a smile. The following week she appeared depressed and vaguely irritable. When questioned, she admitted that she was angry at me. "I noticed Carol turning her head to look at you before, so why didn't you notice?" she said. Then she added, "I got upset on the way home last week, because I kept thinking about what you said. Maybe I see things you don't see, or you see things I don't see." We devoted the remainder of the session to discussing this new insight. For the first time, this caregiver was coming to recognize that her perspective of the infant was not and should not be exclusive; instead, others, such as the therapist, could harbor an independent perception of the infant's status and the relationship she shared with the infant.

The caregiver's comments represented a marked progression in the development of a therapeutic relationship. After this session the caregiver began to abandon her attitude as the ultimate interpreter of the infant's behaviors and started to consider the therapeutic viewpoint. This phenomenon, whereby the caregiver actively and eagerly immerses herself in the therapist's fresh perspective, signifies the middle, or working-through, stage of therapy. Now that her defenses are somewhat relaxed, the caregiver is able to see that others can provide meaningful insight into the infant's developmental processes, motivating her grasp of these insights in order to foster and enhance the baby's future development. During this phase of treatment the caregiver is willing to analyze her own perceptions of the infant and to contrast and incorporate the new perspective that emerges from discussion with the therapist.

The middle phase is, needless to say, a period of extreme and intense emotional and intellectual exertion for the caregiver. It may be argued that at this juncture the caregiver's sense of identity becomes more vulnerable to change, but this is only a transitory state. The caregiver has started to shift her perspective from an egocentric state to a perspective of the infant that embodies the viewpoint of the other, initially represented by the therapist and then eventually by the other caregiver. This shift is necessary for the caregiver to begin negotiating *equidistance* between her perceptions and the perceptions of others. Only when the caregiver can contrast the infant's perceptions from other points of view will she be able to understand and incorporate an integrated perspective of the infant. Indeed, unless the caregiver can conceptualize the infant from various perspectives, she will subsequently have difficulty in allowing the infant to explore and master burgeoning developmental capacities and, ultimately, in allowing the infant to exercise these skills in an autonomous fashion. During this phase, therapeutic techniques such as contrasting the past with the present, reconstruction, confrontation, interpretation, and counterprojection are particularly useful for acquainting the caregiver with insightful viewpoints about the infant.

The intensity of the relationship eventually diminishes in intensity as the caregiver begins, in a seemingly spontaneous fashion, to assert new perspectives and opinions about the infant's development. Now, however, the caregiver has a more balanced and integrated perspective for the following reasons: It is devoid of the anticipatory anxiety the caregiver previously experienced at the prospect of discovering new milestones, the developmental progression of the infant no longer causes a resurrection of the caregiver's own childhood conflict, and the caregiver has now learned to integrate new perspectives of the infant into her own representations in a way that does not threaten her pivotal role as the infant's main nurturer. The increasing ability of the caregiver to blend the various interpersonal and intrapersonal perceptions allows her to better predict and thus master the implications of developmental change.

THERAPIST: How did you feel about the changes you experienced during your pregnancy?

CAREGIVER: I had a difficult time adjusting to the pregnancy because the physical changes happened so fast that my mind couldn't react to them before more changes occurred. Both the physical and emotional changes were stressful. When I thought about how my body was changing and how my moods always changed, I felt helpless. I would just sit with my husband and cry.

THERAPIST: How do you feel about changes that take place now, after your child's birth?

CAREGIVER: Now if I feel stressed or my mood changes, I try not to act depressed in front of the baby. She picks up on my moods very easily. I have to be careful not to let my stress rub off on her and make her feel stressed.

THERAPIST: How do you know when she is picking up on your moods and feels stressed?

CAREGIVER: Sometimes if I'm in a bad mood she will be very fussy. She whimpers and waves her arms, but she doesn't want her bottle and she won't take a nap. She just picks up on how I'm feeling—sometimes I feel like whimpering! But now I've noticed that she isn't as sensitive to my moods as she used to be. I think she realizes that it is okay for her to be happy even if I'm not in a good mood.

It should be pointed out that therapists can expect this three-staged process to ensue when they deal with fairly adaptive parents. In certain instances, however, therapists will encounter caregivers with varying degrees of psychopathology who exhibit different observable patterns from the inception of treatment. For example, some caregivers will begin to transfer conflict onto the therapist from virtually the first session, indiscriminantly regressing or lapsing into maladaptive modes of behavior. For these caregivers it is almost as if the infant has usurped their role as the dependent individual. Such caregivers seize on the therapist as a new parental figure who will enable them to recapture their dependent status. When treating such caregivers, the therapist must work to strengthen the identity of the caregiver, so that she can minister to the infant in an adaptive fashion. Yet another variation on this theme occurs with caregivers who display a kind of obsessional attitude regarding the infant that precludes them from responding in a spontaneous fashion. In these cases, the caregiver will often cling to the role of a controller who is, despite this rigid stance, seemingly able to interpret and predict all facets of the infant's development.

Caregivers who move to the second phase of treatment too quickly because of the intensity of their interpersonal reactions, need help in establishing a secure, well-defined sense of self, which in turn permits them to relate to their infants without feeling that interaction represents a merging of boundaries and thus a loss of self. With such caregivers the therapist is encouraged to exhibit a high degree of structure and, whenever the opportunity arises, to intervene by interpreting their interaction with the infant and the therapist.

CONCLUSION

Caregiver–infant intervention moves along a well-delineated pathway, whereby the therapist may anticipate different phases of the treatment and apply specific techniques appropriate to these phases. Observation and inquiry dominate the first stage of the treatment as the therapist becomes more familiar with the caregiver's status and her capacity to predict the infant's upcoming development. Eventually, such inquiry yields to validation and the therapeutic pause, whereby the caregiver begins to relinquish earlier defenses and to characterize what for her is the central conflict in the relationship with the infant. Above all, this form of dyadic treatment strives to integrate the objective perspective captured in the infant's developmental growth with the subjective dimensions of the caregiver's own perceptions.

Dyadic treatment, then, takes a predictable course as the caregiver becomes increasingly attuned and sensitive to the infant's developmental trends. This sensitivity is heightened as the caregiver comes to understand that the subjective impressions of the infant transpiring within the dyad may be insufficient for a comprehensive understanding of his developmental experiences. As this realization becomes more apparent, the caregiver begins to focus on the therapist's insights. In turn, the therapist's task is to elucidate objective developmental trends for the caregiver and help her integrate perceptions of these trends into the daily experience with the infant.

This process is lengthy and arduous; during treatment the therapist will require a diverse array of techniques that sensitize the caregiver to the infant's needs and heighten her ability to predict his developmental transformations. The therapist can rely on several techniques for achieving these goals. Because dyadic therapy, by definition, highlights the primary relationship between caregiver and infant, diverse interventions may help the therapist enhance the communicative skill of both mother and infant.

Chapter 9

Strategies for Enhancing Previewing Through Representational Exercises

INTRODUCTION

Researchers have determined that during interaction within adaptive dyads, caregivers tend to manifest a series of subtle behaviors that provide rhythm and fluidity to the exchange. These subtle cues, often referred to as "intuitive behaviors," include visual contact, vocalizations, and appropriate holding behavior. In addition, adaptive caregivers also display a tendency to *preview* imminent developmental trends to their infants. That is, such caregivers seem acutely sensitive to infant manifestations and use their perceptions of infant behaviors to represent or envision upcoming developmental and interpersonal changes. Subsequently, the caregiver converts these representations into actual behavioral episodes or *rehearsals* that introduce the infant to the sensations of the new developmental milestone.

Thus, adaptive interaction between caregiver and infant appears to rely on the caregiver's heightened sensitivity or awareness, which enables her to experience the infant's perspective and to predict the contours of developmental growth. This sensitivity emerges in an especially compelling manner through the caregiver's representational capacities. *Representation* here refers to the ability to envision or imagine on the stage of active consciousness the infant's current developmental status and to compare this image with expectations of future growth. In this sense, representations are fantasies that contain specific information about desired future outcomes. It appears that adaptive caregivers engage in this process intuitively and are often unaware of the degree to which they are continually *predicting* the emergence of new skills on the part of the infant. In contrast, one feature that appears to characterize caregivers who have dysfunctional relationships with their infants is their seeming inability to predict or envision future developmental change through representational exercises. For such caregivers it is almost as if the future is a blank slate upon which they cannot imagine imposing their hopes for the future. As a result, therapy that promotes representational skills in maladaptive mothers and enhances representational capacities in adaptive mothers is likely to benefit the dyadic relationship. Learning these skills will enable maladaptive mothers to predict future outcomes and acquire a better sense of control and competence in guiding the interaction with the infant. Moreover, because representation intensifies the ability to predict developmental change, such mothers are likely to experience a new sense of mastery in the relationship, which they may also share with the infant. But this form of treatment may also benefit caregivers who are already fairly competent in their nurturing and representational skills. After learning how to engage in representational exercises in a more systematic way, such caregivers are likely to acquire more profound insight into the infant's developmental processes. This more refined level of insight can be directly applied to the behavioral exchange with the infant.

Representational techniques offer unique psychological advantages for both the therapist and the caregiver who are attempting to achieve a greater degree of rapport with the infant. First, the imagery generated during representational exercises is not confined by the ordinary rules of space, time, and motion, or by linear logic. Thus, caregivers can shift from one event to another, linking ideas in a freely associative manner with regard to a specific content. Anticipations about future events can be brought into the present, as the caregiver begins to experiment with different kinds of behavioral responses. Representation is also a highly flexible way to express ideas, because the therapist can suggest new situations, alternatives, concepts, and actions. Moreover, engaging in imagery is safe, in that patients can experiment with ideas and behaviors without incurring the risk of consequences. This quality of experimentation, particularly regarding future endeavors, makes representational exercises appropriate to the setting of dyadic treatment, in which the therapist is attempting to promote previewing behaviors and to instill more accurate and adaptive perceptions concerning infant development.

The therapeutic attraction of representational exercises lies in two qualities that are embedded in this technique: the ability to formulate predictions and the capacity to exert a measure of control over upcoming events. Researchers have now confirmed that many forms of depression result in the subjective experience of powerlessness and uncontrollability. The individual is caught in an inexorable tide of uncontrollable events and is helpless to stop or deter the onslaught. Strategies that enable the individual somehow to impose control and purpose, and to exert the potency of his or her will, have often been successful in remitting the depressive affect. Representational exercises are analogous to these depression-lifting strategies. They provide a domain that liberates the caregiver from the constraints of time and space. Within an atmosphere of guidance and support, the therapist directs the caregiver first to envision the spectrum of infant development and then to intercede as a primary actor in determining the fate of the infant as well as the imminent direction of the dyadic relationship. As a result, principles of prediction and control are instilled in the caregiver, who is empowered to act on her newly revived skills by devising previewing exercises.

This chapter outlines a roster of representational exercises that the therapist can use during dyadic therapy. As will be seen, the goal of these exercises is twofold. First, the therapist encourages the caregiver to use mental representations to gain greater familiarity with the infant's current developmental status and the extent of his communicative abilities. Second, these exercises promote skills of prediction and control while encouraging previewing behaviors that help the caregiver understand imminent developmental change and the implications of such change on the dyadic relationship.

MENTAL REPRESENTATION

Using the most expansive definition, representation refers to the perceptual capacities that allow the individual to envision a past, current, or future event or object in the absence of that event's or object's direct external stimulation. Representations contain a heterogenous array of affective, verbal, and visual imagery concerning the specific meaning the individual attributes to the events or objects. In this sense, representations are full-fledged fantasies that are richly endowed with all of the sensory elements that make fantasies such compelling and complex diversions.

There are a number of factors to consider when evaluating representations. First, even when the therapist directs the creation of images, the individual may still direct the images generated and elaborate on content of the representation. These elaborations have therapeutic significance and warrant greater investigation because they provide access to the patient's interior reality. Research by Spanos (1971) and Kazdin (1979) has clearly demonstrated that better responses to imagery may be obtained when subjects actively elaborate suggested scenes. This exercise enables the therapist to develop an understanding of the caregiver's style of representing information. In addition, the caregiver may form images that differ from the therapist's intent, providing further insight into the caregiver's preoccupations.

The ability to represent is comparable to forming composites of experiences rather than merely pictorial images of events. In addition, pictorial images can be constructed simultaneously while formulating new interpretations and then discarded at the end of such processes. As a result, researchers generally concur that equating representations with the process of generating a "mental image" is not adequate to describe the complexity of how individuals generate internal representations. Rather, they have suggested that the so-called *propositional network theory,* which considers data structuring as a main element of internal imagery, may have more value in explaining the nature of representations derived from the external world (Elliot & Ozolins, 1983). In this sense, representation may be considered an *active* process of construction and reconstruction, rather than merely a passive review of material.

All of these investigations, however, recognize one significant fact: Representation appears to be the mechanism whereby individuals process images and information about the most important events in their lives. The representations of the caregiver concerning the infant, therefore, are highly significant when the therapist is probing the caregiver's awareness of infant developmental trends. From such representations the caregiver formulates impressions about the overall course of infant development and about imminent developmental events, and ultimately designs previewing behaviors to forge an adaptive relationship that enhances infant maturational capacities. The caregiver's representations will enlighten the therapist about how the caregiver will predict and then control the future course of her relationship with the infant.

Other researchers, most notably Singer (1971), Tower and Singer (1981), and Anderson (1978) have approached imagery from a different level, commenting that the main function of such imagery is to process sensorimotor input. Singer has suggested that a series of well-established images become ingrained in memory over time, so that the individual accumulates a blueprint of increased complexity. In this fashion, automatic behaviors are emitted without conscious effort while the processing of new information is taking place on a different level. For example, an individual can drive a car along a familiar route while maintaining a conversation. Debate still exists as to whether representational imagery is a *digital function,* in that cognitive processes generate complex images in an abstract or symbolic form, or whether representation is an *analogic* form of communication. By analogic is meant that the individual actually perceives the representation on a sensory level (e.g., through sight, smell, sound, taste, or touch). The imagery would thus be analogous to the content of the material being imagined. Representation is the initial step taken by the caregiver in the *previewing* process, and previewing exercises incorporate analogic forms of communication that enable the caregiver to enact through behavioral ministrations with the infant in the present. Previewing exercises also represent events that have not yet been encountered and thus incorporate a digital form of communication. It is probable, therefore, that both digital and analogic aspects of communication are utilized during representational exercises.

Researchers such as Piaget and Inhelder (1971) have written about how the individual synthesizes the imagery generated during representation. These researchers have divided imagery into two categories: reproductive imagery and anticipatory imagery. *Reproductive imagery* refers to a concrete photographic image that transpires when the subject experiences an event and, subsequently, replicates the event in memory just as it occurred in reality. *Anticipatory imagery* involves manipulation or alteration of the image. Through anticipatory imagery the subject can generate novel scenes and behaviors. As the infant begins to manifest behaviors indicating an upcoming behavioral milestone, for example, the caregiver transforms her perceptions of these manifestations and recombines them to generate new images that delineate the infant's future development and the effect of such future development on her relationship with the infant. By relying on representations, the caregiver generates scenarios that anticipate imminent changes in the dyadic interaction and, in turn, uses these predictions to devise previewing exercises that acquaint the infant with upcoming developmental and interpersonal changes.

This description of the representational process suggests that caregivers whose capacity to represent is hindered by conflicts may be unable to provide their infants with an adequate degree of previewing to stimulate future developmental achievement. It becomes incumbent upon the therapist to discern relatively early in the treatment the degree to which the caregiver can create vivid, clear, and sensorialy rich representations of upcoming developmental and interpersonal changes. Therapists should explore whether the caregiver can generate increasingly complex representations to help the infant coordinate previous and imminent experience so that developmental and interpersonal change becomes predictable and, to a certain degree, controllable. From such predictions the caregiver and infant can begin to rehearse future changes together in the form of previewing exercises. Thus, the therapist should explore the caregiver's representational skills throughout the treatment.

Therapists should also be especially attuned to the relationship between internal representation and external perception in the caregiver and should observe behavioral sequences between mother and infant to evaluate the status of interaction within the dyad. This type of objective assessment should be performed at each session. Once therapists become familiar with conducting an objective assessment, they should probe the caregiver's subjective impressions of behavioral sequences with the infant. The interacting of infant and caregiver during sessions enables the therapist to compare almost instantaneously the objective interaction with the caregiver's subjective impressions. Therapists can thereby discern how these subjective impressions are converted into interpersonal manifestations.

A consciousness of imagery is another dimension pertinent to the evaluation and assessment of the caregiver's representational capacities. Data reviewed by Singer (1974) and Tower and Singer (1981) indicate that the therapist should not assume the caregiver's awareness of representational ability. Most likely, representations exist whether she is aware of them or not. Data suggest that representations are continually being generated and processed, and that under certain conditions individuals can learn to become more attuned to these processes. Dyadic therapy in which the caregiver is instructed to be sensitive to her representations and to relate them to the therapist verbally is one method for reinforcing such awareness. In the optimal situation, however, the caregiver will be cognizant of her representations concerning the infant, will reflect on these representations, and will use them to formulate previewing exercises that she enacts during interaction to enhance the infant's developmental potential.

Thus a number of especially important issues should be considered when assessing representational abilities. Is the caregiver representing spontaneously or does she have to make a significant effort to do so? Does the caregiver display flexibility and diversity in her representations? What is the relationship between the representations and the external perceptions from which the representations are derived? What objective and subjective impressions of the dyadic relationship does each representation convey? Is the patient conscious of the representational process? Does the capacity to represent improve if the patient is encouraged to generate imagery? How does the caregiver transpose her representations into previewing exercises? How does the caregiver's emotional status affect representational and previewing processes? Is the caregiver aware of the interpersonal implications of future developmental outcome?

A highly adaptive caregiver may accumulate a repository of representations that she subsequently may experiment with, rearrange, and use derivatively to generate new representations. In addition, such caregivers will be likely to express enjoyment at their capacity for predicting the future course of infant development and to voice feelings of control concerning the dyadic interaction. In less optimal circumstances, the caregiver may represent the infant in a concrete fashion but be less able to generate abstract representations. The therapist should encourage such caregivers to discuss developmental milestones attained by the infant and should also explain the phenomenon of precursory changes—those changes in infant behavior that suggest imminent acquisition of a new skill. After several weeks, most caregivers will become more adept in their observations and will begin to disclose information voluntarily about the infant and the infant's development.

CAREGIVER: Now that he is walking, it is very hard to talk to him. I am just afraid that his speech is going to fall behind.

THERAPIST: What strategy do you think you should use?

CAREGIVER: Maybe I should just follow him everywhere he goes (anxious).

THERAPIST: Would you feel comfortable doing that?

CAREGIVER: No—not really.

THERAPIST: It might be interesting for you to speak to him while he is walking. You might point out objects and pronounce their names. That way he can integrate walking with talking.

CAREGIVER: Should I let him go around the house when he wants?

THERAPIST: If you guide him. How would you feel trying these exercises with him?

CAREGIVER: I would like to try doing them.

THERAPIST: Can you make some predictions as to how he may respond to you?

CAREGIVER: (Practices with infant pointing at new objects) The only thing I've gotten so far is a headshake "yes" that he wants me to open a box for him, instead of him throwing it at me. He imitates me. I nod my head "yes," and he nods his head.

THERAPIST: How do you interpret this reaction?

CAREGIVER: I think he likes this exercise.

In other cases, the caregiver's representations concerning her infant may be overtly hostile and aggressive. For example, one caregiver in treatment reported a recurrent daydream in which she and her infant were taken hostage. Although she managed to escape, the infant did not—nor did the caregiver attempt to rescue the infant. As a consequence, the infant was shot by the kidnappers. Another caregiver in treatment reported that she occasionally imagined her infant was laughing at her when she wasn't looking at him. Thus, when exploring the representational abilities of the caregiver, therapists should discern whether the caregiver's representational disclosures suggest an adaptive, maladaptive, or somewhat less than optimal perspective on the infant's development. Moreover, therapists should observe carefully the immediate implications that such explorations may have in the dyadic interaction and should determine whether any discrepancies exist between the caregiver's representations and her overt behaviors with the infant.

Although the preceding examples of maladaptive representations may be extreme instances of hostile representations, adaptive caregivers may also have periodic representations tinged with ambivalence about their infants. One such mother commented that she had envisioned the experience of abusing her infant. She reported extreme anxiety concerning this representation but eventually disclosed it to the therapist. This reaction is not uncommon in adaptive mothers, who are ultimately able to confide their fantasies—even negative fantasies—about the infant to the therapist and thereby deter possible enactment of the representation. Such mothers should be encouraged to disclose all representations. By having the caregiver engage in this activity, the therapist gains insight into the caregiver's overall thought processes and the flexibility with which she represents the infant's development and the continually changing relationship with the infant that results from these developmental processes. From such disclosures the therapist can determine which representational exercises will be most beneficial for the caregiver.

THE CONCEPT OF REPRESENTATIONAL EXERCISES

One of the therapist's first tasks in helping new mothers relate to their infants and interact in a more adaptive fashion is to educate caregivers about the role of representational exercises. The goal here is to enable caregivers to represent and ultimately experience the world from the perspective of the infant. Accessing a patient's representations is highly beneficial during intervention because imagery techniques help patients gain insight into their own deep and previously hidden motivations. In addition, representational techniques give the patient free rein to anticipate upcoming events and to rely on therapeutic support to effect changes in behavior that will result in more adaptive outcomes. Sherman and Fredman (1986) have outlined a catalog of representational strategies that may be used effectively during therapy, including *association, construction, completion,* and *expression.* During association patients are asked explicitly or implicitly to respond to a word, image, idea, or story. During construction exercises patients devise their own stories, fantasies, and family sculptures. The actual content of the construction will be the patient's own invention, although the fantasy will be a direct response to a request by the therapist. Completion exercises require the patient to finish a cue suggested by the therapist, such as a sentence. Therapists may also ask patients to finish a story or contribute to a fantasy or daydream initiated by the therapist, group, or other family member. When relying on expression exercises, the therapist allows the patient free expression in play, arts, crafts, writing, drama, puppetry, or dreams to represent herself and her experience in any way she sees fit. Patients can also be asked to select and bring in important pictures from the family album or to recall early memories.

An understanding of the potency of representational techniques indicates why these strategies have been such productive tools for diagnosis and treatment resulting in adaptive changes (Morris, 1970). Essentially, it is useful to think of representations as the exercise of the imaginary capacities. As Sherman and Fredman (1986) observe, these imaginary techniques have long been used by family therapists who have relied on the imagery evoked by family photographs, puppetry, poetry readings, writings, imagery, and metaphor to heighten perceptions concerning behavior among family members. In this context, representations refer to individuals (e.g., the infant), events, and experiences (e.g., developmental change) that are real or imaginary. In generating these representations, the caregiver experiences perceptions from some or all of the five senses. Moreover, as Araoz (1982) has noted, creating a representational image is more experiential than critical, more subjective than outer-reality oriented, and more primary process than secondary process thinking. Therefore, during representational exercises the caregiver will be accessing so-called primitive thought processes, which operate on the deepest level of perception. Needless to say, access to these processes is extremely helpful to the therapeutic effort because it enables both therapist and caregiver to bring to the surface the caregiver's deepest perceptions concerning the infant.

Describing the process of representation in greater detail, Sherman and Fredman (1986) have commented that individuals *create* images of themselves in the world and guide their actions according to such images. These images not only capture the meaning of past experiences, but also lead to the *anticipation* of future events. Examination of the representational disclosures of patients in psychotherapy has identified three processes that transform experience into an image that differs from original reality: *generalization, deletion,* and *distortion* (Bandler & Grinder, 1975). Generalization is the process of extrapolating one aspect of an experience and using it to represent the entire experience and all other experiences in the same category. As an example, a couple whose first child was born with a congenital defect would decide not to have any more children because they have come to believe all their progeny would suffer from the same defect, despite medical evidence to the contrary. Deletion is the process by which individuals selectively pay attention to certain aspects of experience while excluding other details. For example, a depressed individual who imagines that her entire life is a failure and that she can do nothing worthwhile, despite previous successful romantic and professional experiences, is engaging in deletion. Finally, distortion is the process that enables individuals to transform their experience of sensory data. Distortion occurs when an artist alters a landscape based on his own impressions.

Throughout this chapter, the phrase representational exercises is used to describe a technique that appears to be particularly useful in conducting dyadic therapy involving a caregiver and infant. Representation encompasses more than the ability to maintain already-experienced images in consciousness. It also includes the capacity to rely on images of earlier experiences to formulate new images about the future. Thus, a caregiver with a 4-month-old infant may be asked to represent her perceptions of her infant when he was 2 months old, as he is currently, and how he will be when he is 6 months old. The first two representations will depend on the caregiver's sensitivity to infant manifestations, as well as the sharpness of her recall, whereas the last representation—involving an image of what the infant will be like in the future—requires the caregiver to devise a new, not yet experienced image based on predictions of upcoming development.

This last form of intervention, involving the representation of future interaction with the infant, challenges the caregiver's skills to their fullest capacity. Not only must the caregiver envision the nature of the infant's upcoming skills, she also must formulate an image of how her relationship with the infant will change as a result of his maturational abilities. Representational exercises *heighten* the caregiver's own sense of attunement both to infant manifestations and to expectations concerning interpersonal changes in the relationship with the infant. By representing these changes, the caregiver assesses her sense of control and mastery over the dyadic relationship, which will tend to infuse the interaction and be conveyed directly to the infant. Moreover, representational exercises also allow therapists to *prepare* caregivers for events that often disrupt dyadic rapport, such as developmental transitions, separation, and the evocation of the caregiver's memories concerning past experiences with her own caregiver. Finally, representational exercises heighten the caregiver's perceptions of the infant's experience. The rapport that adaptive caregivers share with their infants emerges, in part, because of their acute sensitivity to the infant's experience. They not only can empathize with the infant, but can also imagine the infant's perceptual experience from his perspective. This refined level of sensitivity enables the caregiver to control the course of the infant's development, while infusing the infant with feelings of mastery about the future.

The following discussion outlines a series of representational exercises that can be integrated into the treatment protocols of caregiver–infant dyads.

Representing the Infant's Arrival

Helping new parents acclimate to the birth of an infant can be immensely gratifying for the therapist. Interventions to help expectant parents prepare for the infant's arrival may be most effective when the therapist works vicariously with either one or both of the caregivers. Preparation for the infant's arrival is crucial for a variety of reasons. First, a new birth may herald a resurrection of childhood conflicts in the parents. In some cases, an impending birth triggers memories of a mourning cycle because it threatens the marital relationship. Parents may also be reminded of childhood memories that involved their own scapegoating within or exclusion from the family unit. In addition, the parents may feel that the infant's arrival in the family will shatter their own intimacy. Patterns of privacy may be disrupted, and the infant's schedule looms as an unpredictable intrusion on the patterns of interaction the caregivers have established. Moreover, the imminence of the infant's birth causes the caregivers to reevaluate their preparedness for assuming the parental roles, which can arouse feelings of uncertainty. Thus, the new birth will be traumatic because it may disrupt modes of interaction to which husband and wife have grown accustomed. If the caregivers experience the resurrection of earlier memories and anxiety concerning their own future relationship, it may ultimately be problematic for them to establish a positive bond with the infant. More often than not, caregivers bring unresolved conflict(s) of previous relationships into the interaction with the infant. The therapist's task in this situation is to clarify the family and individual case history of each new parent when preparing the caregivers for representing the infant's arrival.

Caregivers should be asked to represent how they believe the arrival of the infant will change their lives and, in this regard, should be asked to describe specific changes in daily routine and the like. As the caregivers become more adept at engaging in these representations, the therapist can begin probing deeper issues, such as the awakening of conflict that the baby's birth presents. As these conflicts are explored, the therapist should first allow the caregiver to express anxieties or negative fantasies and then encourage the caregiver to devise more adaptive predictions.

THERAPIST: What changes in daily routine will the baby have on your life and your husband's life?

CAREGIVER: (Deep sigh) In some ways I don't look forward to it. All my friends tell me I'll be up all night feeding a crying baby and I don't think my husband will be much help.

THERAPIST: Sometimes it takes some time to get used to the baby's schedule, but most of the mothers who see me say that after a while they get used to it and are able to predict when the baby will need to be fed.

CAREGIVER: Do you think so? But then, of course, sometimes I think of other things . . .

THERAPIST: Can you tell me what other things you think about?

CAREGIVER: I . . . I am . . . well, what if the baby is born with some kind of defect or . . . worse?

THERAPIST: Many of the women I have spoken with voiced the same concern. In fact, it seems to be quite common for expectant mothers to have those concerns.

CAREGIVER: My obstetrician says everything is fine. But I just can't help imagining . . .

THERAPIST: What do you imagine?

CAREGIVER: Just . . . that the baby will have some sort of defect.

THERAPIST: It probably will help you to focus on what the obstetrician has said. That is objective evidence that your pregnancy is going well. Also, you shouldn't be afraid to express your fears. But you should recognize that they seem to be the kinds of common trepidations most women undergo. By focusing on those fears too much though, you may prevent yourself from preparing for the arrival of a healthy new baby, which is the most likely outcome.

CAREGIVER: You may be right. I didn't think about it like that before.

Representing the Somatic, Socio-Affective, Cognitive, and Motivational Dimensions

This representational exercise emphasizes an awareness of the various modes of expression the infant uses to communicate subjective states. An understanding of these dimensions helps the caregiver better understand the world from the infant's point of view. To help caregivers comprehend the infant's communicative cues, the therapist should ask the caregiver to describe the infant's facial expression, vocalizations, gestures, and body movements, and to contrast them with their own observations. After each such description the therapist should probe more deeply, encouraging the caregiver to provide a multidimensional (somatic, socio-affective, cognitive, and motivational) characterization that captures the complexity of the infant's response. If, for example, the caregiver comments that the infant is expressing "happiness," the therapist should ask the caregiver to describe the various components of the infant's facial expression. Is the infant partially smiling, smiling with ambivalence, or displaying a full smile? The infant's simultaneous vocalizations need to be described as well. Is the infant laughing or squealing? Arm gestures may be characterized by the infant's displays of clapping and flapping, whereas a description of posture would focus on whether the infant is erect or is jumping up and down. By characterizing the infant's socio-affective skills in this manner, the therapist conveys to the caregiver that each discrete affect (e.g., happiness) correlates with numerous dimensions (e.g., proximity-seeking), and that socio-affective cues can be differentiated and then integrated to ascertain the infant's overall mood.

Similar exercises help the caregiver characterize the cognitive dimensions of the infant's experience. During the first months of life when the infant cannot yet communicate through language, cognitive capacities can be addressed derivatively by describing the infant's socio-affective responses. Cognitive processing requires the ability to engage in comparative analysis of the different stimuli that confront the infant, and to rely on immediate and remote memory. Cognitive processing also enables the infant to formulate a behavioral strategy for achieving control by perceiving a cause–effect sequence or relationship between stimuli.

Researchers such as Blass, Ganchrow, and Steiner (1984) have demonstrated how affective expression and contingency learning are interrelated during infancy. Infants as young as 2 hours old were gently stroked on their foreheads during 18 two-minute conditioning trials. Following the stroking sessions, each infant received a dose of intraoral sucrose. Members of a control group received sucrose in each trial but were not stroked. Following the trials, infants in both groups were exposed to 9 one-minute extinction trials in which they were just stroked. The infants in the control group showed no evidence of conditioning. Members of the experimental group, however, emitted more head orienting and sucking responses during the stroking sessions and showed a classic extinction function to head stroking during extinction trials. In addition, 7 of the 9 infants in the experimental group cried during the extinction trials, compared with only one of the 16 infants in the control group. Taken together, the data from Blass et al. indicate that disruption of a contingency relationship—and thus of the infant's expectation of experiencing a future contingency (e.g., head stroking while feeding)—produces negative affect.

For caregivers to formulate, interpret, and represent the infant's motivational patterns, then, they must interpret somatic, socio-affective, and cognitive signals. Thus, it is important for the caregiver to understand that the infant's development represents a dynamic process requiring the *coordination* of numerous skills to achieve a sense of coherence. This representational exercise focuses on the caregiver's ability to guide the infant toward coordinating diverse developmental phenomena.

Once the caregiver becomes attuned to the notion of perceptual coordination and its role for overall adaptive maturation, the therapist should encourage representations involving the discrete behaviors that promote adaptation in several of these domains. For example, the therapist might ask the caregiver to imagine an interactional sequence in which the infant's somatic, socio-affective, cognitive, and motivational dimensions are stimulated simultaneously. As a result of engaging in this representational exercise, the caregiver will come to recognize that while singing a song to the infant, she needs also to attend to the gestures she is exhibiting. By being aware of all of these domains of functioning, the caregiver will gradually learn to coordinate interactional behaviors. Coordination is especially important because it promotes self-regulation and thus the experience of internal control. For example, the therapist should ask the caregiver to interact with the infant and describe the particular affects the infant is expressing, and then ask the caregiver what thoughts she believes the infant is processing during that particular interaction. Moreover, the infant's cognitive patterns may be tapped by focusing on such dimensions as attention and concentration span. The therapist should ask questions such as the following: What emotions is the infant expressing? What kinds of events tend to evoke them? How long was the infant able to pay attention to and concentrate on the ministrations? Was the infant shifting attention while the caregiver tried to engage him? The following dialogue suggests how the therapist can guide the caregiver in this representational exercise:

THERAPIST: How would you describe his mood right now?

CAREGIVER: Right now? (Turns baby to her, places him on shoulder to burp him) Right now he's in a good mood (confident).

THERAPIST: How would you describe his behavior when he is in a bad mood?

CAREGIVER: He whines or he's bored or looks tired.

THERAPIST: (Shows infant a teddy bear he has not seen before) Can you give me your impressions of what the baby is feeling now?

CAREGIVER: (Looks at infant's face and strokes the back of his head) Umm . . . I think he's excited and curious, because he raised his eyebrows and made his "happy noise."

THERAPIST: What is he thinking?

CAREGIVER: He's probably thinking about how this stuffed bear is different from all his other bears and stuffed animals.

THERAPIST: Is there anything in his response that captures your attention?

CAREGIVER: Yes, he's reaching out with his hand to grab the bear. I think he recognizes what fur looks like now and likes it because it feels soft to touch.

Representing the Infant's Temperament

The term *temperament* refers to the individual's behavioral style. Researchers now concur that temperament is constitutional and is discernible shortly after birth. An excellent starting point for acquainting caregivers with the skill of representation is for the therapist to inquire about the infant's temperament, because most caregivers harbor some basic perceptions about the infant's constitutional disposition. Therapists may first wish to introduce caregivers to the nine dimensions that make up a temperamental profile, as outlined by Thomas and Chess (1977): the level and extent of *motor activity;* the *rhythmicity, degree of regularity of function* exhibited during eating, elimination, and between the cycles of sleeping and wakefulness; the *response to a new object* or *person;* the *adaptability of behavior* to changes in the environment; the *threshold* or *sensitivity to stimuli;* the *intensity* or *energy level of responses;* the infant's *overall mood,* such as pleasant or cranky, friendly or unfriendly; the infant's *degree of distractibility;* and the infant's *attention span* or *persistence.*

Researchers in the field of temperament have found that the nine basic temperamental traits or dimensions may be grouped into constellations, or clusters. These syndromes of temperamental type have been correlated with different affective profiles. The three main temperamental types identified by Thomas and Chess are "easy," "difficult," and "slow to warm up." Infants with easy temperaments are characterized by rhythmicity, regularity of function, and easy responses. Infants with difficult temperaments tend to withdraw from new stimuli, show low adaptability, negative mood, and irregularity. Finally, slow-to-warm-up infants manifest a quiet disposition and tend to be slow in their ability to adapt to new stimuli and circumstances. Once the caregiver has described her infant's behavior with regard to each dimension, she should cluster the categories of temperamental dimensions in order to describe the infant as having an *easy, difficult,* or *slow-to-warm-up* temperament. In addition, the caregiver should provide a description of her own temperamental status and comment on whether she feels her temperament is well-suited to the infant's temperament.

THERAPIST: Can you describe the baby's temperament?

CAREGIVER: What do you mean by temperament?

THERAPIST: Your baby's overall disposition. Is she calm or excitable, does she appear to be very active, does she show regularity in her daily cycles of sleeping and waking, and in her eating patterns? If you had to characterize these types of qualities, how would you describe her?

CAREGIVER: I guess she's pretty active and she has a good disposition. She responds well to new people, as if she welcomes them, but she doesn't get overly excited with them.

THERAPIST: The combination of qualities you are describing is usually referred to as an "easy" disposition. Would you agree with this characterization?

Representing Cross-Modal Abilities

The capacity for transferring sensory impressions from one perceptual modality such as seeing to another perceptual modality such as touching is known as *cross-modal* functioning and provides insight into how the infant coordinates diverse perceptions impinging from the environment. Researchers have focused on cross-modal functioning in infants to determine the level of perceptual processing during early life. For example, neonates with a mean age of 72 hours have been found to be able to discriminate and imitate happy, sad, and surprised facial expressions (Field et al., 1982). Thus, as early as the neonatal stage, the infant appears capable of storing abstract representations of the visual images of objects or events (Meltzoff, 1981). Such representations are then compared against the infant's own proprioceptive feedback that derives from his own facial movements (Meltzoff & Moore, 1977; Reissland, 1988). This finding indicates that the infant can *transfer* experiences perceived in one modality into other modalities, e.g., from visual to facial movements. Transferring information from one mode to another permits the infant to identify the variant and invariant features of objects, and thus to convert temporary mental representations into stable schemes (Piaget, 1952; Trad, 1990).

One of the most important achievements for any caregiver is to represent how the infant acquires information about the external world and coordinates it through cross-modal functioning. Cross-modal integration refers to the variety of skills that assist the infant in integrating diverse sensory perceptions and formulating an integrated view of a particular stimulus. To represent cross-modal abilities, the caregiver needs to represent each discrete sensory mode through which the infant perceives information. For example, certain cues, such as the caregiver's vocalizations, are conveyed to the infant audiovisually (i.e., the infant often both hears the sounds and sees the caregiver's face—particularly the lips—as she is emitting the vocalizations), whereas other cues, such as the caregiver's stroking of the infant's face, are experienced through the perception of touch. Caregivers should be encouraged to represent how the infant assembles and integrates this complex network of perceptions.

To represent cross-modal abilities, the therapist should encourage a series of exercises and should begin by instructing the caregiver to focus on one of the infant's perceptual capacities, for example, hearing. The caregiver should be asked to represent what she thinks the infant hears and then to describe the infant's experience when hearing a particular familiar vocalization. Once she has achieved this, the caregiver should be encouraged to represent another of the infant's perceptual capacities, such as touching or smelling. After the caregiver has represented each of the five perceptual abilities, she should begin to represent the ability to transfer information perceived from one perceptual mode to another perceptual mode. The therapist can then ask the caregiver to engage in an interactive sequence with the infant and subsequently to describe how the infant experienced and represented the various perceptual cues that occurred during the sequence.

THERAPIST: (Therapist, engaging infant in several minutes of play, shows infant a mobile swirling around, makes clicking noises, and gently strokes infant's head.) Can you describe your infant's perceptions? For example, what was she hearing, seeing, and sensing?

CAREGIVER: I know she heard the clicking noises, because she picked up her head and watched you. She especially likes it when I make those noises with her. She was also watching the bright colors on the mobile. I've noticed she's attracted to sharp, bright colors. Oh, and I guess, she liked the feeling of being stroked on the back of the neck. She really likes it when her father or I do that.

Representing Transitions

The goal of this exercise is to assist caregivers in representing the infant's *sense of continuity*. Transitions are contained in virtually every interaction the caregiver has with the infant. It is vital for the caregiver to communicate awareness about transitions between states—such as playfulness, alertness, and drowsiness as well as between interactions—and, in turn, to convey the notion that these states can be regulated in a smooth fashion so that stimulation does not disrupt the infant's physiological or motivational status. Once the caregiver conveys these perceptions during interaction, the infant will be supported in regulating his own state changes.

The caregiver's gestures when holding the infant are an example of representing transitions. An adaptive caregiver will engage in play sequences with the infant and then gradually curtail the episode of play, lowering the intensity of the emotions displayed and supporting the infant in his effort to make the transition to another state, such as sleep. Characteristically, such caregivers will not guide the infant through behavioral states abruptly, but rather will use their sensitivity to provide appropriate levels of stimulation for the infant.

The development of an appropriate interactive style during transitions is an area in which the therapist's modeling behavior can assist caregivers. If, after observation and assessment, the therapist recognizes that the caregiver is failing to recognize the infant's thresholds of stimulation, the therapist should model a more attuned response and then ask the caregiver to initiate this behavior during an interactive sequence. Caregivers can also benefit from observing videotapes of themselves during dyadic exchange. Such recordings are particularly persuasive in conveying how the caregiver may be violating the infant's regulatory capacities by subjecting him to a deluge of different states without establishing a smooth transition between them.

During the first few months of life, for example, the infant will obviously require a greater degree of assistance—both physical and psychological—to regulate transitions. As time goes on and the infant's regulatory skills become more sophisticated, he will experience greater flexibility when interacting with the environment. Only by being acutely sensitive to this incremental developmental progress through continual representation will the caregiver be able to provide the proper level of stimulation for the infant. The therapist's task, then, is to enlighten the caregiver with respect to the infant's need for structure and to ensure that the caregiver's interpersonal behavior conforms to the infant's developmental level. The following vignette is an example of this form of adaptive structuring:

THERAPIST: (Hands infant to caregiver)

CAREGIVER: (Before placing infant on her lap, caregiver lifts infant to establish eye contact and then smiles directly at her. Infant smiles back and, with her mother's help, sits down on her lap. Caregiver holds infant firmly, but allows her enough space to turn around and gaze at room. Infant stands up on her mother's lap and caregiver slowly loosens her grasp until her hands are barely grazing the infant's back. The infant is thus able to stand without feeling as if she is going to fall, because her mother's arms still surround her, offering a supportive but nonintrusive structure.)

Representing Intention

Intentionality is one of the most fundamental concepts new caregivers can acquire during therapy designed to promote adaptive development. Intentionality may be defined as the mental state that attributes purpose and meaning to behaviors (Shultz, 1980). Intentionality is, essentially, a determination to act in a certain way or to bring about a certain state of affairs. In addition, intentionality refers to the caregiver's perception that infant behaviors are purposive, that these behaviors are designed to communicate a message and attain a variety of goals. Indeed, once the caregiver has grasped the notion that the infant's behaviors are intentional, rather than arbitrary or due to reflex, she will begin representing the infant as an individual with his own unique personality and desires.

To help caregivers represent intention, it is advisable to ask questions such as, "What do you think the infant was trying to convey to you when he gestured like that?" "What do you think he was trying to convey by smiling or crying?" These questions serve several purposes. They alert the caregiver that the infant is indeed demonstrating an implicit "intention" within each communicative gesture and manifestation. As a result, the caregiver begins to adopt the infant's perspective to gain more insight into his subjective perceptions. Furthermore, the caregiver gradually relates to the infant as an individual with his own unique needs and desires. In addition, however, these inquiries stimulate the caregiver to begin observing the infant more closely, to evaluate the sometimes nonapparent intention underlying each behavioral manifestation. Finally, questions such as these motivate caregivers to be more alert to the infant's intentions and more adept at evaluating their own intentions during interaction with the infant. This awareness is crucial, because the intentions of both members of the dyad are inextricably intertwined. Just as the infant's intention to elicit a particular response will affect the caregiver, so too will the caregiver's intentions affect the infant's responses.

If the therapist encourages the caregiver in these representational exercises, gradually the caregiver's perceptions of the infant's motivations become more objective and astute. Moreover, the more sophisticated the caregiver's skill in examining the infant's intentions, the greater her ability to make appropriate attributions to infant behavior.

(In middle of session, infant stirs from her nap and stretches her arms. Caregiver gazes in infant's direction and then removes a bottle of milk from her tote bag.)

THERAPIST: How did you know she was hungry?

CAREGIVER: Oh, I recognize that gesture with her arms. We signal each other. Whenever she wakes up and stretches her arms like that, I know she wants to be fed.

(Seven-month-old infant begins making crawling gestures in the direction of caregiver.)

CAREGIVER: (Clapping hands excitedly, sits on knees facing infant) Ooh! Yes, come on . . . I know you can do it! You're almost walking! (Moves to greet infant, picks him up, then hugs him)

THERAPIST: Do you think your infant interacts differently with you when you are feeling depressed?

CAREGIVER: Yes.

THERAPIST: Can you describe how his interactions change at those times?

CAREGIVER: (Smiling) He just laughs as if to make me laugh and come out of my depression. He's got these noises and sounds.

THERAPIST: Do these interactions snap you out of the depression?

CAREGIVER: (Nods, smiling broadly) Yes.

THERAPIST: Do you think he does it intentionally, to pull you out, or do you think it's by accident?

CAREGIVER: It seems like it's on purpose, like he calls me, laughing instead of whining.

Representing Mastery

Among the therapist's primary goals is to encourage the caregiver's awareness of the subtle changes in the relationship that are caused by the infant's increasing developmental skills. This awareness enables the caregiver and infant to develop a sense of *mastery* over the changes in the relationship precipitated by development. When the caregiver is not asserting mastery over these interpersonal changes, both dyadic members may experience somatic (e.g., lethargy), socio-affective (e.g., withdrawal), cognitive (e.g., confusion), or motivational deficits (e.g., lack of interest).

To avert this outcome, the therapist can instruct the caregiver in representational exercises that focus on predicting mastery outcomes. One such exercise involves asking the caregiver to imagine how she might interact with the infant when the infant has mastered a future developmental milestone. For example, if the infant seems on the verge of crawling, the therapist might ask what images come to mind when the caregiver represents the action of crawling, how the caregiver envisions the infant will begin to crawl, and how the caregiver thinks the action of crawling will change their relationship.

It is usually beneficial to ask a *trio* of questions that range from general perceptions about the developmental milestone itself, to more specific perceptions about how the infant will exhibit the milestone, to the perceptions the caregiver harbors about her response when the milestone is achieved. This latter query and its response have the highest predictive value, because they enable the caregiver to communicate to the therapist perceptions about her own development in terms of the relationship with the infant.

These perceptions can offer the therapist myriad insights into why the evolving relationship with the infant is occurring in a particular fashion. By disclosing these representations, the caregiver will have the opportunity to understand her contributions to the interaction from different perspectives.

CAREGIVER: I always imagine that she's going to do things faster than she does them.

THERAPIST: Can you give me an example?

CAREGIVER: I thought she was going to crawl. We kept saying "Any day now" because she would get up on all fours and rock, and we would say "Oh, by next week she'll be crawling" and it took her longer than that. Now that I have become more aware of her developmental changes, I'm more attuned to when new behaviors will actually start emerging.

Representing Developmental Transitions

Transition in this context refers to the changes in the infant's level of functioning during the time that a developmental milestone is beginning to consolidate. To concentrate the caregiver's attention on developmental transitions, it is best to isolate a particular milestone and ask the caregiver a series of questions about how she believes the infant experienced the milestone and how she felt when she first witnessed the infant displaying the precursory changes that indicated the milestone was imminent. Inquiry involves asking the caregiver what thoughts, memories, or feelings come to mind when reflecting on a particular milestone that the infant has already mastered. One caregiver in treatment reported that she had been told by her own father that she both walked and talked at a very early age. This caregiver had expressed fear several times that her own infant's development was delayed, and it was only after reflecting on her own past history and what she had been told about it that she was able to understand her difficulties in accepting her infant's pace in acquiring new skills. The therapist may, for instance, periodically play tapes of previous sessions so that the caregiver becomes familiar with the dramatic developmental changes that the infant has demonstrated over time.

Thus, this representational exercise not only permits the caregiver to gain familiarity with precursory changes, but also allows the infant to attain developmental organization during transitional states.

(The caregiver has reported to the therapist that the infant has demonstrated kicking gestures and will probably begin crawling soon.)

THERAPIST: How do you feel about Johnny's emerging crawling skills?

CAREGIVER: It's exciting, in a way, because I've seen so many changes in him since he was born, but crawling is a real change. And it's also a little frightening.

THERAPIST: How is it frightening?

CAREGIVER: Because, I guess, when he starts crawling he could move out of my sight . . . and even get hurt. (Anxiety enters the caregiver's tone. After a brief silence) I also want to convey to him how excited I am about his progress.

Representing the Caregiver's Past Interactions

This exercise encourages the caregiver to focus on the memories of past interactions that are elicited during the interaction with the infant. Latent conflicts that may hinder the caregiver's ability to interact adaptively with the infant can be explored through such exercises. As a result, the therapist begins to recognize how previously unresolved conflict has infiltrated into the interaction with the infant. Before adaptive exchanges can occur, earlier conflicts must be disentangled and divorced from the interaction between caregiver and infant. Unless the caregiver becomes aware of conflicting past situations, she may continue to superimpose vestiges of unresolved conflict on the interaction with the infant.

CAREGIVER: In my relationship with my parents autonomy has been an issue with me before.

THERAPIST: What comes to mind when you think of autonomy?

CAREGIVER: I guess there was a separation that I never dealt with. I grew up on my own. I had no rules—nothing. I was just so angry at the world. I said to them, "I don't want to have anything to do with you anymore."

THERAPIST: How did you react emotionally?

CAREGIVER: I withdrew from them. I didn't want to have anything to do with them. There was no communication. I was on the street, failing in school and trying different drugs.

THERAPIST: Do you see separation as a problem you never dealt with effectively?

CAREGIVER: Yes.

Representing Boundaries

A common theme that arises during caregiver–infant therapy concerns *boundaries*. By boundaries is meant both the physical and psychological barriers that exist between the infant and the caregiver. Perhaps one of the most difficult tasks for the infant during these first years is developing coherence despite developmental growth. Although this achievement may be difficult for the infant, it is equally problematic for the caregiver, who must relinquish aspects of an enormously rewarding relationship to foster the infant's growth.

Two anecdotes gleaned from the treatment of mothers and infants will elaborate how the theme of boundary development can arise in therapy. The first incident occurred several months into treatment when the caregiver of a 6-month-old girl commented that sometimes she felt exhausted when caring for the child. "This morning, for example, I was trying to clean the house so I could be on time for the session. In the middle of all this, the baby started crying and even though it really hurt me not to go to her, for the first time I felt, 'Look, kid, you're on your own. Mommy has needs also and this time you'll just have to wait for a minute.'" In expressing these sentiments, the caregiver conveyed her feelings of guilt when she realized that, for the first time, she had put her own needs ahead of those of the infant. Yet, as the session progressed, the caregiver voiced the view that perhaps it was important for the infant to learn that her needs would not always be attended to immediately.

The second anecdote pertaining to boundaries involved a more intimate issue. In this instance, the caregiver of a 6-month-old baby boy noted that every so often the infant would awaken in the middle of the night and she or her husband would bring him into their bed. "At first my husband and I enjoyed this, because it seemed to calm him down. But now when we bring my son into bed, he kicks me and pulls my hair. I also feel inhibited about sex when I know he's awake in the other room or with us," the caregiver commented.

CAREGIVER: We just got him a new crib.

THERAPIST: What triggered this decision?

CAREGIVER: I guess we realize that he's older now and needs more of his own space. Also, we stopped bringing him into bed with us. Even though we go to him when he cries, we try to comfort him but keep him in his crib. I think it's important that he learns he has his own space that is separate from ours.

THERAPIST: How does your decision make you feel?

CAREGIVER: Actually, I like it, because now I'm beginning to see him as an individual with his own personality.

Representing Feelings After Separation

One irony of development is that despite the intense intimacy that evolves between caregiver and infant, separation is an inevitable sequela of maturation. Indeed, the first 2 years of life may be summarized by noting that the infant and caregiver grow close in order to be able to grow apart. Separation in this context refers to the representation of the infant's capacity to exercise developmental skills independently from the caregiver. Separation can be highly traumatic for the caregiver, particularly if the caregiver has established a rapport with the infant, because it may break the continuity of the relationship. For some caregivers, separation threatens to change and perhaps obliterate an interaction that has been highly intimate, gratifying, and rewarding.

Separation can be equally traumatic for a maladaptive caregiver whose relationship with the infant has been less than harmonious. In these instances, both caregiver and infant experience a loss: The infant will be ill-equipped to embark on an independent relationship with the environment and others, whereas the caregiver may experience a sense of alienation.

For all of these reasons, it is vital to assist caregivers in representing feelings associated with separation. To do this, the therapist should help the caregiver view separation as an integral part of the dyadic relationship that correlates with virtually every developmental change. In fact, separation is an overall reaction that systematically occurs whenever the infant and caregiver experience a change in their relationship precipitated by the emergence of new developmental precursors or the consolidation of a developmental milestone. Every developmental change provides the infant with greater degrees of autonomy.

Thus, the caregiver should be coached to examine and represent her reactions to separation as an inevitable correlate of development that occurs even before the infant's birth. To help the caregiver achieve this ability, the therapist should encourage the caregiver to make predictions about future changes and ask her to describe the likely impact of each new milestone on her relationship with the infant. Thus, caregivers should describe general feelings about separation, perceptions of how the infant will respond to separation, and perceptions of their own prior experiences with separation. This exercise assists the caregiver in understanding the issues that affected her during separation from her own caregiver.

THERAPIST: Can you tell me about some of the developmental trends you've noticed in the baby in the past few weeks?

CAREGIVER: Now she is crawling. She is able to crawl a few feet on her own before she turns back to make sure I'm there.

THERAPIST: How do you feel about these changes?

CAREGIVER: Sometimes it's frightening because I realize just how quickly she is growing up. But I try to let her know that I'm proud of her also.

THERAPIST: How do you do that?

CAREGIVER: I talk to her, encourage her when she is crawling. That way she knows from the sound of my voice that I'm always with her.

As a second step, the caregiver should envision the different possible outcomes that could result from separation from the infant. The therapist should attend to the caregiver's descriptions with great care, because it is necessary to help the caregiver place these descriptions in perspective. The therapist should recognize that the caregiver, particularly a caregiver who has an adaptive relationship with the infant, may suffer intense pangs of anxiety during periods of separation. It is particularly important for the therapist to help the caregiver alleviate this anxiety. Unless the caregiver explores and learns to dispel such anxiety, it is likely that negative feelings could be transferred to the infant during periods of interaction. In turn, the infant may be unable to overcome the distress aroused by these debilitating feelings, thus hindering him from exercising the developmental skills necessary for separation.

THERAPIST: It is common for the infant to bring objects to the caregiver to share them with her and then to go back and explore the world. The more they can explore and the more they can separate and come back and check with their caregivers, the more secure the representation of the caregiver is.

CAREGIVER: Like peekaboo?

THERAPIST: Yes . . . it's like a version of peekaboo behavior. During peekaboo the infant explores his new understanding that even when he covers his eyes and the caregiver is out of sight, she will still be there when he uncovers his eyes.

Representing the Infant in His Absence

This representational exercise is of crucial importance, because it focuses on what is often the most threatening implication of the developmental process. Specifically, this exercise requires that the caregiver maintain an internal image of the infant when he is absent. As an example, one adaptive caregiver in treatment expressed feelings of hopelessness while she was weaning her 6-month-old infant. Once she expressed these emotions, therapy focused on isolating the source of the depression. Ultimately, the caregiver determined that her depression stemmed from two sources. First, she felt upset that her weaned infant would no longer be dependent on her for nourishment and the unique physical closeness that is a part of the breastfeeding experience. Thus, weaning symbolized separation. Equally as disturbing to this caregiver, however, was the realization that, with the advent of weaning, the infant's development was moving inexorably forward. In other words, the weaning experience had emphasized the rapid pace of change. Moreover, the caregiver had become increasingly aware that her control over the progression of developmental processes was relatively minimal.

To assist this caregiver in overcoming her depressive feelings, the therapist devised a series of representational exercises that focused on asking the caregiver to envision the infant displaying several developmental milestones prior to the weaning. For each milestone represented (e.g., the infant gazing directly at the caregiver, the infant playing with the caregiver, the infant holding objects by herself, the infant being breastfed), the caregiver explained how she felt, particularly when she recognized that, by engaging in the skill, the infant was displaying a growing form of independence and autonomy with implications for the caregiver's role and her relationship with the infant.

After several rehearsals of such representational exercises, the caregiver was able to see the infant's overall development from a new perspective. She now viewed it as a process and perceived each incremental achievement in the infant's development as having two outcomes. First, the caregiver recognized that with developmental change came achievement, which the infant experienced in the form of mastery and competence. Second, however, the caregiver now possessed more adaptive insights about the reasons for the separation caused by the inexorable pace of development. That is, the caregiver was now emotionally prepared to deal with the interpersonal implications that the infant's burgeoning somatic, socio-affective, cognitive, and motivational skills had on the dyadic relationship.

Once these goals were achieved, the therapist designed therapeutic strategies to help the caregiver conceptualize development as a positive phenomenon whose repercussions could be adaptively integrated into the dyadic relationship. For example, the caregiver began to discuss the infant's upcoming attendance at preschool the following year, and she was able to share her sense of pleasure and enthusiasm because the infant would be exposed to new challenges that would help her learn even more complex adaptive skills. In turn, these new skills would enlarge the content and quality of the dyadic relationship.

This representational exercise helps caregivers place development in an appropriate perspective and recognize the periodic feelings of separation and loss that are inevitable in the developmental process. For these reasons, it is imperative that the therapist work through any emotional ambiguities that the developmental process can arouse by encouraging the caregiver to practice these representational exercises.

(Therapist 1 takes infant out of the room)

THERAPIST 2: How do you feel about not having him in front of you?

CAREGIVER: Umm . . . Fine.

THERAPIST 2: Can you represent images of his face or his gestures or his behavior without having him in front of you?

CAREGIVER: It takes a while before I can do that.

THERAPIST 2: Can you remember how he looked a few minutes ago?

CAREGIVER: Yes. I do that sometimes when I'm away and he's someplace else.

THERAPIST 2: You try to remember something about him?

CAREGIVER: Yes.

THERAPIST 2: What happens when you try?

CAREGIVER: I feel guilty for not being able to do it right away.

THERAPIST 2: What do you mean by "guilty"?

CAREGIVER: I think I should really remember him . . . what he looks like.

THERAPIST 2: Because?

CAREGIVER: I don't know why.

THERAPIST 2: Well, let's try to think why.

CAREGIVER: I guess . . . because he's my son.

THERAPIST 2: You think that he should be present all the time, at least in your mind?

CAREGIVER: Basically, yes.

Representing Reunion

Just as it is vital to encourage the caregiver in representational exercises involving separation, it is equally important to emphasize the significance of *reunion episodes*. To represent reunion adaptively, however, the caregiver must first come to terms with the implications of separation. She must accept separation as an inevitable aspect of the infant's growth and development, rather than as an effort on the infant's part to reject the caregiver. The therapist should instruct the caregiver to represent reunion episodes as ultimate forms of adaptive interaction. Reunion provides an unparalleled opportunity for sharing and mutual exchange within the dyad and allows the infant and caregiver to become "acquainted" all over again.

CAREGIVER: (Describing feelings when she picks infant up from day care) I'm always happy to pick her up. I know day care is good for her, because she is with other children and she learns all sorts of new activities. Besides, I get time to myself. But I can't help it . . . I really look forward to picking her up. She's always so happy to see me . . . and I'm happy to see her. It's a very good feeling when she runs to greet me.

CONCLUSION

The preceding discussion has focused on an innovative technique for conducting therapy with caregivers and infants. This form of therapy, which relies on instilling the principles of adaptive caregiving through representational exercises, has been shown to be effective both with caregivers who already display a degree of skill in dealing with infant development and with maladaptive caregivers whose capacity to engage in sequences of harmonious interaction is impaired.

One reason this form of treatment is so effective in ameliorating interactional failure within the dyadic relationship is that it relies on enhancing the fundamental skills, referred to as *intuitive behaviors,* that virtually all caregivers possess. Intuitive behaviors that fall into this category include eye contact with the infant, vocalization behavior, appropriate holding gestures, and feeding competence. In addition, this chapter has posited yet another form of behavior encountered in adaptive caregivers that has not been previously commented upon. This behavior is referred to as *previewing* and encompasses the caregiver's intuitive perceptions about imminent developmental achievement and her capacity to introduce the infant to upcoming changes in an appropriate fashion. Therapy utilizing representational exercises emerges from the matrix of previewing behavior. This theory of treatment may be summarized as follows: Previewing behavior tends to be prominent among adaptive caregivers, and infants exposed to previewing exercises tend to thrive and achieve developmental milestones at an appropriate pace with minimal difficulty. Therefore, encouraging caregivers to use their representational skills to engage in previewing exercises heightens the rapport within the caregiver–infant dyad.

Perhaps the most effective way of coaxing forth previewing behavior is to bolster skill in representing a variety of interactions with the infant. Thus, the therapist should guide the caregiver through a range of representational exercises, beginning with representations of discrete function and moving on to more complex representational skills that implicate more sophisticated abilities—such as the capacity to represent developmental transitions. Finally, the caregiver is challenged to engage in representational exercises that may evoke conflict from her own past, which, in turn, may be detrimentally affecting dyadic interaction. In this category are such exercises as the ability to represent caregiver past memories, separation, and reunion episodes. Once the caregiver has progressed to this level, it is likely that she will have gained facility in evoking representational images.

In addition to fostering the caregiver's skill in representing developmental change, however, this form of treatment also emphasizes direct application to the therapeutic and interactional milieu. Only by testing the results of the representational exercises during exchange with the infant will both caregiver and therapist be able to gauge whether interactional impasses are beginning to recede and development is proceeding along a more adaptational pathway. The therapist can assess the caregiver's progress by evaluating the degree of previewing behavior that begins to emerge during dyadic interaction. Previewing encompasses caregiver skill in anticipating imminent developmental achievement and subsequently introducing the infant to these milestones at an appropriate pace. Thus, the degree of previewing behavior the caregiver exhibits in the dyadic exchange provides a barometer for gauging how effectively the representational exercises have promoted adaptive patterns in any particular dyad.

The therapist should periodically raise a trio of questions about each developmental milestone that the caregiver is representing. These questions focus first on the caregiver's overall view of the milestone. For example, when does the caregiver think most infants begin to crawl or walk or talk or feed themselves? The second query addresses the developmental progress of the caregiver's own infant. The therapist might ask, for instance, when the caregiver believes her infant will begin to show signs of crawling, how she will feel when he exhibits these behaviors, and how she thinks the infant will feel when he has achieved the milestone. A third inquiry challenges the caregiver to describe her perceptions of her own achievement of these particular milestones during her own infancy and childhood. This latter query is particularly revealing, because it often encourages the caregiver to explore her past and to deal with latent conflicts within the therapeutic setting.

As a final note, it needs to be emphasized that representational exercises present a flexible therapeutic approach. Therapists need not perform every single representational exercise or even engage in these exercises in the order presented here. Rather, this chapter has sought to provide overall guidance in initiating adaptive dyadic interaction to promote harmonious development, and therapists should feel free to use these representational techniques in a flexible manner.

PART FOUR

Applying Previewing During Dyadic Intervention

Chapter 10

Stages in the Caregiver–Therapist Relationship

INTRODUCTION

Seasoned clinicians are accustomed to charting the changes in the therapeutic relationship that occur during each patient's treatment process. Thus, most practitioners recognize that during the initial phase of therapy patients often resist the therapist's interventions and retreat into their own complacent haven of interpretation. This stage is referred to as the stage of *assertiveness*. As patients become more receptive to the therapeutic process, the initial resistance yields. Patients begin revealing uncertainties and doubts about their previously impermeable facade of self-assurance. An *alliance* fueled by a sense of trust then emerges. As the treatment progresses, patients enter into a highly charged relationship with the therapist that is referred to as *working through* and that reveals a full panoply of previously undisclosed experiences. Fueled by the interactions with the therapist, patients begin to reevaluate their sense of self based on a newly constructed scheme of interpersonal relations. Finally, as patients become adept at contrasting the therapist's perspective with their own, treatment enters the stage of *resolution*. A successful treatment allows these stages to evolve smoothly without precise points of demarcation. Astute clinicians will recognize the transitions between these phases of treatment and will adapt their strategies accordingly.

Interestingly enough, these treatment phases are not unique to individual psychotherapy but are, in fact, present during virtually all forms of treatment that last for more than a few sessions. Thus, treatment stages also emerge when therapy involves a group, a family, or a dyad, such as a caregiver and infant. In addition, therapeutic formats involving more than one individual, such as dyadic therapy, may result in an even more complex version of the stages in the therapeutic relationship because the therapist has an opportunity to witness not only the caregiver's relationship with the therapist, but also the caregiver's relationship with the infant.

By observing how the patient behaves with another individual and transfers emotion to that individual, the therapist can obtain enhanced insight into any conflict that may intrude on the patient's relationships. This is particularly the case with dyadic therapy because, in most instances, the therapist will be observing a relatively new and fresh relationship that is evolving between mother and infant, in which debilitating patterns of exchange have not yet become entrenched. As a result, the therapist can witness conflict as it first surfaces and begins to insinuate itself into the relationship and can observe the initial behavior patterns that can lead to debilitating interpersonal patterns if left unchecked.

From working with numerous caregiver–infant dyads, I have observed firsthand the stages of the therapeutic relationship that occur within the setting of dyadic treatment. Although the stages within dyadic treatment can be readily delineated, however, they are not identical to the stages of individual therapy because the infant's presence provides another readily available object on which the caregiver can superimpose conflict. The infant's presence and the caregiver's shifting attention toward the development of the infant signify other factors to which the therapist must be attuned during dyadic treatment.

Moreover, in addition to discerning the precise therapeutic stages that occur during dyadic treatment, my work with caregiver–infant pairs has also revealed that these stages are manifested by different behaviors, depending on whether the caregiver is classified as being adaptive or maladaptive. Adaptive caregivers—who may be defined as those whose interpersonal interactions with the infant promote development in a positive fashion—exhibit a flexible ability to relate to the therapist. In contrast, caregivers classified as maladaptive—those with histories of psychopathology—show an impaired capacity to relate to other individuals, including the infant. As a consequence, the stages of the therapeutic relationship tend to be less distinctive. In addition, researchers have recently determined that a form of short-term psychotherapy that relies on representational techniques may be beneficial in the treatment of mother–infant dyads. Because this treatment is short-term, the therapist must be particularly sensitive to changes in the therapeutic relationship.

In this chapter, I will examine in greater detail the stages of treatment encountered during dyadic treatment involving a caregiver and infant. The key features of each stage will be highlighted to assist therapists in recognizing and monitoring treatment progress. In addition, this discussion will alert therapists to the ways in which these treatment stages will differ depending on the caregiver's level of adaptation. Because adaptive and maladaptive caregivers display different responses to therapy, it is important to chart how these divergent responses manifest themselves in the patient's attitude both toward the therapist and toward the infant. Recognizing these differences enables the therapist to diagnose potential conflict and to devise strategies for fostering adaptive interaction within the dyad.

FORGING A THERAPEUTIC ALLIANCE

After only a few weeks in treatment, caregivers of infants often display remarkable changes in their attitudes toward their babies and in the way that they envision or represent the dynamic contours of the infant's current developmental status and imminent maturational change. These changes affect four essential domains of interaction, each of which will eventually exert a dramatic impact on both members of the dyad. The four areas include how the caregiver relates to the infant during sequences of interaction; how both caregivers relate to one another; how the caregiver relates to the therapist; and how the therapist continues to introduce treatment techniques that foster developmentally enhancing behaviors within the dyad.

One reason these changes occur is that the caregiver has entered into an alliance with the therapist whereby productive work designed to enhance the interaction with the infant can proceed. For such an alliance to occur, however, the caregiver needs to be in what Paolino (1981) has referred to as a "state of readiness." This state of readiness enables the caregiver to understand, both cognitively and emotionally, the intervention process and to manifest a capacity for constructive psychological and behavioral change as a result of that understanding. This state of readiness has also been described as the capacity for psychological mindedness and insight by Appelbaum (1973), who identified three subcategories of this quality. First, Appelbaum notes, psychological mindedness is the capacity to perceive the connection between thoughts, feelings, and actions. This entails a perceptive skill involving the tendency not to project or externalize the inner self onto environmental objects. The capacity of the patient to understand the meanings and underlying causes of experience and behavior is the second feature of psychological mindedness. Appelbaum views this ability as a cognitive skill. Here, the patient must want to pursue an understanding of the causes of specific thoughts, feelings, and actions. Finally, Appelbaum points to the capacity to direct inward, meaning the ability to reflect on one's own psychic perceptions and, through introspection, to attribute organization to these representations.

Caregivers who enter treatment with these basic skills will likely be inquisitive about the nature of their interaction with the infant and the causes of various interactional behaviors. For these caregivers, motivating insight through the use of previewing exercises is generally a relatively easy task. In addition, the caregiver will be likely to view the therapist as a supportive partner who guides the direction of insights. When the caregiver possesses this attitude of psychological mindedness, establishing a therapeutic alliance should be a fairly natural occurrence that occurs within the first few sessions.

Previewing is one strategy that the therapist may use to encourage the caregiver's state of psychological mindedness. Previewing refers to the wide variety of manifestations a caregiver engages in during dyadic interaction to acquaint the infant with imminent developmental change and its likely effects on the dyadic relationship. It encompasses such caregiver–initiated activities as the ability to represent upcoming change; the ability to devise behavioral exchanges that permit the infant to coordinate precursory behavioral manifestations as well as to rehearse future skills; and the intuitive skill of returning the infant to his current developmental level after a previewing exercise. In addition, previewing also includes all of the infant behaviors that convey to the caregiver an eagerness and readiness to experience upcoming developmental change.

To comprehend how previewing emerges from within the dyadic interaction, the therapist can observe how the caregiver is attuned to the behavioral manifestations of the infant almost immediately after his birth. From such interactions the caregiver's anticipations about future infant development will begin to influence the current relationship. Illustrations of these predictions or expectations are abundant. The caregiver may, for example, notice that the infant is attempting to raise his head and extend his arm to reach for a particular object or that the infant has started to exhibit signs of anxiety in the presence of a stranger. From such behaviors the caregiver predicts which developmental skills are on the verge of consolidating in full-fledged form. Thus, the caregiver will represent the image of the infant holding up his head independently or may envision the infant's distress when confronted in the future by a stranger.

Once the caregiver begins to represent developmental skills, she will move to the next step—devising specific behaviors that acquaint the infant with the interpersonal implications of such developmental achievement. For example, placing the infant's hand around a spoon, supporting the neck of an infant who is attempting to raise his head independently, exercising the limbs of an infant in gestures that simulate crawling, and engaging in eye contact while the infant experiments with a novel situation are just some illustrations of how adaptive caregivers expose infants to the visceral and subjective sensations of an upcoming developmental milestone.

Finally, adaptive previewing requires that the caregiver recognize when the infant has had sufficient exposure to the imminent developmental change and is ready to return to his previous status. The adaptive caregiver will then gradually taper off the previewing exercises. Thus, adaptive previewing has three main components. First the caregiver represents or envisions imminent developmental trends based on her perceptions of current infant manifestations; next, she converts these representations into interpersonal exercises in specific skills that can be introduced to the infant during sequences of interaction; third, she allows the previewing experience to subside, permitting the infant to return to his earlier level of adaptation. If the caregiver lacks any of these components, it is recommended that therapists attempt to foster these skills.

Beyond the process of previewing, dyadic therapy is unique for a variety of reasons that affect the stages of treatment. Among the outstanding features of dyadic treatment is its ability to incorporate an *objective reality* into the caregiver's perspective. This objective reality occurs largely because the therapist and caregiver focus attention on the infant's developmental changes. These manifestations embody an objective reality because they can be observed, reported, and validated by the therapist, caregiver, and to a certain extent the infant, within the therapeutic situation. In this respect, dyadic therapy requires that the therapist use techniques such as physical examination and manipulation with the infant, strategies normally relegated to the purely medical model, in combination with more traditional psychiatric techniques such as observation. The therapist should also be aware, however, that dyadic therapy encompasses a *subjective reality* that is more traditionally dealt with in other therapeutic situations. Most notably, therapists will rely on the caregiver to report the subjective impressions she harbors about her infant's development and about her attitudes toward these changes. Moreover, at least initially, the caregiver will function as an interpreter of the infant's behaviors, describing to the therapist how the infant uses social cues and other behavioral manifestations to communicate a particular state or message. These descriptions of the infant's status offered by the caregiver are subjective in nature.

CAREGIVER: When I first became pregnant, I wanted a baby boy . . . Then I had amniocentesis and was told the baby was a girl.

THERAPIST: How did you feel when you found out you were pregnant with a baby girl rather than a boy?

CAREGIVER: Fine. All I really wanted was a healthy, happy baby. And now I am so happy I have her.

THERAPIST: Do you think she is aware of your happiness?

CAREGIVER: Yes. She's happy and she's healthy (smiles and talks to her baby).

THERAPIST: How do you know that she feels happy?

CAREGIVER: Because when I give her a kiss, she smiles at me, and then she laughs, and then she plays with me. It is like a chain reaction . . . one nice thing after the other.

Often it is not sufficient to address a specific behavioral limitation the caregiver manifests on the surface because the interactional impediment is, in actuality, only a symptom disguising a more general problem of identification, self-concept, or object relations. To discern whether this is the case, the therapist should institute specific techniques at the beginning of treatment to convey to the patient that the therapeutic milieu is an open forum for discussing and resolving conflict (Luborsky, 1984). The following guidelines are useful in establishing this atmosphere of alliance. First, the therapist should listen carefully to the caregiver's problems and urge the caregiver to cast these dilemmas in terms of goals. This technique can be readily applied to caregiver–infant intervention; for example, the therapist can ask the caregiver to state several goals for her interaction with the infant. A caregiver may wish to learn how to respond more effectively to her infant's cries, may wish to begin weaning the infant, or may need advice for coping with periods when she is separated from the infant. Whatever the articulated problem, however, the therapist should continually strive to place it in the context of the dyadic relationship while urging the caregiver to confront and address the challenges posed by the infant's changing development.

Luborsky's expressive approach also helps to solidify the *therapeutic alliance*. This approach may particularly benefit dyadic treatment, since caregivers often enter treatment hoping to find an environment where they can freely express their most intimate perceptions about their relationship with their infant. The first phase of the approach involves *observation* and *listening*. Above all, the therapist needs to convey a posture of receptivity and empathy to both the caregiver and infant as individuals and to the dyadic relationship itself as a self-contained entity. *Understanding* eventually follows as the therapist acquires a more profound sense of how certain dynamics influence the interaction with the infant and of how the caregiver's manifestations either promote or impede adaptive development. *Responsivity* characterizes the third stage, meaning that the therapist tells the caregiver some of what he or she understands about the problems being confronted. In the dyadic context, this form of responsivity requires the therapist to disclose insights about the caregiver's perceptions and behaviors and to share perceptions concerning the interaction transpiring within the dyad. After the therapist has disclosed his or her impressions of the dyadic interaction, it is important to convey eagerness to learn more about these and other issues. Thus, returning to an observational and listening stance will make the therapist continue to focus on the processes of development, which are continually unfolding for the infant and the caregiver.

Luborsky's model has particular value in dyadic treatment. Essentially, such treatment is unique because the therapist is witnessing two significant relationships: first, the relationship between the therapist and caregiver; second, the relationship between the caregiver and the infant. Indeed, dyadic therapy presents the therapist with a situation that is generally not encountered in conventional individual treatment. With dyadic therapy, the therapist has an unparalleled opportunity to witness, firsthand, how conflicts are acted out either within the therapeutic relationship or, alternatively, during interaction with the infant.

STAGES OF THE THERAPEUTIC RELATIONSHIP

As a preliminary matter, the therapist should be sensitive to the caregiver's continual response to the infant's developmental changes. The child's presence and his growth often become the primary focus in the life experience of first-time caregivers, at least until the infancy period has ended. In particular, when the infant is on the verge of reaching a new developmental milestone, the caregiver's attention may be diverted from the therapeutic relationship. Moreover, the emergence of certain developmental milestones in the infant can also affect the caregiver's attitude to the therapist. For example, if the infant manifests a "social smile" directed at the therapist, the caregiver may become eager to transfer positive feelings to the infant. On the other hand, an exhibition of "stranger anxiety" on the part of the infant may cause the caregiver to withdraw somewhat from her relationship with the therapist. As a consequence, the therapist must be mindful of how the infant's developmental course overlays the therapeutic relationship evolving between mother and therapist.

More precise descriptions of the therapeutic relationship as it unfolds during dyadic treatment are appropriate at this point. Stage 1 of the therapeutic relationship during dyadic treatment is the period of *assertiveness*. During this time the caregiver perceives and describes the infant in operational terms and tends to manifest an almost limitless knowledge concerning the infant's developmental processes. This stage is generally evident during the introductory sessions with the patient; however, it may linger for a longer period. The following exchange, indicative of Stage 1, occurred during an intake interview:

THERAPIST: How are you adjusting to the baby's arrival?

CAREGIVER: Very well. He has a very pleasant disposition. His feeding schedule is regular, he hardly ever cries, and he's very responsive when my husband and I play with him.

THERAPIST: Did the baby's schedule require any major changes in your schedule or your husband's schedule?

CAREGIVER: Not really. We prepared a lot, especially me. I read everything I could get my hands on, so now I feel like I know what I am doing. Sometimes I even think I know more than my pediatrician (laughs a little uncomfortably). Of course, I don't mean the specific medical things, but just about everything else I'm pretty much up on.

THERAPIST: Can you describe how the baby responds to you.

CAREGIVER: Well, for example, whenever he cries, I know exactly what he wants. . . . It's strange; I always seem to know.

THERAPIST: So he's communicating with you in that way. How else does he communicate?

CAREGIVER: (Forcefully) Yes, I always know just what he wants.

Stage 2 of the therapeutic relationship is the stage of *assessment*. During this phase, the patient relinquishes the authoritative, omniscient posture exhibited during Stage 1 and gradually begins to share and explore uncertainties and insecurities with the therapist. During this phase the patient comes to view the therapist as possessing a different and informative viewpoint with respect to the infant's growth and behavioral manifestations.

The caregiver may also display a new eagerness to disclose information about herself. The following example illustrates this stage:

THERAPIST: Since you started treatment do you feel any changes have occurred in your perceptions toward yourself or the baby?

CAREGIVER: Being able to talk about my feelings.

THERAPIST: Can you give me an example?

CAREGIVER: When we talked about fantasies (laughing), it was the first time I said that Sharon wasn't as pretty as I had hoped she would be, and that I hadn't said so to anyone . . . (trails off, looks down at baby as if embarrassed).

THERAPIST: How did you feel after you said that?

CAREGIVER: (With a short-lived smile) It made me feel a little guilty, and it was kind of a relief that I had finally said it.

Typically, at this second stage the caregiver has established a genuine alliance with the therapist.

Stage 3 of the therapeutic relationship is a period of *coalescence, convergence,* or *working through*. During this phase, which lasts until the resolution of conflict, the therapeutic relationship is at its most intense. Occasionally, this phase of the therapeutic relationship is characterized by an idealization of the therapist, whom the caregiver has come to view as a virtually infinite repository of wisdom about the infant's development and interpersonal issues. During this period, the therapist's attitudes and neutral perspective are absorbed avidly by the caregiver.

This phase of the treatment has also been referred to as the period of "working through" the patient's underlying conflicts, in an attempt to establish greater psychological equilibrium. During Stage 3 the patient's interaction with the therapist seems to become most intense. Unconscious derivatives relating to the caregiver's unresolved conflicts tend to emerge at this juncture, and the relationship between patient and therapist is at its most heightened level. Although therapists have long been familiar with the intensity of this phase, different theorists have attributed varied meanings to the significance of the working-through period. For therapists with a traditional psychoanalytic background, the working through signifies that point in the treatment when the defensive operations are sufficiently relaxed so that instinctive wishes can emerge in an undisguised fashion. Such instinctive wishes are expressed by the patient in dreams and fantasies whose symbolism suggests the strategies whereby the patient has previously kept forbidden wishes from intruding on the conscious thought processes. These phenomena manifest themselves at this time because the patient has come to transfer conflict onto the neutral figure of the therapist.

In contrast, therapists with an interpersonal background view Stage 3 as a time of intense collaboration between therapist and patient. During this time, the patients reevaluate their behaviors in a more objective light and begin to make certain modifications in interpersonal behavior. From the inception of treatment therapists working with caregivers strive to achieve this motivation to modify interactional patterns by sharing diagnostic formulations about development and its potential interpersonal outcomes and proposing that caregiver and therapist embark upon a goal-oriented journey. The period of most intensive collaboration occurs during the working-through process, as the caregiver relinquishes common patterns of maladaptive interaction. The interpersonal approach is pertinent in this regard because of its alertness to the patient's phenomenology (Cooper, 1989). This emphasis on phenomenology enables the therapist and patient to better understand the implications of the patient's unique experience with significant others.

The therapist must use all the stages of the treatment to attain insight into the caregiver's relationships—not merely her relationships with the infant and therapist. For example, during Stage 1, the therapist would inquire in depth about the caregiver's relationships with members of her family, her experiences during marriage and pregnancy, and her evolving relationship with the infant. These inquiries acquaint the therapist with the patterns that typify the patient's interaction with others. The therapist should be prepared to encounter some resistance when the caregiver adopts the highly assertive stance. During Stage 2, as the caregiver becomes more comfortable with the therapeutic process and as defensive operations dissipate, the caregiver begins to focus on the more intimate aspects of interpersonal relationships. This second stage of the treatment will likely be characterized by reports about how the infant's presence and his developmental progress have affected the caregiver's other relationships, such as her relationship with her husband. In some cases, however, the caregiver will offer these disclosures somewhat tentatively.

As the caregiver proceeds to the working-through phase, she provides details about these relationships more frequently, often disclosing dreams and fantasies whose symbolism indicates how areas of conflict may be eroding significant relationships. The sessions now focus almost entirely on how the caregiver relates to the significant people in her life. Change is problematic because abandoning stereotyped modes of interaction with others arouses anxiety until new interactional skills are developed, rehearsed, and consolidated. An alteration in interpersonal skills necessitates experiencing new emotions, cataloging new perceptions, learning new skills, and significantly, reporting new fantasies and new dreams. In dyadic treatment, this is likely to mean that various dimensions of the caregiver's relationship with the infant will change.

As with the other phases of treatment, Stage 3 is influenced by the events that transpire within each individual involved in the relationship. As a consequence, the way that the caregiver evaluates her own actions, as well as those of others, will inevitably alter her interactions with others. By understanding the impact of experiences with significant people in her past, the caregiver acquires a more profound understanding of how she has become the person she is and why she has evolved a particular sense of self. During Stage 3, the caregiver's gradual acceptance of transformation allows her to begin modifying the distortions brought from previous relationships. Insights penetrate more incisively into interactional patterns (Fromm-Reichmann, 1960; Singer, 1968). This quality of the working-through stage does not preclude the possibility that sudden awareness or flashes of insight can occur early and forcefully in the treatment. Singer has suggested that the working-through period may represent a time during which the patient tests the sincerity and candor of the therapist. In this sense, the phase signifies a time during which a trusting and an empathic relationship emerges between the therapist and the caregiver.

Stage 3 has particularly significant implications for dyadic therapy involving a caregiver and infant. To resolve conflict, the caregiver's own early childhood memories involving her primary relationship with her caregiver need to be resurrected, because this first relationship serves as a paradigm for the later relationships in the caregiver's life, particularly the relationship with the infant. The new relationship evolving between caregiver and infant provides the most important stimulus for evoking such material from the caregiver's past. Not surprisingly, whatever weaknesses or vulnerabilities troubled the caregiver's own primary relationship with her mother often replicate themselves during the exchange with the infant. The therapist will have a direct opportunity to observe and understand the extent to which the caregiver inculcates the infant with these maladaptive patterns. As a consequence, during Stage 3 the therapist not only obtains insight into the caregiver's conflicts but also can witness how she transfers these conflicts to other relationships, such as the relationship with the infant.

The extent to which the insight gained by the caregiver during the working-through period realigns interpersonal patterns with the infant will determine the nature of the psychological change effected by the treatment. Any understanding or new awareness attained through intervention must be tested and retested by the caregiver in new configurations and contacts with other experiences (e.g., the relationship with the infant). Thus, therapeutic insight creates repercussions in the patient's life that reverberate through all of the patient's relationships.

Stage 3 is distinctive, because the caregiver experiments with various new interactional patterns with the infant, often in the presence of the therapist. The defensive operations will be more relaxed by this stage of the treatment, so caregivers tend to disclose intimate information about how they represent the infant, what hostilities they harbor toward him, and how they will accommodate the changes that emerge in their relationship as a result of the developmental processes. It is not unusual for the caregiver to dominate the session by providing an abundance of information, by disclosing dream material, and by revealing "secrets" that she has kept in diaries. By coaching the caregiver to become actively engaged in the complex process of evaluating earlier interactional patterns and realigning them into more adaptive patterns, the therapist actively participates in the caregiver's efforts to forge more attuned patterns of interaction with the infant.

During Stage 3, therapists may also encounter a problem highlighted by Tenzer (1984), who observes that virtually all theorists writing about the working-through phase have commented on the patient's need for repetition. This need is grounded in the notion that just because a patient apparently accepts an interpretation in one session does not mean that at the next session she will necessarily recall or even recognize this interpretation, let alone generalize it to new behavior. One reason for this repetition, according to Tenzer, may be that it is extraordinarily difficult to detach the self from firmly held belief systems and ingrained patterns of behavior. The individual perceives what makes sense and what fits. Initially, what must be is simply perceived as what is, however contradictory the evidence. Only after numerous repetitions that enable the caregiver to understand the relationship from different perspectives is there sufficient accommodation to allow for a different point of view. This notion may apply especially to caregivers in treatment, who are accustomed to viewing the infant from a particular perspective. Only after the therapist has repeatedly attempted to convey a different perspective can the caregiver begin to acknowledge different strategies for dealing with the relationship with the infant.

The following exchange occurred during the working-through stage of treatment involving the mother of a 9-month-old daughter:

THERAPIST: We were talking during the last session about how you felt when you saw that your daughter, Jessica, was able to crawl.

CAREGIVER: Yes, I remember that.

THERAPIST: Did any other thoughts come to mind reminding you how you felt at those times?

CAREGIVER: Scared . . . it frightened me. I thought she would crawl away when I wasn't looking.

THERAPIST: And what would have happened?

CAREGIVER: She would have gotten lost, I guess or even hurt . . . I don't know, I'm not sure.

THERAPIST: I've noticed that you watch her very carefully when she moves away from you.

CAREGIVER: Yes, I do . . . You know, it's funny, but when you said that I remembered something that happened to me when I was very young . . .

THERAPIST: Can you tell me about that memory?

CAREGIVER: I was older than Jessica, maybe 3 years old. My mother took us shopping. . . . It was me and my brother. And I guess she was paying so much attention to my brother who wanted some candy that she forgot about me. I must have wandered off and went to another aisle in the store. When I turned the corner of the aisle, I wasn't looking and accidentally bumped into a shopping cart and hurt my head. I started crying and finally my mother came. I think I was very angry because I couldn't understand why she always paid so much attention to my brother. I was even smaller than my brother and my mother didn't even notice me until I had wandered away and got hurt.

Stage 4 of the therapeutic relationship, which I have referred to as the period of perspective taking, represents a modification of the intense atmosphere that dominated during Stage 3. By this period the caregiver not only adopts a neutral stance when considering other perspectives (e.g., the therapist's perspective) but also begins to assert her own, new perspective about the infant's status. In other words, the caregiver is no longer as engrossed in the therapist's viewpoint. Now she is able to interpret the therapist's comments with heightened sophistication and objectivity, without returning to the previous distorted perceptions about her infant or about her relationship with the infant.

During this period the caregiver expresses opinions that reflect her own fresh perspective, which has emerged because previously suppressed conflict tracing back to the caregiver's childhood has now been brought to consciousness and resolved. I have observed that during the period of perspective taking the caregiver often experiences a feeling of mastery as she considers the possibilities posed by the infant's development. She now views the infant as a unique and distinctive individual.

The conversation with the mother who was upset about her daughter's crawling behavior emerged again a few sessions later.

CAREGIVER: You know, I realized something after I told you the story about getting lost in the supermarket.

THERAPIST: I remember we spoke about your memory of that incident a few sessions ago.

CAREGIVER: Well, I think I understand that what I was doing wasn't fair to Jessica.

THERAPIST: Can you explain?

CAREGIVER: I guess I was taking something that happened to me, a bad experience from my own childhood and imposing it on my relationship with Jessica, like imposing a burden unnecessarily. Maybe I was so concerned about Jessica's crawling because I did not want her to get lost and be hurt the way I was. I especially don't want her to feel that I am not paying attention to her . . . the way my mother made me feel. But Jessica is not me and I'm not my mother. It wouldn't be fair to prevent Jessica from doing what she wants to do and is ready to do, just because something once happened to me a long time ago.

Stage 5 of the therapeutic relationship represents freedom from conflict and *conflict resolution*. The caregiver is now confident in attributing her own meanings and interpretations to the infant's behaviors. She can predict future changes better and is comfortable in sharing insights with the therapist. The following therapeutic exchange reflects this conflict-free stage:

CAREGIVER: I make sure my baby sees her grandparents at least once a week. In many respects, my mother is like a second set of hands for me.

THERAPIST: Like a resource for you.

CAREGIVER: Yes. I know I can leave the baby with her and run out and do something. We spend weekends together and chat on the phone. She's going to be 70 this year (with pride), but you wouldn't know it. My mother is so tuned in to this kid that it's incredible. She also has a comment for everything that's going on. She guesses what Carol is feeling, what Carol is saying; and she really is sensitive and doesn't miss a thing. I now see my mother in a positive light, whereas before I viewed her negatively.

STAGES OF THE THERAPEUTIC RELATIONSHIP FOR ADAPTIVE AND MALADAPTIVE CAREGIVERS

Just as the therapeutic stages emerge during the treatment of virtually all dyads, so too do the stages acquire different nuances depending on the caregiver's level of adaptation. It is particularly important for the therapist to be aware of these differences for several reasons. First, noticing the phases of treatment and how the caregiver interacts with both the therapist and the infant facilitates diagnosis. Beyond diagnosis, however, dyadic therapy strives to modify maladaptive patterns and to instill skills that will lead to optimal interaction between caregiver and infant. The more rapidly the therapist can discern maladaptive patterns, the more adept he or she will be at initiating techniques to help the caregiver surmount these patterns and devise more appropriate methods of interaction. In particular, the therapist can rely on previewing techniques to create a more developmentally adaptive relationship within the dyad. Before doing this, however, the therapist must become familiar with the types of responses evinced by both adaptive and maladaptive caregivers during treatment.

It is helpful, therefore, to examine how these stages emerge. For example, with adaptive caregivers during Stage 1, operational descriptions and authority are common and almost rampant. One adaptive caregiver I worked with insisted, during our first session, on reciting for me the litany of all possible reasons for her infant's crying episodes. When I suggested additional reasons, the caregiver dismissed my comments as nonapplicable or irrelevant. At times during this first session, I felt as if I were receiving a lecture. The caregiver interpreted my queries as threats to her self-image of being an adaptive and nurturing mother. In contrast, another caregiver I treated, who was maladaptive, displayed a different kind of resistance during Stage 1 of the treatment. This mother seemed reticent to discuss the infant in my presence. During Stage 1, then, adaptive caregivers are prone to portray an authoritarian stance, whereas maladaptive caregivers may be overtly resistant to any discussion with the therapist or may hesitate to engage in interaction with the infant.

Example of an Adaptive Caregiver During Stage 1

THERAPIST: At times, when the baby has felt uncomfortable, have you been able to identify why she felt uncomfortable?

CAREGIVER: Oh, sure. Always.

THERAPIST: Can you give some examples . . . when you were able to discover what was bothering your baby and when you just couldn't determine why she was upset?

CAREGIVER: I don't think there was ever a time when I couldn't figure out what was bothering her. She's not a fussy baby, she's pretty easy. So when something is bothering her, I usually know what it is right away.

Example of a Maladaptive Caregiver During Stage 1

THERAPIST: What have you noticed about your baby? I know you are a first-time mother and you said he is a good baby, but can you say anything else about him?

CAREGIVER: (Turns in seat to look at baby, pauses for a few minutes, thinking) Um, he's mellow. (Smiles, shrugs) He doesn't say much. He gets bored a lot . . . I guess he's like me.

In my experience, during Stage 2 of the therapeutic relationship adaptive caregivers voluntarily begin to disclose intimate aspects of their interactions with the infant and to solicit the therapist's advice more openly. Adaptive caregivers appear to show a new receptivity to the therapist's observations and insights and display an eagerness to listen to the therapist's interactions. In contrast, maladaptive caregivers continue to display resistance during this period. In those moments when therapists offer suggestions, maladaptive caregivers accept the advice unenthusiastically or without comment.

Example of an Adaptive Caregiver During Stage 2

CAREGIVER: I knew that babies were attracted to faces, but she's not interested in mirrors yet. When will that happen?

THERAPIST: Do you know when she's going to be interested in recognizing herself in mirrors?

CAREGIVER: (Excited) No, but I'd love to find out!

THERAPIST: At approximately 18 months.

CAREGIVER: (Grins and hugs baby as if in anticipation) I was debating whether to put them in her crib. I have a few toys with mirrors and I was wondering if I should put them into the crib for her yet. I guess I'll just wait a few months.

Example of a Maladaptive Caregiver During Stage 2

THERAPIST: You had said earlier that you first wanted to breastfeed. Was that something that you accidentally fell into or you really thought about it and planned for it?

CAREGIVER: I wanted to try it.

THERAPIST: What motivated you to do so? Mothers have shared with me a wide variety of reasons. What were your thoughts?

CAREGIVER: I figured it would be easier. For example, when you get up in the middle of the night it is easier just to breastfeed than to get up and mix the formula and all that.

THERAPIST: Some mothers tell me that they intuitively feel that breastfeeding brings them closer to their child in some way. I was wondering if you had felt that way?

CAREGIVER: Yeah, I heard that. I heard that breast milk is definitely healthier (shrugs). It probably is, but . . . um, it's whatever you're comfortable with. I figured I'd give it a shot (defensive). There's always the formula anyway.

THERAPIST: But besides the milk being healthier, did you feel in any way that it might be a means for bonding of you and the infant, that it might bring you closer in some way.

CAREGIVER: No. I didn't think about that.

Stage 3 of the therapeutic relationship, the working-through period, is highly distinctive with adaptive caregivers. In the ones I treated, a feeling of heightened emotion became apparent. At this time, observations about the infant's development are actively solicited, and the caregivers are willing to contrast the therapist's observations with their own. Moreover, there is a significant increase in the observational material that caregivers bring into the sessions. They report on situations with spouses that occurred during the week, on new behaviors observed during interaction with the infant, on various experimental responses that have been attempted with the baby, and on displays of interaction that have occurred in the therapist's presence. Now that they are more attuned to maturational trends, these caregivers seem energized by the possibilities of their infant's development, as if they were becoming fluent in an exciting new language. They also seem to depend on the therapist's guidance for providing sophisticated interpretations of infant behavior. Finally, adaptive caregivers during this phase are actively seeking to establish and maintain equilibrium in their relationships with their spouses, children, and other members of their families.

Example of an Adaptive Caregiver During Stage 3

CAREGIVER: So now you know what new skills she has been demonstrating this week, a lot of noises.

THERAPIST: You mean more babbling.

CAREGIVER: Louder, louder, much louder than before. When she started to babble she started on one level, and now her voice goes higher. It's as if she's exploring different notes. It's funny. I love watching this, listening to this. She's gone through a phase where the noises she was making seemed to be an octave higher and over the last week she's gotten louder.

THERAPIST: What else?

CAREGIVER: Um . . . Friday night she was very, very loud and the both of us, my husband and I were just laughing. It was just so funny, watching her babbling and talking. My mother arrived Saturday in time for lunch, and it's as if the baby knew exactly what she was doing. She was showing off. The minute she saw Grandma, she started making the noises from the night before. I wonder sometimes if she knows that she's doing something and saying "Look what I can do now."

Maladaptive caregivers also display a shift in attitude during this period, although it may not be as pronounced as it is with adaptive caregivers. Maladaptive caregivers continue to convey a detached and guarded stance toward the therapist, although intermittently they comment that sessions are helping them. They are also more cognizant of the infant's developmental progress and appear pleased when the therapist comments on specific developmental changes from week to week. For instance, in one case I was treating, when I commented that the infant's manual dexterity in gripping toys and other objects seemed more advanced, the caregiver nodded and smiled, remarking that she too had witnessed this change. Nevertheless, her skills at both identifying signs of infant development and encouraging their manifestation seemed wooden unless I modeled behaviors with the infant using previewing skills. The primary difference between the adaptive caregiver and the maladaptive caregiver during the working-through phase, then, appears to be that with maladaptive caregivers intuitive nurturing behaviors seem remote, although they begin to emerge. To evoke intuitive responses in a maladaptive caregiver, it is necessary for the therapist to engage in repeated modeling with the infant and to demonstrate for the mother appropriate behaviors through previewing exercises.

Example of a Maladaptive Caregiver During Stage 3

CAREGIVER: If it's a question of getting into the baby's rhythm, it means that I have to be with him all day. It changes all the time.

THERAPIST: Can you explain what you mean by . . . "it changes all the time"?

CAREGIVER: Well, now that he sleeps for longer periods of time, I have to get accustomed to timing changes. He'll fall asleep at 9 when it used to be at 11. (Proud) I can tell better when he's cranky and tired.

THERAPIST: (Approving) So now you feel you can anticipate his mood changes and take care of him before his mood becomes uncontrollable?

CAREGIVER: Most times I do . . . I guess.

A significant difference between adaptive and maladaptive caregivers is the degree to which they can predict the infant's behavior. Often adaptive caregivers, with relatively little encouragement or instruction, will spontaneously make predictions about the infant's development and other facets of the infant's interpersonal behavior. Maladaptive caregivers, however, are more reticent to engage in such predictions and, indeed, appear unable to predict adaptively infant behavior or the future course of the infant's development.

Stage 4 of the therapeutic relationship emerges smoothly and uneventfully in the case of the adaptive caregivers. In fact, the transition to this stage is nearly imperceptible. As adaptive caregivers achieve this phase of the therapeutic relationship, it becomes clear that they are beginning to assert a new, more objective perspective on both their own behavior and the infant's developmental trends. This perspective is uncontaminated by previous misconceptions and conflict stemming from their own earlier development. For example, the following comments of adaptive mothers in treatment make clear that they view their infants as individuals in a state of continual change. One mother shared with me that her infant's energetic disposition now pleased her, although when she entered treatment she had been upset by what she had characterized as her son's hyperactivity. "He's so eager to learn new tricks and I try to invent new games to play with him," she said. Several months earlier this same caregiver had noted that her son had inherited her husband's "volatile and hyperactive" disposition. Now she appeared to have relinquished these negative attributions and substituted a fresh interpretation of the infant's behavior.

Example of an Adaptive Caregiver During Stage 4

THERAPIST: Can you explain what you mean when you say that your baby thinks you're a part of her?

CAREGIVER: It means that she has come to believe I am an emotional extension of her.

THERAPIST: Could you elaborate more on your observation?

CAREGIVER: I'm watching her learn how to roll over. She moves on her stomach in what my husband and I call the Sphinx position, arms stretched out, head raised (demonstrates). It's very funny to watch, because she'll kick and she'll wiggle back and forth until she's halfway over but she doesn't know to push herself with one hand. I can almost feel how it feels for her when she cannot complete what she wants to accomplish on her own. At those times I try to help her by supporting her body.

Example of a Maladaptive Caregiver During Stage 4

THERAPIST: What kind of mood has Stevie manifested for the past few weeks?

CAREGIVER: He's pretty good. I don't know how babies are . . . this is my first one . . . I don't know what else to tell you. Sometimes though he gets upset stomachs and then he gets cranky.

THERAPIST: How do you know when he has an upset stomach?

CAREGIVER: You can hear his stomach rumbling and he kind of cringes.

THERAPIST: What do you do at those times?

CAREGIVER: When he gets out of control and starts crying, I just hold him and don't listen any more. Sometimes when I get frustrated I just leave him in the crib alone. That seems to help him . . . I know it helps me.

Finally, Stage 5 of the therapeutic relationship is the period of *conflict resolution*. The caregiver has now worked through conflict deriving from her own earlier life history or from some "mismatch" between her personality and the infant's disposition, relying on a fresh, neutral perspective to gain new insight into her interaction with the infant. The caregiver is now ready to bring spontaneity into the dyadic relationship. For adaptive caregivers, this is a time of newfound confidence when interpersonal changes precipitated by the infant's development can be shared openly and enthusiastically with the therapist. Often they describe such progress in minute detail. During this phase of treatment the therapist introduces previewing exercises that acquaint the infant with imminent developmental change, and the caregiver engages in them with renewed vigor. Previewing exercises will now serve as a vehicle for continuing and solidifying a more optimal relationship between caregiver and infant. Moreover, because the caregiver will have resolved any residual conflict intruding on the dyadic relationship, her attention will now turn to the infant, who will be viewed as a developing individual with his own unique personality. This fresh perspective helps the caregiver assume the role of active supporter and participant in the emergence of developmental trends. This period is also marked by an emotional exuberance on the part of caregivers, who appear to delight in the very phenomenon of developmental growth and change that is now so evident in their infants. Furthermore, they are able to talk about and to devise previewing exercises spontaneously with skill and enthusiasm.

The period of conflict resolution is also notable for the maladaptive caregivers, who show heightened enthusiasm coupled with a newfound understanding of developmental events. Therapists need to work with maladaptive caregivers intensively during this phase of the treatment. Because maladaptive caregivers may experience developmental transitions as a form of loss, they require continual guidance to participate adaptively in the infant's development. Representational exercises that enable the caregiver to envision developmental trends in a predictable fashion are recommended here, as are videotapes depicting infant growth and appropriate caregiver–infant interaction. The therapist may also rely on modeling strategies, whereby therapist and infant engage in a behavioral exchange in the caregiver's presence, and the caregiver is subsequently asked to imitate this behavior. The primary difference between adaptive and maladaptive caregivers at this point is that maladaptive caregivers lack the intuitive skills for guiding the infant in his efforts to acclimate to the demands of the environment and to learn from the dyadic interaction. In some cases, even when conflict has been resolved, maladaptive caregivers still evince deficiencies in fundamental nurturing capabilities. The therapist's didactic interventions, coupled with a special emphasis on previewing exercises, can help such caregivers overcome these deficits and create a more optimal atmosphere for both the interpersonal exchange and the infant's development.

Example of an Adaptive Caregiver During Stage 5

After resolving the caregiver's ambivalence with regard to breastfeeding, she and the therapist had the following exchange:

THERAPIST: In what ways did having the baby change your life?

CAREGIVER: At times people say that they have a baby to save a marriage and it winds up being just the opposite: Having a baby creates stress that makes life difficult and strenuous for both parents. I thought it would create a lot more stress in our lives. But the stress doesn't seem to be there. Exhaustion, at times, yes . . . frustration at times, yes . . . but other than that, it's like a whole new world that my husband and I have to share, and I think that's just terrific. I didn't expect it to be so rewarding. I didn't expect the closeness.

THERAPIST: So you thought it was going to be a problem?

CAREGIVER: I did not expect the emotional bonding between the baby and me to be as strong as it is. Now that I am so much more aware of the developmental processes and the new skills she keeps demonstrating, I'm even more excited and feel even closer to her.

THERAPIST: Can you tell me more about the "bonding" you mentioned?

CAREGIVER: The closeness between the baby and myself, and now I see it between my husband and the baby.

THERAPIST: Can you define what you mean by "bonding"?

CAREGIVER: Sure. It's . . . it's a feeling. It's a feeling of "connectedness." I think of nursing more than just feeding her. People often say to me, "Oh, she's eating again," but she may be sleeping or just resting, lying in my lap or whatever. It's a kind of comforting togetherness. If she is in any kind of discomfort, it's painful for me. When she had her first shot, I left the room and when she started to cry it was so painful to me inside because I knew that her leg hurt. It's a very strong type of feeling.

Example of a Maladaptive Caregiver During Stage 5

After resolving her impulsive urges to get pregnant again, the mother of a 3-month-old infant made the following disclosures:

THERAPIST: Do you feel that you and your baby are sharing a more relaxed relationship now?

CAREGIVER: Yes . . . I guess we've gotten used to each other. I kind of like having him around now.

THERAPIST: Can you explain what you mean?

CAREGIVER: I think I understand him more . . . I can sometimes see things from his point of view . . . and I feel we are communicating, even though he can't talk yet.

THERAPIST: How do you communicate?

CAREGIVER: The way he moves his body . . . or, now I look at his face more than I used to and I can understand what he wants.

THERAPIST: It sounds as if you have developed a kind of language, even though you don't use words.

CAREGIVER: Yes, that's exactly what it is like . . . as if we have a special language and I now know when to use it.

Therapy with caregivers and their infants should also address the seminal characteristic of their relationship—the sense of perpetual transition and transformation as the developmental processes unfold. In addition, caregivers need to recognize that the continual transformations in their relationship with the infant that result from the infant's acquisition of new developmental skills represent a kind of emotional double-edged sword. On the one hand, the caregiver celebrates the infant's ever-expanding ability to exert mastery over the challenges posed by development; on the other hand, with each incremental achievement, the relationship moves away from the nurturing embrace of the caregiver toward independence. It is only when the caregiver adjusts to this dynamic of continual change that an adaptive relationship can ensue.

Despite successfully traversing the five stages of treatment, some caregivers may still have problems as a result of the emotional implications raised by the ever-changing pace of development. Even in the most optimal dyadic relationship developmental change means increasing autonomy and independence for the infant, which, in turn, can represent for the caregiver a loss of the intimacy she had shared with him until then. This perceived loss may trigger feelings of despair and depression because the caregiver is reminded of earlier episodes of loss in her own life or because she feels threatened by the infant's progress toward autonomy. Feelings of loss often arise during periods when the infant achieves key developmental milestones that signify burgeoning independence. Some obvious examples include weaning behavior, the advent of crawling, or walking behavior. The caregiver fears that the infant's evolving autonomy will disrupt the dyadic rapport. To diagnose such states, therapists should keep in mind the four major deficits associated with depressive affect: affective, cognitive, motivational, and self-esteem deficits. The therapist must encourage the caregiver to reveal more about past experiences, future events, or dreams involving the theme of loss. Previewing exercises also help to pinpoint the origin of such emotions, as does free association. Once these techniques have been used, it is necessary to help the caregiver understand how these

Table 10–1. *Stages During Dyadic Therapy*

Adaptive Caregiver	Maladaptive Caregiver
Stage 1—Assertiveness	
Caregiver displays operational and concrete knowledge and appears to be lecturing therapist with her encyclopedic knowledge.	Caregiver appears unaware or detached.
Caregiver actively interacts with infant.	Caregiver displays minimal interaction with infant.
	Responses to therapist's queries are perfunctory and wooden.
Therapist interventions are resisted or are not invited.	Constricted affect is constantly displayed.
Stage 2—Assessment	
Caregiver shares developmental phenomena with therapist in authoritative fashion but also begins to disclose more intimate issues concerning doubts and uncertainties about the infant's development and their implications for the marital relationship.	Resistance continues, although caregiver begins to make comments when therapist interacts with infant and to show interest in observing such interactions.
Caregiver begins to solicit therapist's opinion.	
This atmosphere allows therapist to begin predicting the emergence of future conflict.	
Stage 3—Working Through	
Caregiver shows intense emotional response to therapist, who is now viewed as an idealized object and a resource of information about infant development.	Although attitude toward therapist continues to be detached, caregiver appears more interested in observing interaction between therapist and infant. These behaviors are modeled by caregiver in tentative and hesitating fashion.
Caregiver encourages therapist to interact with infant while observing avidly.	Caregiver is beginning to work through her conflict.
This period represents apex of therapeutic relationship and working through of conflict.	Caregiver solicits therapist's opinion about marital issues.

Table 10–1. *(Continued)*

Adaptive Caregiver	Maladaptive Caregiver
Stage 4—Perspective Taking	
Caregiver begins to exercise her ability to adopt the perspective of infant, views infant as having an independent viewpoint.	Caregiver gradually comes to see infant as an independent entity with his own viewpoint.
Stage 5—Conflict Resolution	
Caregiver's main conflict has been identified and resolved. She is now able to understand motives and meanings of infant's behaviors without imposing her own point of view.	Caregiver shows growing awareness of infant's status as an individual, coupled with diminished tendency to impose meaning on infant's behaviors. Prediction of an interactional conflict(s) depends on degree of caregiver's psychiatric disturbance.

deficits may impinge on current and future interaction with the infant and have a detrimental effect on his adaptation. Eventually, by encouraging caregivers to view the full implications of development—in both its positive and negative aspects—the ambivalence recedes and the caregiver emerges with a more profound understanding of how to promote adaptive growth in the infant.

Table 10–1 summarizes the differences between adaptive and maladaptive caregivers at the different stages of the therapeutic relationship.

ESTABLISHING A THERAPEUTIC ALLIANCE

Perhaps the most intense period of treatment occurs during the third stage, or working through, of the conflict, after the caregiver has come to trust the therapist and begins to reveal intimate details of her psychological experience, particularly in the form of dream material and reveries. These disclosures signify that the caregiver is beginning to reassess her relationship with the infant and adopt a more objective perspective concerning infant development and her relationship with the infant. Excerpts from the following case history involve a primiparous pregnant woman in her 6th month of pregnancy. The patient had an earlier history of psychiatric disturbance dating from her adolescent years and had been under the care of a psychiatrist intermittently since then. She had completed half of her college education toward a nursing degree and had married at the age of 25. She became pregnant at the age of 27 and had been referred to prenatal counseling by her regular therapist, whom she saw on a weekly basis, because it was felt that she might benefit from speaking to a therapist who specialized in prenatal issues and that she might eventually enter a psychotherapy group for pregnant women.

The first time the therapist saw the patient, she displayed a negative reaction. This reaction emerged most forcefully when she compared the therapist with the psychiatrist she saw on a regular basis.

THERAPIST: Can you describe your feelings about the baby?

CAREGIVER: Well, I was thinking maybe I'd like a girl, because I think it would be easier to take care of a girl.

THERAPIST: You think girls are easier to take care of than boys?

CAREGIVER: I guess so. With girls, you can dress them up in fancy clothes and they behave better.

THERAPIST: Any other thoughts about that?

CAREGIVER: Um . . . yes . . . but I don't think I should tell you, because you are not my doctor yet. I don't know if you will be my doctor. I already have a doctor. First I have to see if I like you.

THERAPIST: I understand.

Although this patient displayed obvious resistance during the first encounter, she ended the session by commenting that she had started to keep a journal about her experiences during the pregnancy. The therapist suggested that she might consider bringing the journal to upcoming sessions. During the next few sessions, the patient always arrived promptly and reported on the occurrences of the previous week with particular emphasis on her physical and emotional status. At the beginning of the third session, she commented that the therapist looked "really nice today." Thereafter at each session she expressed a greater feeling of rapport with the therapist, remarking for example, that the therapist seemed "like a good listener" and had "a kind face." Although the patient did not bring the journal she had mentioned at the first interview to the sessions, she began to disclose more details of her personal life. For instance, she devoted an entire session to relating how she had met and married her husband. At another session, she described her childhood relationship with her father and her paternal grandmother. The patient's mother had died when she was 6 years old, and she spoke at length about various "lady friends" her father had invited home as she was growing up.

Beginning in approximately the 4th month of treatment, the patient asked if the therapist would be interested in hearing some of her dreams.

She had reported previously that since becoming pregnant, she had experienced difficulty in falling asleep at night and dreamed profusely. When the therapist asked if she could relate some of the dreams, however, she commented that she couldn't remember. Nevertheless, shortly thereafter the caregiver seemed eager to share these dreams and fantasies. The first such dream was notable in that the patient had begun to predict or "preview" what her relationship with the infant would be like. As a preface to the dream, the patient explained that she had been dozing in bed, waiting for her husband to return from work. Her husband had started working a night shift recently, and the patient told me that he was rarely interested in having intercourse with her, even when she initiated intimate behaviors. As a result, she reported, she had begun having fantasies about having sex with a woman. "I guess I could control a woman more easily," the patient told me. Before she actually fell asleep, the patient fantasized about having sex with her girlfriend. In the dream, both women wound up pregnant.

CAREGIVER: I dreamed that my girlfriend just had a baby, and I just had a baby. We gave birth at the same time. My girlfriend was breastfeeding her baby, and I was breastfeeding my baby. But I didn't have any milk. Then I realized I didn't have any bottles of milk either, because I wasn't planning to use any. Maybe I could improvise and add sugar to some milk.

THERAPIST: You became concerned because you didn't have any milk?

CAREGIVER: Yes, then the baby didn't want the milk.

THERAPIST: You mean he turned away from the breast.

CAREGIVER: Yes.

THERAPIST: How did the baby show you that he didn't want the milk?

CAREGIVER: By turning away. But I knew the baby was hungry.

THERAPIST: What made you aware that the baby was hungry?

CAREGIVER: I just . . . I knew the baby was hungry.

THERAPIST: How did you know that?

CAREGIVER: Because I hadn't fed that baby for a month or two weeks.

THERAPIST: So part of the dream was that the baby was hungry, because you hadn't fed him for a long time?

CAREGIVER: Yes.

THERAPIST: So you put him near your breast? And then what happened?

CAREGIVER: And then I put my nipple in the baby's mouth and he pushed it away.

THERAPIST: How did you feel?

CAREGIVER: I felt paranoid, and scared. I began to think very fast because I knew the baby was very hungry . . . it hadn't eaten for a long while. I was trying to think of things to feed the baby. I think I borrowed a baby bottle from a friend or my sister-in-law. I put some milk in the bottle and then I added some sugar.

THERAPIST: Why do you think the baby rejected your breast?

CAREGIVER: I don't know. (Patient then changes that subject and mentions a television show she has seen about a woman who can't become pregnant and is "deceived" by a fertility doctor who promised help.)

This dream, reported during the 4th month of treatment as the patient was entering the working-through phase, is significant because of the wealth of information it conveys about how the patient views her interactions with others. Initially, it will be remembered that the patient said that her prenocturnal reverie involved reflections about having sex with her husband. She complained that she could not control her husband sexually and therefore she had sought to initiate a sexual liaison with her girlfriend, whom she believed she could control sexually. Despite this liaison, both women had become pregnant and gave birth. Pregnancy and the birth process may here signify events that the caregiver believes are beyond her control. The patient can, however, control the infant in the dream to a certain extent by withholding food. But the infant eventually overcomes this interaction by "rejecting" the patient's breast and turning away from the nipple. The patient then becomes "paranoid" and is forced to improvise by borrowing a baby bottle from her sister-in-law.

Thus, the theme of how to control others in her life is preeminent in this caregiver's patterns of interaction. Significantly, in the dream she has begun to anticipate or preview how this form of behavior will be carried out in her relationship with the infant. Later in the session, the patient returned to the dream about breastfeeding as she discussed the physical changes she had undergone during her pregnancy. Throughout the treatment, these physical complaints had been raised frequently by the patient. In the following dialogue, however, the changes of pregnancy are linked, for the first time, to the theme of rejection.

CAREGIVER: If I had known what being pregnant was really like, I would have prepared myself. Because I like to drink champagne, I would have drunk a lot before I got pregnant. That way, when I became pregnant, I wouldn't have missed it so much.

THERAPIST: Did you drink champagne before you were pregnant?

CAREGIVER: Yes. But I wasn't addicted. I think it's the most terrible addiction; worse than cigarettes. I can't deal with the high.

THERAPIST: How many months or weeks prior to becoming pregnant did you drink champagne?

CAREGIVER: I guess a few weeks. I think I may become an alcoholic after I have the baby (laughs nervously). Because every time I open the refrigerator I see champagne. This baby is going to turn me into an addict!

THERAPIST: I don't understand how the baby is involved?

CAREGIVER: Oh, I'm not blaming the baby. I'm just saying that the baby is part of me.

THERAPIST: So after the baby is born, you will drink champagne again?

CAREGIVER: I guess. I have this idea that I have been sacrificing the whole time I am pregnant. I want champagne, but I can't have it because I am pregnant. So now I keep fantasizing about having champagne right after the baby is born.

THERAPIST: Do you think you will be able to care for the baby if you drink champagne after it is born?

CAREGIVER: Well, that's the thing. I think the baby will be a little drunk while I'm breastfeeding.

THERAPIST: Have you thought about the implications this may have for the baby's health and well-being?

CAREGIVER: No, it is definitely not good for the baby . . . and I think that the baby would know it and not want to be breastfed.

THERAPIST: Do you think that's why the baby turned away from your breast in your dream?

CAREGIVER: Yes, I think so.

THERAPIST: Because your breasts were filled with something like champagne?

CAREGIVER: (animated) Yes, yes . . . that's what I meant to say, but it didn't come out clearly because of my dream.

THERAPIST: So you think the baby is aware of some of the things you fantasize about?

CAREGIVER: Yes, even though the baby is in my stomach. The baby knows I was thinking about champagne. I know it sounds silly, but I think the baby is aware of me like I'm aware of him. The baby is probably saying, "I'm going to get Mommy. I'll get back at her. I'm not going to drink her milk if she is going to have champagne because I know that is what she really wants."

THERAPIST: It sounds as if you are angry at the baby because it has changed your life, even before it has been born.

CAREGIVER: Yes, the baby makes me feel paranoid.

THERAPIST: About what?

CAREGIVER: About everything! I feel so paranoid about life. Being a woman and having a baby in my body. You start really feeling like a woman. You start getting paranoid. The baby starts making me feel and think about loss, death, grief, unhappiness. I could have a miscarriage or the baby could be born stillborn or I could die . . . you know, all the thoughts that go through your mind when the baby is inside of you.

THERAPIST: It sounds like you feel you don't have control over these thoughts.

CAREGIVER: I don't have control, and it messes me up both mentally and physically at the same time. It's like I'm dead already and the baby is alive inside of me, and everyone thinks the baby is more important than I am and isn't that concerned about me any more and my needs. That's why I want to have the champagne, because it's something I want, even if it's not good for the baby. No one understands, not even my husband. He thinks I should be happy about the baby, but I'm not . . . all that's happened is it's changed me and made me think about all the terrible things that could happen to me.

During this session many of the patient's innermost fantasies were disclosed, including her deep-seated resentment at the baby for forcing her to undergo the developmental changes associated with pregnancy. The patient also revealed her perspective on relationships in this sequence when she expressed her desire to indulge in champagne drinking, despite knowing that such behavior would be detrimental for her prospective relationship with the baby.

Her comments also reveal that she is aware of the changes that the new relationship with the infant will impose on her. This relationship has already caused her to feel "paranoid" by forcing her to think about death and loss, has caused her to "sacrifice" by giving up the pleasure of drinking champagne, and has created divisiveness in her relationship with her husband, who cannot understand what it feels like to be pregnant.

From such revelations the therapist can begin to work with the caregiver to resolve the inherent conflict in her relationships with others. Often the nature of such conflict will not become apparent until this stage of treatment, when the patient has begun to divulge dream and fantasy material. The therapist needs to be patient and receptive until reaching this point in the treatment. During Stages 1 and 2—the periods of assertiveness and assessment and the beginnings of more intimate disclosures—the therapist should help the caregiver relinquish insecurities that prevent her from disclosing information, fantasies, and free associations, so that they can forge a more intimate relationship. Stage 2 is marked by the disclosure of intimate material, generally pertaining to the caregiver's fantasies about the baby and her relationship with her husband. Not until Stage 3, however—the working-through period captured in the preceding dialogue—does the caregiver begin to reveal an abundance of unconscious residues in the form of dreams and other fantasies. To prepare the caregiver for this phase, the therapist should comment early on that he or she would welcome the disclosure of dream material. This request can be repeated intermittently, although the caregiver should not be pressured to disclose such material. As can be seen with the preceding excerpts, the caregiver will reveal her unconscious thought processes in the form of dreams when she feels comfortable about doing so. At that time, the therapist can help the caregiver in working through the conflict that has surfaced.

A vital component of short-term psychotherapy, and indeed all psychotherapy including dyadic treatment, is the transference phenomena evoked in the patient. Transference may be considered one of the main features of treatment that motivates change in the patient. According to Worchel (1986), the transference must be experienced in terms of past relationships, and a prerequisite of analyzing the patient's transference is the analysis of any resistance to treatment. Worchel advocates that a "breakthrough" into the unconscious processes of the patient occurs as a result of the patient's direct and living experience of feelings in the transference, and in particular, his or her relationship with the therapist. In virtually every case, the transference relationship begins to be evoked during the initial interview. Although each patient brings potential transference feelings from the beginning of the treatment, however, often it is only after the therapist systematically challenges the patient's resistance that these feelings emerge on the surface of the interaction. Among the therapist's principal aims, therefore, is to mobilize transference feelings and bring them out into the open discussion of the session.

The therapist can begin this process once the patient has made an opening statement. Worchel notes that the therapist may then immediately begin probing to make the patient examine the content of what he or she is saying and to give specific details. Eventually, the patient will make a comment that enables the therapist to probe for the actual emotion awakened by the transference. Many patients strive to evade the full impact of their feelings and, as a result, the therapist's task remains to probe more deeply, continually applying pressure to the resistance. Confronted with such pressure, the patient grows alarmed that his or her most painful areas will be explored and often resists further, becoming evasive through such defenses as vagueness, distancing, and rumination. According to Worchel, the therapist should continue challenging these defenses, and it is likely that the patient will become even more resistant. As the patient's resistance grows, transference feelings move to the forefront in the form of anger. Worchel explains that the resistance intensifies because of the need to avoid and conceal painful feelings. The therapist can now confront the patient with these evasive tactics, pointing out that they represent an attempt to defeat both the therapist and the patient's own avowed goal of seeking help. Eventually, Worchel notes, most patients are able to experience and acknowledge their feelings, and when this occurs, they almost inevitably experience great relief with an increase in motivation in the therapeutic alliance. Progress in the treatment is now possible, permitting an examination of other areas of the patient's life, past and present, in a more objective and meaningful manner.

A transference reaction evolves in a similar fashion during dyadic treatment where, more often than not, the caregiver will be displacing experiences deriving from her own childhood onto the person of the therapist. As in the model for analyzing the transference described by Worchel, therapists conducting dyadic therapy should attempt to engage the patient from the outset of treatment and to probe more deeply when encountering resistances. It is important to remember, however, that dyadic therapy differs from individual therapy because of the infant's presence. Any resentment or anger the caregiver is experiencing toward the therapist can be displaced by the caregiver onto her relationship with the infant. Thus, when conducting dyadic treatment, therapists should be cautious about challenging the caregiver's resistances too forcefully before she is ready to work through her conflict.

CONCLUSION

This chapter has attempted to delineate the five stages encountered during the therapeutic relationship when treatment focuses on a caregiver–infant dyad. Stage 1 is the period of assertiveness. During this introductory phase of treatment the caregiver often resists the therapist's insights. Stage 2 is the period of assessment. At this time, the patient begins to question uncertainties and insecurities that arise in her relationship with the infant and, at times, with the other caregiver. Stage 3 is the period of "working through." This phase of treatment is characterized by intensity. During this time, the caregiver is likely to disclose dream material and other fantasies spontaneously as her alliance with the therapist heightens and she begins to work through conflict stemming from an earlier period of her own development. Working through such conflict diminishes the likelihood that emotional residue from earlier relationships will intrude on the relationship with the infant. Stage 4 is the phase of involvement. During this period, the caregiver begins to understand the infant from different points of view, including that of the therapist and the infant. This new perspective is possible because the caregiver has resolved earlier conflict that threatened to interfere with or contaminate the interaction with the infant. Stage 5 is the phase of conflict resolution. It is marked by an invigorated interactional exchange between caregiver and infant. Previewing exercises will now take place frequently, as the caregiver gains confidence in introducing the infant to imminent developmental trends and to her own role in guiding the infant toward adaptive development. Moreover, as was pointed out, the infant's development can itself affect the therapeutic relationship between therapist and caregiver.

Although this chapter highlighted the key features of each of these phases, it also noted that the therapeutic relationship would differ somewhat depending on whether the caregiver was adaptive or maladaptive. In addition, discussion focused on how these therapeutic transitions affect the caregiver's relationship with both the therapist and infant, and how the therapist can help the patient overcome conflict to facilitate progress in the treatment and to instill previewing behaviors that reflect the infant's imminent developmental changes.

Chapter 11

Applying the Principles of Dream Interpretation to Dyadic Intervention

INTRODUCTION

The use of patient dreams and other fantasies during the psychotherapeutic process first gained popularity through the work of Freud (1900), who viewed such material as a valuable source of insight into the patient's *primary thought processes*. Freud defined the primary thought processes as the unconscious wishes of the patient, which are disguised and censored by the waking mind, making them virtually unintelligible and inaccessible during ordinary conscious disclosure. Through the revelation of dream material and its subsequent exploration, the therapist can discern the nature of the conflict troubling the patient. Because the patient's innermost desires and fears surface so forcefully in dreams, the therapist can use these fragments from the domain of the unconscious to pierce the veil of defense mechanisms that ordinarily shield and disguise the patient's unresolved conflict.

Although dreams therefore have enormous value during therapy with an individual patient, their therapeutic use with a caregiver–infant dyad is equally potent for several reasons. First, dreams use the process of *regression,* which enables the patient to reenact early developmental periods in life and derive *latent/unresolved conflict* from them. According to Freud, by deciphering the symbols embedded in the dream, the therapist and the patient can together understand key events from the patient's past. When the therapist is working with a caregiver–infant dyad, it is probable that a given pattern of maladaptive behavior that is overtly enacted in the mother–infant interaction derives from unresolved conflict in the caregiver's past. Thus, encouraging the caregiver to disclose dream material assists the therapist in uncovering areas of latent/unresolved conflict that are likely to intrude on the dyadic relationship.

The dream material of a new mother is also likely to contain content concerning the mother's unconscious attitude toward the birth of the child and his arrival into the household. For example, the birth of an infant may potentially usurp the caregiver's role as a prominent figure in the life of her husband and family. The caregiver's role as mother challenges her resources in the sense that she will now be primarily responsible for the life of another fragile human being who, at least for the first several years, will be almost entirely dependent on her. Caring for a newborn is not only physically exhausting but is also psychologically draining, simply because the caregiver has far less time to address her own needs. For these reasons, the caregiver may come to resent the intrusion that the infant poses to her previously independent status. Because resentment toward the infant is socially unacceptable, however, it is unlikely that the caregiver will express these feelings openly. Instead, feelings of resentment and hostility toward the infant tend to emerge in dream material that captures the caregiver's most profound emotional response to the infant.

Moreover, although the disclosure of dream material with an individual patient enables the therapist to discern unconscious conflict, in dyadic treatment the therapist obtains the additional benefit of being able to observe how the conflict is enacted in the relationship with the infant. The therapist can use the caregiver's dream material as a paradigm for dissecting domains of conflict and can then test the accuracy of these interpretations. In this manner, the conflict extrapolated either from the dream or through direct observation can be cross-validated in a manner not feasible in individual therapy. With individual patients, the therapist must wait for the patient to recount an event that occurred and then connect perceptions derived from the patient's dreams with the patient's *narrative* of real-life events. During dyadic treatment, however, the therapist can directly *observe* not only how the caregiver portrays conflict but also how she enacts such conflict in one of the seminal relationships of her life—the relationship with the infant.

Because dream material offers such a powerful tool for highlighting the contours of the caregiver–infant relationship, therapists are advised to encourage caregivers to focus on this material and should express an interest in listening to dreams and other fantasy material even during the initial interview. Therapists should request that the caregiver discuss any fantasy or dream material which has surfaced. It is often easy to obtain such material because the dramatic body changes that accompany pregnancy frequently arouse long-buried fantasies that surface in dream imagery. New mothers may be more hesitant about disclosing such material during the initial interview. However, if therapists inquire about dream material in a nonthreatening fashion after noting factual data, the caregiver will often be less reserved about revealing dream material and other fantasies. Therapists should also mention that the discussion of dreams is an integral part of the treatment and should suggest that caregivers write down their dreams and bring these reports to sessions for insight into their relationships with their infants.

Therapists have a twofold goal in using dream and fantasy material during dyadic treatment. First, the caregiver's reports will guide therapists in formulating a diagnosis regarding dysfunctional patterns of interaction within the dyad. By deciphering the predominant symbols and themes in the dream, therapists can begin to assess the nature of the conflict troubling the caregiver. Subsequently, by observing the dyadic exchange, therapists can validate their impressions. Beyond its diagnostic value, dream material also allows the therapist to engage in several direct treatment techniques. As will be discussed later in this chapter, once the therapist has identified a key conflict through the fantasy and dream material, he or she has several alternatives. First, the caregiver should be persuaded to *free associate* and try to *interpret* the dream material herself. Through free association, the caregiver will often be able to explore the genesis of the conflict inherent in her behavior and to understand how this conflict is interfering with her relationship with the infant. In such instances, the exploration of dream material results in insight that enables the caregiver to begin modifying her behavior. In other cases, the caregiver will not be able to attain insight from the disclosure of fantasy material itself, and the therapist may choose to rely on a different model of intervention (e.g., modeling) to correct apparent interactional deficits that are attributable to the caregiver's conflict. The effects of modeling can be dramatic because the caregiver will observe directly how the therapist initiates adaptive interaction with the infant and can then replicate this interaction in the therapist's presence. Successfully performed modeling can thus assist the caregiver in bypassing the exploration of unconscious data if she is not yet equipped to deal with it in a direct manner.

Previewing is a third technique the therapist can employ to diagnose or *predict* conflict when analyzing the caregiver's fantasy and dream material. It may be a particularly useful tool for helping the caregiver to explore conflict because this process challenges the caregiver to confront some of the more fundamental issues that awaken latent/unresolved conflict. As an example, previewing encourages the caregiver to deal with the issue of separation from an intimate other, particularly the separation that comes with developmental growth, a key theme often found in the associations, dreams, and fantasies of patients. Caregivers are not immune to this event, and in fact, issues of separation may cause conflict in the interaction with the infant. Although the caregiver may initially resent the intrusion posed by the caregiving experience, she gradually comes to expect the infant's dependence on her. Numerous caregivers I have treated have commented that the nurturing period spanning the first 2 years of life was one of the most gratifying they had encountered, especially because of the intimate relationships shared with the infant. The child's rapid and somehow uncontrollable development in the direction of autonomy, however, often challenges the rapport of this relationship. This trend toward autonomy can leave the caregiver feeling depleted and lonely. Such emotions often trigger the caregiver's early feelings of separation stemming from her own childhood.

One way to prevent the emotional upheaval of these events from hampering the relationship is to have the caregiver preview the infant's future development by assessing any material, including dreams, that provides a forum for addressing her anticipations about the future. Previewing consists of having the caregiver represent an upcoming developmental trend and describe the interpersonal implications of such change. The caregiver is also encouraged to formulate interpersonal manifestations that introduce the infant to the upcoming developmental change and to demonstrate these behaviors with the infant while the therapist observes the exchange. The therapist then notes the rhythms of the caregiver's behavior and her ability to support the infant's efforts toward autonomy.

These techniques—free association and interpretation of dream material, modeling when areas of potential conflict prevent further exploration, and previewing—represent some of the ways that the therapist can use fantasy and dream material in treating caregiver–infant dyads.

EXPLORING THE ADAPTIVE FUNCTIONS OF DREAMS

Before examining how dreams can further patient insight during dyadic treatment, it is important to understand the role that dreams play in our psychological functioning. Freud (1900) noted that at the core of the dream is a dream-wish that can be interpreted in two ways: first, as a wish originating in the patient's unconscious; second, as a compromise wish that is constructed from the unconscious wish. It is the first kind of dream-wish, however, the unconscious wish, that Freud (1900) viewed as the force motivating the construction of dream material.

Although wishes belonging to the unconscious mind may be the preeminent force behind dreams, other kinds of wishes also contribute to the construction of dream material. Within this category, Freud pointed to wishes that are aroused during the day but left unfulfilled; wishes that arise during the day but are repudiated and repressed, in the sense that they are driven from the preconscious to the unconscious; and wishes arising during the night that are stimulated by bodily needs. Freud cautioned, though, that although these other categories of wishes might contribute to the dream, without the wish from the unconscious the dream cannot be formed. Freud stated, for example, that the unconscious wishes are always on the alert, ready at any time to find their way to expression when an opportunity arises for allying themselves with an impulse from the conscious and for transferring their own great intensity onto the latter's lesser one. Moreover, Freud (1900) noted that a wish that is represented in a dream must be an infantile one. In the case of adults, it originates from the unconscious; in the case of children, where there is as yet no division or censorship between the preconscious and unconscious, it is an unfulfilled, unrepressed wish from waking life (Nagera et al., 1969).

Nagera et al. note that it is important for the therapist to focus on the latent dream content. These researchers point out that the latent dream content consists of dynamically unconscious wishes, latent dream thoughts, and sensory excitations. Dynamically unconscious wishes or id impulses are prevented by internal censors or ego defenses from reaching consciousness or even preconsciousness during waking life. Indeed, several such wishes may be present in the same dream. Freud observed that dreams often have more than one meaning. Not only may they include several wish fulfillments one alongside the other, but a succession of meanings or wish fulfillments may be superimposed upon one another, the bottom one being the fulfillment of a wish dating from earliest childhood. According to Nagera et al., latent dream thoughts include current preconscious preoccupations and wishes or indifferent impressions of waking life that have retained some cathexis during sleep, and preconscious thoughts that are linked with earlier experiences. Sensory excitations enter dreams when somatic sources of stimulation during the night, such as thirst or sexual excitation, fit in appropriately with the ideational content derived from the dream's psychical sources. All of these components combine in the dream. Moreover, the fulfillment of a wish is in the latent content of every dream, a general rule that also includes those dreams manifesting unpleasant or anxiety-provoking content.

It is also important to understand the role that censorship plays in dreams. As Nagera et al. explain, dream censorship controls the expression of unconscious wishes pressing toward consciousness and thereby threatening to wake the sleeper. The state of sleep makes possible a partial relaxation of the censorship because unconscious wishes can no longer find expression through action. Freud's (1900) explanation of this process was that the state of sleep makes dream formation possible because it reduces the power of the endopsychic censorship. For Nagera et al. the unconscious impulse uses this nocturnal relaxation of the defenses to force itself into consciousness with the dream. Nonetheless, the ego's defenses during sleep are not entirely obliterated, but only diminished. As a result, the forbidden wish being expressed in the dream remains disguised and unrecognizable. A final observation concerning the nature of dreams is that they rely on the patient's skills in representing images. Representation in the dream work, according to Nagera et al., modifies thoughts and impulses so that they can be represented—usually in visual form—as part of the manifest dream content.

These phenomena are useful when devising techniques for eliciting and analyzing dreams in caregiver–infant intervention. During such treatment, the caregiver will generally be eager to share dream material with the therapist, particularly after a therapeutic alliance has been established and after the therapist has suggested bringing such material to sessions for discussion. In listening to and interpreting such material, the therapist should bear in mind that the dream will contain a hidden wish deriving from the caregiver's own infantile experience and also that the dream is likely to have implications for her relationship with the infant. Thus, the therapist should exercise particular caution when interpreting the meaning of the dream: If the true meaning of the dream is too threatening for the caregiver to deal with, the therapist's premature analysis and interpretation could result in hostility that becomes displaced onto the infant. The therapist should use the dream as a vehicle for understanding the caregiver's own most intimate perceptions and conflicts and should attempt to discern how these conflicts have insinuated themselves into the caregiver's relationship with the infant. Rather than analyzing the dream directly, a more efficacious strategy may involve addressing issues of conflict and dysfunction that are evident in the dyadic exchange because these conflicts are emblematic of the conflict that has emerged through the caregiver's dream. Finally, representational capacities are a prerequisite for the ability to dream, so the therapist should encourage the caregiver to engage in all forms of representational exercises.

Freud (1900) commented that therapists should "disregard the apparent coherence between a dream's constituents as an unessential illusion" (p. 449). In other words, Freud was aware that the true meaning and significance of the dream lay beyond its surface structure or its *manifest content*. One technique for delving beyond the manifest content of the dream, first advocated by Freud, involves having the patient free associate to the images contained in the dream. This form of free association, Freud believed, allows for the revelation of the meaning hidden in the dream's symbols and imagery. The dream constitutes a residue of what the patient intends to signify or convey, with its manifest content disguising a more profound *latent content*.

Freud also advised that to discover what a particular dream means, the therapist needs to consider several factors. First, it is necessary to examine the circumstances that provide the occasion for having or relating the dream. For example, what kinds of precipitating experiences did the patient have that day before falling asleep? Or, what important issues were raised in the session before the patient communicated the dream? As posited by Kohut (1977), the therapist's knowledge of the patient's key conflicts and concerns are further clues for discerning why a patient has seized on a particular dream construction. Second, what kinds of symbolic transformations were chosen for constructing the dream? Third, what is the nature of the system that is responsible for the ultimate transformation of these symbols? Fourth, what intentions may underlie a particular presentation in symbolic form? In other words, what has motivated the particular meaning the patient has given to the symbol?

Along these lines, Edelson (1973) has posited that the way that the patient describes the dream—the very structure of the patient's language—communicates almost as much as the hidden symbolic content. On occasion the symbols or images are relatively understandable and may derive from thought processes that are fairly close to consciousness. In these cases the therapist may understand the implications of the dream fairly rapidly without much need for free association exercises on the part of the patient. Nevertheless, the patient may need time and encouragement to recognize and assimilate the content of the dream and to accept its implications with respect to her emotional state. It may require several sessions before the patient can interpret the message she has conveyed in the dream and begin formulating strategies to modify her behavior.

More recently, researchers have underscored the *adaptive* functions achieved by dreaming (Bradlow, 1973; Erikson, 1954; Kohut, 1977). Fosshage (1987) for example, has stated that to perceive dreams as being primarily adaptive, it is necessary to reexamine the nature of the primary thought processes. Fosshage defines the primary thought process not as a primitive form of mental representation, but as a form of cognition that relies on sensory images; such images serve an integrative role. Eisnitz (1987) has emphasized that in dreaming the dreamer essentially regresses in the service of self-representation. Virtually all dreams, whether they represent some reconciliation with a developmental event or effort to work through a conflict, possess the capacity for revealing unresolved conflict.

Once dreams are perceived as serving the adaptive function of attempting to resolve conflict, the distinction between manifest and latent content becomes unnecessary. Fosshage's view of dreams as part of an adaptive, integrative, and creative function emphasizes the clinical benefit of their manifest content. Foulkes (1985) is another researcher who believes dreams are mental acts organized both at a *momentary* level and on a *sequential* level. According to Foulkes, dreams are organized in the form of a narrative or story in the same manner as much of our waking experience. Although the narrative organization may break down, Foulkes notes that most transitions in dreams preserve either the characters, the setting, or both. Some therapists tend to deemphasize this aspect of dream imagery, focusing on the disorganized, regressive, and disguised qualities of the dream, instead of on the more coherent and organized thematic content.

This discussion has highlighted some general conceptions and theories related to interpreting the dreams of patients in treatment. Freud distinguished between the manifest content of the dream and its more hidden aspects, which are communicated in symbolic forms. This latter feature of the dream is referred to as its latent content. Many researchers have advocated free association for ascertaining the meaning of the latent content. There are, however, other useful techniques for interpretating the meaning of the dream. For example, the therapist should attend to the particular nuances of the language the patient uses in describing the dream and the circumstances surrounding it. In addition, although Freud stressed that dreams allow access to primary thought processes and therefore emerge from the unconscious of the patient, recent theory suggests that dreams may involve thought processes that are more accessible to the patient's awareness. As a result, therapists should ask patients to speculate on the meaning of the dreams that they relate. The following illustration indicates how the patient may already possess some awareness of the conflict revealed in the dream material:

CAREGIVER: I had a dream that I was teaching my baby how to walk. We were walking outside near a hospital. He lost his balance, fell, and hit his head on the sidewalk. I rushed him to the hospital, and a doctor operated on his head. He had to get many stitches. Later on the nurse brought out two babies. One was on top of the crib and one was underneath. One of them was my baby, and he was naked. I couldn't tell if the other one was a boy or a girl. I asked the nurse why my baby was able to have a baby for me.

THERAPIST: How do you feel about this dream?

CAREGIVER: I thought it was unrealistic that my baby gave birth to his own baby. Of course, that couldn't happen in real life.

In this case, the caregiver had formed a close and intimate relationship with her 14-month-old infant. She was able to preview the infant's upcoming developmental trends and, until several weeks prior to the disclosure of this dream, had appeared to delight in her infant's achievements. Frequently she had commented that having the baby had changed her life for the better, given her new purpose and meaning, and allowed her to enjoy the kind of intimacy and closeness she had not previously experienced in her relationships. Nevertheless, when the infant began to exhibit signs of full-fledged walking behavior, an irritability surfaced in the caregiver, who complained that the baby was becoming too independent and that such behavior was not good for him. Without acknowledging her fear of losing the intimate relationship with the infant directly, the caregiver unexpectedly began to speak about having another baby. This dream suggests that the caregiver is cognizant, on some level, of the ambivalent feelings she harbors concerning her infant's burgeoning autonomy.

OVERCOMING THE RESISTANCE FOR EXPLORING DREAMS

Although the analysis of dreams can provide compelling insights into the unconscious struggles troubling the patient, dream material itself is not free from the taint of complex symbolic constructions that cloak their meaning. The many symbols inherent in dream material that disguise the meaning of the dream have been referred to as resistances (Gillman, 1987). Some resistances are inherent in the construction of dreams. Rothstein (1983) has described this process as an assimilative effort in which defense mechanisms modify the process that makes the content of unconscious processes become available. This assimilative effort results in the manifest dream that the patient reports to the therapist, whereas the disguises shield the dreamer from an awareness of the conflicting elements that lie underneath it.

Gillman (1987) has pointed out that resistance affects how the patient discloses the dream material. For example, some patients will save a dream until the end of the session, thereby precluding meaningful discussion about it. Other patients will resist free association to the imagery contained in the dream. Thus, therapists need to attend not only to the content of the dream, but also to the circumstances surrounding its disclosure.

The following case history embodies these principles. Gina, a 28-year-old securities trader, was referred for treatment by her gynecologist, who cited the patient's ambivalence about whether to continue her pregnancy. She had had three previous abortions, despite adequate knowledge of birth control techniques, one during her first marriage and two during a 4-year relationship preceding her recent remarriage. She was adamant in her view that she did not want children: "My husband knew this before we got married," she repeated several times during the first interview. An ostensibly confident woman, Gina appeared unsure and defensive only when discussing pregnancy and childrearing. On those two issues, she told the therapist, she felt she was being "attacked" constantly. She explained that her earlier marriage had ended because her first husband had wanted children and she had not. Now 6 months into her new marriage, she had discovered that she was pregnant and had become deeply concerned, actively considering an abortion although her husband had mixed feelings about terminating the pregnancy. "This is a nightmare! It feels like my first marriage all over again!" she said angrily.

When the therapist asked to discuss the reasons she was opposed to having a child, she first mentioned her fear of the pain of childbirth. On further consideration, she added that her own mother, an alcoholic, had not been a particularly nurturing parent, and Gina felt that she might not be able to nurture her child because of her own childhood experience. Finally, she mentioned the pressure of her job, stating that she thought that the stress she faced at work would have a "negative effect on a fetus." When the therapist observed that her statement implied a capacity for nurturance, Gina responded angrily that anyone could be nurturing for 5 minutes at a time, "even my mother."

In the third session, Gina complained of a nightmare in which she and her husband were shopping at a department store. "I'm wheeling this huge shopping cart as if we were in a supermarket, but in fact it was a very expensive and exclusive shop." In the dream, Gina does not want to shop, but her husband insists that they continue. As they go from department to department, her husband piles items—clothes, jewelry, groceries—into the cart, despite Gina's protests that none of the articles are things she wants or normally wears. "As I see my husband doing this, I get more and more anxious. I don't know how we're going to pay for all this junk—that is, how I'm going to pay for it; somehow I know my husband doesn't have his credit cards and it's all going to go on my account. Finally, I can hardly see over the top of the cart, it's piled so high, and still Harry keeps throwing things on it. I stop pushing the cart and begin crying and all the women in the store start staring at me and shaking their heads." Pressed for her opinion on the meaning of her dream, Gina said she thought it referred to investment pressures she had been experiencing lately. "I need to get control of things again," she insisted.

During the fourth session, the patient related a dream she had had the night before the session. In the dream she was seated in a nonsmoking car on a commuter railroad train into the city. As she sat reading her newspaper, the train went through a tunnel. While they were traveling through the tunnel, the lights in the car went out and everything was pitch black. When the train emerged from the tunnel and she could see again, Gina found herself unwittingly among smokers in a smoking car—a situation ostensibly repelling to her. "I hadn't moved, but suddenly everyone around me was puffing away. It was disgusting, but after a minute I sort of gave in and lit up a cigarette too."

When the therapist asked if Gina could relate her feeling about cigarette smoking, she responded that she had never tried tobacco, that both of her parents had been heavy smokers and she was afraid of getting "hooked" herself. Upon further inquiry, Gina admitted that as a teenager she had tried marijuana twice but stopped after the second time, fearing that she would become addicted, because addiction "runs in the family. . . . The second time I tried it (marijuana) I came home stoned, and Mom was drunk, and I guess being high made it [her mother's inebriation] seem even worse than usual. Mom was really out of control. I realized that I just couldn't take the risk of smoking pot and winding up like my mother."

After discussing these associations with the patient, the therapist interpreted the first of these dreams as a reaction, not only to the pressure to have a child, but to a perceived pressure to change, to be transformed unwillingly into another person as a result of the pregnancy. The articles that her husband has pressed on her are not what she would choose for herself; instead, these items may burden her and change her into someone else. In addition, Gina realizes that not only is she under pressure to change, she is the one who will have to "pay" for the unwanted transformation. Unable to vent her rage at being transformed against her will, the patient's reaction is to cry hopelessly; but this crying itself draws the attention, and implied censure, of other women in the store. These women, who presumably are shopping at the same "store" of their own volition, condemn Gina for her unwillingness to participate, to become a mother. That the patient, despite being "very careful about birth control," had already had three abortions and was anticipating a fourth, indicates that her avowed opposition to childbearing is fueled by more ambivalent emotions than she admits. Finally, some symbols of the dream are suggestive: the wire shopping cart into which the articles are piled is reminiscent of a cage; and the clothes and objects are thrown untidily into the cart, creating a heap of "things" that Gina plainly cannot control. Control, by the patient's own admission, is an issue of considerable importance to her. The imagery of the dream also suggests that Gina may be perceiving the infant as a creature who will be overly dependent on her and who will further deplete her resources on all levels. It is Gina who is pushing the cart that becomes heavier and more unwieldy with each purchase her husband tosses on the pile. Symbolically, Gina is here projecting that she will shoulder the physical burden of childbirth, a burden of which her husband is oblivious, at least in the dream.

In addition to interpreting the dream's symbols, the dream itself can be used to predict how Gina would interact with the infant if it were born. For example, the manner in which Gina perceives and reacts to dependency needs in the dream predicts how she might experience her own infant's dependency needs. A predominant theme in the dream is Gina's anxiety and concern, indicating that she is anxious and concerned about the implications of others' dependency needs for her own autonomy. It appears she believes that if she gave birth, the infant would infringe on her own independence.

In the second dream, transformation imagery is even more striking, as is the link to addictive behavior, which the patient fears is her familial legacy. While commuting to work, Gina emerges from the tunnel (which may symbolize the experience of giving birth) only to find that she has become an "addict," a characterization associated with her own mother. Despite the disgust she feels for cigarette smoking, Gina does not resist when she finds herself surrounded by smokers and subsequently begins to smoke, as if the mere fact of the transformation she has undergone in the dream has undermined her ability to engage in free choice. This imagery is more potent because of Gina's memory of smoking marijuana and seeing her mother intoxicated, and her subsequent fear not only of becoming addicted, but also of being out of control. The dream further shows how Gina has symbolically represented the end of her pregnancy through abortion. An inappropriate affective tone suffuses this dream, because although Gina is initially "disgusted" when she finds herself in the smoking car at the end of the tunnel, she almost immediately joins the smokers by "lighting up." This behavior evidences a wish to identify with the aggressor. Used as a predictor, the dream suggests that Gina might retaliate against what she perceives to be the depleting dependency needs of the infant. She would be manifesting inappropriate aggressive behaviors through her identifications with previous aggressors.

Although the intensity of Gina's ambivalence at the prospect of motherhood is uncommon, the emotion itself is not. Bardwick (1971) has addressed the high incidence of ambivalence about pregnancy and the changes this ambivalence causes in young women. At the same time, this patient has a strong sense that childbearing and raising a child is still, despite the increasing incidence of women working outside the home, a primary focal activity for women. Sherwen (1981) notes a clear split between dependence and independence in the fantasies of pregnant women; perhaps this perceived split extends even to women confronting the options of parenthood or abortion. Benedek (1959a) has noted the extent to which parents of both sexes identify with their own parents. A feature of this patient's second dream is the fear that in becoming a mother, a woman is doomed to replicate her own mother's life.

The depth of this patient's ambivalent feelings about motherhood made it clear that the pregnancy was evoking a serious conflict in Gina. It was suggested that Gina continue in therapy to define and resolve the issues of control and family history that colored her perception of motherhood. Because ambivalence dominated her behavior, it was apparent that she was not yet emotionally equipped to cope with the conflict aroused by pregnancy itself. The therapist was also advised to encourage the patient to continue reporting her dreams. This technique would make it possible to closely monitor the patient's perception of the conflict aroused by dependency feelings as well as her ability to acknowledge and eventually resolve this conflict.

DREAM IMAGERY DURING THE VARIOUS PHASES OF MOTHERHOOD

Dream Imagery During the Prenatal Stages

There is a growing body of literature on the perceptions and fantasies of pregnant women concerning their unborn children. This research also explores the relationship between these antenatal fantasies and the subsequent ability of mother and infant to bond securely after the birth. Exploration of dreams improves the therapist's ability to predict the nature of the patient's unresolved conflict. Caplan (1959) analyzed the fantasies of expectant mothers and sought to correlate types of fantasies with corresponding trimesters of the women's pregnancies. The first stage in Caplan's scheme spans the time from conception until the mother perceives the infant's movements in utero at approximately the 4th month of gestation. During this period, the gain in body weight and swelling of the breasts revive adolescence-related fantasies about body changes. As the second trimester approaches, the prospective caregiver begins to acquire a more realistic perception of the unborn infant as an independent being. Fantasies at this time may be diverse and unusual. The infant may be represented as a dirty or shameful object that the mother needs to expel or as a parasitic creature gnawing from within. Expectant mothers can also experience the fetus as devouring, attacking, or destroying during this period (Ballou, 1978;

Benedek, 1970a, 1970c; Pines, 1972; Raphael-Leff, 1980). According to Caplan, the final trimester is typified by mood swings that range from pleasure at the prospect of the impending birth to anxiety that the fetus might die during childbirth or fantasies that the infant may be born damaged or deformed.

Other researchers, most notably Coleman (1974), have noted that during pregnancy women are apt to become fascinated by dreams and fantasies, as if searching for omens or predictions that will assuage their questions and anxieties. Such fantasies may also have a specific effect on the postnatal relationship of mother and infant. For example, Condon and Dunn (1988) have found that a strong prenatal fantasy of the baby can cause parental disappointment if the real neonate varies too much from the *fantasy baby*. Parents with less structured fantasies about the unborn child, and parents whose real baby is a close match to the fantasy child, are much more likely to be content with their infant after the birth.

In women whose prenatal dreams and fantasies focus on the development of a relationship with the unborn child, evolution of a secure and flexible bond with the child is likely. These women are using fantasy material to preview an adaptive relationship with the infant. But what about those women whose emotional dysfunction hampers the ability to forge an adaptive relationship with the infant? If, as Kestenberg (1956) and Benedek (1959a) suggest, motherhood is itself a developmental phase, it follows that caregivers whose histories indicate unresolved emotional issues and troubled early development may find motherhood to be a period of turmoil.

The dreams of pregnant women are likely to be highly revealing to the therapist, because certain key issues that disrupt or at least challenge the patient's view of herself dominate during pregnancy. For example, as noted earlier, the change in the woman's physical appearance is likely to cause some realignment in body image—with either a positive or negative result. So too will the pregnant woman be treated differently by others, including her husband and family, as she traverses the rite of passage from being an independent female to assuming the role of mother. Each of these transitions affects perceptions of how she views herself and her personality. Because these images are seminal to the individual's self-image and self-esteem, it is likely that dream imagery will reflect abundant information about how the pregnant mother is coping with these changes. As will be seen in the dreams of the following two patients, self-representations tend to become distorted during pregnancy. In the first case, the patient dreamed that she was in a ruined, dilapidated house, whereas in the second dream, images of a dead dog and a burning cigarette predominated for the patient. Therapists working with pregnant women need to be alert to the ways in which their patients' dreams reflect self-representation and should attempt to determine the predictive value of the dream material.

In addition to modifications in self-representation, pregnant women also commonly report separation themes. As a transitional event pregnancy would likely evoke previously suppressed memories of separation episodes. Some of these dreams represent a belated attempt by the patient to master the trauma of the anxious and depressive affects aroused by prior experiences with loss (Myers, 1987). Myers' findings are, in many respects, analogous to those of Caplan (1959), who observed that pregnancy tends to unleash past memories associated with change in object relations (e.g., loss). These feelings of mourning and loss come with the pregnant woman's recognition that her body will now bear the indelible mark of motherhood and that she will no longer be merely a daughter dependent on her own mother; now she will be a mother in her own right, responsible for nurturing her infant. The woman's independent status and her ability to rely on others are therefore "lost" to a certain extent as she assumes the motherhood role and accountability for the infant's dependency needs.

The imagery of separation that can occur with the evolution of pregnancy is somewhat less obvious. As will be seen in the first dream discussed in the following paragraphs, during the 9-month gestation period expectant parents begin to develop an attachment to the unborn baby and to fantasize about the infant's personality. By the time delivery approaches, the expectant mother often has difficulty relinquishing this fantasy baby with whom she has had an imaginary relationship for the past several months. Moreover, the birth itself is likely to evoke images of separation and mourning that are reminiscent of the separation experiences in the caregiver's earlier life (Pines, 1972). These issues trigger memories of how the expectant woman perceives her own mother dealt with her during infancy and childhood.

As with other dream images explored in this chapter, it is important for the therapist working with pregnant women to attempt to isolate these themes of separation and loss from the fantasies they report. By identifying the caregiver's conflict in dealing with her changing self-representation and the sense of separation that accompanies the developmental processes, the therapist can help her explore and resolve ambivalent feelings that threaten, before the baby is born, to intrude into the later interaction with the infant.

Catherine, the first of two expectant mothers whose dreams are examined here, had no history of psychiatric dysfunction but was referred to therapy because of her increasing anxiety about her unborn baby. The patient and her husband had waited until their finances and careers were firmly established before starting a family. Even at that point, it had taken almost 3 years for Catherine to conceive. At the time of her first session, Catherine was 38 years old and 6½ months into her pregnancy. Although she had experienced some spotting during the first trimester, all indications were that the fetus was healthy and that the remainder of the pregnancy and delivery would proceed without problems. Despite these assurances,

Catherine's apprehensions for the fetus's health increased as her pregnancy advanced. She had discussed leaving her position as vice-president of a construction supply firm to minimize the stress of her job and any potential danger to her unborn child. She often characterized her fantasies as containing "ridiculous anxieties," but she was not able to minimize their impact on her state of mind. The patient told the therapist that the day before her first session she had been deeply disturbed by a greeting card she had seen by chance. "It was white, with a splashy red heart on it, but it made me think of blood on bandages and I felt this sudden panic that I was going to miscarry." This brief fantasy had disturbed her so much that she had to go home for the rest of the afternoon. Her husband, she noted, was sympathetic to her distress but did not share her fears or understand her anxieties. She reported that he continued to remind her of the obstetrician's assurances that the pregnancy was proceeding normally.

Two of Catherine's dreams offer particular insight into her anxieties. In the first, related during her seventh meeting with the therapist, she described being in an old tumbledown house, a ruin that looked familiar to her. When pressed to explain this sense of familiarity, Catherine suggested that it might be the house in which she had spent the first 6 years of her childhood. Exploring the wreckage, Catherine felt compelled to go deeper and deeper into the house, until she felt severe pains in her abdomen. When she looked down, she saw that "her belly had swollen enormously," to twice the size it had been a moment before. As the pains grew more severe, she kept crying out that it was too early to have the baby, that it was not time yet. Then she suddenly awoke. Catherine reported that she had been agitated and disoriented for several minutes after waking from the dream.

In a dream related during the next session, Catherine returned to the ruined house. This time she went to the basement and began looking for something that would help her identify the house as the one in which she had lived. Finally, on a high shelf in a corner, half hidden by boxes and debris, she saw one of her old childhood dolls, which was torn, dirty, and missing a leg. Catherine reported that when she tried to reach for the doll she felt a sharp pain in her belly again, and that the harder she reached, the greater her pain. Then she felt a shoving sensation behind her and turned to see a doctor pushing her from behind and her husband pulling from the front, trying to get her to leave the basement. "I kept telling them that I couldn't leave without the doll, but they didn't seem to hear me," she added. When asked to identify the doctor pushing from behind, Catherine hesitated. "At first I thought it was my obstetrician, but then I thought maybe it was you," she said, referring to the therapist.

Dreams have a distinctive place in the process of reconstruction because they often reevoke our earliest and most emotionally laden experiences (Dowling, 1987). Among these early experiences are instances of utter helplessness and dependency. They are traumatic in the sense that they contribute to the structuring of our personality, the genesis of psychopathology, and the organizing and clustering of our seminal experiences. It is not unusual, then, that during periods of stress and uncertainty in our adult lives we tend to recollect such helpless episodes through our dream material. By formulating a strategy for overcoming this primal, infantile helplessness, we may discern a means of extricating ourselves from the current crisis.

Both of Catherine's dreams are set in a context from the patient's childhood: the house in which she spent her earliest years. Significantly, in both dreams the house is in ruins; it is not a place to which she can return. As if to underscore the idea that her past is lost, Catherine's pains occur only as she tries to establish a more substantial link to the past by exploring the ruins of the house. Both dreams end with the imminence of birth and Catherine's panicked sense that the event is arriving too soon; in both dreams the house may also symbolize her fears of physical trauma and the destruction that the childbirth can precipitate. In the second dream her husband and doctor (variously her obstetrician or the therapist) may be helping her to leave the house while Catherine protests that she cannot leave without the doll. Perhaps leaving with the doll is the only way that the patient believes she can rescue herself and gain control of her past. Additionally, by removing the doll from the wreckage, Catherine may be attempting to reassure herself about the safety and health of her unborn child. That both husband and doctor are in the house with her indicates her awareness of their support; this is particularly important because the patient had expressed some anxiety that her relationship with her husband was undergoing stress as a result of the imminent arrival of the baby.

Catherine's symbolism of a dilapidated house may have further implications for the unborn baby. The ruined house suggests that Catherine may perceive her uterus as being unprepared and somehow inadequate for the transformations necessary to nurture the developing fetus. When used as a predictor for how Catherine may interact with the infant, the dream suggests that this expectant mother fears that she will be unable to respond in an emotionally positive fashion to her infant, because she herself has not experienced sufficient differentiation and the transformation necessary to become a full-fledged nurturing figure. The presence of the doll—as well as her husband and doctor—in her second dream, indicates that Catherine is attempting to resolve how she will negotiate a triangular relationship once the baby is born and how the birth will affect her relationship with others, most notably her husband. The "push and pull" imagery implies that the triangular configuration evokes a sense of conflict. Moreover, the image of the doll with the missing limb may be a predictive metaphor, suggesting that if the conflict of negotiating a triangular relationship remains unresolved, Catherine may be at risk for treating the infant like an inanimate object whose needs she will not meet adaptively.

Ostensibly this expectant mother was eager to make "any and all sacrifices" to assure the welfare of her unborn child—even to the point of leaving her job, which was not deemed medically necessary. But there emerges in the dream a countervailing emotion of resentment at having to make these changes. Catherine's anger is so potent that she fears it will destroy the baby. To defuse this rage against the infant—which cannot be acknowledged consciously because it is "unacceptable"—the mother believes that she must leave behind all traces of her past; it is as if she were saying "I must give up everything of my old life to be transformed into a good mother."

The material presented by the second pregnant woman is also noteworthy. Loretta was 22 years old and in her 3rd month of pregnancy. She had been seeing a therapist on a weekly basis for 14 months for treatment of her schizoaffective disorder. Her therapist had referred Loretta for a special evaluation to ascertain the patient's overall perceptions of the pregnancy. At the time of the first session, the mother–infant therapist noted a significant inability on the patient's part to discuss or make predictions about her unborn child. A voluble and fluent speaker, Loretta's responses were frequently combative or defensive, except when she specifically discussed her unborn child. At those times her demeanor appeared calm and unconcerned. Direct questioning proved unsatisfactory with this patient, but when she was permitted some control over the discussion, the expectant mother provided enthusiastic responses. She spoke vividly of a delusional episode she had experienced during adolescence and indicated that during that episode she had possessed the ability to "control other people's thoughts." When asked to explain this process she said, "I could control what my father was thinking. I knew just what he was going to say to me, and I could make him say those things just by thinking about them. Whenever that happened, I knew I was controlling his thoughts."

Over the course of several sessions, Loretta described three "special" dreams she had had in sequence since learning of her pregnancy. In the first dream, she described an attempt to remove her wedding band. "I couldn't get it off," she said. "My hand had gotten too fat." In the dream, she finally succeeded in removing the ring and placed it in a drawer in her bureau. Later in the dream, she looked for the ring but could not find it. "I could have sworn that I opened the drawer and put it in there because that's where I keep all of my jewelry. When I asked my husband where it was, he said to me, 'Loretta, it's on the floor, it fell on the floor.' But I said, 'No, it can't be on the floor, because I know I put it in the drawer.' But when I went and looked, I saw my husband was right, it was on the floor." In her second dream, the expectant mother reported that she got up from her bed to get a hanger from the closet. "I got the hanger, twisted it, then put it on the floor under the bed. It was as if I had to do that; it was almost like a compulsion. I've seen movies where pregnant women want to kill their babies and they gave themselves abortions with hangers." In the third and final dream, Loretta was staring up into the sky and saw her dog, who had died several years before. She then "smelled something burning" and realized that she had "left a cigarette burning"; at this point Loretta woke up. When asked to give more details about the dream, Loretta added that when she smelled the cigarette, "I looked up at the sky, and this time there was something wrong with it. I could see the dog's spinal cord, legs, head, two front teeth, and tail. The parts were all mixed together, and the dog was deformed."

The conflict implicit in all three dreams, evoked by the pregnancy, is dramatic. The representation of loss and mutilation—of losing the ring, of the hanger (suggesting abortion imagery), and of the hurt or diseased dog (evocative of the unborn child)—is particularly striking. The dog imagery, which continued in her discussion of the pregnancy, is intriguing not only because it provides some insight about Loretta's *representations* regarding the fetus but also because it demonstrates her perceived fear of giving birth to a damaged child, her own personal transformation as a result of the pregnancy, and her fear of becoming a mother. Later in the session, Loretta confided, "I have to sleep on my back now, and I think I must be snoring, because I wake up to the noise and I know it is not my husband. I sound just like my dog used to sound." In later sessions, Loretta remarked that she had never expected that pregnancy would "change" her so much. When the therapist asked what she had expected, the patient answered evasively, "I don't know" or "I can't think about it."

Various studies, along with anecdotal accounts (Adams-Hillard, 1985; Condon, 1986, 1987a, 1987b; Gelles, 1975), have suggested that the psychological urge of the pregnant woman to assault the fetus is not rare. Although her dream representation allowed Loretta to vent some of the fears and conflicts she felt toward her pregnancy and her unborn child, the imagery is thinly veiled and indicates a far less adaptive response to ambivalent emotions than Catherine's emotionally harrowing, but successfully dissociated, dreams. Thus, Loretta's struggle to rein in her destructive wishes remains a seminal issue requiring intervention and continued support through therapy.

The sequence of Loretta's dreams is notable because the theme of confusion and misperception dominates. For example, Loretta is mistaken about where she has placed the ring and forgets about the burning cigarette. These events indicate that Loretta harbors anxiety that the infant may be "misplaced" like the ring or may be "damaged" like the dog in the sky. The symbolism here also suggests that Loretta may be seeking to disguise the hostility she feels for the unborn infant. The compulsion to twist the hanger, the dropped and misplaced ring, and the burning cigarette are all symbols of overt carelessness and destruction that may indicate Loretta would be prone to hurt the infant if she felt it were a creature beyond her control.

Dream Imagery During the Postnatal Stages of Motherhood

The birth of a child, the end of a 9-month wait, and, theoretically, the resolution of parental fantasies about the unborn infant also have significant meanings for the caregiver. Both woman and fantasy baby are transformed; the expectant mother becomes a mother; the fetus is at last an infant. But they are also separated: mother and child are no longer one physical unit, united in one body. In addition, parents who have invested considerable energy in the representation of a fantasy baby may confront, in the neonate, the loss of that imagined and already-loved child (Condon & Dunn, 1988). The parents may therefore need time to grieve for the fantasy that has been lost and to adjust to the reality of the infant who has actually become a part of their family. This relinquishment of the fantasy baby for the real baby is only the first of many separations and realignments in the family's relationships. Every developmental milestone that occurs thereafter is, in effect, a reminder that the infant, to thrive and prosper, must continue to pull away and separate while continuing to change.

Of all the dream imagery discussed in this chapter, perhaps the most fascinating to examine is the imagery described by caregivers during the postpartum period. The dreams and fantasies that predominate during this period are particularly compelling because the therapist has the opportunity to compare the content of the dream material with the real-life functioning of the caregiver during interaction with the infant. In this respect, the dreams reported by new mothers have an even more compelling predictive value than the dreams of pregnant women. Although the therapist can predict some conflict that will eventually emerge during caregiver–infant interaction when assessing a pregnant woman's dreams, validating these predictions is not possible until after the infant is actually born. With new mothers, however, once the therapist identifies conflict buried within the dream content, he can almost immediately evaluate how this conflict manifests itself during the exchange with the baby.

In the first of the following cases, the caregiver was struggling with feelings of loss and separation triggered by the emergence of weaning behavior in her infant. This mother's dream emphasized images of loss and separation and was an evocation of previous life events that had caused unresolved conflict. In the case of the dreams of the second caregiver, images of violence and hostility dominated in her dream and the therapist interpreted this imagery as reflecting the caregiver's anger and hostility toward her infant. In both instances, disclosure of these dreams allowed the therapist to predict domains of conflict and to help the caregivers devise strategies for resolving the conflict.

The following case report deals with a caregiver who shared a highly empathic and affectionate relationship with her infant son. As becomes clear through the dream material, however, the professed intimacy of the dyad actually disguised the caregiver's fears regarding issues related to her son's dependency. These fears became apparent to the therapist when exploring the patient's dreams. In analyzing such dreams, therapists are urged to use caution because the caregiver may not be equipped to deal with the full implications that emerge from the dream material.

A 3-month-old infant was brought to the clinic by his mother, a 23-year-old woman with a master's degree in political science. The mother was courteous and sympathetic and displayed positive affect during interaction with her infant. She shared a dream she could "never understand." Soon after she began telling the therapist about the dream, she added important material that she believed was pertinent to the dream. "In the dream," she said, "my husband and I had bought a miniature version of our own car customized in the form of a very soft pillow. The shape and colors printed on the fabric of the pillow imitated the fabric of a real car. We bought the pillow to keep the baby company when we were away from him," the mother told me. "In the dream," she continued, "I realized suddenly while I was walking in the street that my son's car pillow was being driven. I followed it, and when it stopped for a red light, opened the passenger door and sneaked inside. As I closed the door, I panicked, realizing that there was no driver. Instead, there were a few layers of fabric on the driver's seat. With my left hand, I tried to get rid of the fabric while supporting myself with my right hand on the dashboard. I eventually managed to throw the fabric into the back seat. After trying to manipulate the car's controls, I realized that it was driven by remote control. It then occurred to me that my son must have a very advanced mind to be able to operate a car by remote control. Even I couldn't understand how to operate the car. Next, I tried to stop the car. I pressed the brake, but it didn't work. I pressed the accelerator, but it didn't work either. Then I got desperate and pressed both at once. The car skidded 180 degrees and began traveling in reverse. Then the direction changed about 30 degrees. I was very frightened. I knew the car was no longer under control."

For a moment, the patient appeared to be in a trance. She looked at the therapist and said, "No one had control. I was frightened because the car was going backward over a hill and I knew it was close to the end of it. When I realized this, I began to sweat heavily. I pulled my hair and thought I was going to die. The car ran into a fence at the end of the hill. It flipped backward from the hill down, stopping, oddly enough, in the center of a fire station. When it hit the floor, it bounced back, lying upside down. As I managed to climb out, the fire department personnel formed a fencelike circle around me and the car, getting closer, closing the circle. They smiled, held out their hands, and asked if I was all right. With hesitation I told them I was. Soon I turned, pointed to the car sorrowfully, and told them the car was damaged beyond repair. They raised their eyebrows in question; their faces became paperlike and rigid. They asked whose car it was. I felt like a thief. 'It's my son's,' I said, 'and worse, he's going to know that I ruined the controls of his car.' I was beside myself with the possibility of telling my son what I had done . . . that the car was beyond repair. Then I woke up, and I remember feeling sad and disappointed."

Exploration of the patient's dream revealed that the pillow represented her wish to be in close proximity to her son when he slept, to be with him always, thus preventing any form of separation. "He would have 24-hour companionship," as the patient once commented. The dramatic process in this dream obscures her motivation to remain close to her son and control his development.

In the next two dreams the caregivers were, through their dream material, enacting feelings of helplessness evoked by the realization that they could not control the emergence of autonomy in their infants. Both of these mothers were displaying a tendency to cope with imminent separation in a dramatic fashion that most likely replicated the trauma associated with their own experiences of past separation. The therapist's task was to assist the caregivers in devising more adaptive means for dealing with their infants' development and the interpersonal implications triggered by such maturation.

These cases involve two primiparous caregivers. The first, Jill, entered treatment when her daughter was 4 months old, citing her wish to better understand her infant's developmental processes and the upcoming weaning process. Her interaction with the infant was characterized by attunement (Stern, 1985) and reciprocity (Brazelton, Koslowski, & Main, 1974), and by a high degree of skill in previewing developmental milestones (Trad, 1990). The caregiver had breastfed the infant from birth, and early in the course of treatment volunteered that her interaction with the infant, Mimi, particularly during breastfeeding episodes, was one of the most rewarding experiences of her life. When Mimi reached 8 months of age, Jill mentioned her plans to begin the weaning process. Initially, her expressed attitude about this event was wholly positive, but during the following month, the caregiver became increasingly withdrawn and subdued. Questioned about her daughter's progress at weaning and her own feelings about this process, Jill admitted that Mimi had several times rejected her breast in favor of a bottle and that this previously anticipated milestone had begun to "affect" her deeply. She then addressed the topic directly, noting that her life had been "deprived of meaning" and that she tried to hide her sense of hopelessness from the baby but did not believe she was doing very well. "I just feel empty. I don't feel Mimi is mine anymore." In addition, the caregiver admitted that because she had had several distressing dreams during the past weeks, she now found it difficult to fall asleep; her resulting exhaustion further augmented her sense of frustration and helplessness.

Shortly after the first time her infant rejected the breast in favor of a bottle, Jill experienced the following dream. She was driving through the neighborhood in which she had been raised as a child. Passing neighbors' houses, Jill suddenly recalled an old friend whom she had not seen or heard from in many years. She explained that her friend's father had died unexpectedly and that the whole family had moved away immediately after the funeral. In the dream the memory moved her deeply and she suddenly missed her friend very much, but in relating the dream later, Jill expressed considerable surprise that the memory of this friend had surfaced.

During the same session in which Jill revealed her dream, the caregiver mentioned that she had decided to have a cyst removed from her left hand in the next week. She had had the cyst for a number of years, but it had begun to bother her only recently. She complained that the cyst was particularly troublesome when she checked the temperature of her infant's bottle. Her doctor, she explained, "would just lance the cyst"; her description of the process was unusually graphic. "If it's only fluid-filled, he will simply drain the liquid out," she finished, adding that this minor surgery "would not" inconvenience her for more than a day or two.

Jill's dream clearly recalls an episode of loss, paralleling the current loss being experienced as a result of her infant's weaning. Through her dream, the caregiver reviewed an earlier event that had triggered feelings of loss and depression. But when her infant turned away from the breast, signaling a loss of the intimacy that Jill prized, Mimi also triggered the caregiver's anger at the rejection. Unconsciously, she may have felt that her daughter was ungrateful and unappreciative of their previous closeness and intimate relationship. To isolate her anger, Jill focused her attention on a cyst, which became essentially a symbol of the breast. Like her breasts, the cyst was fluid-filled, and like the breasts, it had been a part of her for a long time but had only recently become troublesome. By draining the cyst, the caregiver was by extension draining and drying up the source of nurturance. In addition, lancing the cyst may have symbolized a way of punishing herself for experiencing anger at what she perceived to be Mimi's rejection. This anger could not be expressed overtly by the caregiver, who also felt deep affection for her infant.

Jill overcame her depression by discussing her previous experiences with losses and by refocusing her attention on her daughter's emerging developmental skills. Because she had found a creative method for defusing the aggression and anger evoked by her infant's weaning and could participate in and enjoy her daughter's subsequent growth and development, Jill was able to continue her adaptive relationship with her infant. The therapist here reinforced for the caregiver the notion that the infant's growth did not necessarily mean a change in the intimacy the dyad had shared and that, in fact, as the infant matured and gained new skills, they could share more intimate experiences.

Whereas Jill was able to resolve the conflict aroused by the separation implicit in the weaning process, Corinne, a 22-year-old caregiver with a history of psychotic episodes dating from adolescence, had fewer adaptive resources for dealing with the anxiety aroused by separation. During her adolescent episodes of psychosis Corinne had heard voices instructing her to "hurt herself." On one occasion she made several cuts on her wrists with a razor blade. Since that time her self-destructive impulses had been largely under control. When her infant was 2 months old, Corinne arrived in treatment. Her interaction with her infant was mechanical and seemingly without affection. Corinne seldom made eye contact with her son, rarely vocalized when interacting with the child, and initially appeared to possess only a limited repertoire of responses to meet his needs. As treatment progressed, however, her nurturing skills improved considerably.

Six months into treatment, when her son was approximately 8 months old, Corinne appeared at a session with a severe burn on the left side of her face. Questioned about the scar, she reluctantly reported that she had "accidentally" burned herself with some kitchen chemicals. She veered away from the topic, but when the session was nearly ended she volunteered a dream in which imagery of self-destruction was striking.

In this dream, Corinne was playing in the garden of her grandfather's house with her son. Suddenly, she and the baby were taken hostage. One of their captors began to stab the baby repeatedly, so that blood spurted out everywhere. While this was happening, the caregiver saw a chance to escape and began to run as fast as she could. Only when she thought she had run far enough to be safe did she remember that she had left her baby behind; with this realization she awoke in a state of agitation. As if to underscore the content of the dream, Corinne immediately stood and began assembling her belongings to leave, smiling deprecatingly at the therapist and saying, "I guess we're done for today!" At the next session, when questioned about this dream, Corinne insisted that she had almost forgotten it, could not recall any details, and refused to speculate on its meaning.

Corinne's reluctance to discuss the dream and her later forgetfulness suggest that she had some awareness of her hostile feelings. For example, the hostility that suffuses Corinne's dream is directed against the infant; there is no symbolic surrogate. Corinne's abandonment of the infant is extremely specific as well. Finally, the coincidental timing of the dream with the incident in which she "accidentally" burned herself is striking. In fact, Corinne's "accidents" may be representative of those destructive impulses that were not sufficiently neutralized by her depressive dissociation. The burn incident and the kidnapping dream occurred when her 7-month-old son was rapidly achieving a developmental milestone (i.e., crawling) that underscored his separateness from her. This juxtaposition suggests the caregiver harbors a significant repository of anger at her son's imminent developmental achievement and concomitant separation from her. An earlier accident is also revealing when viewed in this light. Corinne had burned off some of her hair while lighting her stove, necessitating a new and severe haircut: At the time of this incident, the patient's 6-month-old infant had just begun to sit up unassisted.

Corinne's attempts to hurt herself signify her struggle to manage the anger evoked by her perception of losing control over her infant's burgeoning development. Symbolically, she seeks to leave her infant before he can leave her. In the same way, the abandonment of her son in her dream is not only a sign of her anger but also of her desire to escape before he can hurt her further by his increasing autonomy. Corinne's inability to dissociate fully from her destructive urges threatens to emerge in her interaction with the infant, further compromising her already minimal ability to nurture her son. Continued treatment to help the caregiver overcome these destructive impulses was therefore recommended in this case.

USING DREAM IMAGERY TO EXPLORE THE THERAPEUTIC RELATIONSHIP

The therapeutic relationship that evolves during dyadic treatment involving a caregiver and infant can be particularly intense because focusing on the caregiver's alliance with the infant tends to implicate her relationship with her own caregiver. Moreover, in dyadic treatment the therapist serves as an authority figure who can provide knowledge about childrearing techniques and about the processes of normative development. Finally, as a third person interacting with the caregiver and infant, the therapist provides a new and more objective perspective from which to analyze the behavior of the dyadic members. As a result, it is not unusual for caregivers or expectant mothers entering treatment to establish a strong alliance with the therapist and to *transfer* feelings relating to earlier childhood conflict onto either the figure of the therapist or the infant.

Thus, therapists should be sensitive to the potency of the response they can evoke during dyadic therapy. One way in which this highly charged response may reveal itself is in the form of dreams. This phenomenon is not so unusual considering that even in individual treatment the patient's dreams often convey the contours of a highly charged transference relationship to the therapist. It is now accepted that caregivers who are undergoing treatment along with their infants tend to resurrect previous conflict they experienced with their own mothers (Ascher, 1985). In fact, the caregiver's relationship with her own nurturing figures becomes a pivotal issue that often dominates dream imagery in these cases. It is almost as if, until the caregiver has resolved the conflicts she encountered during her own nurturing years, she will be unlikely to devise a viable and adaptive model for nurturing the infant. The following case report describes a dream of a caregiver being seen in treatment with her infant. Not unexpectedly, this patient depicts the therapist as a nurturer, partner, and lover. As such, this patient appeared to be representing various conflicts that stemmed from the important relationships in her life, including the relationships with her own mother and her husband as well as her relatively new relationship with her infant.

The patient began treatment in the first month of her second pregnancy, having given birth to a daughter one year earlier. Her own mother died several years ago. During her mother's final illness the patient was prevented from visiting the hospital and previously reported to the therapist that since then she has felt a mixture of lingering regret and bitterness about not being able to "say goodbye." During the past several months the patient's father has invited her to attend various social and business meetings with him; she has told the therapist that she becomes very uneasy during such events, attributing her discomfort to a fear of getting too close to her father and reawakening sexual fantasies. The patient notes that this must be the real reason why she declines her father's invitations, although she reports that consciously she only feels annoyance at her father who, even 2 years after her mother's death, seems immersed in a perpetual ritual of grieving. She reports that she angrily wants to tell him, "Why can't you be stronger and go on living your life?"

A few months after treatment started, the patient reported the following dream. "My father called last night. He tends to call me every other night even though I have told him that my new job leaves me drained during the week and that there is no need for continually calling me. I feel he is treating me like a little girl, making sure I'm home safe by 10 PM. When he called last night, he said he had been trying to get through for a while but that the line was busy. This comment always annoys me further, because it's as if he wants to know who I was talking to and why I was on the phone. I feel this is an invasion of my privacy. Last night he began rambling on as usual. I know he just needs to talk, and his questions about me are just an excuse because he is lonely, but I was abrupt nevertheless.

"After we got off the phone, I was lying on the bed watching the news. I was very tired and knew I would go to sleep right after the news ended. I was just lying on my back, slouching against my pillow and weaving a shawl for my daughter. I began feeling bad that I had been so abrupt with my father. Then I remembered my mother and how nasty she was to me right before she died. Feelings of anger rose up in me, but I fought them down. Although I am angry with her, I know I must somehow resolve these feelings. Then I fell asleep.

"In the dream you [the therapist] are there. It's as if I'm waking up in a clean open space. As I come to consciousness I see we are in a room. The walls are painted white or some other pastel color like pink, but I don't feel confined at all. In fact, the atmosphere in the room is pleasant and cheerful. It is almost as if the room had a mood of cheerfulness. We are close to each other and we feel very comfortable. Then I see you are holding me, but your touch is so gentle I almost don't feel your fingers or they feel like . . . whispers . . . that's the word that comes to me. The light in the room is gradually increasing and I am aware that the sun is filtering through the window. There are delicate curtains on the window that I know are there to protect us from too much sun. I seem to be reclining on my back and I can see your face, sometimes in profile, sometimes your full face. Then, you start touching my belly softly with your palm, as if you are patting the baby. Your hand feels warm and slightly firm. You seem to be concentrating. At first I think, oh good, he wants to have sex, but then I become anxious, maybe you will think I am too fat and that's why you're feeling my stomach, and I also feel guilty because of my husband. I know I care for him very much even though he seems to have become more distant with this second pregnancy. Suddenly, I am not afraid because I know why you are touching me. You are feeling me to see if I am hungry or full. You are not concerned about my pregnancy. When I realize this, I feel very good inside because I now understand that you really care about me. I want to tell you this in words, but then I realize we don't need words, we are communicating on a very deep level. It is as if the messages I am sending to you have no thoughts, only feelings. The picture becomes clearer now and I see you are cradling me in your arms like a baby, we are in the face-to-face position. Slowly you begin bringing your face closer to me. The top half of my body is nestled against your chest. I am blissfully comfortable. Your coming closer makes me feel good, you continue to feel my belly very softly, each touch feels like a soft, delicate little drop, just for me. It swathes me like a blanket. I want the feeling to go on forever. Then the alarm goes off. I wake up but immediately want to continue the dream. I try to recapture this wonderful, almost indescribable feeling that I experienced when you were touching me."

This dream combines a variety of images and reveals the potency of the transference relationship that can arise between patient and therapist during dyadic treatment. In the dream, the caregiver has cast the therapist in a variety of roles. First, the dream has overt sexual connotations and indeed, at one point in the dream the caregiver believes that the therapist wishes to have sex. These fears are allayed, however, when the caregiver realizes that the therapist's true motives in the dream are to offer nurturance and that the therapist is concerned about whether the caregiver is "hungry or full." Portrayed in this capacity, the therapist has himself assumed the role of caregiving figure. The therapist's behavior here, however, is in sharp contrast to the caregiver's own parents: Her mother was nasty to the caregiver and then died before the caregiver could say good-bye, whereas the caregiver's father bothers her with annoying phone calls and attempts to intrude on her privacy. In addition, the therapist in the dream is genuinely concerned about the caregiver. Unlike the caregiver's husband, he is not "distant" as a result of the pregnancy; and unlike her father, he does not ramble on in meaningless conversation, but instead communicates with the caregiver on an extremely profound level. The therapist also uses soothing gestures to "cradle" the caregiver in his arms and "swathe" her body "like a blanket." In essence, the caregiver's dream material has transformed the therapist into an ideal nurturer. Finally, the dream suggests that the therapist has knowledge of the caregiver's pregnancy and the experience she is undergoing and is, on a certain level, an authority figure with regard to childbirth.

Through this dream, then, the caregiver is beginning to raise and deal with some of her unresolved conflicts. Her unsatisfactory relationship with her father is managed by creating the image of the ideal father through the therapist. The therapist's nurturing skills also appeared to assuage some of the pain the caregiver had experienced from being deprived of her mother's affection. Moreover, the caregiver's depiction of the therapist in the dream suggests that she is attempting to formulate an image of an adaptive parent that she can emulate once her child is born.

CONCLUSION

The case studies in this chapter suggest that themes of self-representation and separation are implicit in the experience of motherhood and becoming a mother; that the changes necessary to create and nurture the new infant evoke intense emotions, including happiness, anger, fear, depression, and loneliness. In each case presented, the therapist may ask, what are the transformations in self-representation? From daughter to mother? From career woman to mother? From dependency to autonomy? And in each case the therapist may ask, what is to be lost here? A satisfying and rewarding career? A fantasy baby? A sense of self? The sense of controllability? The intimate and proprietary relationship between mother and infant? Despite the ideal facade frequently depicted for motherhood, it is hardly surprising that a condition capable of creating so rich and intense a bond can also have a dark and sinister side.

In the dreams and fantasies of Gina, Catherine, and Jill, the imagery is vaguely repugnant: the railroad car choked with cigarette smoke, the ruined house, the cyst. These images resemble many of the foreboding objects that are part of dream landscapes in the lives of individuals who experience transformations. The repugnancy of these images is clearly distanced from the dreamer; even Jill regards the cyst on her hand as something alien that must now be excised. In contrast, the dreams of Loretta and Corinne contain imagery that is not fully dissociated: the dismembered dog and the baby who has been brutally stabbed. In addition, both of these caregivers evidenced inappropriate affect when relating their dreams, as if they were less than comfortable with what these fantasies revealed about their own roles as expectant mothers. This too is in direct contrast to the psychic distancing felt by the other patients described.

"I wish I'd had a year or two to get used to what being pregnant was going to be like," Loretta had said, early in her therapy. "I knew about most of the things that would happen to my body, but I don't think I really accepted them beforehand. And I didn't know how much my mind would change: how I'd feel about what was happening to my body, the baby kicking, how much I can't control what's happening to me. It's hard to make the adjustment." This woman's statement is applicable to any of the women whose histories are reported. Because motherhood is a dynamic process with virtually unceasing change, flexibility and the ability to deal with these transformations and concomitant separations are necessary characteristics for adaptation. It is perhaps inevitable that maternal hostility will be evoked frequently during the process of pregnancy and childrearing because of the intensity of the relationship between mother and child, but if the caregiver learns how to represent and discharge feelings of abandonment and hostility symbolically, she may resolve these negative emotions without disturbing her relationship with the infant. Caregivers who cannot sufficiently manage and repress their feelings of hostility are at risk of discharging these feelings randomly on themselves or on their children. As a result, the dreams and fantasies that these women experience may clearly indicate the internal struggle wrought by the transformations that attend the mother–child relationship.

The dream imagery discussed here also suggests how the therapist can predict or focus on a troublesome area of conflict that is threatening to intrude on the dyad's adaptive interaction. With certain caregivers, disclosure of dream material coupled with free association exercises are sufficient to provide insight for modifying behavioral patterns toward the infant. In other cases, the therapist may wish to use modeling behavior after fantasy and dream material has been revealed or may wish to ask the caregiver to provide her interpretation of what the dream signifies. Finally, encouraging the caregiver to represent and subsequently preview the interpersonal implications of upcoming developmental trends is a further technique for predicting and/or resolving the conflict that emerges in the context of development.

The therapist must also explore how some of the major themes that are present in dream imagery are operating in the fantasies of the expectant mother or new caregiver. Most significantly, how is the patient resisting the psychological conflict embedded in the dream and what defensive operations are shielding the true nature of the conflict from the patient's awareness? In addition, what evidence does the dream offer of the caregiver's self-representational status? Have the pregnancy and the imminent or newly assumed role of mother affected the woman's self-image and self-esteem? Does dream material reveal ambivalence about separation, either from the fetus through the act of birth or from the infant as he develops in the direction of autonomy and independence? Finally, how can the therapist predict the course of future interaction based on the conflict inherent in the caregiver's dream and fantasy material? Each of these issues must be dealt with for the patient to obtain the full therapeutic benefit of the dreams disclosed during sessions.

Chapter 12

Resistance, Transference, and Countertransference

Mechanisms That Hinder Previewing Abilities

INTRODUCTION

This chapter examines the concept of *resistance,* a frequently discussed psychotherapeutic phenomenon. Within the context of individual therapy, resistance has traditionally included all of the patient's manifestations that disrupt, impede, or interfere with treatment. At the root of resistant behavior lies the patient's fear of revealing primary conflict while remaining defenseless to confront the aroused anxiety. In dyadic treatment, resistance functions in a similar manner, in that the caregiver uses various strategies to deflect attention from the problems that have led her to seek treatment with her infant. Her motives, however, may be unique. In many cases, she is attempting to stave off the infant's future development as well as the effects of such development on her relationship with the child. That is, during caregiver–infant therapy, the caregiver may resist *previewing future developmental outcomes* that involve herself and her infant because she fears that the infant's growing autonomy will change and alter their intimate relationship, from which she derives enormous emotional benefits. This chapter will explore the distinctive manifestations and motives that lie behind such caregiver resistance.

In addition, although therapists are relatively familiar with the forms of resistance used by patients in individual treatment, the behaviors caregivers may employ to avoid therapeutic progress are not as commonly known. As a result, one section of this chapter will provide a catalog of the typical behaviors used by resistant caregivers in dyadic treatment. This catalog will enable therapists to recognize when resistance threatens to impede progress.

Moreover, therapists should administer the techniques for interpreting resistance very carefully when treating a caregiver and infant. In dyadic therapy resistance needs to be dealt with in a particular manner, to allow the treatment to progress without disrupting the caregiver–infant relationship. Through confrontation the therapist may run the risk of having the caregiver retaliate against the infant. Individual therapy allows the patient to act out dysfunctional behavior with the therapist, but in dyadic therapy the caregiver may introduce maladaptive behavior into her interaction with the infant which can have devastating effects on his development. With this in mind, the chapter provides productive strategies for handling resistance within the context of a mother–infant relationship.

THE EMERGENCE OF RESISTANCE DURING DYADIC INTERVENTION

Resistance is a common theme in the literature. A variety of definitions have been offered for this phenomenon, including Greenson's (1967) comment that resistance is all those forces within the patient that oppose the procedures and processes of treatment, and Sandler's (1973) view of resistance as those forces within the patient that oppose the treatment process. Langs (1973) has contributed to the notion of resistance by noting that it consists of devices that the patient uses to interfere with the progress of treatment and to prevent the emotional expression of potentially disturbing derivatives of conflict-related fantasies.

Resistance impedes the progress of dyadic therapy in a similar way. During the treatment of a caregiver and infant, resistance represents all of those behaviors displayed in the therapist's presence that indicate the caregiver's reticence to disclose inter- and intrapersonal processes while interacting with the infant or to permit the therapist to participate in the dyadic interaction. Resistance may therefore assume the form of verbalizations, physical behaviors, or attitudes that permeate the therapeutic atmosphere and create an invisible barrier against spontaneity in the exchange.

Resistance during dyadic therapy may have underlying motives that differ from the motives found in individual therapy. In essence, resistance develops when the caregiver fears previewing future developmental outcomes with the infant because the interaction with the infant has potent implications for her. One such implication is that the caregiver realizes the infant is rapidly acquiring developmental skills that will eventually enable him to assert his autonomy and independence. In other words, continued interaction and encouragement of infant skills will lead to an inevitable separation between caregiver and infant—or so the caregiver believes—and a loss of the intimate dyadic relationship in which the infant is dependent on the caregiver. Thus, the infant's development may arouse *feelings of loss* and attendant *depression* that the caregiver will attempt to stave off through resistance.

The infant's continual development may also awaken other kinds of loss in the caregiver. As an example, if the caregiver herself experienced deprivation during infancy and childhood, the feelings associated with those past episodes are likely to be aroused when the infant undergoes the particular developmental phase at which the caregiver experienced such early deprivation. Once again, feelings of depression may surface, causing the caregiver to change her interaction with the infant and to resist exploring the source of the conflict with the therapist. Finally, the infant's development will remind the caregiver that she is a provider who is responsible for the infant. Many caregivers find this prospect of responsibility frightening and will attempt to avoid confronting its implications in any way possible.

There are, then, many reasons why caregivers in therapy with their infants are likely to show resistance. The therapist who encounters such resistance should, therefore, first attempt to assess the caregiver's motives by asking, "Why is the caregiver seeking to avoid the implications of the infant's development?" By phrasing the question in this manner, the therapist can better ascertain the genuine motive behind the resistance.

Seligman and Pawl (1983) have discussed various impediments to the formation of a working alliance in infant–parent therapy and have focused on transference reactions in particular as both an impediment to and an opportunity for progress. According to these researchers, the caregiver's past history and conflicts, as well as the basic scope of her personality, may prevent her from providing optimal care to the infant. Moreover, reawakened memories of difficult childhood experiences cast a shadow on the caregiver's relationship with her child and will often also cause her to view the therapist as a potentially bad, or at least not-so-good, parent. As a result, the therapist becomes a convenient object upon whom to foist negative transference feelings such as defensiveness, wariness, covert aggression, and avoidance, which are warded off as the caregiver simultaneously expresses a desire for the therapist's help. Thus, it is ironic that the same problems for which the caregiver seeks help are those very conflicts that may impede the therapist from providing help.

Seligman and Pawl explain, for example, that the optimism engendered by the prospect of a supportive relationship with the therapist is often inextricably bound up with the caregiver's expectation of disappointment and rejection, parallelling her own tendency to juxtapose love and withdrawal with unreliability, unavailability, rejection, and other forms of psychopathology. The caregiver does not wish to replicate her own painful childhood experiences with her infant, but she is at a loss to devise adaptive strategies that will help her overcome her own developmental deficits. Many parents, therefore, must distance themselves from the therapist through such maneuvers as missing appointments, not hearing what is said, and not saying what they mean. Greenson (1967) notes that the forms these impediments take are as varied as the forms of defense and resistance that have been discussed so thoroughly in the literature.

Many caregivers are prone to an impulsive *acting-out* style of coping which may further complicate resistance to dyadic treatment. This behavior precludes or delays the establishment of a trusting and collaborative alliance with the therapist—a prerequisite for appropriately managing counterproductive expressions of deprivation and anger. Such cases may be especially difficult for therapists who are committed to attempting to help the infant even when the caregiver seems unwilling or unable to forge the basic working alliance required to use this help. Indeed, the therapist must be wary of establishing an alliance with the infant that excludes the caregiver.

To overcome resistance the therapist may need to tailor the approach to the caregiver's particular psychopathology. For instance, with a suspicious or paranoid mother, caution and factual information, along with emphasis on the caregiver's control of treatment procedures, may be indicated. A passive and dependent caregiver would require the rapid establishment of a consistent, regular structure that highlights the therapist's reliability. With a repressive and intellectualizing caregiver, the therapist might spend hours listening to the details of her work or home life, employing the language of emotion only when confident that this will not excessively threaten much-needed defenses.

The concept of resistance proposed by Greenson (1967), views this phenomenon as a counterforce within the patient operating against the progress of the treatment, the establishment of a transference relationship with the therapist, and the procedures and processes used by the therapist to move the treatment forward. Resistance during dyadic intervention is a phenomenon that the therapist observes to be operative within the patient, rather than an observable phenomenon that is a consequence of a two-party interaction. Thus, the therapist needs to be vigilant about detecting when resistance threatens the therapeutic alliance. Freud (1900) outlined several different forms of resistance, including (a) repressive resistance, (b) the transference resistance, (c) the resistance due to secondary gain, (d) the resistance caused by the repetition compulsion, and (e) the resistance created by the need to punish oneself. According to Davis (1989), resistance to the awareness of transference occurs when the patient is commenting about a relationship outside of the treatment setting but is unconsciously alluding to the transference relationship. For example, a mother may be talking about how her husband or infant does not understand her and is unconsciously perceiving that it is in fact the therapist who does not understand her. Resistance to the resolution of transference occurs, according to Davis, when the patient wants to continue to gratify her impulse in the transference rather than relinquish it. This manifests itself clinically when the patient does not consciously express all her transference feelings. Freud allows the resistance to increase and heighten so that the therapist can more easily confront the patient and clarify the problem. Silence is thereby one of the best technical interventions for increasing the resistance sufficiently to focus it on the patient. Nevertheless, this strategy must be used with caution during dyadic therapy because a caregiver may act out her anger at the therapist during her interaction with the infant.

MANIFESTATIONS OF RESISTANCE

Cataloguing the kinds of interpersonal behaviors that fall under the rubric of resistance is not difficult. Most therapists would list such behaviors as the formation of mental blocks, verbal attacks, expressions of a desire to terminate treatment, and confused sessions in which the patient ruminates, digresses or expresses extreme doubt. As Langs (1973) cautions, any of these behaviors may arise continually throughout the treatment. When resistance is operating, the therapist should assess the situation and understand its context, as well as the unconscious meanings that are being expressed by the patient's manifest and latent behavior.

In dyadic therapy, however, resistances may appear in several unique guises. The therapist should be particularly alert to situations in which the caregiver becomes overly *self-absorbed, emotionally detached, and/or apathetic,* and *fails to predict and preview* the infant's developmental changes to the point where she excludes or ignores the infant or denies that any such change is occurring. By demonstrating this behavior, the caregiver may be resisting interaction with the infant. To test whether such behaviors are present, the therapist can ask the caregiver to describe imminent infant developments or to represent and describe sequences of future interaction with the infant. If the caregiver expresses no psychological curiosity about the infant's development or cannot talk about her interaction with the infant, some form of resistance is likely. In other instances, resistance may take the form of canceling sessions or challenging the therapist's interventions with the infant in some fashion. Examples of the latter include coming to sessions and discussing information that the pediatrician or someone else has provided about the infant. Through such behavior the caregiver is tacitly attempting to convey that the therapist is not an authority about the infant and therefore need not be listened to or followed.

Another form of resistance occurs when the caregiver forges an intense transference relationship with the therapist at the expense of consolidating a strong relationship with the infant. By focusing attention on the therapist, the caregiver manages to avoid confronting the implications aroused by interaction with the infant. Although it is important for the caregiver to establish a transference with the therapist, this transference should ultimately enable the caregiver to explore and progress in a relationship with the infant that promotes development. When the caregiver's reactions to the therapist are overly intense and fused, they may hinder bonding with the infant. In this fashion, the caregiver manages to manipulate her relationship with the therapist to exclude the infant. Therapists should be alert to this form of a transference relationship because it will frustrate the treatment.

The Transference in Caregiver–Infant Therapy

Although the treatment of mother–infant dyads within the therapeutic setting is unique for a variety of reasons, perhaps the most noteworthy aspects are the reactions that occur in this situation. In essence, the *relationship* that the patient establishes with the therapist is mandatory for the patient's progress. By forging a therapeutic bond with the therapist, the patient begins to reveal the roots of suppressed childhood conflict that have resulted in a pattern of adult behavior. The therapeutic relationship provides a safe haven for resurrecting these long-buried and suppressed emotions and enables the therapist to understand the origins of the patient's conflict. The therapeutic relationship also serves the equally significant function of providing an impetus for *change* because after gleaning the nature of this relationship and its potency, the therapist can begin to offer interpretations of behavior that eventually lead to insights on the part of the patient. From such insights the patient begins the painstaking process of modifying behavior patterns, attitudes, and expectations.

But the therapeutic relationship in caregiver–infant treatment poses different problems that the therapist must deal with before genuine progress can transpire. In such a situation the therapist is operating at both an advantage and a disadvantage. The advantage is that the nature of the patient's transference will become apparent dramatically and almost immediately by observing her interactions with the infant. During individual therapy it may take a long time for the therapist to discern the type of relationship the patient has sought to create within the therapeutic milieu. But when seeing a caregiver–infant dyad for treatment, it may be possible to kaleidoscope identification of the transference bond into just a few sessions. The therapist can observe in vivo how a particular caregiver transfers affect by observing how she interacts with the infant and, in particular, how she previews upcoming developmental events to him.

To tease out the contours of the transference, the therapist should rely on two separate skills: *direct observation* and *inquiry* about subjective representations of the interaction. Direct observation of the caregiver–infant dyad enables the therapist to assess the level of intuitive exchange between the pair. During the first few sessions mothers may be reticent about displaying overt interaction in the presence of the therapist, and this hesitation may actually indicate that the caregiver recognizes the potency of the exchange and is reluctant to share this intimate relationship in a still unfamiliar environment. But as the weeks progress and the caregiver acclimates to the therapeutic milieu, picking up the infant and displaying sequences of interaction should become routine.

When exhibitions of interaction initiated by the caregiver do not evolve, the therapist should interpret the *resistance* that prevents the caregiver from establishing a positive relationship with the infant and, in turn, from ministering to his needs effectively through previewing behaviors. These cases will be more problematic to treat, and the therapist will need to review the therapeutic relationship. Once the therapist has forged a bond, this relationship may serve as a *model* of interaction to superimpose on the caregiver–infant relationship.

Early in the treatment caregivers may also display what Malan (1979) has referred to as *unconscious communication*. Malan notes two key signals that the patient is engaging in unconscious communication. First, the caregiver, often with an abrupt shift in subject, speaks with evident interest and spontaneity about a topic whose relevance is not immediately apparent.

Second, the therapist who analyzes this sudden shift in the conversation will discern a clear parallel with some other subject whose relevance and emotional significance are much greater.

An example will illustrate this behavior. One caregiver I had treated for 2 weeks began her third session by noting that she was annoyed at the erratic patterns of her 6-month-old son. Suddenly, she abandoned this topic and began to complain vociferously about her mother-in-law who, she informed me, was always calling or dropping by at unpredictable times, disrupting the caregiver's schedule. It was not difficult to discern that the caregiver's real anger was toward her son and his "unpredictable" feeding schedule but that she did not yet feel comfortable sharing these negative emotions with me. This anecdote emphasizes that the therapist must be ever vigilant about analyzing the caregiver's reactions and unconscious communications. Early analysis of the transference in dyadic treatment is especially crucial because the caregiver may be conveying negative predictions to the infant that will interfere with adaptive development. The therapist can provide interventions at an earlier point in the treatment process to avert maladaptive interactions.

Whenever episodes of overt interaction occur, the therapist should be especially aware of assessing nuances of behavior and evaluating the intuitive response elaborated on in earlier chapters. For example, the therapist should observe whether the caregiver is adept at holding the infant and providing adequate stimulation. Evidence of visual and vocal cuing will also be either apparent or absent during these interludes, and the therapist should judge whether the caregiver is making eye contact and providing the kind of auditory response that is appropriate to the infant's regulatory capacities. Failure to manifest these behaviors may signify that the caregiver is not sufficiently exposing the infant to previewing.

The therapist is trying to discern, through intuitive antennae and an awareness of the most subtle communicative signals, how the caregiver and infant are experiencing one another on every level. Encompassed within this definition is how the caregiver conveys predictions about the future to the infant. Is this a relationship in which the caregiver intuitively senses that the infant needs to be held, fed, or have his diaper changed? Can this caregiver differentiate the infant's signals so that an almost imperceptible network of messages passes between the pair? In contrast, does the caregiver appear oblivious to the infant's myriad signals, or is she grafting her own agenda onto the infant instead of trying to discern his true needs? A third alternative is also possible: The therapist may get the distinct impression that the caregiver is conveying hostility or some other negative emotion to the infant. This negativity will become evident when the infant displays irritability and discomfort in the therapist's presence and the caregiver appears reluctant to comfort the child. It is crucial to observe both the outward behavior of the dyad during interaction and the more subtle predictive messages being conveyed between the pair. These subtle messages become understandable only when the therapist has become attuned to the caregiver–infant relationship.

The importance of having the therapist independently evaluate the transference between infant and caregiver is illustrated in a study by St. James-Roberts and Wolke (1988) that sought to detect whether independent investigators evaluate infant temperament differently from the infants' caregivers. Significantly, there were discrepancies in the temperamental assessment of these two groups. Maternal assessments were internally consistent but were weakly explained by infant constitutional factors. One explanation for these discrepancies is that caregivers transfer discrete expectations to their infants and attribute a particular meaning to a given response. Therapists must, therefore, assess infant response independently and subsequently clarify the caregiver's interpretation and responses to the infant.

In a related study, Oates and Forrest (1984) determined that a majority of caregivers have unreliable memories of their pregnancies. This research team asked a group of 47 mothers to recall the details of their child's birth and of any child-rearing problems by conducting a questionnaire approximately 5 years after the birth. When the mothers' responses were compared with documented hospital records, it was found that they overestimated the length of pregnancy and the number of neonatal problems, and could not accurately recall other objective data, such as obstetric complications. Only half of the mothers could recall birth weight accurately. These findings substantiate the report of St. James-Roberts and Wolke and underscore the need for the therapist's careful observation of the relationship between caregiver and infant.

Yet another element contributes to profound understanding of the dynamics that unfold during a treatment session—the therapist's countertransference experience in the presence of a given caregiver–infant dyad. Countertransference responses refer to the range of affective responses that the therapist experiences with the patient. When treating caregiver–infant dyads, the therapist is likely to have a response to both members of the pair. It is vital for the therapist to acknowledge these feelings and determine their source so that they do not contaminate the relationship being forged during the therapeutic encounter.

Definition of Transference. Broadly defined, transference refers to the process of bringing unconscious wishes to the surface. As a consequence, once the transference is called into action, primitive prototypes from the patient's past resurface and are experienced with a strong sense of immediacy. These powerful, often long-buried, memories from childhood are then transferred to the new object. LaPlanche and Pontalis (1973) define the transference as the terrain on which all basic conflicts and dilemmas play themselves out. In this sense, the establishment, modalities, interpretation, and resolution of the transference define the patient's cure. Through the transference relationship the patient is not only *resurrecting* but ultimately *resolving* conflict rooted early in life.

The transference enables recognition of how a particular patient forges relationships and clarifies the significant factors in that patient's current and past relationships. When Freud (1895a) spoke of transference, he was referring to a mode of displacement that allows expression of unconscious wishes in masked or disguised form through the material (e.g., behaviors, dreams, etc.) furnished by the unconscious and preconscious residues. Freud described the transference as occurring when the patient transfers unconscious ideas onto the therapist and referred to transference as a new edition or facsimile of the childhood impulses and fantasies that are aroused and made conscious during therapy. Transferences, according to Freud, have the peculiarity of replacing some earlier person with the person of the therapist. In other words, the therapist comes to play the role of a parental figure.

Through the transference, the patient revives and experiences the relationship to parental figures in a characteristically ambivalent fashion. Thus, in treating a caregiver–infant dyad, the therapist should be aware that the caregiver will eventually begin displacing the suppressed wishes of childhood onto both (caregiver–infant, caregiver–therapist) or either relationship. In an ironic twist of fate the caregiver may even begin to identify with her own caregiver and transfer onto the infant those feelings she experienced as a child. One way for the therapist to detect whether this is in fact occurring is to observe the previewing behaviors the caregiver is engaging in with the infant. From the contours of such exercises, the therapist can discern the maladaptive representations that the caregiver harbors about the infant's future development.

The transference may also be described as a suppressed wish, whose content appears in the patient's consciousness without any memories of the surrounding circumstances that would mark it as having recurred in the past. The wish that was present then is now linked to the infant or therapist, an object(s) with whom the caregiver is legitimately concerned. Reduced to its essentials, then, Freud viewed the transference as a particular instance of *displacement of affect* from one psychological situation onto another. Moreover, the mechanism of transferring onto the person of the therapist is triggered precisely at the moment when particularly profound repressed memories are in danger of being revived and revealed. Viewed in this light, the transference appears as a form of resistance while, at the same time, it verifies the proximity and potency of unconscious conflict. Thus, the transference aids in understanding and ultimately overcoming patient resistance, in that it is particularly hard to admit the repressed wish when this acknowledgment has to be made to the person the wish involves.

One last descriptive term is useful at this juncture, *transference neurosis*. According to psychoanalytic theory, transference neuroses allude to an artificial neurosis into which the manifestations of the transference tend to become organized. The neurosis is built around the relationship with the analyst. Working through the transference neurosis safely and resolving it by placing it in the perspective of childhood helps the patient relinquish the neurosis. The energies dissipated by the resolution of the transference neurosis attach themselves to individuals and activities in the patient's present-day life. The patient can then make an emotional investment in areas of legitimate productivity, as well as in areas previously viewed as being unimportant. Beyond this, however, during the treatment of caregiver–infant dyads the contours of the transference relationship assume an additional dimension. It is likely that the caregiver not only will establish a transference relationship with the therapist but also may display a transference bond to the infant. The therapist, in these instances, should be particularly attuned to indicia of displaced affect transferred onto the baby.

To ascertain the nature of the caregiver's transferential relationship with the infant, it is also necessary to explore how the infant is perceived within the context of the family. The family and its unique dynamics are so fundamental to the child's development that the therapist can comprehend the dyadic interaction between caregiver and infant only by considering the entire family unit. There are some common aberrational patterns that occur within the family to which the therapist should be alert (Lask, 1982). For example, in situations of caregiver–infant coalition, one parent might psychologically attack the other, using the infant as an ally. *Triangulation* occurs when both parents use the infant in a kind of psychological tug-of-war, each attempting to win the favor of the child at the expense of the other parent. Another common pattern discerned by Lask is that of the *go-between*. In this configuration, the infant may serve as a kind of messenger to transmit messages between the parents, who are essentially noncommunicative with one another. Finally, Lask outlines the pattern of using the infant as the *whipping boy* to ventilate anger and hostility that one parent cannot express directly to the other parent. These patterns originate in the caregivers' own infancy and are revived when they become parents. It is only by closely observing dyadic interaction and analyzing the caregiver's transference reactions to the infant that the therapist can determine whether these aberrant patterns are being instilled within the particular dyad in treatment.

Variations of the Transference. Gilman (1986) has defined both a *mirror transference* and an *idealizing transference*. According to this researcher, the mirror transference stems from a period during childhood when the patient needed approval and acknowledgment by the person of reference—usually the primary caregiver—who, in this context, becomes a "mirror." Retrospectively, the caregiver reacted to the infant's needs in a mal-adaptive fashion. When a caregiver resurrects a mirror transference during dyadic therapy, she usually needs to be reassured by the therapist's acknowledgment and approval. But if she experiences the analyst's intervention as being inadequate, disruptions will immediately surface and the caregiver will lose the feeling of security that she had maintained until then. Therapists should be alert to mirror transferences because the caregiver who feels inadequate may transfer these unresolved feelings to the infant and consequently fail to stabilize an adaptive relationship with the baby. Similarly, a sense of fusion with a person of idealized strength and composure emerges in the idealized transference. Here the issue is the mobilization of the parental images in the therapy.

A familiarity with these nuances is particularly crucial when the therapist is treating a caregiver–infant dyad, because any transference that develops between the caregiver and therapist could very likely parallel the same phenomena in the caregiver–infant relationship. This occurs because, during the development of a therapeutic relationship, the caregiver will dredge up long-buried experiences of childhood conflict, which she then transfers to the therapist. Yet, the therapist comes to signify a kind of substitute parent and so the patient endows him or her with an inordinate amount of authority. Because the caregiver will scrutinize each comment or behavior, therapists should use utmost caution to avoid rendering unfounded interpretations—such interactions will often be transferred to the infant.

In certain cases the patient fashions a unique kind of transference tinged with negative or even hostile emotions that, as a consequence of its potency, leads to negative countertransferential reactions in the therapist (Anzieu, 1986). The combination of a negative transference/countertransference phenomenon then creates a repeated and prolonged situation that Anzieu refers to as a *paradoxical communication* emanating from childhood trauma and conflict. What is significant in these cases is that the therapist unwittingly collaborates in the patient's goal of sabotaging the treatment because negative countertransference feelings block productive work. The therapeutic situation here inevitably leads to failure, which is conveniently dubbed a negative therapeutic reaction. According to Anzieu, it is only through knowledge of the main types of pathogenic communication used in therapy that the therapist will be able to realign the transference, maintain a neutral stance, and help the patient work through the situation. Besides its clinical and technical aspects, the paradoxical communication also entails numerous theoretical implications about the genesis, functioning, and deficits of the patient's ego. Thus, if such a transference should occur, the therapist may use it for gaining further insight into the caregiver's inner life and the conflict she is striving to avoid confronting, particularly in the context of her interaction with the infant.

The Countertransference

If the therapeutic relationship is such a powerful tool during care-giver–infant therapy, the therapist's own countertransference is equally significant and cannot be ignored. Countertransference has been variously described. Bollas (1983) and Pick (1985) have referred to it as a continuous internal response by the therapist to the patient's presence. Briefly, the countertransference captures the therapist's own personal reactions to the patient because patients can and do arouse the therapist's deeply suppressed emotions. Dyadic therapy, especially, may arouse countertransference feelings emanating from the therapist's own childhood. These emotions need to be carefully examined so that they do not interfere with the treatment.

To utilize the countertransference to the fullest advantage in a therapeutic setting, the therapist should reflect for a moment to determine what evoked a particular emotion and the memory associated with it. In performing this self-analysis, the therapist will often gain additional insight into the patient's conflict.

Several categories of countertransference occur frequently when the therapist is treating a dyad: feelings of envy, feelings of exclusion, overidentification, and overintellectualization. Feelings of envy are likely to surface when the caregiver engages the infant in play. As an observer, the therapist may suddenly yearn for the security of the intimate relationship unfolding in front of his or her eyes. These feelings may be especially acute in therapists who have no children. Feelings of exclusion are also typical during such play sequences, and if these feelings are particularly intense, they may stem from a childhood experience of sibling rivalry, during which the therapist felt the caregiver favored a brother or sister. It is particularly important for the therapist to be cognizant of the prevalence of these feelings and to guard against allowing them to enter into the therapeutic relationship in the form of inadvertent comments or remarks. The therapist's behavior should also convey a stance of participant observer (Sullivan, 1953). As noted before, if the therapist inadvertently permits envy or exclusion to impinge on the caregiver–infant relationship, the caregiver is likely to absorb these emotions and superimpose them on the dyadic exchange.

Guy, Guy, and Liaboe (1986) have commented that pregnancy and parenthood bring in their wake profound physical and psychological changes. These changes have a particularly significant impact on both male and female therapists, as well as on their patients. As noted by Deutsch (1944), pregnancy creates significant disturbances in the psychic balance of all women, reactivating early conflicts and causing intense introversion, time-limited regression, and identification with the fetus. There may be emotional changes, fatigue, and a growing sense of vulnerability.

During dyadic therapy part of the therapist's task is to explore the caregiver's experience during pregnancy and to examine the emotions that were aroused by the impending birth. For both male and female therapists, this aspect of the treatment may result in strong countertransference feelings. For example, female therapists should be aware of how they feel about the birth process in general. If the female therapist is childless, she may experience jealousy because the patient has successfully carried an infant to term and given birth. Male therapists may experience similar ambivalence and jealousies. The point is not that these countertransference reactions will impede treatment, but rather that it is incumbent on the therapist to examine his or her own feelings about parenthood before engaging in this type of therapy.

Other common countertransference responses involve overidentification and overintellectualization. In the case of overidentification, it is almost inevitable that the therapist will experience some desire to regress when in the infant's presence. As long as the regression is mastered and used in the service of adaptation, this form of countertransference reaction may be highly productive. For example, if the therapist engages in baby talk with the infant, it may assist the caregiver in developing the skill to respond adaptively to the infant. Moreover, such exercises may provide the therapist with a more profound awareness of the infant's perceptions regarding the caregiver. Overintellectualization, however, should be avoided. Displays of overintellectualization, in the form of clinical or technical language or a lack of spontaneity and affect, generally stem from the therapist's insecurity with the role of a parental figure. To avoid these reactions, the therapist must confront his or her own feelings of incompetence and master them.

This section has proposed various ways in which the caregiver uses the dyadic treatment milieu to resist therapeutic efforts to enhance her interaction with the infant and her perceptions of his development. The therapist will occasionally encounter a caregiver who overtly resists the infant by pleading an inability to represent his development or to focus on the interaction with him. Such caregivers may assert that the infant arouses virtually no response for them. Other caregivers express resistance by forming a unique and potent transference bond with the therapist that virtually ignores the infant's presence. In some cases, the caregiver will become overly self-absorbed or will form an exaggerated alliance with the therapist that effectively prevents her from devoting energy to and bonding with the infant. In other cases, the caregiver will deflect negative feeling onto the person of the therapist either by idealizing others, such as the pediatrician, while suggesting that the therapist is somehow less than competent with respect to matters involving the infant, or by developing a paradoxical transference in which the therapist appears in an extremely negative light and is even verbally abused. All of these strategies divert the caregiver's attention from the relationship with the infant and his development, thereby increasing her resistance to the treatment. The therapist who is alert to these forms of behavior should be able to identify episodes of resistance that threaten to intrude on the progress of the treatment.

Another common form of resistance is the patient's use of seductive strategies toward the therapist to deflect attention from her own inner conflict. These strategies provide caregivers with a technique for resisting the implications of the treatment. Langs (1973) referred to these types of fantasies when he noted that reactions to the therapist range from those that are primarily determined by relationships and experiences with other significant persons in the patient's life—transference reactions—to those that are primarily determined by the actual behavior, communications, and attitudes of the therapist—nontransference responses. In almost all situations patients' reactions are based on a mixture of both, although one type of reaction tends to predominate. Beyond these basic transferential fantasies, patients have at their disposal seduction fantasies that function as a form of resistance by diverting the therapist's attention from the problems that have drawn them to therapy.

Overt seduction fantasies can also emerge when the caregiver personifies the therapist as a sexually desirable individual in either dream material or directly expressed fantasy. Nor does the gender of the therapist matter for the purpose of these fantasies. What is important is that the patient envisions the therapist as the object of sexual desire. He or she may be represented as a lover or as the ideal and all-loving parent the caregiver never experienced. As a result, the genuine motive of the fantasy is exposed—both caregiver and therapist become entangled in deciphering the nuances of these feelings, once again diverting attention from the exchange with the infant.

In dyadic therapy two particular kinds of seduction fantasy tend to dominate. First, the caregiver may express, either overtly through behavior or less overtly through dream material, that she wants the therapist to be her caregiver and to gratify her needs. This fantasy allows the caregiver to avoid the responsibility of caring for the infant, because in essence she desires to be an infant herself. In another common caregiver seduction fantasy the caregiver wants to nurture and care for the therapist, who is envisioned as being deficient or emotionally needy in some fashion. Caregivers who are susceptible to the former fantasy will often portray themselves as being helpless, inept, or victimized, to arouse the therapist's sympathies. On the other hand, if the caregiver wishes to nurture the therapist, she will emphasize flaws in the therapist's appearance or behavior that presumably only she can correct. Both of these attitudes distract attention from the caregiver's relationship with the infant and his developmental progress.

Therapists need to be alert to these signals, because it is relatively easy to be seduced psychologically and to become entangled in such diversive tactics. To defuse these fantasies, the strategy of focusing on the arena of interaction is highly recommended. Here the therapist initiates interaction with the infant to reinforce the purpose of treatment for the caregiver. As with the earlier forms of resistance mentioned, shifting attention away from the focus of inappropriate affect is generally sufficient to convey in a nonthreatening, supportive manner that the therapist will not tolerate and will challenge any strategies that evade the main purpose of treatment.

Resistance can also arise in the form of representational deficits on the part of the caregiver. One goal of dyadic therapy is to enhance the caregiver's capacity for representing her infant's developmental status and for using such skills to derive predictions about the infant's future maturation and its effects on her relationship with him. Some caregivers will not, however, be able to represent their infant's development. This inability to describe the infant's prevailing developmental condition or to formulate projections about future change may be due to resistance or may be attributable to a cognitive or emotional deficit.

To cope with this kind of manifestation, therapists should engage in modeling techniques and then begin providing their representations about the infant. Subsequently, the therapist can encourage the caregiver's own capacity for representation by guiding her in formulating descriptions that focus on infant somatic manifestations, cognitive and socio-affective cues, and the infant's motivational attitude. If the caregiver attempts to divert attention from the representational exercises, the therapist should supportively focus on the infant's developmental status and on the caregiver's response to various forms of developmental change. In this fashion, it is possible to overcome the inability to engage in representational exercises and previewing behaviors—whether due to a representational deficit or to actual psychological resistance on the part of the caregiver.

While overcoming the caregiver's resistance, the therapist should also be alert to the awakening of any countertransference feelings. Caregivers who are responding adaptively to the infant but, at the same time, resist working with the therapist to encourage such a response, may awaken a negative countertransference because the treatment is likely to awaken in therapists emotions relating to their own early childhood experiences. If the caregiver is responding maladaptively, the therapist may experience a negative response because he or she recognizes, on some deep level, the extent of the caregiver's dysfunction and is angry at it or disgusted by it. We all tend to want to imbue mothers with positive attitudes, so even professionals trained to recognize the cause of such maladaptation may experience a negative response. Therapists must analyze these feelings, work through them, and ensure that they do not intrude on the dyadic treatment.

THERAPEUTIC METHODS FOR APPROACHING RESISTANCE

There is virtually no dispute in the psychiatric literature about the necessity of overcoming the resistance before treatment can continue. Theorists uniformly believe that this is an essential step to progress and have recommended a variety of strategies for overcoming resistance. Langs (1973), for example, advocates a two-step approach. First, it is essential to *interpret* the resistance for patients by using plain language rather than technical terms to make them aware that they are being defensive and blocking the work of the treatment. The therapist should directly point out to patients how they are accomplishing this blockage—whether it is by rumination, acting out, avoiding a specific topic, being remote, producing confused dreams, or avoiding their inner fantasies. These are merely several ways in which resistance can surface. Langs adds that from the sequence and context of the material the patient presents, the therapist should, whenever possible, make conscious for the patient the general strategy that is engendering the blockage. As an example, the therapist may be able to point out that the patient, while discussing his or her mother or father, has been remote, unclear, or otherwise unproductive. Moreover, this level of *confrontation* should somehow indicate to the patient the cost of the resistance, including the disruptive effects these behaviors have on the treatment. The therapist may, for instance, mention that the patient is not making progress in using the sessions to overcome problems or that symptoms remain unchanged as a result of this resistive behavior. Dispensing uncritical reminders can help motivate the patient to examine and consciously modify resistances while unconsciously producing derivatives that will illuminate its repressed aspects.

As a second step, Langs advocates establishing and interpreting from the patient's associations the nature and form of the resistance, its unconscious meanings, and its roots. According to Langs, this is the crux of the therapeutic work that leads to resolution of the resistance. This strategy also enables the patient to understand the ways that he or she deals with interpersonal stress as well as the underlying motivations for the resistance.

Although this form of confrontation and clarification may be appropriate in treating an individual patient, it is best to avoid confrontational techniques in caregiver–infant dyadic therapy. Such confrontation can lead to *parallel process/acting out* behavior or to the arousal of negative emotions that the caregiver may manifest during behavioral exchanges with the infant—either in the therapist's presence or after the session has ended. The therapist should be continually mindful that treatment strategies will likely have overriding repercussions for the dyadic interaction. As a result, *clarification* is a more appropriate, less challenging technique to use when encountering resistance in dyadic therapy.

The first step in clarification involves discerning whether the caregiver is resisting interaction with the therapist or the infant. Depending on who is being resisted, the caregiver will tend to focus attention on the other person. For example, if the caregiver resists interaction with the infant, it is likely that she will devote her energies to interacting with the therapist. If, on the other hand, she fears the potency of the transference with the therapist, she will direct attention to the infant. Thus, the first step in clarifying a resistance is ascertaining which individual the caregiver is resisting. Once this has been determined, the therapist's task is to redirect the caregiver's attention toward the person she is resisting. If the caregiver is avoiding the infant, for example, the therapist should redirect attention by independently beginning an interaction with the infant that will gradually cause the caregiver to focus attention on the infant. Conversely, where the caregiver appears preoccupied with the infant at the expense of the therapist, the therapist should gently enter into the dyadic exchange to redirect the caregiver's attention. Such redirection serves the same purpose as confrontation but is less threatening. When the therapist redirects the focus of attention and interaction, the caregiver is provided with subtle insight into the nature of her resistance.

CAREGIVER: (Caregiver hands infant to the therapist at his request. Therapist plays with infant, rocking him on his lap, talking to him.) Anyway, Dr. T, Danny gives me freedom, and that's what I like about him. And he gives me independence too. He makes me want to achieve more in life. He makes me want to be successful. (Therapist continues to vocalize with the infant and rock him on his lap. Caregiver becomes irritated.) Dr. T, you are not listening to me! Can you repeat what I just said to you?

THERAPIST: You said he gives you independence and makes you want to be successful.

CAREGIVER: Well, the baby also gives me independence and reliability. . . . (Therapist continues to vocalize with and rock the infant.) Dr. T, you are not listening.

THERAPIST: He's teaching you independence and reliability. Why do you have the impression that I'm not listening to you?

CAREGIVER: (Surprised) Because you seem like you're focusing more on the baby. Danny . . . (Caregiver reaches for infant.) Come to Mommy.

Confrontation should be avoided for another reason besides preventing the caregiver from engaging in a parallel process of acting out negative response with the infant. Resistance is essentially an unconscious response, in that it derives from a deep level of perception. One of the goals of dyadic therapy is to make the caregiver more aware of and attuned to her own levels of intuition, particularly those perceptions that affect interaction with the infant. Thus, by redirecting the caregiver's attention subtly to the object she is resisting—be it the infant or the therapist—the therapist provides the caregiver with an intuitive communication about her own behavior that enables her to better understand her interactions.

The therapist who pursues the strategy of redirecting the caregiver's attention will generally find that the resistance eventually diminishes and recedes. Evidence of such remission occurs when the caregiver can freely return to the person she has originally resisted. For example, assume in the preceding dialogue that the caregiver's resistance was directed toward the therapist. The therapist sensed this resistance from the caregiver's overt behaviors and other manifestations and, as a consequence, focused his attention on the infant. Following the therapist's lead, the caregiver began to interact with the infant in a spontaneous manner. Gradually, however, as this interaction with the infant continued, the caregiver's resistance and anxiety receded and she was able to return to the therapist's inquiries without feeling threatened. It is at this juncture—when the caregiver returns to the person she has initially resisted—that the therapist should delicately probe the contours of the resistance. This can be done in a nonthreatening manner by making a comment such as "I noticed that earlier you became apprehensive or anxious when I raised the topic of your husband's feelings about the baby's erratic feeding schedule." This comment should be open-ended, so that the caregiver does not feel compelled to respond. Often the caregiver will be able to respond and will then provide the therapist with information about the resistance. At other times, however, the caregiver will not respond to the therapist's inquiry but will merely listen and reflect on it. This response may be adequate depending on the caregiver, and the therapist should not probe further. Clarifying the issue of resistance for the caregiver in the form of a nonthreatening inquiry when the resistance has abated and the caregiver has redirected attention to the object initially being resisted is generally sufficient to enable the caregiver to begin reflecting on the motives for her behaviors.

A vital factor to consider in interpreting resistance during dyadic therapy involves the infant's reaction to the caregiver. It is important to note how the infant, who represents such a potent *transference object,* serves as a projective mediator through which caregivers express their feelings about themselves, their early objects, and the therapist. By speaking about the infant or even through the infant, the caregiver may express feelings and ideas that would otherwise be too threatening either to her self-esteem or to the therapeutic relationship. For example, Seligman and Pawl report on a case in which during an early stage of therapy, the mother responded to the therapist's announcement of his upcoming vacation by turning to her 6-

month-old daughter and commenting, "I guess he doesn't like us any more." When the therapist interpreted this comment as an expression of the caregiver's current feelings of rejection, she remembered her own mother's abandonment of her when she was 3 years old. This realization in turn led to a greater understanding of the caregiver's reluctance to become dependent on the therapist. Thus, attention to the caregiver's resistance may create an understanding of the correlation between the transference to the therapist and the potential transference with the infant. This observation enables the therapist and caregiver to move from reflection in one relationship to reflection on the relationship with the infant, thereby gaining an unusual degree of progressive insight.

Caregiver reactions to offers of help by all kinds of professionals are determined by their personalities and unresolved conflicts and will be expressed in transference reactions. The psychological orientation of infant–caregiver intervention encourages extensive exploration of these reactions. One method is the *deflection of attention* (Seligman & Pawl, 1983). This approach provides the caregiver with a nonthreatening way of experiencing anxiety, appreciating its source, and better appreciating the insights and psychological guidance offered by the treatment. In addition, slowly focusing attention on the resistance manifestation helps the caregiver to clarify confusing emotions of helplessness, anger, guilt, frustration, and anxiety that may infuse her relationship with her infant, and helps her to relate these feelings specifically to the resistance.

Davis (1989) advocates dealing with resistance through inquiry that involves exploring the patient's difficulties and the ability to respond. When resistance surfaces, the therapist should rapidly identify and clarify the defenses and should attempt to acquaint the patient with the defenses that have impeded functioning. This approach may be helpful in certain cases of dyadic therapy; the therapist, however, must be continually aware that techniques attempted with the caregiver may be enacted with the infant and have repercussions for the caregiver–infant relationship. Thus, caution is advisable when devising a strategy for coping with the resistances that arise during treatment.

CONCLUSION

This chapter has addressed the phenomenon of resistance during dyadic therapy with a caregiver and infant. Resistance involves all of the caregiver's strategies—whether in the form of fantasies or overt behaviors and comments—that prevent examination of the interaction and relationship between the caregiver and infant. The prevalent resistance manifestations in dyadic treatment have been discussed, and therapists have been offered a two-step technique to counter the caregiver's resistance effectively, without damaging the often fragile relationship between caregiver and infant. This technique involves a form of clarification, whereby the caregiver's attention is diverted to the person—either infant or therapist—who is not being resisted. Gradually, as the caregiver regains awareness, she will be able to return to the resisted person. At this juncture, it becomes appropriate for the therapist to address the nature of the resistance through open-ended and supportive inquiry. The chapter has also explored some highly potent forms of resistance, including seduction fantasies whereby the caregiver attempts to entangle the therapist in interpersonal issues that once again divert attention from her interaction with the infant. When encountering this form of resistance, the therapist should strive to redirect the caregiver's attention, so that the scope of treatment addresses the caregiver–infant relationship and the implications of maturational change.

Chapter 13

Applying the Principles of Modeling and Psychoeducation to Dyadic Intervention

INTRODUCTION

Modeling behavior, as an intervention strategy, has been variously defined. On a fundamental level, modeling involves the depiction or simulation of a specific behavior by one individual, who serves as a kind of actor, while a second individual observes and then imitates the behavior. Rutter (1975) has noted that individuals tend to model the actions of others with whom they have shared intimate, personal relationships, and this is particularly true with children, who generally replicate their parents' range of behaviors. Although children may be especially susceptible to modeling, adults who are motivated to change certain behaviors are also receptive to the cues presented by models.

The therapeutic technique of modeling exposes the patient to an individual—either the therapist directly or a videotaped model—who demonstrates the desired behaviors. According to Jacobson (1987), the therapist can engage in modeling in both a formal and informal manner. Formal modeling occurs during task instruction, which requires the therapist to perform the task while verbally describing the behavior and simultaneously modeling the behaviors associated with successful task performance. The therapist and patient then alternately perform the task. At first, the therapist prompts the patient in the performance of the task by expressing positive encouragement. Gradually, however, the therapist fades the instructions to a whisper and then becomes silent. When the patient makes a mistake or is learning a new task, the therapist returns to modeling overt self-instructions and has the patient do the same. Informal modeling generally involves a real-life problem situation encountered during a therapeutic intervention. Jacobson explains, for example, that during the first session the therapist may comment on how disorganized his or her desk is and then express a plan for organizing it better. In subsequent sessions, the therapist would then remind him- or herself of the previous plan to organize the desk. The therapist should present an image of being a coping model rather than a mastery model. That is, when portraying such a real-life problem to the patient, the therapist might display some initial difficulty or concern but would eventually overcome the problem situation effectively. According to Jacobson, this approach enables the patient to identify more closely with the therapist, because the model is fallible and imperfect but nonetheless accomplishes the task at hand.

As Rutter has emphasized, children tend to be particularly susceptible to modeling their parents' behavior. This is not surprising, because the children are exposed to their parents almost continually from birth and are dependent on them for formulating perceptions about the world and life experience. As a result, the intuitive behaviors caregivers manifest toward the infant from birth become significant models for him in formulating his own behavioral code. In this regard, caregiver verbalizations help the child develop language and verbal intelligence. Parents also model appropriate behavior for the child, selectively encouraging or discouraging particular kinds of conduct.

Modeling has also been found to result in other benefits. For example, it can assist individuals in overcoming psychological difficulties such as phobias. Bandura (1982a, 1982b) found that having a phobic individual watch someone else progressively approach and cope with feared objects helped to eliminate the phobia. Modeling can effect changes in the frequency or intensity of previously acquired responses, according to Lavatelli and Stendler (1972). Lövaas (1961) found that children exposed to aggressive cartoons chose more aggressive play subsequently than children who had watched a nonaggressive movie. Lavatelli and Stendler also note that the personality traits of individuals exposed to modeling behavior influences the amount of imitative behavior that occurs. For example, individuals who have low self-esteem or high dependency needs, or those who have been previously rewarded for imitative behavior are more likely to imitate the behavior of a model. Individuals are also more susceptible to imitate a model if they believe there is a resemblance between the model and themselves. Finally, Gewirtz and Stingle (1972) distinguish between different types of modeling. As these researchers explain, after witnessing a model's response, the individual will often exhibit a similar response, which would be termed *imitation*. A behavior is imitative if it matches the model's cues and behavior but is not a response to common stimulus antecedents or environmental constraints. Generalized imitation occurs when many different responses of a model are copied in diverse situations, often absent extrinsic reinforcement. In contrast, Gewirtz and Stingle point out that the term *identification* has generally referred to a person's taking on abstract psychological characteristics of a model, such as attitudes, values, and emotional states, rather than specific behaviors.

These descriptions of modeling suggest its value. The caregiver experiencing difficulty during dyadic interaction is likely to be receptive to techniques that can assist her in developing better strategies for communicating with the infant. At the same time, the infant's developmental status makes him prone to the behaviors of the caregiver. Thus, through modeling techniques, the therapist can effect adaptive change in both members of the dyad.

As noted previously, dyadic therapy involving the caregiver and infant differs from individual therapy in several significant respects. Perhaps the most distinguishing characteristic is the therapist's exposure to two discrete forms of interaction. First, as in conventional psychotherapy with an individual patient, a therapeutic alliance forms between the therapist and patient. The analogue in dyadic therapy would be the relationship between the therapist and caregiver, which personifies the degree of rapport within the therapeutic environment. In addition, as the caregiver begins to manifest transference phenomena, the therapist can determine the nature of any unresolved conflicts that may trouble the dyadic relationship. Second, dyadic therapy permits the therapist to observe directly the relationship between the caregiver and infant. Close exposure to the intimacy of the mother–infant exchange enables the therapist to understand the emotional rapport between the pair and, secondarily, permits validation of the caregiver's verbal reports. That is, during dyadic treatment the therapist will be able to discern whether a congruence exists between what the caregiver says about her relationship with the infant and the actual enactment of the mother–infant exchange. Because of these unique features, dyadic therapy resembles family or group therapy more than individual therapy.

These qualities of dyadic therapy present the therapist with an unparalleled opportunity to gain insight into the psychological status of both caregiver and infant for the purpose of diagnosis. By observing the caregiver–infant interaction, the therapist will be able to implement a variety of interventive techniques. As a result, dyadic therapy provides two simultaneous "Rorschachs" or impressions of the caregiver's interactions and permits the therapist to compare and contrast these behaviors and perceptions to derive the most efficacious models for intervention.

Modeling is a category of intervention that is particularly helpful to the therapist engaging in dyadic therapy and encompasses numerous strategies. A common strategy that promotes a higher degree of dyadic adaptation is observation of the dyadic interaction followed by either replication of the same interaction or substitution of another interaction. For example, if the therapist notices that the caregiver becomes upset and cannot handle the infant when sensitive issues are raised, while the infant simultaneously begins fussing and resisting the caregiver's embrace during these periods, the therapist may volunteer to hold the infant and model comforting interventions. Through such interventions, caregivers are often reassured that effective strategies exist to reassert equilibrium in the interaction. After the caregiver's distress has abated, the therapist would point out that the infant's disruptive behavior coincided with the caregiver's own distress and would suggest the benefits of the modeled behaviors.

Another form of modeling occurs when the therapist initiates contact with the infant to rehearse for the caregiver the various behaviors that may be absent from the caregiver's own behavioral repertoire. In this regard, it is helpful to keep in mind the constellation of *intuitive behaviors* discussed in Chapter 1. From the onset of treatment, therapists should assess the degree to which the caregiver uses intuitive behaviors to engage in adaptive interaction with the infant. For example, is the caregiver maintaining a sufficient amount of eye contact with the infant? Are the frequency and intensity of her vocalizations appropriate for the infant's developmental state? Is the caregiver's holding behavior adaptive? Is she providing the infant with a secure base for exploration? If any of these or other adaptive behaviors are lacking or are muted, the therapist may choose to model the appropriate method of interaction for the caregiver and then to suggest that she replicate the behavior during interactions with the infant. This chapter will discuss in detail how modeling strategies can be an interventive instrument for promoting adaptive rapport within the dyad.

MODELING STRATEGIES FOCUSING ON CAREGIVERS

Parent training incorporates modeling and enhances dyadic interaction as well as family interactions in general (Gordon & Davidson, 1981; Graziano, 1977). This technique highlights those parental skills necessary for teaching attunement and sensitivity to the infant. As the infant's sensitivity becomes more acute, the parent becomes more adept at administering appropriate previewing behaviors.

During parent training the therapist acts as a consultant or advisor to the parents who serve as the primary agents of behavioral change for their children (Tharp & Wetzel, 1969). Thus, the individual who interacts directly with the so-called problem child is not the therapist, but the parent who works under the therapist's tutelage or directive. The therapist teaches the parents to redesign their responses, attuning them to the child's conduct so that they strengthen adaptive and eliminate maladaptive behaviors. This form of treatment mandates an active role for the therapist.

A prominent feature of parent training that is applicable to caregiver–infant intervention is its emphasis on behaviors performed during interaction. According to Gordon and Davidson, the focus of attention is not so much on the particular problem that has caused the parent to seek therapy as it is on the nature of the interaction between the parent and child. Such issues as how effectively the parent conveys appropriate emotion to the child during interaction become highly relevant. The notion is that by realigning the interaction, maladaptive behavior will recede and be replaced by behaviors that encourage adaptive patterns of interaction. Similarly, parent training views problems of development as aspects of dysfunctional interaction. Once the caregiver learns to address developmental issues in a sensitive and attuned manner, many of these difficulties disappear. As maladaptive interaction recedes, it is replaced by a new perspective that enables the caregiver to understand the infant's developmental trends with greater sensitivity and to respond to these rhythms of maturation with appropriate previewing behavior.

As a consequence, the therapist must encourage the caregiver to use her intuitive skills to reinvigorate the interaction with the infant. In this approach the therapist depicts various aspects of development and subsequently speaks to the parent about her representations of her infant's developmental achievements. It is important to emphasize that the therapist interacts primarily with the caregiver who, in turn, interacts primarily with the infant, applying the knowledge she has acquired. This model also encourages the caregiver to use her own skills to observe directly and reinvigorate areas of her own competence. By witnessing how her various ministrations and changed behaviors modify the infant's behavior in a more adaptive manner, the caregiver gains a feeling of mastery over the interaction and develops expectations about future growth. The therapist's goal is to instill the sense that the caregiver can guide not only daily interaction but also the infant's overall development through adaptive previewing behaviors.

As a result, in the *behavioral parent training* model the therapist functions as a consultant to both parents, and the parents serve as the primary paradigms effecting behavior modification for their own children (Gordon & Davidson, 1981). Thus, the individual in direct contact with the infant is not the therapist, but the parent. The therapist assists the caregivers in understanding the ramifications of their actions so that they can redesign and realign their responses to the infant in such a way as to strengthen adaptive behaviors.

Gordon and Davidson recommend that when employing behavioral parent training, the therapist should first conduct an intake interview involving only the caregivers. The goals of this interview are to identify troubled interaction within the marital relationship, to obtain a complete psychological history of each caregiver, and to select tentative targets for behavior modification. It is best to conduct this interview without the infant because his attention-getting behaviors may inhibit information gathering, and/or the caregivers may be reluctant to discuss private matters that bear directly on the treatment. In addition, during the first session the parents will most often attempt to present the infant in a highly favorable light by highlighting the infant's adaptive mechanisms. In contrast to the parents of older children, caregivers of young infants tend to have difficulty identifying areas of conflict during interaction because associating the infant with problematic behavior patterns easily arouses guilt feelings. As a consequence, parents tend to attribute negative interactional patterns to their own deficits or to ignore these patterns entirely. Moreover, if there is a conflict between the parents and their child, the infant's presence during the initial interview serves to reinforce the frequently encountered initial reluctance to participate in therapy.

During the initial stages of the clinical interview, it often becomes evident that the caregivers have difficulty identifying precisely the problems that occur during interaction with the infant. Typically, presenting complaints may be stated by using labels as both descriptors and causes of behavior. For example, caregivers often describe their infants in highly global terms, using words such as "overactive," "difficult," or "negative." When questioned as to why the child "hits" or "screams," the caregiver will often answer by saying, "He's just difficult." These general descriptions provide the therapist with only limited insight, but the caregiver's ability to express these views represents an indispensable "first step" in the treatment. Although it is impossible to probe the infant or young child's behavior in depth during the early interviews, the therapist can observe and measure the caregivers' perceptions. A typical dialogue follows:

CAREGIVER: He is just so difficult to calm down.

THERAPIST: You've indicated that the baby is difficult. Can you describe these behaviors?

CAREGIVER: I feel I can't control him. He always keeps crying, even when I try to rock him.

THERAPIST: Do you feel that when you try to soothe him, you fail to have any effect?

CAREGIVER: Yes, and then when he finally allows me to control him, there is always something else.

A rigorous inquiry process is important to help the caregiver identify any behavioral referents that cause conflict leading to an unsatisfying, maladaptive interaction. Once the caregiver has articulated the difficult behaviors, the next step in the assessment is to analyze the maladaptive interactions by observing each caregiver during behavioral exchanges with the infant.

It is important to remember that the behavioral model requires the therapist to effect changes in the caregiver–infant relationship by working with the parents. The therapist must observe and analyze parental behavior and, significantly, must convey directly to the caregivers any impressions concerning troubled areas of interaction. Subsequently, the therapist can instruct the caregiver in behavior modification techniques that will elicit a more adaptive response from the infant. Although the therapist may occasionally model appropriate behaviors by interacting directly with the infant, the goal is not to usurp the parental role; rather, this technique provides parents with an example of effective and appropriate interaction that they can then transfer to their exchange with the infant. The therapist using this approach monitors progress in the treatment by observing changes in the dyadic interaction between parent and infant.

One of the most frequently cited reasons for caregiver inadequacy in dealing with infants is the caregiver's inconsistent responses, generally typified by an overreliance on noncontingent interaction (Miller, 1975). To rectify this situation, caregivers should receive basic training that enables them to recognize both the occurrence and nonoccurrence of the infant's adaptive or maladaptive behavior. At the same time, parents need to discriminate the aspects of their own behavior toward their children that consist of positive attention, negative attention, and minimal attention. Parent training strives to teach caregivers how to formulate appropriate *matches* between the child's behavior and their own behavior. For example, a typical sequence might involve adaptive and praiseworthy child behavior followed by positive adult attention. The therapist can maximize the likelihood of such appropriate matches and more consistent responses by training the caregiver to observe and measure the child's behavior and to monitor her own responses, which often include insufficiently emphasized adaptive manifestations within the caregiver's own behavioral repertoire. The caregiver must recognize and interpret the infant cues being directed to her attention and to respond appropriately. Although to do this, she needs to be acutely sensitive to the infant's behavior, the caregiver must go beyond these short-lived or transient infant responses and probe more deeply into their implications. For example, what overall mood is the infant experiencing and what kinds of behavioral and affective skills is the infant relying upon to communicate with the caregiver?

During the diagnostic assessment the therapist should begin matching treatment techniques to the individual patient. There are at least four factors to consider before determining the proper strategy. First, it is important to assess the degree to which the caregiver can control social and environmental circumstances. A single mother with three small children may simply not be in a position to alter her social environment sufficiently to resolve the conflict. Secondly, interpersonal problems between parents may preclude their working as a collaborative team to create an optimal environment for the infant. The caregivers' lack of agreement or cooperation with each other in parent training may indicate ambivalent attitudes in their own relationship that interfere with their response to treatment. Such caregivers may experience intense conflicts about any joint decision involving the entire family. Counseling in these cases often can do no more than provide temporary control over the parents' attempts to negate each other's relationship with the infant. Thus, the therapist can deal successfully with the problems that occur during interaction with the infant only after improving the routine communication between the parents.

As a third factor, caregivers are subject to myriad interpersonal factors and maladaptive emotional states, such as depression and anxiety, that can severely limit their ability to benefit from behavioral parent training. When the initial assessment indicates that psychopathology is present, other forms of intervention—such as individual therapy—may be necessary prior to or in conjunction with parent training. As a fourth and final factor, the constitutional resources and innate motivation of the infant may indicate that different forms of intervention would be appropriate. For example, a flawed parental communication coupled with marital conflict may have already impeded the child's maturational skills. In essence, the concept of matching the treatment appropriately to the dyad lies at the core of this form of therapy.

One important aspect of parent training is that it encourages contemporaneous individual psychotherapy if one or both parents should require it. The nature of dyadic treatment is such that the therapist may need to resolve personal conflict before attempting interactive modifications with the infant. The issues that cause psychological maladaptation in the parents can be quite diverse, ranging from family crises to chronic feelings of not wanting to assume the role of a parent and thus resenting the infant. The effective parent therapist needs to be familiar with a wide variety of psychotherapeutic and behavioral strategies—cognitive restructuring, assertiveness training, systematic desensitization, communication skill training—to resolve these complex problems. Parent training provides caregivers with the initiative to administer their own therapy when the therapist is not present or available. Eventually, by learning this approach, parents can successfully handle the problems of childhood before they develop into more negative, coercive types of behavior patterns that have become entrenched in daily interaction and are thus more difficult to eradicate.

The *motivational therapy* model adopts a different approach to the parent. Salzman (1984) posits that because behavioral patterns tend toward stability and rigidity, the parent must have assistance in developing a positive motivation for change. To do this, therapists must increase the caregiver's awareness of her self-esteem by offering positive feedback for the parent's interpersonal capabilities, divorced from idealizations and unrealistic expectations. Only then will the caregiver see the compulsive choices previously fostered by conflict.

INTERVENTIVE MODELING TECHNIQUES

The Role of Video-Recording

Most therapists concur that *video-recording* is a valuable adjunct to the therapeutic process. Videotapes allow both therapists and caregivers to be "observers" and to witness previously hidden and disguised manifestations (McRea, 1983; Ward & Bendak, 1964). In particular, through videotaping techniques, subtle nuances of the caregiver's interaction with the infant emerge more vividly and so directly that they cannot be denied or ignored.

The first issue raised by this technique is how to acclimate the patient to the idea of video-recording as an aid to treatment. The following are some strategies for introducing patients to the concept. First, caregivers should be notified in advance about the potential value of videotape techniques. When raising the issue of videotaping, the therapist should strive to provoke the patient's questions and curiosity not only about how videotaping will supplement the treatment but also about confidentiality issues. It is recommended that the therapist respond patiently and in detail to each query. A caregiver who does not immediately react to the potential use of videotaping may be asked directly about her reactions to being taped in an attempt to bring fears to the surface and to alleviate anxiety (Berger, 1978a, 1978b). Moreover, although most caregivers will not object to being taped, the therapist can use the caregiver's reactions—positive or negative—as material for further exploration. A caregiver's reaction to the introduction of video-recording can, for example, implicate attitudes about trust, as well as paranoid tendencies and grandiosity (Heilveil, 1983). Another technique whereby therapists can introduce patients to videotape is by suggesting the use of videotape over a period of time, thereby allowing the patient to decide flexibly about using it further and to ask gradually as the treatment advances about the benefit of watching themselves interact with the infant. According to Heilveil, this approach gives patients an opportunity to work through their anxieties while maintaining some semblance of control.

If the idea of video-recording is introduced after a therapeutic alliance has occurred, it is rare that patients experience much more than slight initial apprehension—in fact, the "stage fright" reaction is relatively uncommon and may be an indicator of severe underlying anxiety (Heilveil, 1983). Following this phase of brief apprehension, the majority of patients acclimate well to the presence of the camera and even display an eagerness to observe their performance and learn from it.

The therapist should have two primary goals in presenting videotape feedback to the patient. The first is to direct attention to behavioral cues manifested by both caregiver and infant that the therapist deems are important in revealing the nature of the dyadic rapport (Berger, 1978a, 1978b). After pointing out important cues, the next step is to encourage the patient to provide spontaneous explanations when these manifestations become evident on the tapes. Comparing or connecting two events may imply causality to the patient and emphasize her motivations, such as, "Whenever I raise the subject of feeding the baby, you frown and clench your fists. Can you tell me what makes you feel this way?" This form of intervention may contain elements of either clarification or confrontation. Another approach is simply to ask the caregiver to discuss her perceptions of the impressions observed on the videotape. In short, therapists should choose among the numerous interventions available for use within the framework of videotape feedback, based on the requirements and status of the therapeutic relationship during that particular phase of the treatment.

When interpreting videotapes for the caregiver, therapists should be careful not to neglect the more global set of *nonverbal* cues provided by the patient's posture and body language. Characteristic physical positions—sinking into the chair, as if to hide from the world; throwing the chest forward and cocking the head to the side, as if to challenge the world; folding the arms and drawing the face tightly, as if to erect a shield against the world; or hiding the infant, as if to prevent the therapist from noticing any trouble with the baby—are blatant examples of behaviors that may surface. More subtle behaviors are available for observation as well. When observing videotaped dyadic interactions, the therapist should be attuned to the caregiver's bodily gestures toward the infant as well as her intuitive skills.

Besides acutely observing subtle patient behavior in the video-recording sequences, the therapist also can serve a *didactic* function during such episodes by teaching the patient to observe her own responses, as well as those of the infant, closely. In this regard, the therapist should encourage the caregiver to use introspective skills and to make cause–effect hypotheses based on observations of her own behavior. Heilveil (1983) recommends doing this principally through the feedback modeling of interpretations and through observation of the videotape itself.

Significantly, the therapist must remember that a central influence on video-recording the therapist–dyad interaction is the relationship between therapist and the caregiver. The patient's response to the video-recording experience will not only depend on her unique personality and structure of psychological defenses but also on the quality and nature of her therapeutic alliance or rapport with the therapist. Because it is important to keep the therapeutic alliance as a centerpiece of the therapy, the therapist's role may best be construed as collaborative. Nevertheless, an attitude of complete collaboration during videotaping can prevent the therapist from maintaining the psychodynamics of the relationships involved. The therapist and the caregiver together can explore the videotape playback in the same way that they would, perhaps, interpret a dream, or explore home videotapes brought by the caregiver to the therapy session, or discuss a particular interactive sequence with the infant, such as a developmental change. During these episodes of mutual exploration the therapist helps the caregiver overcome resistance to frightening beliefs, attitudes, and feelings and assists her in acquiring an objective view of her own behavior.

At particular junctures in therapy, some caregivers, however, may feel too vulnerable to withstand the impact of watching their dyadic interactions on videotape. The best guide for when not to use videotape techniques remains the therapist's perceptions and intuitions. At other times, it will be necessary to modulate the pace and intensity of the exploratory work until the patient is "ready" for the dramatic revelations that often accompany video-recording. If the therapist does not wish to confront a patient for fear of rupturing a needed defense, then this realization would influence the choice of whether to use videotape feedback at certain points in the treatment. If therapists sense this form of resistance, they can first rely on other means of bolstering the caregiver's confidence to prepare her for videotaping. For example, the therapist might highlight the positive, adaptive aspects of the caregiver's interactions, thereby creating a climate of confidence and trust within the patient–therapist relationship. Videotaping can also be used to point out positive aspects of the mother–infant interaction, infant developmental changes, and so on. In fact, video-recording may be especially suitable for dyadic therapy because the main force motivating treatment is often the expectation that some change can be effected directly within the boundaries of the caregiver–infant relationship. Videotape is a rapid way of pinpointing interactional deficits that can then be corrected through modeling alternate behaviors and providing a new paradigm of interaction for the caregiver.

As a caveat, however, both Berger (1978a, 1978b) and Heilveil (1983) warn that care should also be taken with patients who are extremely depressed or who have a history of depression and/or suicide attempts. Such patients may use their videotaped image to validate an exceptionally poor self-concept. This caveat is especially pertinent in dyadic treatment because depressed caregivers may seize any external cue to rationalize an impaired relationship with the infant and to perpetuate it. As a consequence, although video-recording techniques are valuable adjuncts in the treatment of caregivers who are prepared and equipped to modify their interactional patterns with the infant, videotapes can also be a damaging mechanism that undermines caregiver confidence and self-esteem.

In addition, video-recordings may identify the degree to which the caregiver engages in intuitive behaviors with the infant during dyadic exchange. Videotapes have been especially effective in revealing the intricate nature of facial expression and the correlation of changes in facial expression with emotional change. Videotaping has also been useful for discerning emotional categories of response. This is particularly so in the etiology of emotional display because video captures nonverbal emotional categories that are too subtle for detection during ordinary observation, including individual differences in movement and gesture, eye contact and other aspects of looking, and the manner in which the individual deals with personal space (Summerfield, 1983). In addition, videotaping techniques can disclose other forms of intuitive behavior, such as appropriate vocalization and holding behavior.

One illustration of the insightfulness of video-recording techniques is the Facial Action Coding System (FACS) developed by Ekman and Friesen (1978) to evaluate those subtle muscular changes that constitute facial expression but are imperceptible during ordinary observation. Although a FACS analysis can be extraordinarily time-consuming because it involves frequent reruns and a slow-motion evaluation of each frame of the film, this assessment would not be possible at all without the benefit of videotaping. The FACS allows for a degree of precision and analysis that is lacking in more traditional methods of facial analysis in the context of social interaction. Thus, videotaping yields profound insight into the nature of human interaction that is not generally available with other methods.

Another advantage of video-recording is that it not only permits the "mimicking" or imitation of real life but also provides opportunities to examine the contours of interaction that escape disclosures during normal daily observation. For example, Summerfield (1983) has reported on the insights that may be gained from the use of *more than one camera angle,* from *close-ups,* from *slow-motion frames,* and from other specialized technologies such as *freeze-frames.* This advanced technology permits the observer to visualize phenomena that previously remained hidden from view and often obscured from consciousness. Through these more subtle cues the therapist can gain awareness of the true meaning and import of the caregiver's behaviors toward the infant and of the infant's response to the caregiver.

In organizing the type of social interaction that the therapist may wish to explore with video-recording, Hartup (1979) recommends the following procedure for categorizing behavior patterns. First, Hartup suggests considering the *frequency* of the behavior. Frequency in this context includes the presence or absence of an act and how often it occurs. For example, how common are episodes when the caregiver makes direct eye contact with the infant? *Latency* is another factor to be considered and alludes to the length of time it takes an individual to respond to a situation. Here the therapist would observe how long it takes the caregiver to respond to an infant cue. Hartup refers to the degree of magnitude of the response as the *intensity.* An illustration would be the loudness of voice involved when expressing an emotion or the presence and persistence of gestures that are unnecessary to convey a particular message or emotion. The therapist also should pay attention to duration, that is, the length of time a behavior continues. Duration, as Hartup points out, has two components: the *length* of time taken for the total unit of behavior and the *proportion* of total time taken up by that particular behavior during a discrete episode. For instance, how much time does the caregiver spend smiling at the infant? *Density* involves the amount of time that is devoted to a particular category of behavior. For example, how much time does the caregiver spend holding the infant adaptively or vocalizing appropriately? Finally, the therapist should spend some time concentrating on the *sequences* of the interaction. In this context, sequences refer to the order in which the behaviors occur, and an example might be turn-taking behavior during conversation. Does the caregiver, for instance, provide the infant with sufficient time to respond?

As this discussion suggests, diverse data are ascertainable through videotaping and can be used to accomplish a variety of diagnostic goals with respect to understanding a particular dyad's style of interaction. Dyadic treatment highlights certain unique forms of behavioral exchange between mother and infant, and the therapist needs to focus on these manifestations specifically in devising formats for videotape episodes. As some examples, eye contact, vocalization, and appropriate holding behaviors are key emblems of the degree of adaptive skill permeating dyadic interaction. The therapist may wish to focus on the incidence of these manifestations in videotape episodes and to design techniques, such as freeze-frames and close-up shots, that evidence these indicia of interaction. Other more generalized categories of interaction may include the degree of adequate stimulation the caregiver offers the infant, the extent to which she plays with the infant, and the adequacy of both the contingency and discrepancy experiences she provides for him. The therapist should also be mindful of the caregiver's awareness of developmental trends and of how she facilitates the infant's predictions about future development. These predictive capacities are stimulated to the extent that the caregiver understands infant development and uses this awareness to devise previewing behaviors that acquaint the infant with the interpersonal implications of these trends of imminent growth. The unique advantages of videotape technology allow the therapist to probe the caregiver's previewing skills and witness directly whether such skills permeate the dyadic interaction in either promoting or stifling adaptation. The therapist can also model such interactions, can show videotapes of adaptive interaction, can discuss these videotape models, and can then advise the caregiver in enacting with the infant various adaptive behaviors seen on the tape.

Techniques for Video-Recording

This section will discuss some specific modeling strategies that a therapist can employ with caregivers during dyadic therapy. The camera represents a powerful instrument that is capable of stripping away the layers of defense the patient may bring to treatment. The therapist, while watching a videotape with the caregiver, should carefully observe her responses and later ask the caregiver how she felt about her behavior and if she felt she interacted effectively with the infant. Other topics of exploration can deal with the patient's attitudes about expressing emotional issues to another and her perceived expression of emotions as compared with the intensity shown in the replay. In other words, videotaping allows therapist and caregiver to examine whether the caregiver conveys emotions accurately and how well the caregiver believes she previously conveyed these emotions through behavioral cues. The discrepancies that emerge between appearance and reality may underscore particular communication and emotional deficits the caregiver is experiencing during interpersonal interaction with the infant and/or spouse.

Heilveil (1983) has described an alternate form of this technique. This researcher places a camera directly behind a monitor aimed at a patient who is seated facing the monitor. This creates an interacting mirror or feedback loop. The patient, who is facing only the image of her face, is asked to imagine that the image on the screen is that of another person (e.g., the infant). The patient is then asked to have a conversation with this other person. The therapist, seated outside of the camera's range, discusses the image on the screen with the actual patient. This creates a dialogue through the medium of the videotape monitor and often permits the patient to express feelings she has difficulty expressing directly to the therapist. Goodyear and Parish (1978) have described an interesting variation on this technique. These researchers use this technique, coupled with standard replay, or freeze-framing. At moments when such close-ups or freeze-frames are used, patients are encouraged to express how they feel. This strategy provides the therapist with a kind of "Rorschach" that reveals the patient's emotional state.

Video-recording techniques are particularly useful in dyadic therapy for still another reason. Many of the communicative gestures between the caregiver and infant occur on a microscopic level involving manifestations that are imperceptible during ordinary observation. To outline all of these manifestations comprehensively would be difficult. Nevertheless, they generally encompass the caregiver's eye and body contact with the infant, the full range of vocal communications exchanged between the pair, and the caregiver's overall ability to provide adequate stimulation for the infant. Many of the behaviors that have been referred to earlier as intuitive are encompassed here. Often these behaviors are either not perceptible through direct observation by the therapist or are only apparent in their grossest proportions. For example, the therapist may notice that the caregiver is not supporting the infant's head and neck properly or that a minimal degree of eye contact is occurring, but in fact interpersonal behaviors are also lacking at a much more subtle level. Videotaping, combined with such techniques as freeze-framing, better discloses the full extent of these behaviors.

As a result, video-recording may be especially helpful for diagnostic purposes. The therapist can observe, on tape, elements that are disguised during direct observation. Video-recording permits the therapist to use freeze-frame techniques (Alger, 1978), and the freeze-frame can be a perceptible model for discussing a variety of emotions and behaviors. The therapist and caregiver can return to freeze-frame references continually to discuss how to enhance interactional skills with the infant. The freeze-frame can also be used as a projective technique (Daitzman, 1977). By arresting an image and having the patient tell a story about that image, the therapist acquires insight into the caregiver's inner conflicts and the way that these conflicts may emerge during interaction with the infant. During the early stages of the use of videotape, therapists may find themselves carefully selecting the particular moment of time to be frozen for analysis and discussion. Eventually, however, patients begin to call for a freeze-frame themselves and to volunteer their perceptions concerning their own behavior toward their infants. Whether the freeze is called for by the patient or therapist, however, the best use of the technique is mutual examination and exploration of the distinctive manifestations captured on the tape. Freeze-framing embodies the nuances and subtle expressions of a behavioral sequence, and these subtleties may communicate more about the patient's conflicts than extensive verbal discourse. The freeze-framing technique, which can disclose subtle intuitive behavior, is particularly helpful in dyadic therapy because so many of the caregiver's manifestations occur almost spontaneously at a barely perceptible level during direct observation.

Another videotape technique is a phenomenon referred to as *half and half* (Alger, 1978). It involves separately playing back either the sound or the picture portion of the videotape to accentuate attributes that went unnoticed when all features were played in unison. By highlighting the audio feature alone, caregivers become more attuned to and aware of the emotion conveyed through vocal communication: speech nonfluencies, hesitations, a monotonic rhythm, and other vocalization features become exaggerated. In addition, the caregiver gains sensitivity about the infant's vocal responses. Similarly, viewing only the visual portion of the tape accentuates behavioral manifestations and gestures that would otherwise not be apparent. This technique may be particularly helpful in dyadic therapy where the subtle behavioral manifestations the caregiver exchanges with the infant are of crucial significance in encouraging and reinforcing adaptive interaction. The half and half technique also allows the caregiver to better understand the multiple responses—vocal, physical, and psychological—that she must coordinate to achieve adaptive interaction.

Researchers have noted that video-recording during treatment can result in a dramatic modification in both self-concept and interpersonal behavior (Boyd & Sisney, 1967). This dual level of change—in both the objective perception of self-behavior and the subjective awareness of the motivations for the behavior—is of particular value in dyadic therapy and is another reason for adopting these techniques. In dyadic treatment it becomes vital for the caregiver to understand not only the outward manifestations that may be inappropriate during interaction with the infant but also the subjective feelings that may be motivating these maladaptive behavior patterns.

Once the caregiver has attained these realizations through the use of videotaping, the therapist can begin helping the caregiver to convert maladaptive patterns into more suitable behaviors. Hosford and Mills (1983) have identified some of the adaptive behaviors that can be acquired through video therapy. Among these behaviors are assertive actions that permit the expression of emotion in nonhostile ways (Hersen & Bellack, 1976; Lazarus, 1971; Libet & Lewinsohn, 1973; Rimm & Masters, 1979). Appropriate holding behavior, eye contact, and vocalization behavior may also be encouraged through videotaping. In addition, videotapes can help the caregiver introduce more advantageous rhythms of response into the dyadic relationship. These goals should be kept in mind when formulating strategies for video-recording caregivers and infants. As noted earlier, the therapist engaged in dyadic therapy will be striving to generate a model for interaction that the caregiver can immediately utilize to change interactive patterns with the infant.

Moreover, the therapist relying on videotaping can use one of two basic strategies: Educational videos that depict appropriate modes of interaction can serve as models to guide the caregiver's future behavior, or the therapist can videotape interaction within the dyad directly and play this tape back for the caregiver. When relying on videotapes that use models, the therapist should attempt to locate tapes in which the model resembles the patient in terms of age and background (Kazdin, 1974). It is also recommended that such models show a similar personality and mood (Bandura, 1977a, 1977b).

Three steps are followed during and after viewing such model videotapes. First, the therapist instructs the caregiver to pay particular attention to the important features of the modeled behavior and perhaps to discuss the most prominent qualities of interaction. This directive presumably enables the caregiver to internalize the information and to develop both verbal and visual cognitive representations, which are stored in memory. The therapist should "test" these representations by asking the caregiver to describe what she has observed and how these observations have enhanced her understanding of interaction with the infant. The second step in the videotaping technique is to ask the patient to translate her cognitive representations of the modeled behaviors into actual behavior with the infant. In other words, after observing and discussing an example of adaptive interaction depicted on the videotape, the caregiver should be encouraged to enact this kind of interaction with the infant. Some caregivers may hesitate to do this at first, and in these cases the therapist should first model the appropriate behavior. During such episodes the therapist may also wish to point out directly to the caregiver how such interactions will enhance the dyad's rapport. As a third step, to ensure that caregivers can behave in the manner shown on the videotape once they leave the treatment setting, therapists should encourage the frequent rehearsal of social skills with the infant in two ways. First, the therapist should encourage adaptive interactive sessions during the treatment itself to inculcate the manifestations displayed on the tape. Second, the therapist should encourage the caregiver to discuss how she is using these instructions in interaction to better enhance her behavior with the infant during times away from the session. As with other techniques, the videotape behaviors are eventually transferred to genuine dyadic interaction through episodes of reinforcement.

Self-modeling, a technique whereby videotapes of the caregiver during interaction are later played back and reviewed during treatment sessions, is an approach with enormous benefits. Viewing the "self" as it is depicted objectively is remarkably effective in motivating individual change and may even be a more advantageous tool than viewing models of others engaged in adaptive behavior (Shotter, 1983). Self-observation has distinctive advantages. As Shotter points out, viewing a videotape of the self allows individuals to observe themselves objectively because they are confronting recordings of their own behavior, not the behaviors of other people. This phenomenon enables individuals to observe the self as an object, in much the same way as they observe others. For the first time individuals may be forced to face aspects of their behavior that previously were suppressed or obliterated from conscious perception. Second, videotapes of the self cause a kind of self-conscious reaction. Not only does the person now see herself as others see her, but she also sees the self she has created and portrays to the world, a sense of self-recognition that sparks dramatic change.

For Dowrick (1983) self-modeling has a dramatic effect because it has "no errors." That is, the individual is depicted on the screen, warts and all, and there is no opportunity to hide behind defensive mechanisms or to ignore the potent reality of the behavior. In this sense, self-modeling has a desired confrontational effect that triggers the urge to change and is so useful for dyadic treatment. Once the caregiver recognizes the deficits in her behavior, she can begin to transform the video image into the person she wants to be. In other words, researchers are correct in asserting that videotaping patient interactions and playing these tapes for the patient can have a shocking effect, particularly if the patient has attempted to deny or disguise the existence of maladaptive patterns of interaction. By the same token, once the initial shock has abated, this technique offers the patient an unparalleled opportunity to alter behavior dramatically and, in a sense, to reinvent relationships and recreate more adaptive behavior patterns. This second aspect of video-recording is of principal importance in dyadic therapy. Dyadic treatment strives, above all, to effect changes in the interactive behaviors between mother and infant by realigning the caregiver's perceptions about the developmental course of the infant. Because of its capacity to foster the recognition of behavioral trends and to encourage the modification of particular behaviors and attitudes toward the self, videotaping techniques are ideally designed to achieve this outcome and to do so more rapidly than other therapeutic techniques that rely on introspection and interpretation.

THERAPIST: Was there anything in the tape that felt new to you?

CAREGIVER 1: I had one thought about the piece at the end about giving babies regular milk. Have any of you read anything about that?

CAREGIVER 2: I had a babysitter for my 3-year-old, and I was very conscientious about giving him soybean formula. On his first birthday I told the babysitter, "O.K., you can start giving him cow milk." The sitter told me she had been doing that for six months! And he was fine. Another thing they brought up in the tape was propping bottles. I thought that was a good point because I had to prop the bottles to feed the twins.

CAREGIVER 3: Do you stay with them to make sure they don't choke?

CAREGIVER 2: Yes, absolutely.

PSYCHOEDUCATION

Virtually all caregivers harbor preconceived notions about what happens when a newborn baby enters a family setting, but these general impressions traditionally don't encompass many of the conflicts and areas of turmoil that can accompany the birth of a child. *Psychoeducation* refers to strategies that teach individuals how to acclimate to new circumstances in their lives that may have dramatic psychological effects, such as the arrival of a new baby and the integration of the infant into the family setting. Rather than relying on psychotherapy alone, however, psychoeducation incorporates a didactic function by teaching individuals new skills that will enable them to meet the challenges posed by their circumstances.

Such techniques may be particularly advisable for first-time, new parents, who are often anxious about the changes the new infant will exert on the marital relationship and on everyday matters such as daily schedules, living arrangements, and the division of responsibility between the couple. Psychoeducation offers these parents practical guidelines for adjusting to the infant's presence in the home. Advocates of psychoeducation report that *establishing structure* is critically important because the home environment will be new and alien to the baby, and conversely, the new parents may hesitate to acknowledge and accommodate the changes caused by the new infant. Families can achieve structure by formulating clear expectations for both the infant and themselves, by committing themselves to open communication, and by anticipating and resolving problems effectively. In essence, the parents need to preview and devise strategies for these changes. Therapists can assist families with new infants in negotiating this transition period smoothly through direct advice, as well as through *psychoeducation* geared to enhance the families' communication and problem-solving skills (Bernheim & Lehman, 1985). Psychoeducation techniques facilitate the acceptance of the infant into the family unit so that he becomes an instrument for enhancing emotional rapport instead of an unwelcome intruder who usurps the affection of one or the other parent.

Psychoeducation involves teaching strategies to reduce stress. According to Bernheim and Lehman, one method of staving off stress is to *establish a regular schedule* for the infant with respect to sleeping, elimination, and eating patterns. A truism about virtually all newborns is that their daily schedule—when they eat, sleep, have bowel movements—is likely to be both unpredictable and erratic. This is partly because the infant's physiological mechanisms are only beginning to function and adjust to life outside the womb. Perhaps the best way for the therapist to deal with this unpredictability is to reassure caregivers that, in fact, most newborns manifest somewhat erratic schedules. Reassurance is often sufficient to allay anxiety. The therapist should also stress two other factors. First, even though the initial few weeks or months with a new baby will often be filled with disruption and unpredictability, the infant's schedule will most likely become more regular and predictable as time passes and as the caregivers become more adept at managing him. This gradual adjustment to the infant's schedule should also be previewed. In addition, caregivers should try to discern patterns in the baby's behaviors even in the first few weeks of life. These patterns will enable the caregivers to exert some measure of control over the infant and to begin to experience a degree of competence about nurturing him. The majority of infants, even those whose schedules seem most erratic, are functioning according to some meaningful and coherent biological or rhythmic clock. An infant who awakens crying at 3 o'clock in the morning may initially disturb his parents, but if the infant arises at the same time each morning, the caregivers can eventually discern a pattern and attune their behaviors to those of the infant. The caregivers may agree that on certain nights of the week it will be the mother's responsibility to get up with the infant, whereas on other days, this burden will fall on the father's shoulders. This *delineation of roles* also allows the caregivers to confront the changes the infant's presence has effected in their lives. By becoming attuned to the infant in this fashion, the caregivers are also reinforcing the message that the infant is a predictable being, and they can later reflect this notion of predictability back to the infant during previewing episodes.

Psychoeducation also involves helping the caregivers become attuned to the processes of development the infant is undergoing. Therapists should point out to parents examples of how the infant is attempting to respond to environmental cues and to signal diverse messages. Eventually, parents can report on the strategies they have devised for meeting the infant's needs and for anticipating upcoming changes in behavior that are the product of developmental growth.

Other recommendations include helping parents in *planning ahead and anticipating events* to avoid surprises for both caregivers and infant, and in devising specific strategies to deal with problematic behaviors (Bernheim & Lehman, 1985). Perhaps the greatest risk to a supportive home environment is the family's sense that events are out of control, that they lack the skills to solve problems, that crises cannot be resolved, and that the future has become a threatening, unpredictable event. Such emotions, if allowed to fester, can disrupt the caregiver's locus of control and exacerbate an already tenuous situation. Moreover, these feelings of lack of control will also be conveyed to the infant who will experience the world as an uncontrollable and unpredictable place. Stress levels tend to increase dramatically when caregivers feel they are enmeshed in a situation over which they can exert minimal control and order. It is therefore vital to teach parents how to deal with potential crises before they erupt. Planning ahead is particularly useful because it is important to provide a contingent atmosphere so that the infant will learn to anticipate certain events and to use his skills for overcoming challenges. If the infant's expectations are fulfilled, a feeling of mastery ensues. The caregiver can reinforce this feeling of mastery during previewing episodes. Training the caregiver to visualize how maturational changes will occur in the infant and what it will be like to experience a developmental milestone from both the caregiver's and the infant's perspectives is one technique for instilling feelings of mastery. In fact, *perspective-taking exercises* signify an example of how therapists can help new parents assert a sense of control early in the dyadic relationship. By engaging in such exercises, the therapist can help caregivers modify unrealistic expectations and better anticipate aspects of development that will inevitably occur in their own infants.

To preview effectively, however, the caregiver must first learn to *represent* the developmental changes the infant is likely to experience in the imminent future. Developmental events here refer to major milestones and their precursory behaviors. Some caregivers will demonstrate a remarkable adeptness at representing future behaviors—it is almost as if these caregivers possess an internal blueprint of how their infant's development will unfold over the first 30 months of life. For others, however, representation is initially a more perplexing task. Although these mothers may be able to describe the broad outlines of development, they are unable to perceive subtle changes or to predict which maturational accomplishments will occur next. In such cases, the modeling techniques described earlier in the chapter may be helpful. Other mothers will be unable to connect a particular developmental milestone with the child's chronological age. In these cases, the therapist should rely on videotapes and charts that delineate developmental trends specifically, thereby enabling the caregiver to visualize how her infant's development is likely to progress.

Once the caregiver has learned the phases of development she can move on to actual previewing behavior. This requires applying the newfound knowledge and perceptions to interactional sequences that acquaint the infant with the sensations of the imminent developmental accomplishment. The goal here is to provide the infant with a telescopic view of all the perceptions that he will experience when he consolidates and achieves the upcoming milestone. For example, how will the developmental attainment feel on an emotional level, what thought processes will the infant undergo when the skill is attained, how will the infant's motivation be affected, and what sorts of somatic changes will the infant undergo? The optimal pre-viewing episode enables the infant to experience each of these phenomena and to integrate them into a meaningful representation of upcoming expe-rience. For the caregiver to understand the infant's perceptions during these myriad changes, videotaping and modeling may be helpful. Finally, previewing requires that the caregiver sense when the infant has become satiated with the new experience and wishes to return to his previous developmental level. When he reaches this point, the sensitive caregiver will gradually curtail the previewing and supportively allow the infant to return to his already attained developmental plateau.

The prerequisite for engaging in these previewing exercises is the caregiver's ability to perceive the infant's developmental status objectively. This involves reconciling the caregiver's imaginary perceptions of how the infant will develop with the objective dimensions of the infant's unique personality. Although we all harbor preconceived notions of how babies should behave and develop, each infant is unique, endowed with a particu-lar and distinctive temperament, physiological mechanism, and psychologi-cal attitude that the caregiver must, on some level, recognize objectively and accommodate to adaptively. Related to the notion that each infant is unique is the fact that virtually all new parents must make the transition from the fantasy baby whom they imagined before the birth to the real-life physical entity who has entered the family. This transition often involves a period of psychological mourning during which the caregiver relinquishes the image of the ideal baby and replaces it with the representation of the real baby. In addition, during this period of readjustment the husband and wife must realign their own relationship to accommodate the needs of the infant.

One aspect of adjusting to the newborn's arrival involves *establishing effective lines of communication*. According to Bernheim and Lehman (1985), adequately conveying expectations, emotions, dissatisfactions, aspirations, limits, and plans is especially critical during the period following the baby's birth, and can be communicated in a supportive home environment that reduces stress. Caregivers should be explicit when expressing the develop-mental achievements they expect from the infant and at what time, what behaviors they expect will be disruptive, and what limits they can place on the infant's manifestations. Caregivers may also wish to set aside interactive periods when they focus on discerning changes in the infant's developmen-tal capabilities. For example, specific times should be established for when both parents interact with the infant or when the mother describes the infant's daily achievements to the father. Again, what is important is estab-lishing some degree of regularity and consistency in the daily schedule. It is also recommended that caregivers practice being emotionally calm and supportive with one another. In this regard, *mirroring* can be taught as an exercise that enhances communication while keeping negative emotions in check. Mirroring refers to the caregiver's ability to speak in a tranquil and controlled manner, despite an apparently stressful situation. The other caregiver will then manifest this tranquil attitude back to the first caregiver. Mirroring is actually a form of modeling, whereby one individual displays adaptive behaviors that the other individual replicates. The therapist can teach the caregiver mirroring, and she can subsequently instruct her spouse in this technique. Caregivers must also be cautioned that life with a newborn infant will often fray nerves; it is important for parents from the outset to function as a mutually responsive, adaptive team, in order to overcome any erratic behavior patterns the infant may display.

It is crucial as well for new caregivers to verbalize during treatment the emotions their infant arouses in them, especially feelings of frustration, and to dissipate negative emotions in a productive fashion that does not interfere with the relationship being forged with the infant. These emotions can be particularly debilitating for new parents whose confidence may already be undermined by the infant's erratic and unpredictable schedule and behavior patterns. In fact, in contrast to other forms of therapy, dyadic intervention requires that the caregiver become an active participant in the treatment, expressing not merely her own concerns but the infant's viewpoint as well. Moreover, the caregiver must transfer this stance to the interaction with the infant by becoming sensitive not only to her own perspective on events but also to the infant's emotional and psychological experiences. Although adults can be reflective in their relationship with others, this kind of introspective approach is not appropriate during interaction with the infant, who is not yet ready to communicate verbally. Instead, he requires overt stimulation and participation, often in an almost exaggerated fashion, to provide him with the sense that the environment is both contingent and predictable and that the caregiver will fulfill his needs. Caregivers must learn to express their feelings to one another in a concise manner that incorporates suggestions for positive action.

When modeling techniques are not yielding results, another developmental method for helping caregivers negotiate the transition to parenthood utilizes direct *exploratory psychotherapy*. This strategy encourages the caregiver to air her innermost feelings about whether the real infant has met the expectations of the idealized infant imagined prior to the birth. One such mother I treated had an infant with colic. The caregiver complained that the infant cried uncontrollably for up to 4 hours each day. Although her pediatrician had assured her that there was no physiological abnormality, this mother was at a loss to explain why her infant was incapable of being comforted. As treatment progressed in a secure environment, she voiced her feelings of profound disappointment and anger at the infant to the therapist. This caregiver revealed that her colicky infant was not the pleasant, tranquil baby she had envisioned during her pregnancy. Once these feelings emerged and were expressed directly in a nonjudgmental setting, the caregiver was better equipped to abandon her earlier disappointment and to begin learning the most effective strategies for coping with her child. Moreover, during treatment she was also able to examine the issue of how her husband had adjusted to the entrance of the infant into the household. An exploration of this period of adjustment is vital for caregivers whose infants have a physical abnormality or display a difficult or slow-to-warm-up disposition. Unless the caregivers reconcile whatever feelings of resentment, disappointment, or anger they are experiencing, they will be unable to learn how to preview adaptively. Realignment of the marital relationship to reflect the infant's presence is also a crucial component of this process, and the therapist should explore whether the infant's arrival has caused resentment or discord between the husband and wife.

THERAPIST: I know there were some physical problems when the infant was born. Can you tell me about that?

CAREGIVER: Well, he was born prematurely and then the doctors discovered a problem with his heart. As a result, he had to remain in the hospital for a while. It was very stressful for me and my husband.

THERAPIST: Can you tell me how you felt during this period?

CAREGIVER: I was exhausted the entire time. I spent hours at the hospital and then I would just go home and collapse . . . and I guess I was also disappointed.

THERAPIST: Disappointed in what way?

CAREGIVER: I guess because . . . because I sort of expected him to be . . . almost perfect. At least that's the way I envisioned him while I was pregnant, and it was kind of a shock when he was born with a defect. It was so unexpected. The doctor told us throughout the pregnancy that the baby was fine. So to learn about this terrible defect after the birth caused my husband and me to question ourselves and our own relationship. Had we done anything to cause the baby's problems? There was even a period of time when I guess, in thinking about it now, we blamed the baby. We also went through a period when we questioned our own relationship in the marriage.

THERAPIST: How do you feel about that now?

CAREGIVER: I think I have adjusted. I've learned to accept the baby for who he is . . . he has his own special personality, but it took time. After a while, with your help, I learned that he was able to respond to me and that his development was continual and within the normal range. So I guess I have become both more receptive and accepting.

Another form of modeling technique that the therapist can use involves infant massage to stimulate flexibility of the infant's limbs and to promote the caregiver's attunement to the infant's physiological perceptions. Basic massage in preterm infants has been found to stimulate growth and enhance performance on the Brazelton Neonatal Assessment (Scafidi et al., 1990). This strategy, whereby the therapist massages the infant and then encourages the caregiver to model the behavior, may be particularly advantageous for caregivers who lack the capacity to represent infant developmental trends.

THERAPLAY

A treatment referred to as *theraplay* has evolved from the work of clinicians with severely emotionally disturbed children. Theraplay seeks to ascertain whether an adaptive "match" exists among family members with respect to the degree of stimulation that is provided. As explained by Jernberg (1979), theraplay adopts an assertive approach to handling maladaptive behavior. When the child is behaving in a maladaptive or uncooperative fashion, the therapist will respond with a kind of vigor and intrusiveness not encountered in other treatments, for example, by forcing eye contact or physically blocking the child's pathway. Theraplay focuses on the intimacy between child and therapist. The emphasis of the approach is to address the behavior directly while ignoring the bizarre, the past, and fantasy. The therapist initiates, structures, and takes charge of the session; perhaps as a consequence of this heightened degree of intrusiveness, more resistance and even temper tantrums are encountered than with other forms of treatment.

The underlying premise of theraplay is that adaptive infants undergo a particular kind of nurturing experience with their caregivers. Eventually, the infant comes to welcome the clarity, security, and predictability offered by these stimulations that provide structure and organization, thereby enabling him to feel he is living in a predictable world. Such nurturing interactions are meaningful for both mother and infant and are necessary to adaptive exchange. Sometimes, however, environmental factors or factors inherent to the constitutional endowment of the infant intrude on the achievement of this kind of relationship.

With respect to constitutional factors, Jernberg (1979) focuses particularly upon infant temperament (Thomas, Chess, & Birch, 1970) and the work of Fries (1944), who characterized infants as being of either "high" or "low" activity level. Theraplay seeks to clarify the infant's temperament and to ensure that the caregivers appropriately match their infant's temperamental needs. In addition, theraplay considers the views of Bergman and Escalona (1949), which propose that babies have a protective barrier against stimulation. Some infants have a "thin" protective barrier, causing them to be overexcitable. At the opposite end of the spectrum are those infants with a "thick" protective barrier, which leads to underexcitation. In between is a group of infants who have a barrier of intermediate strength. According to the theories of theraplay, if the match between the infant's needed level of stimulation and the level provided by the caregiver is not adaptive, maladaptive patterns will erupt among family members with repercussions for other family relationships. To remedy this mismatch of stimulation levels, theraplay adopts a series of strategies within the family context. For example, both parent and child will be asked to tell one another's fortunes. This exercise forces family members to make predictions about one another's behavior and brings to awareness their engrained assumptions. The therapist can ask other family members to predict the infant's behaviors in the future and to describe what their changing relationship with the infant will be like. Thus, theraplay forces a kind of emotional confrontation among family members, while urging them to predict future behaviors and to respond adaptively.

Each strategy discussed in this chapter relies on some form of modeling whereby the therapist presents the caregivers with a paradigm of adaptive interaction—through direct interaction with the infant, videotaping techniques, exploratory psychotherapy, psychoeducation—and then encourages the caregivers to compare their behaviors with the models of appropriate interaction. Following this comparison, the caregivers will be directed to engage in more adaptive interactions with the infant. These techniques have often resulted in dramatic change because the exposure to a model provides caregivers with an ascertainable image of behavior toward which they can strive.

CONCLUSION

This chapter has described various techniques that may be efficacious in helping the therapist to motivate the caregiver in such skills as representation, previewing, and intuitive techniques. These behaviors may be encouraged through modeling in the form of video-recording, which vividly depicts actual interactions and demonstrates how the caregiver can modify her own behavior along adaptive lines.

Two different kinds of video-recording can be used. First, the therapist can rely on general tapes that portray models demonstrating adaptive forms of interaction and ask the caregiver to imitate various behaviors depicted in the tapes. A second method involves taping the caregiver herself during interaction and then, as the caregiver and therapist observe this tape, discussing ways to improve or enhance dyadic rapport. These self-modeling tapes derive their effectiveness primarily from encouraging the caregiver to view her interaction with the infant directly and to confront deficit or maladaptive behaviors. Researchers have found that such confrontational modeling techniques often help patients to modify their behaviors. This outcome of modification in the context of an interpersonal interaction makes self-modeling an advantageous technique for dyadic therapy.

Candid discussion between therapist and caregiver, when coupled with modeling strategies, is another means of enhancing dyadic interaction. Often caregivers need to talk through problems with an objective observer and listener who will not offer judgmental opinions. The therapist, who should approach each dyad with a fresh and open perspective, represents just such a figure. Moreover, as the treatment continues, the caregiver will turn to the therapist as an individual who has expertise in working through the difficulties encountered during dyadic interaction. To supplement the therapist's role as an authority figure, direct interaction between therapist and infant is encouraged. The therapist can use such interaction to present the caregiver with a model of interaction that is often less threatening than a videotape model.

Beyond these skills, the therapist's presence and encouragement empower the caregiver with feelings of mastery and competence. Once she attains these feelings, previewing can be encouraged, particularly if the therapist refrains from too much direct interaction with the infant and acts as a vehicle through which the caregiver vicariously exercises her skills. In other words, it is often important not to intervene directly in the dyadic exchange by interacting with the infant. Rather, the therapist should, relatively early in the relationship, instill the principle that it is the therapist's role to provide appropriate models of interaction, whereas it is the caregiver's role to initiate, monitor, and modify behavioral exchange with the infant. She is the individual who controls the infant's level of adaptation and who stimulates his skill in predicting future interaction. By adopting this stance and by using the techniques of modeling mentioned earlier, the caregiver will leave treatment with the confidence that she possesses the skill to guide interaction with the infant in an adaptive fashion.

PART FIVE

Applying Previewing During Nondyadic Approaches to Dyadic Intervention

Chapter 14

Applying Principles of Family Therapy to Dyadic Intervention

INTRODUCTION

The preceding chapters have focused on the dyadic model as a treatment strategy that can have significant ramifications on the efforts of both the caregiver and infant to achieve optimal mental health. Nevertheless, although dyadic treatment can be successful when only the caregiver and infant receive therapy, it may also be advantageous to include other family members in the treatment whenever possible. Or, if other family members are unable or unwilling to attend treatment, the therapist may still integrate some family therapy strategies in the context of dyadic treatment.

The reasons for transplanting some techniques of family therapy into the dyadic model are manifold. As has been noted, when mothers embark on the task of nurturing their infants they often replicate the behavioral patterns and attitudes to which they themselves were exposed during childhood. Although a skillful clinician can eventually detect these patterns through both observation and psychotherapeutic inquiry, enormous benefits may result when the entire nuclear family attends treatment and the therapist can observe these behavior patterns directly. This approach often facilitates enacting certain seminal behaviors, allowing the therapist to diagnose with a greater degree of precision such phenomena as patterns of attachment, the intergenerational transmission of psychopathology, patterns of triangulation, and the ability of family members to communicate intimacy and to achieve autonomy. Moreover, techniques of family therapy may disclose subtle patterns of interaction that are less susceptible to diagnosis when only the mother and infant are being seen for treatment. For example, in some families one child, who is tacitly designated as the "scapegoat," absorbs and subsequently manifests extreme psychopathological behavior while bearing the blame for the family's dysfunction. The other family members then attribute all deviant behavior to this individual. The scapegoating process is generally complex, however, and customarily implicates virtually all the other members of the nuclear family. Exposing this process and its psychopathological underpinnings requires an understanding of interaction within the entire family. Moreover, recent research has demonstrated that because the subjective perceptions of both parents in the family insinuate themselves into patterns of family interaction, it is necessary to understand the dynamics of the entire nuclear family before effective diagnosis and treatment can occur. Family therapy can also provide specific insights into the origins of caregiver deficits that preclude rehearsing adaptive previewing exercises with the infant. The therapist thus can view the mother–infant dyad more comprehensively and can detect and assess dysfunctional patterns as well as disclose adaptive behaviors such as previewing.

This chapter will highlight the fundamental theories of family therapy and will attempt to extrapolate various diagnostic and therapeutic techniques that therapists may use analogously with caregiver–infant dyadic therapy. Neither the infant nor the caregiver approaches the dyadic relationship with a *tabula rasa* or "blank slate": The caregiver brings to the relationship her years of experience from her own family of origin, whereas the infant's compelling constitutional endowment binds him to the caregiver like a psychological umbilical cord. The strategies used by family therapists may provide another opportunity for instilling principles of adaptive *previewing* within the dyad. As a diagnostic aid, previewing offers a technique for predicting interpersonal conflict; at the same time, therapeutic previewing exercises may modify behavioral patterns to achieve more adaptive responses. Just as previewing can be integrated into dyadic treatment to enhance the therapist's awareness of conflict between caregiver and infant and to realign the patterns of communication, so too can previewing techniques assist the therapist conducting family treatment. In the context of family therapy previewing may offer an innovative diagnostic aid and treatment approach. A thorough understanding of the unique contributions of family therapy will provide indispensable assistance to the therapist attempting to analyze the complex and often challenging relationship between mother and infant.

APPLYING THE PRINCIPLES OF FAMILY THERAPY TO DYADIC INTERVENTION

Adaptive development is to a certain degree contingent on the quality of the infant's *previewing* experiences. When administered correctly, previewing reinforces the family's sense of identity because it encourages the infant's developmental autonomy, sense of self, and independence from the family unit while reinforcing the sense of intimacy and rapport among family members. This dual image—of infant autonomy juxtaposed against the continuity of the relationship of parents and infant—is fundamental to the notion of previewing that fosters the infant's ability to balance his individuality within a relational bond. However, the infant will not be exposed to this kind of adaptive perspective within the family unless the caregivers—both mother and father—were themselves exposed to a family that promoted autonomy and self-identity in a supportive atmosphere. In the event the caregivers did not receive such exposure, treatment relying on one or several of the following approaches may be necessary to realign the patterns of family communication and to instill patterns of adaptive development. By examining the theories and applications of family therapy in depth, this chapter seeks to marry the principles of family intervention to the techniques of dyadic treatment.

Although a marital unit consisting of a husband and wife may technically be a "family," it is only with the birth of a child that our conception of a family, as a social and psychological reality, seems fulfilled. Indeed, the word *family* implies a complex series of relationships between individuals within a particularly designated group and among all those group members as an entity. For example, dyadic relationships exist between husband and wife, mother and infant, and father and infant. Yet, the notion of the family also attributes an overall process of interaction to this group of individuals that binds the family into a cohesive whole. Viewed this way, the family becomes an extraordinarily complicated entity that is influential in both establishing an individual's identity and developing the individual's ability to function in a social setting. How do individuals learn to fulfill their needs for autonomy and independence while still maintaining the often demanding relationships that sustain the integrity of the family unit? As formidable an accomplishment as this may appear to be, the majority of families negotiate a balance between individual and group needs that fosters nurturing patterns of interaction while promoting differentiation of the individual family members.

Despite examples of adaptive family functioning, however, in many families patterns of interaction go awry and dysfunctional or maladaptive behavior becomes the glue that binds these families together. In the past two decades, a form of psychotherapy that addresses issues concerning the dynamics of the family has developed. *Family therapy* attempts to approach the family from a variety of perspectives. One perspective, the *systems* approach, strives to understand how families convey or suppress emotional messages and develop a complex series of relationships based on such affective communications. This approach posits that when emotional expression is avoided because of the painful feelings evoked, individuals tend to manifest potentially detrimental behavior patterns, such as *triangulation* and *scapegoating,* that allow them to circumvent genuine communication. After a while, such behavior patterns become ingrained in the family's customary method of operation. In these cases, psychopathology subverts the overall emotional expression within the family. The effect of such interpersonal strategies is devastating because, as the children in the family develop, they transmit the legacy of dysfunctional emotional expression intact from one generation to the next.

The *structural* approach examines such phenomena as role-playing and the formation of alliances among family members. This orientation also examines how individuals within the family derive a sense of identity as a result of the experiences they endure with the authority figures, generally the parents, in the family. The outcome of these interactions is that children tend to replicate the parental models they encountered in their own childhoods as they become parents. Once again, a new generation is created to perpetuate the old patterns of alliance that led to dysfunction.

Two other popular perspectives adopted by family therapists are the *problem-oriented* and the *functional* approaches. Advocates of the problem-oriented approach highlight one particular conflict that the family is experiencing, often the conflict that has brought them to treatment. Using this conflict as a paradigm, the therapist first encourages family members to define and explore its contours and then implements behavior modification techniques that assist the family in gradually solving the problem. The rationale in this approach is that the family creates a blueprint of behavior for resolving future disputes more adaptively. The functional approach, on the other hand, adopts a global perspective and attempts to rectify dysfunction in overall patterns of interpersonal behavior. When using the functional approach, the therapist strives to create a state of equilibrium such that the family members can express and share an appropriate amount of intimacy while simultaneously receiving encouragement for autonomy and independence. Beyond these traditional techniques researchers have begun to apply principles derived from fields such as *attachment theory* to elucidate familial patterns of interaction. Among these the *family narrative* approach seeks to examine the subjective perceptions of the parental figures deriving from their own childhoods. These narratives offer insight into behaviors currently being enacted within the family.

These various approaches to family therapy provide unique and valuable contributions to the field of caregiver–infant therapy for a wide variety of reasons. First, although dyadic therapy consisting of a mother and infant highlights the seminal relationship between this pair, the mother–infant relationship cannot and should not be viewed in isolation from the rest of the family. The patterns of interaction in both caregivers' families of origin will have an indelible effect on how each parent interacts with the infant. Indeed, it may be argued that it is impossible to fully understand the dyadic relationship without exploring these past interactional patterns because, as numerous researchers have pointed out, caregivers tend to replicate the experiences and interactional configurations to which they were exposed as children. Moreover, the parents' relationship with each other will also exert a strong influence on family dynamics. The notion here is that interpersonal exchange—whether adaptive or dysfunctional—has its origin in the experiences of infancy.

For these reasons a therapist treating mother–infant dyads should at least be familiar with the diagnostic and treatment techniques offered by family therapy. These principles can be valuable even if only the mother and infant attend sessions, because the therapist can still explore the endowment of interactional experience the mother has inherited from her family of origin and can use this information to better understand the attachment between mother and infant. In other cases, the mother may be encouraged to bring additional family members to sessions either periodically or on a more regular basis. From such sessions the therapist can gain insight into the dynamics operating within the whole family. The principles of family therapy, then, enhance the benefits of dyadic treatment.

OVERVIEW OF THE STRATEGIES OFFERED BY THE FAMILY THERAPY APPROACH

Family therapy has gained widespread popularity during the past two decades. One factor motivating interest in this intervention is that many of the obstacles encountered by patients in their interpersonal relations appear to stem from misalignments in communication, imbalances in affective expression, and dysfunctional patterns of behavior that originated in their families of origin. Therapists have found that many of these interpersonal pathologies—which inevitably surface to haunt individuals as they strive for autonomy from their families—can be rectified if the family of origin is *reassembled* and the dysfunctional behaviors are expressed and *worked through* in the context of family. By correcting these dysfunctions in family interaction, individuals are often liberated from psychological obstacles that have prevented their pursuit of a new generation free from dysfunction. The strong influence family therapy can exert on an individual's capacity to build an optimal family structure makes this form of treatment particularly appropriate for altering maladaptive patterns within a caregiver–infant dyad. The premise is that dyadic failure may be due, in large part, to the replication of conflicts the caregivers experienced within their own families of origin. Moreover, because the infant's adaptive development derives from the internalization of the perspectives of both the mother and father, understanding the interaction within the context of the caregivers' families of origin has the utmost significance. For these reasons, the principles espoused by family therapy become a useful tool for the therapist conducting dyadic treatment.

Learning about these principles, however, requires a discussion of the various approaches to family therapy.

Insight–Working Through Approach

The Insight–Working Through Approach to family treatment, as described by Feldman (1979) is a highly interactional strategy that relies heavily on strategies involving confrontation and subsequent interpretation. Confrontation in this regard refers to the process of encouraging family members to cope directly with some dysfunctional aspect of their behavior. The numerous techniques for accomplishing this goal include verbal feedback, family "sculpture," spatial manipulation, and videotape playback.

Verbal techniques may be the most direct means of achieving a direct confrontation of conflict within the family. One researcher has advocated that the therapist adopt an assertive posture by calling attention to the inefficiencies, inappropriate behavior, and the defeating effect of certain defenses (Ackerman, 1966). Ackerman further notes that therapists should provoke the family members' defenses by exposing dramatic discrepancies between the family members' rationalizations and their subverbal attitudes. In other words, if the parents are treating one child as a scapegoat, the therapist may aggressively challenge the rationale for this behavior and seek to ascertain the real underlying perceptions of the family members regarding the need to use the child as a foil to disguise their emotional conflict. Bell (1961) encourages family therapists to verbalize their observations on the current status of family interaction and in particular on the specific events that occur during therapeutic sessions. Zuk (1971) recommends that the therapist expose and otherwise resist the family's efforts to deny or disguise conflict. Confrontation for Satir (1967) involves demonstrating to family members how they actually perceive others. As one example, when a family member says that another family member who is depressed "looks fine," the therapist might counter with the verbal remark that the depressed individual really "looks upset and hurt." Verbal confrontation in this fashion challenges the perceptions of the family members.

In addition to relying on strategies of verbal confrontation, Feldman (1986) also recommends what has been referred to as experiential confrontation. Experiential confrontation has also been referred to as family sculpture. During episodes of family sculpture relationships are portrayed in space and time so that events or attitudes may be perceived and experienced simultaneously (Duhl, Kantor, & Duhl, 1973). Family sculpture begins when the therapist asks family members to portray their perceptions of the family in action, rather than to describe these perceptions in words. As a consequence, the therapist establishes a scenario within which all family members are confronted with a new experiential awareness of the family system. Moreover, acting out these perceptions in front of the therapist forces family members to acknowledge his or her more neutral response to these representations.

A family sculpture episode begins when the family members are asked to think of the spaces between people as representing emotional closeness. Feldman (1986) then notes that the therapist asks one family member to be a sculptor and to position the other family members in space in terms of their relationships to one another and to the sculptor. As the sculptor begins to position people, the therapist asks a series of clarifying questions, such as "How do you see the other family members not only in relation to yourself, but also in relation to one another? How does the mother relate to and touch the father? Does the child only touch the father through the mother?" When other family members attempt to interject their perceptions of the situation by noting, for instance, "No, that's wrong. That's not how it really is," the therapist freezes the family members in their positions and reminds them that all members will have a turn to position the family as they experience it. Through this technique the therapist underscores the notion that there are numerous perceptions of reality in all families and that each person's perception of reality merits attention and consideration from other family members. At the conclusion of a sculpture exercise the therapist and family discuss what their family sculptures have revealed, and they attempt to integrate the total experience.

Minuchin (1974), another prominent family practitioner, has described a variation on experiential confrontation that he refers to as "manipulating space." Essentially this technique consists of positioning family members in ways that either strengthen or weaken particular subsystem boundaries. Minuchin observes that if the therapist wants to create or strengthen a boundary within the family, he can bring members of a subsystem to the center of the room and have other family members move their chairs back so that they can observe but cannot interrupt. If he wants to sever contact between two family members or to defuse a situation of intense enmeshment, the therapist can physically separate these family members or can position himself between them and act as an intermediary. Spatial manipulation, according to Minuchin, carries with it the potency of symbolic simplicity. What Minuchin calls the "graphic eloquence" of the spatial manipulation conveys the therapist's message.

Confrontation between family members may also be sparked by videotape playback, which Alger (1973) has described as a form of introducing system-specific feedback into the therapeutic sessions that allows the therapist to implement immediate corrections and alterations in behavior patterns. During this process family members can resolve to devise new strategies for achieving more adaptive goals. Alger has delineated four techniques for using videotape playback with families in treatment. First, a family session may be recorded and then replayed in its entirety immediately following the session or immediately prior to the next session. An arbitrary segment of several minutes of a session, chosen at random, may also be recorded, and then the remainder of the time during the session is devoted to analyzing the behaviors revealed during the playback review. The playback review should be limited to those segments that the therapist has selected as being particularly meaningful or insightful. Specific replay during a session should be available to family members on an informal basis. That is, the therapist or any family member should feel free to interrupt a session at any time and request an instant replay of a particular segment. Family members should be encouraged to do this particularly when they perceive a discrepancy between the verbal comments of other family members and behavioral manifestations that have emerged during interaction.

Although confrontation is a seminal aspect of the insight-oriented technique, confrontation alone is insufficient to motivate permanent change among family members. Interpretation, whereby family members acknowledge and work through conflict, is also essential for a genuine re-structuring of the family's relational patterns. As Feldman (1986) points out, interpretation is a concept that originated in the psychoanalytic approach to treatment. Moore and Fine (1968) have noted that interpretation is a form of intervention whose goal is to achieve therapeutic results by enhancing the patient's perception of himself through an awareness of psychological content and conflict that has previously been suppressed, denied, or otherwise avoided on a meaningful level. Dynamic interpretations refer to psychological forces that produce a particular effect on the mental life of the individual at any particular time, whereas genetic interpretations indicate or clarify the connections between past mental states and present ones.

In family therapy, however, interpretations have a broader definition. Bell (1961) has outlined four varieties of interpretation, referred to as reflective, connective, reconstructive, and normative. Reflective interpretations are, in effect, equivalent to confrontations. The therapist here may directly change the patient's comments. Corrective interpretations are therapist comments that direct the family member to previously unacknowledged links among acts, events, attitudes, and experiences. Of special significance in this regard are unrecognized reciprocal behaviors between family members. Here the therapist matches role with role, feeling with feeling, and perception with perception. In reconstructive interpretations the therapist recalls the history of the family, its relationships, and its peculiar or unique methods of interaction. The reconstituted past then serves as a context for interaction in the present. The therapist using normative interpretations compares the behavior of the family in treatment with behavior patterns in adaptive families. Bell warns that the therapist should rarely use this latter form of interpretation because family members may view such statements as a directive to simulate certain behaviors.

The Insight-Working Through model of family therapy is especially useful for therapists treating dyads because this paradigm encourages family members to disclose their subjective perceptions, to acknowledge the implications of these perceptions, and to resolve any discrepancies between outward behavior and internal perception. This process enables parents to attain a more objective perspective that is uncontaminated by conflict and, in turn, allows them to view infant development in a new light. Indeed, if the confrontation and interpretation aspects of this model are successful, the parents should be motivated to apply their new perspective in previewing imminent developmental events for the infant.

Systems Approach

The Systems Approach posits that individuals have a tendency to become affectively *enmeshed* in emotionally charged problem situations (Kerr, 1981). This enmeshment triggers other imbalances within the structure of the family, disrupting the state of dynamic equilibrium that is most conducive to adaptive development. Such emotional entanglement can emerge in several characteristic patterns. *Triangulation,* which is one such pattern, occurs when excessive emotional tension exists between any two family members and one of them seeks to dissipate the tension by creating a triangle that involves a third family member. For example, a mother may displace an excess of emotional energy onto the infant, causing the father to experience rejection. The father may then displace feelings of resentment onto the infant, in effect coercing the mother to act as mediator. If, however, the mother comes to the infant's defense, the father is once again left out of the emotional relationship. In essence, triangulation represents a strategy whereby family members avoid and postpone dealing with conflict in a direct fashion and instead circumvent emotional issues by dissipating the emotion. Although some degree of triangulation may be advantageous for diluting powerful feelings that have been aroused, in general, such patterns of interaction thwart adaptive development because triangulation prevents family members from confronting and addressing emotional conflict. Instead, they displace emotional energy in the effort to entangle another family member in the conflict. Thus, family members perpetually avoid the core of the conflict by engaging in a kind of emotional displacement that resembles musical chairs.

Proclivities toward triangulation also interfere with the caregiver's ability to preview upcoming development to the infant. When tendencies to triangulate exist, the caregiver will devote energy to circumventing emotional chaos rather than to focusing on and representing imminent developmental achievement. As has already been discussed, previewing adopts a prospective perspective, whereby the caregivers provide representations and interactions that foster future development. If emotional conflict has enmired the family members in maladaptive patterns, it will hinder the motivation to preview.

The Systems Approach proposes that the family's emotional process enables family members to deal with conflict and its emotional residue (Kerr, 1981). When tension is exacerbated within the family, family members engage in four basic strategies for dissipating such tension: (a) creating emotional distance, (b) becoming conflicted or enmeshed with one another, (c) compromising individual functioning to preserve group harmony, or (d) aligning with another family member to form a triangle. Each strategy provides temporary relief by dissipating the emotional residue associated with the conflict. Moreover, each of these dysfunctional patterns of interaction tends to become entrenched for two reasons. First, these patterns enable family members to avoid confronting genuine issues and to generate instead pseudoconflicts that divert attention from the underlying true conflict. Thus, the family can continue to derive whatever gratification the maladaptive behavior provides, while circumventing the real problem. Second, these strategies exacerbate the tension that is creating imbalance within the family structure. As a result, the strategies must be perpetuated to stave off further strife.

Systems theory also proposes a *family projection process*. This process refers to the way in which parents transmit the incapacity for dealing with emotional conflict to their children. Families that rely on triangulation to circumvent emotional issues become *undifferentiated*. This means that the dynamics developed by the family stifle individuation and autonomy and promote a sense of fused identity. Such families deal with emotional conflict by submerging it in complex emotional interactions—such as triangulation—that dilute the identities of individual family members but cause them to remain dependent on one another to perpetuate strategies that circumvent conflict. The family projection process fuels this dynamic. In this context, individuals may be viewed as existing on a scale of *self-differentiation*. At the lower end of the scale are individuals whose dominant style of relationship is enmeshment. Individuals at the upper end of the scale have the capacity to maintain individuality and togetherness in balance; such family members are individuals in their own right as well as effective and cooperative team players within the family. *Emotional cutoff*, another concept associated with systems theory, refers to the way that individuals commonly deal with enmeshment in their families of origin. By relying on this strategy, individuals insulate or sever themselves emotionally from the rest of the family. As an alternative to enmeshment, emotional cutoff allows the family member to distance himself from the conflict at the expense of severing the emotional bond with the family. Finally, the *multigenerational transmission process* refers to the transmission of maladaptive strategies from one generation to the next. As a consequence of such activity, family members from both generations remain undifferentiated, reinforcing the emotions associated with fusion. *Scapegoating* is another common strategy of families that tend to be undifferentiated. This phenomenon occurs when a conflict threatens to disrupt the relationships between family members; to dissipate the tension, they devise a dramatic alternative by choosing one family member to play victim. In turn, the victim becomes the repository for all the family's rage and confusion. The overwhelming result of absorbing all this negative emotion generally is disruptive behavior. In effect, the scapegoat incorporates and then manifests the controversy that threatens the family because he is enmeshed in the conflict. Like a self-fulfilling prophecy, the scapegoat enacts the battle on a miniature scale, thereby enabling other family members to avoid dealing with the real implications of the emotional upheaval. Unfortunately, the scapegoat selected by family members is often the most developmentally immature member of the family. Infants are prime candidates for scapegoat status because they lack the ability to assert their own independence and are almost entirely dependent on other family members for emotional support. Each of these strategies precludes adaptive previewing because the caregivers generally lack the skill to represent nonconflicted exchange with the infant in the future and to predict development adaptively.

Systems theory can also explain how psychological symptoms within the family may be converted into somatic symptoms that affect primarily one family member, such as a child. One family I treated was experiencing a crisis that appeared to center around the failure of a $2\frac{1}{2}$-year-old to become toilet-trained. Although the child's behavior was the focus of the family's attention, in fact when the family was viewed as a whole, other significant interactional symptoms began to emerge. It is important to recognize that symptoms affecting one family member actually serve a function within the family system itself. As some researchers have noted, the underlying interactional conflict—for example, marital discord—is detoured and foisted onto one family member who absorbs and exhibits the conflict. Often the infant or young child in the family becomes the center of the strife and shows localized symptomatology that actually indicates generalized dysfunction within the family unit.

In this situation the therapist's first goal is to diagnose the nature of the conflict by examining the family's patterns of interaction and considering the degree of engagement or disengagement among family members as well as the extent of overly enmeshed relationships. Based on the premises of systems theory, lack of differentiation among family members is a sign of dysfunction, because this phenomenon indicates that family members are unable to assert their individual personalities and needs.

With respect to treatment, the therapist's overall goal will involve liberating the infant or young child who has been chosen as the family's scapegoat. Through previewing, the therapist can begin exploring the representational patterns of individual family members. In addition, because it adopts a prospective approach, previewing exercises allow the therapist to ascertain how family members will respond to upcoming crises in development. The therapist can use this material to analyze the family's current crisis and to help family members assert adaptive patterns. Moreover, previewing acts as a preventive intervention by helping family members modify their dysfunctional behaviors before another developmental crisis occurs. Previewing also enhances insight into functioning between generations in the same family. An underlying premise of this therapy is that intervention cannot occur without considering at least two generations of the family because conflict becomes entrenched within one generation and is subsequently transmitted to another generation. Similarly, previewing interventions should also focus on evaluating at least two generations of the family. This approach will disclose how representational patterns have been maintained across generations and how each generation has continued to enact dysfunctional patterns. Beyond the diagnostic advantages of previewing, this technique also enables family members to understand and acknowledge, perhaps for the first time, the intergenerational transmission of conflicted behavior.

Systems theory, then, strives to understand the emotional underpinnings inherent in the relationships between and among family members. An underlying premise is that virtually all families use these strategies for coping with emotional issues. The therapist's task is to *predict* the degree to which such strategies will suppress the evolution of the infant's autonomous patterns. After identifying these behaviors, the therapist can work with the family to instill better techniques for coping with emotional issues and eventually for using previewing to deal with conflict more adaptively.

Structural Approach

The Structural Approach views the family as a cohesive unit of interrelationships among individual members (Aponte & Van Deusen, 1981). Three dynamic processes influence the family structure: *boundary formation, alignment,* and *power.* The boundaries within the family consist of those rules and regulations that dictate which family members serve as authority figures and which roles are assigned to other family members (Minuchin, 1974). Such rules govern who is "in" and who is "out" of significant family interactions. In effect, the family boundaries delineate the allotment of authority to each family member. Alignment refers to the joining or opposition of one family member to another in performing a task and in this regard resembles triangulation (Aponte, 1976). *Joining* concerns behaviors whereby the therapist reinforces areas of family strength, rewards, and affiliates with each family member; complements and supports threatened members; and explains problems. When joining is used, the therapist must alternate between engagement and disengagement (Kauffman & Kauffmann, 1979). This intervention includes fostering *coalitions* and *alliances* among family members. Coalition is a process of joint action taken by two family members against a third family member, whereas alliance is the union of two family members who have a common interest not shared by a third family member (Haley, 1976). In an adaptive family, for example, the marital coalition serves as the strongest and most resilient alignment in the family; the intactness of this relationship predicts the generational boundary between parents and child, as well as the equilibrium in other areas of communication (Glick, Clarkin, & Kessler, 1987). In contrast, other configurations are encountered in malfunctioning families. For example, families whose marital coalition is relatively weak or absent tend to have strong alliances across the generations and sexes with a relative absence of other effective channels for forging an emotional bond. Therapeutic techniques that enable the family to deal with these malfunctions include *reframing, enactment,* and *focusing* (Minuchin, 1974). During reframing, the therapist identifies the family's typical mode of response or "frame" and then counters with a competing view, called a reframe. Such a therapeutic strategy models a more relaxed, less constricted view of the world and the events of mundane family life. Enactment involves acting out the family's interpersonal problems during the therapeutic session. Enactment enables the therapist to observe the interpersonal behaviors in the problem sequence instead of dealing with the censored or distorted versions of each family member. Focusing refers to sifting through the abundance of irrelevant material provided by the family members and coaxing them to concentrate on genuine issues. According to Aponte and Van Deusen (1981), patterns of harmony or mutual opposition develop in many of the activities pursued by family members and justify the existence of another significant element— power—within the family structure. Power has been defined as the relative influence each family member exerts on the outcome of an activity. Family members manifest power by the way they actively and passively combine so that the intentions of one or more members prevail in determining the outcome of any given activity.

The Structural Approach requires the therapist to assess each of these factors to diagnose the level of adaptation. In an optimal situation boundaries will provide clear delineations that influence family members' roles and their expectations for one another's behavior. Family members will be differentiated and yet will have strong ties uniting them. Adaptive families' boundaries tend to be flexible rather than rigid. Under these circumstances the family moves away from previously determined roles and allows other family members to experiment with different forms of autonomy. This flexibility fosters such activities as previewing, which requires that both caregiver and infant experiment with predicting and rehearsing imminent development. *Actualizing* family transactional patterns is a technique advocated by Minuchin (1974). This researcher notes that patients usually direct their communications to the therapist. Although this approach obviously makes sense in the individual treatment format, it is generally not as effective in family treatment. Instead, the therapist should supportively guide the family members to speak to one another rather than to the therapist and to enact transactional patterns rather than to describe them. Moreover, as Minuchin cautions, unless therapists adopt the stance of neutral observers, they run the risk of being triangulated into patterns of family dysfunction. Davenport and Adland (1985) and Szapocznik, Perez-Vidal, Hervis, Brickman, and Kurtines (1990), for example, have pointed out that patterns of *denial* and *dependency* frequently arise in the family context with greater potency than in individual treatment because family members can effectively use one another as shields against the therapist's scrutiny. With respect to resistance, Szapocznik et al. advocate that the therapist adopt a firm attitude that mandates participation by all family members involved in the presenting problem. Denial and dependency, two common pitfalls to progress in family therapy, can be dealt with more gradually through previewing exercises that disclose potential conflict and reveal how these behaviors preclude adaptive interaction. Above all, the therapist must avoid becoming involved on an emotional level with these potent issues and should instead encourage family members to enact their drama.

Problem-Centered Approach

The pivotal goal of the Problem-Centered Approach is to identify a particular problem within the family and to design strategies for alleviating that problem (Epstein & Bishop, 1981). This approach hypothesizes that highlighting one distinct conflict and instructing the family in methods to alleviate such dysfunction will enable family members to apply these strategies in other areas of conflict. Such strategies depend less on family dynamics than on the use of astute interventions as models to effect changes in patterns that impede adaptive development and preclude emotional communication among family members (Erikson, 1954; Stanton, 1981). In this fashion the Problem-Centered Approach produces transitions in behaviors or alternative patterns that help family members to approach life's challenges more adaptively (Haley, 1976).

A benefit of this approach is that it enables the family not only to overcome a particular problem affecting family equilibrium but to use the strategies found effective in solving that problem as a paradigm for resolving other family conflicts. A further benefit is that the family will likely derive feelings of success and accomplishment in a relatively short time, and these positive emotions may be an impetus for rectifying other areas of disequilibrium within the family structure. The problem-oriented focus can foster previewing because it heightens the family's feelings of competence and mastery. Once the family comes to understand that problems can be solved and that their solution will result in feelings of positive emotion, family members will be more inclined to look to imminent developmental events with a sense of anticipation and will seek to devise strategies for competently managing future events.

Functional Approach

Just as the Problem-Centered Approach adopts a kind of microcosmic approach to resolving family dysfunction, the Functional Approach adheres to a more *macrocosmic* perspective. Functional therapy strives to analyze the general interpersonal manifestations of family members within the context of the family unit (Barton & Alexander, 1981). The functional model posits that the various behaviors of the individual are meaningless in isolation. Instead, the individual's actions should be conceptually integrated with those of other family members into a chain of behaviors directed toward some overriding family goal. Urdang and Flexner (1972), proponents of the functional model, have commented that individuals should be viewed as being in a state of submission to a continuing action or series of actions wherein they create and respond to the dynamics of an interpersonal environment. Barton and Alexander observe that the functional family model targets the nuclear family as the optimal arena within which to evaluate the dynamics of the interpersonal processes. Understanding these dynamics enhances an understanding of previewing manifestations within the family, which rely on the processes of interpersonal communication between caregiver and infant.

As a result of this emphasis on interpersonal behavior, the functional therapist scrutinizes general modes of communication among family members, particularly, how family members convey intimacy, a desire for emotional distance, or an equilibrium point between these two states through their verbal and physical behaviors. The goal of this treatment is for family members to achieve adequate intimacy while maintaining sufficient distance to reinforce their autonomy and independence. Once again, this approach is likely to enhance previewing behaviors because it instills a balance between interactional behaviors and autonomous responses, and provides motivation to help family members look to the future with optimism.

THERAPIST: (To father) Do you see your baby differently when you carry him than when your wife carries him?

FATHER: When she has him, I want to hold him. Both of us aren't used to having him yet. We still feel a lot of excitement. (Mother talks quietly to infant.) So when she's got him and I haven't seen him, I want to get him, play with him, spend some time with him. Is that a form of jealousy or competitiveness?

MOTHER: We don't fight for the baby.

THERAPIST: (To mother) How do you see the baby when you hold him compared to when your husband is holding him?

MOTHER: When I hold the baby, I feel an innate bond. I want to teach him things to develop his mind so that he will feel important and have the confidence to deal with problems. When my husband holds the baby, they have fun together. He's teaching the baby how to walk and do other physical activities. But when I'm holding the baby, he's more quiet. We sit and listen to music or have baby talk episodes with each other. Maybe I think my time with the baby is more important than my husband's time with the baby. Maybe that's why we fight sometimes.

Contextual Approaches

The Contextual Approach is a comprehensive relational technique whose ultimate goal is to integrate the significant orientations of psychotherapy (Boszormenyi-Nagy & Ulrich, 1981). This technique relies heavily on goal setting. The essential goal is a *rejunctive effort,* meaning that it is possible to balance parental roles by encouraging open negotiation on significant issues, exploring family loyalties and legacies, and undoing stagnant behaviors. This strategy assists families in becoming more directed and adaptive. The therapist engages in *siding,* whereby he earns the trust of each individual family member in turn. Siding occurs as the therapist encourages all family members to express their views, urging more hesitant members to voice their views along with more dominant family members. During episodes of siding, the therapist is free to relate actively to each family member, as long as he or she is cognizant of what is being displaced onto the figure of the therapist and of the countertransference feelings that such displacements evoke. Siding with family members is not the same as joining the family, in that the therapist continues to maintain an independent status at all times. Contextual therapy also involves the phenomenon of *decoding.* Decoding refers to the translation of verbal communications between family members that may contain disguised emotional cues. In general, then, the contextual technique requires the therapist to function as a kind of intermediary among family members.

Siding and decoding involve previous conflicts that have created developmental impasses among family members, but therapists may also use siding techniques to explore and predict family issues that have not yet reached the crisis stage. That is, the therapist can instruct the family members in previewing techniques and can then work with the family in representing and enacting scenarios that may occur in the foreseeable future. These sequences help both therapist and family members foreshadow areas of potential strife and devise strategies for overcoming such inchoate conflict before it causes dysfunction. During previewing, the therapist can use siding and decoding strategies to reassure family members and to help them avoid the emotional evasion and subterfuge that have caused past problems. The Contextual Approach also considers the family's past as a "legacy" that has generated expectations motivating the behaviors of family members. In addition, the therapist may evaluate family loyalties and "splits," particularly if they have caused malalignments within the family structure (Boszormenyi-Nagy & Ulrich, 1981).

Symbolic-Experiential Approach

This approach assesses family tolerance to individual members and their unique behavioral styles, as well as the family as a whole (Whitaker & Keith, 1981). In the Symbolic-Experiential Approach the symptoms of the family members are *redefined* as efforts for growth designed to extricate the family from its conflict. The therapist here exaggerates the symptoms to encompass the entire family, thereby exposing their absurdity. *Modeling* fantasy alternatives to real-life stress is another strategy that can be used. For example, the therapist might ask a patient who has attempted suicide to imagine that when she became suicidal she was going to kill the therapist rather than act destructively against herself. Although this may seem an extreme technique, teaching the use of fantasy expands the family's emotional life without the threat of real violence or real acting-out within its confines. The family here can experiment with emotional issues in the safe and monitored environment of the treatment setting. Other techniques include *separating interpersonal stress from fantasy*. As an illustration, the patient who has attempted suicide can be encouraged to imagine that if she died her husband would remarry, and to anticipate the length of the mourning period and her husband's life thereafter. These contextual techniques are often effective in motivating family members to deal openly with conflict. The innovative use of symbolism and fantasy incorporated by this technique helps to motivate behavioral change in another way as well. Symbolism and fantasy, it should be remembered, often involve representations about the future. These strategies thereby encourage caregiver and infant or any two family members to engage in previewing exercises for issues that have not yet reached fruition. Thus, because the Symbolic-Experiential Approach can implicate fantasies about the future, thereby embracing potential conflict, this technique holds promise for resolving family disputes before they have caused dysfunctional behavior patterns. In addition, this approach makes family members more receptive to previewing behaviors designed to anticipate and assert mastery over imminent developmental events.

Attachment Approach

Another approach to family treatment advocated by such researchers as Byng-Hall (1990) and Stevenson-Hinde (1990) recommends applying *attachment* theory to the family context. These researchers accept the premise that every relationship affects every other relationship and that therefore the nature of the attachment between two members in the family may influence the quality of all other attachment relationships within a circumscribed family unit. According to these researchers, an adaptive family provides a secure base for all of its members, such that each individual is part of at least one securely attached relationship and facilitates or at least tolerates the secure attachment behavior in other relationships within the family. In contrast, in dysfunctional families the bulk of emotional energy appears centered in one relationship. This lopsided relationship tends to contaminate other relationships in the family, leading to inappropriate and even psychopathological responses that stifle independence and generate an enmeshed style of interaction. In particular, the caregiving relationships between parents and children represent paradigms of interaction that are replicated in other family relationships.

Defined broadly, attachment behavior refers to any form of behavior that predictably results in a person attaining or maintaining proximity to and/or communication with some other individual (Stevenson-Hinde, 1990). Moreover, not all the behaviors a child directs to a parent are attachment behaviors; rather, attachment manifestations surface more clearly during conditions of uncertainty, fear, separation, and illness, which exaggerate the bond between the individuals. Byng-Hall (1990) has reviewed various families clinically and found that four particular kinds of dysfunctional relationships tend to function in the family context:

1. Turning to an inappropriate attachment figure.
2. Competition for an attachment figure.
3. Defensive responses to attachment cues.
4. Anticipation that losses similar to those in the past will recur.

In explaining these four disturbed attachment patterns, Byng-Hall (1990) notes that when a child encounters a situation in which the caregiver is either avoidant or unavailable, the child may turn to an inappropriate family member for guidance. A common example of this situation occurs when there is marital discord and a parent turns to a child for support, thereby subverting the typical pattern in which the adult, by virtue of knowledge and experience, establishes the standard of behavior for adaptive exchange and provides a secure base for the child during episodes of uncertainty or extreme challenge. Moreover, Byng-Hall notes that when one child in the family comes to be designated as a "parent" to his own parents, it impairs the child's relationship with other family members, who may become resentful because of this particular alignment. In addition, such a child must formulate his own perceptions of imminent developmental achievement because the parent will be unavailable to play the role of supportive partner.

Another distortion of adaptive attachment patterns that tends to disrupt the family's normal equilibrium is competition for an attachment figure, which occurs when an individual feels insecure, ignored, or neglected in the caregiving relationship. Such family members may make an extreme attempt to capture the attachment figure and to exclude others from gaining access. Competition for an attachment figure often manifests in the form of a jealous, clinging child or an overly possessive spouse who cannot tolerate his mate's attachment to other family members.

Two other attachment patterns that are transmitted across generations and disrupt the equilibrium of the family unit are the defensive response to attachment cues and the anticipation of losses. Defensive responses occur if members of the grandparents' generation responded defensively to attachment cues either by ignoring them or rejecting them, thereby failing to establish a reliable model for parents when establishing attachments with their children. Indeed, the only available model avoids the experience of a loving relationship because of the expectation that such a relationship will fail. These parents may disrupt or sever the normally occurring attachments that evolve within the family because of the distress evoked by emotional intimacy and its potential loss. Byng-Hall (1990) refers to a related phenomenon as the anticipation that losses similar to those of the past will recur. Under this scenario unresolved traumas in the parents' past may cause them to organize family behavioral patterns to avoid the painful consequences of an anticipated repetition of loss. The goal of emotional avoidance then becomes a self-fulfilling prophecy. Such parents may also behave unconsciously in a way that actually recreates the maladaptive behavior and the trauma. The traumatized parent will not uncommonly attempt to coerce his spouse into adopting particular roles in these enactments that interfere with normal parenting. Often, the timing of the anticipated repetition of the catastrophe is based on anniversaries of the trauma or a stage in the family life cycle similar to that during which the catastrophe occurred.

The studies of Stevenson-Hinde and Byng-Hall indicate that the Attachment Approach may yield diagnostic insights into the structural alliances and relationships that characterize a particular family unit. Once therapists understand how attachment patterns have gone awry or have distorted the patterns of adaptive development, they can devise techniques to provide a secure base and a stable attachment relationship, so that family members can create more adaptive attachment patterns.

Family Narratives Approach

Many of the preceding techniques yield substantial insight into how families function and how maladaptation is manifested through self-defeating or nonproductive behaviors. The Family Narratives Approach advocated by Sherman (1990) explores deviant family behaviors through a different strategy, which relies primarily on exploring the *subjective perceptions* or private, internal impressions that family members reveal in their narratives about past events. According to Sherman, family narratives offer a window for viewing aspects of past and present family relationships. Sherman notes that the internal processes govern external behavior through the representations of events and family relationships stored in memory. Relying on Reiss's (1989) model, Sherman recommends considering two perspectives in the family evaluation: *practicing,* which refers to the objective behavioral displays of family members; and *represented family perspectives,* which refers to the subjective perceptions of family members about one another.

The represented family perspectives attempt to sample an individual's internal representations of significant family relationships. Through interviews with the parents the therapist elicits the internal representations of relationships of the earlier caregiver generation. In other words, how does the mother represent her relationship with her own mother? The therapist then correlates these perceptions with the type of attachment relationship the mother shares with the child. As Reiss (1989) has emphasized, virtually all earlier approaches to the study of the represented family have highlighted dyadic relationships and have looked almost exclusively to mother–infant pairs. In contrast, Sherman argues that it is often useful to conceptualize internalized representations of larger family configurations, such as triadic groupings, or to conceptualize representations of the whole family. The clinician uses the parents' disclosures of subjective perceptions to determine whether *parallel relationships* are transpiring within the family relationship. This approach, then, relies on representations from the past to elucidate the present patterns of interaction.

From the previous discussion it is clear that most forms of psychotherapy share certain principles, such as establishing an optimal patient–therapist relationship; guiding the patient to more adaptive behavior patterns that will realign interpersonal relationships; and, especially when infants and young children are involved, stimulating behaviors conducive to adaptive development and communication. Family therapy incorporates many of these principles, but it does so within the context of the entire family unit. Therefore, the goal of family therapy is to improve overall family functioning (Glick et al., 1987). Dyadic therapy, as discussed in the preceding chapters, strives to enhance the relationship between caregiver and infant and, in particular, to promote previewing behavioral skills that prepare the infant for imminent development. Previewing represents a unique form of interaction between caregiver and infant that enables the infant subjectively to perceive a sense of mastery over upcoming maturational achievements while still maintaining a sense of continuity in the relationship with the caregiver. Thus, the caregiver who previews must subjectively represent imminent development and imagine herself as an integral aspect of the infant's experience. Moreover, caregivers must also be able to envision what their future relationship with the infant will be like and how that relationship will be modified by his burgeoning autonomy. Infants too need to acquire a perspective about their future growth and its implications for the dyadic rapport. Will infant autonomy threaten the caregiver or will she respond by representing the future adaptively? Family strategies may yield productive insight into the caregiver's competence during interaction with the infant.

The various family therapy techniques may be integrated with previewing strategies to enhance family development. In general, therapists should adopt an eclectic perspective by using techniques that are most applicable to the family's conflicts and should coordinate these strategies with the principle of previewing.

As an example, the Systems Approach elucidates the mechanisms whereby the family generates alignments, triangles, and scapegoating strategies to avoid emotional conflict. Adaptive previewing cannot occur if one of the caregivers harbors emotional conflict. As a consequence, a therapist relying on the Systems Approach should first explore the maladaptive configurations that have prevented the free expression of emotion by encouraging family members to express their perceptions of seminal family events. The birth of a newborn or the child's entrance into kindergarten are two such events, but virtually all seminal family experiences or indeed the ordinary events of daily life will lead to numerous subjective perceptions. After exploring these perceptions, the therapist can move to the perceptions of past experiences that have evoked conflict within the family. This strategy will, in effect, help family members to preview while they simultaneously probe areas of conflict and bring these problematic domains into consciousness.

Adopting Sherman's (1990) Family Narratives Approach offers another vehicle for coordinating family therapy with previewing strategies. As noted, the narrative technique encourages caregivers to reflect on their own childhood experiences and to share, within the context of the family, stories that were told about them in their own families of origin when they themselves were children. This technique relies heavily on the parents' representational skills by introducing them as a primary focus of the treatment. Once the parents have divulged their representations, the therapist attempts to discern patterns that the caregivers are replicating with their own children. By carrying this strategy one step further, the therapist can also instruct caregivers in previewing exercises that acquaint family members with future events. For example, after the caregivers have divulged their narratives of childhood experiences, they would be encouraged to discuss these stories and to compare apparent similarities between their subjective memories and the attributions made to their children. Integrating their narrative about the past with present representations about their children's behavior helps many parents to identify patterns that were previously hidden in unconscious memory. The therapist can then encourage previewing behavior by eliciting representations about future interpersonal changes between caregivers and their children. This combination of strategies will likely result in the acquisition of insight at a more rapid pace than would otherwise be possible and will provide family members with the skills necessary to direct their future interactions more adaptively.

It is now well accepted that attachment behaviors play a vital role in our interactions with others. Researchers such as Byng-Hall (1990) and Stevenson-Hinde (1990) have applied the principles of attachment theory in the family context to facilitate the working through of maladaptive alignments and dysfunctional patterns of interaction. This approach offers the therapist unparalleled insight into how relationships that preclude adaptive interaction become ingrained within the dynamic of the family. Once again, the use of previewing strategies with this model can result in a more profound understanding of the mechanisms that have disrupted adaptive interaction and can also aid in the development of more positive approaches. To apply this technique, the therapist would first evaluate the straightforward patterns of interaction and attachment within the family and subsequently would use representational strategies to discern why family members have adopted these configurations. Previewing exercises may then be introduced to encourage the representation and, eventually, the manifestation of more adaptive attachment patterns (e.g., proximity seeking and social referencing). In addition, family members would be encouraged to predict attachment behaviors that would be more conducive to family integration as well as autonomy. The following goals should serve as an overriding theme with any of the preceding strategies.

It is vital for the therapist to *support* the coping mechanisms that the family possesses (Glick et al., 1987). No matter how profound the degree of malfunctioning, every family has some level of psychological health that should be encouraged and actively promoted within the therapeutic arena. Empathic listening, direct sharing of the therapist's concerns, positive feedback concerning the use of the family's adaptive behaviors, discussions of parenting alternatives (e.g., comparing discipline styles or helping the family to make difficult decisions) are all techniques driven by this principle. In this way the therapist communicates an adaptive model of mood and tempo within an atmosphere of interpersonal acceptance (Patterson, 1982).

This approach also strives to evaluate the degree of adaptive previewing within the family. Adaptive previewing occurs when one or both caregivers subjectively represent the contours of imminent infant development and subsequently initiate interaction with the infant to introduce upcoming maturational skills. These supportive ministrations enable the infant to internalize an adaptive mode of interaction.

CONCLUSION

This chapter has introduced the theories of family therapy by providing a synopsis for each of the models of family treatment currently being used in clinical settings. Family therapy elucidates the dynamics underlying interaction among family members and, in this respect, can provide indispensable information for the therapist conducting treatment with a caregiver and infant. Although in some cases family members will be willing to participate in the dyadic treatment by attending sessions on either a regular or periodic basis, in other cases family members may be hesitant about becoming involved in the therapeutic process. Nonetheless, family therapy techniques can still clarify the underlying conflict or ambivalence that derives from the caregiver's patterns of behavior. These patterns originate in her own family of origin and affect her interaction with the child.

The techniques of family therapy offer clinicians a wide variety of creative options for use in dyadic treatment. This chapter has described nine of these approaches. The Insight-Working Through Approach advocates the use of verbal confrontations or physical sculpturing to challenge family members to face inherent conflicts that have previously been manifested surreptitiously. Subsequently, the therapist provides interpretation to help family members acknowledge the more objective view of their interaction that emerged during confrontation.

The Systems Approach hypothesizes that family dysfunction is caused by the avoidance of affective expression. Rather than engaging in a direct emotional dialogue, family members instead rely on techniques that disguise or undermine genuine emotional expression, including triangulation, scapegoating, and patterns of undifferentiation. Each of these phenomena represents a vehicle whereby the family members subvert the true meaning of their feelings by displacing emotional content onto others. As a result, the family exists in a state of emotional stagnation that precludes adaptive communication. Moreover, family members remain mired in the past and cannot deal adaptively with upcoming events because they are perpetually trying to stave off conflict. Thus, developmental previewing is generally absent from such families. The therapist must sever these maladaptive bonds by causing family members to cope with emotional issues directly before he or she can implement a new perspective that deals with the future objectively.

The Systems Approach also posits that to understand the dynamics of family interaction and to assert appropriate interventions, the clinician must evaluate at least two generations of the family. To this premise it may be added that previewing strategies offer valuable assistance in both the diagnosis and treatment of dysfunctional patterns that have been transmitted across generations. Previewing is advantageous because it discloses representational patterns and the subsequent enactment of behaviors. By evaluating representations and their prospective enactment, the therapist can ascertain why certain patterns are being replicated within the family structure, as well as the purpose these behaviors serve. Interventions can then help family members preview in a more adaptive fashion that surmounts earlier patterns of dysfunction, thereby severing the process of transmitting conflict to a future generation.

The Structural Approach, which represents a kind of variation on the Systems Approach, analyzes allocations of power and authority among family members. The notion here is that emotional conflict has caused family members to somehow displace emotion inappropriately, resulting in an upheaval in the adaptive patterns of equilibrium that should exist.

The Problem-Centered Approach offers another perspective. Here family members dissect a specific problem that appears to have caused dissension. The theory is that by solving this particular problem, family members will develop a paradigm for conflict resolution that can be used to prevent future problems. In contrast, the Functional Approach adopts a more global perspective, emphasizing general patterns of interactional behavior that have been transmitted from generation to generation, finally becoming embedded in the very persona of the family.

The Contextual Approach adopts the global perspective of the Functional Approach but engages the therapist in the process of "siding" with each member of the family in turn and "decoding" or deciphering the position of that individual within the family unit. The Symbolic-Experiential Approach adopts a more psychoanalytic approach by urging family members to explore their fantasies or subjective perceptions of their role in the family unit.

The Attachment Approach emphasizes the emotional bonds between two or more members of the family and seeks to clarify how caregivers replicate patterns of interaction within their own families of origin. Finally, the Family Narratives Approach encourages the exploration of the history of the family and in particular of the caregivers' relationship with their nuclear families to elucidate the intergenerational transmission of conflict.

Until family conflict—whether it stems from marital discord, triangulation, scapegoating, or the intergenerational transmission of conflict—is resolved, the family members cannot develop methods for effectively representing and dealing with the future, and developmental previewing will not occur.

Chapter 15

Applying the Principles of Group Therapy to Dyadic Intervention

INTRODUCTION

Because dyadic therapy involves the diagnostic evaluation and treatment of two individuals—a caregiver and an infant—and their relationship to one another, the principles underlying this form of therapy, in many respects, reflect the principles in group psychotherapy, an approach that has become popular during the past few decades. As a result, therapists involved in dyadic treatment can benefit from the insights and methods of group therapy and may apply these techniques analogously to the dyadic setting. Among the primary characteristics of group therapy are its variety and its flexibility. Sessions generally consist of members sharing their experiences. Group members receive encouragement and support in an atmosphere that allows for the catharsis of previously painful events, memories, and experiences. Although the emphasis in such groups is on sharing experiences and providing support, there is also a focus on educating the group in new, more adaptive patterns of interaction.

Group therapy yields techniques that are especially appropriate to the setting of caregivers with their infants. First, the caregivers in dyadic groups have undergone a similar experience that includes the wish to become pregnant, pregnancy, the act of giving birth, and adjustment to the arrival of a new infant in the household. These common experiences provide caregivers with a wealth of information to share in the group setting. In addition, because the infants in the group will probably be of different ages, caregivers will be able to offer each other insights and recommendations for dealing with various developmental milestones. A caregiver who is experiencing difficulty during the weaning process may, for example, derive useful advice from a member who dealt with a similar situation a few months or weeks ago. This format is also particularly appropriate for dispensing educational information to new caregivers. Equally as important, because the infants in the group are likely to be at varied developmental stages, caregivers will also obtain a realistic impression of how development proceeds. The variety of different infants and interactional styles will underscore that maturation and dyadic rapport are unique for each individual dyad, but that, at the same time, particular trends in development are consistent and predictable. As a result, dyadic therapy relying on the group therapy approach enables caregivers to *preview* the developmental pace of their own infants.

The group format is also appropriate for conducting psychoanalytically oriented treatment. This form of treatment encourages development of a *transference relationship* between the therapist and group members; the emergence of a transference is used primarily to explore and resolve conflicts rooted in the childhood of the group members. Analyzing the transference relationship with the therapist may be of great value because the therapist can experience directly the conflict emanating from the caregiver's past. The therapist can also explore the degree to which the caregiver is transferring inappropriate affect and behavioral patterns deriving from her past to the infant.

Other phenomena associated with psychoanalytically oriented therapy are also applicable to treatment of dyads. For example, it is not uncommon for caregivers in dyadic treatment to refer to dyadic memories from their own childhood. One caregiver in a group I was leading seemed overly anxious when her infant began crawling; it was as if she wished to prevent her child from experiencing this developmental milestone. When questioned by the other mothers in the group, the caregiver spontaneously related a memory from her own childhood in which she had wandered away from her mother in a store and became frightened. The evocation of this memory provided the mother with insight into her own behavior.

The psychoanalytic approach encourages the therapist to focus on the variants of transference that can arise within the group. Essentially, three types of transference relationships occur in this format. First, the members of the group will each develop a *transference to the therapist* similar to the transference in individual therapy; the patient uses the person of the therapist as a neutral figure upon whom to displace unresolved conflict emanating from early seminal experiences. Second, group members are apt to develop a form of *peer transference* toward other members of the group. Finally, each individual group member will manifest a *transference relationship with the group* as an entity. These diverse forms of transference yield insight into the kinds of interpersonal conflict each caregiver is experiencing, and the therapist needs to be alert to these phenomena. Moreover, caregivers of new infants who enter dyadic treatment are often eager to explore a wide range of issues, and virtually all new caregivers express interest in the appropriate behavior manifested by the infant at certain developmental stages. In this sense, therapists can describe behaviors that are likely to surface at a particular age or developmental period or can respond to questions in a kind of "Q and A" format. In fact, synthesizing a brief "Q and A" sequence into each session encourages caregivers to develop a positive transference to the therapist, who functions as a repository of information and embodies a source of objective knowledge about infant development.

A final contribution of group therapy is that it is an appropriate setting for activities. Group members select an activity, gradually work through the decision-making process, and cooperate in attempting to accomplish a joint task. This aspect of treatment may also be adapted to mother-infant psychotherapy, whether the therapist is seeing a dyad alone or a group of caregivers with their infants. For example, caregivers can use sessions to identify problems and share strategies that are most efficacious in successfully mastering an activity or accomplishing a particular goal.

As a consequence, creative dyadic treatment strives to adopt techniques that are most appropriate to the concerns the caregivers as a group bring to sessions. As is apparent from the preceding discussion, the therapist may draw on eclectic strategies in fashioning a therapeutic course that will benefit any given mother–infant dyad or a group of dyads.

DEFINING THE GOALS FOR GROUPS COMPOSED OF DYADS

One factor that distinguishes group therapy from individual treatment is that the group can articulate shared objectives to attain during treatment and can subsequently use the group format to "work through" and accomplish these goals. Of course, individual psychotherapy also requires the patient to set goals. From the outset of treatment in a group setting, however, the added dimensions of mutual support, educational guidance, and the sharing of experiences through interpersonal exchange motivate group members to express their concerns more forthrightly and to strive for a sense of accomplishment that is consensually validated by other members of the group and the therapist(s).

Commenting on the group's ability to channel the direction of treatment toward concrete goals, Binder and Smokler (1980) have indicated that in contrast to individual psychotherapy, which highlights self-analysis and the attainment of insight through the exploration of conflict, group therapy focuses on others' behavior patterns and resolves aberrations in these patterns by interpretation with the therapist as well as the other group members. Among the most common goals in the dyadic group format are the following:

1. Enhancement of interpersonal skills that promote mastery during the exchange with the infant.
2. Enhancement of caregiver knowledge of infant development in the somatic, socio-affective, cognitive, and motivational domains.
3. Resolution of any conflict in the caregiver evoked by the infant's needs for both independence and dependence.
4. Enhancement of the caregiver's capacity to predict imminent development and to represent such development as it will occur in her infant.
5. Enhancement of the caregiver's skill in previewing imminent development to the infant.

The group facilitates accomplishing these goals because it provides the individual caregivers with a variety of perspectives that they can use to synthesize a more coherent and objective view of their interactive behavior (Imber, Lewis, & Loiselle, 1979; Waxer, 1977).

Among the factors inherent in group therapy that allow achieving these goals is the sense of *universality*. According to Yalom (1975), universality refers to the release from interpersonal alienation many patients experience when they first enter treatment. Learning that others share a similar plight or confront identical anxieties operates as a catharsis, liberating patients from the sense of alienation they feel when they believe they are the only ones with such problems. Group therapy is also unique, according to Yalom, because it enables patients to *impart information* to one another in a nonthreatening atmosphere. Both of these factors help the members mutually work through and resolve conflict. For several reasons the group format represents an optimal environment to overcome the effects of conflict. First, within the group caregivers will be exposed to a diverse spectrum of infant developmental events. Some infants will be crawling, others will grasping objects, and still others will be neonates just beginning to respond to the stimulation of the external world. Moreover, caregivers in groups are also likely to encounter diverse infant temperamental styles. Some infants will display "easy" dispositions, with regular and predictable responses. Other infants will be more lethargic and "slow-to-warm-up" to the world's stimulation. Finally, it is almost inevitable that some infants will be "difficult," in the sense that they become easily irritated or are quick to cry. In addition, a variety of attachment styles will also be represented. The spectrum can range from clinging infants to infants who mingle readily with strangers. Also, exposure to a group reinforces for caregivers that development proceeds at different paces for different infants. Caregivers will also be able to witness how other mothers engage in previewing exercises that introduce the infant to achievements on the next developmental horizon. A group format is also advantageous, Yalom has noted, because it enables patients to experiment with various forms of *imitative behavior*. By imitating the behavioral manifestations displayed by other group members, each caregiver explores behavior patterns that may have impeded the emergence of a mutually harmonious interpersonal exchange. Through imitation, the caregiver can actually experiment with these impressions almost immediately to enhance the rapport with the infant. Within a dyadic group the opportunities for imitation are even more abundant because each member's interaction with her infant provides a model for the other caregivers.

Another phenomenon that plays an active role in groups is that members tend to *replicate* the primary family structure within the group setting. That is, certain members will adopt a "mothering" role, whereas others will function in the role of the child. Within this format, the group tends not only to replicate early familial conflict, but to reexperience and renegotiate aberrational patterns more adaptively. The group, therefore, can enhance the patient's relationships by dynamically addressing the unfinished business of the past that haunts the caregiver's daily life and hinders a full-fledged adaptive exchange with the infant. Precisely because the caregiver will endow the therapeutic relationship with these familial qualities, previous conflict from the caregiver's own family history will tend to appear more rapidly. The therapist can then guide the direction of the treatment to facilitate working through this conflict. All of these issues combine in achieving the overriding goal of dyadic treatment: an optimal rapport between caregiver and infant that will continue to foster adaptive development.

GROUP COMPOSITION

How does a therapist organize a group and choose those caregivers who will benefit most from this form of therapy?

It is important to screen each caregiver thoroughly before introducing her into group therapy. Such screening requires that the therapist acquire a comprehensive history of the caregiver's family background, including childhood, adolescence, and adult experiences prior to giving birth. Events that led up to the pregnancy, the experience of the pregnancy, and the postpartum history of the caregiver, as well as a complete medical history, are also essential. The therapist should assess how the caregiver interacts with the infant and perceives the infant's development and should evaluate the flexibility of the caregiver's interpersonal approaches. Does the caregiver vacilate between adaptive functioning and disturbed interaction, as is the case with many borderline patients?

A thorough screening of each caregiver during a series of comprehensive interviews is necessary for two reasons. First, the therapist should assess each dyad referred to group therapy both cognitively and affectively to determine the goals of the treatment for that individual dyad. It is helpful to understand the caregiver's defensive structure, especially the extent to which she uses denial and projection (i.e., attributing one's own emotions to significant others). Ego strength, ego flexibility, and the status of primary ego functions, such as reality testing and frustration tolerance, should also be evaluated. The same is true of the caregiver's focal problems. For instance, the nature of the caregiver's dependency needs are important factors to clarify before introducing the caregiver into a group setting. Such a screening may require several meetings to evaluate the caregiver's problems, needs, potential, and expectations about treatment.

Second, pretreatment screening is necessary for deciding whether a caregiver will benefit from group treatment and what kind of group model would be appropriate. If the decision is to place a caregiver in a psychoanalytically oriented group, it is necessary to choose a suitable group. For example, an active, articulate, and fairly adaptive caregiver will become restless in a group consisting primarily of dependent, silent, and passive members. Or, a relatively adaptive caregiver who engages her infant easily may feel uncomfortable in a group of caregivers with previous psychiatric histories who have difficulty interacting adaptively with their infants.

Although it is not essential or even desirable that group members have similar socioeconomic background, age, and similarity of life experience, at least some commonality among the members tends to stimulate their bonds of alliance (Poey, 1985). Common interests, not unexpectedly, enable group members to feel more comfortable about sharing intimate aspects of their lives. As evidence of this phenomenon, a variety of researchers have reported on successful group formats with mothers who shared a particular characteristic. Friedlander and Watkins (1985), for instance, had success with a support group designed for the parents of mentally retarded infants and young children; Ballinger, Smith, and Hobbs (1985) instituted a group for mothers from low socioeconomic backgrounds; whereas Holman (1985) reported progress among a group of caregivers diagnosed with borderline personality disorder. This homogeneity among the caregivers creates a less threatening atmosphere within the group and stimulates the feelings of cohesiveness and peer transference that are so vital for achieving progress.

BUILDING A WORKING ALLIANCE

One of the fundamental components of productive group therapy is an atmosphere of trust and candor that permeates each session, motivating members to confront their own problems and to support other group members. When the group consists of caregivers and their infants or toddlers, this kind of productive atmosphere often emerges spontaneously after several sessions, because the caregivers are eager to share perceptions about the continually transforming states of their infants. Indeed, such groups are conducive to building a working alliance precisely because all members share the common experience of raising an infant. Issues such as erratic sleeping schedules, changes in the marital relationship with the advent of the infant, and the onset of weaning patterns, are likely to interest virtually all group members. In addition, because it is likely that the group will be diverse in terms of the infants' developmental skills, caregivers will not only be able to share experiences, but will also be able to observe how others resolve particular interactional problems and to preview or anticipate how they will experience a particular developmental milestone with the infant.

It is not enough, however, merely to discuss the goals of the group. Rather, the therapist's aim is to clarify a contract with the group. *Contracting,* as the term is used in group therapy, refers to an activity that occurs early in the group during which the members articulate and confirm the basic aims of the group (Fried, 1971; Poey, 1985). Contracting requires that the group struggle together to conceptualize and circumscribe each member's symptoms while resolving to correct or alleviate these symptoms as a united and committed team. In many respects the specific goals articulated during the contracting exercise are not as relevant as that the group members and therapist have agreed to dedicate themselves to a mutual endeavor. Moreover, contracting suggests that not only will group members strive for their own achievement of these goals but that they will also attempt to assist others members in realizing these goals. To reinforce such contracting, both the therapist and group members should articulate the terms of the contract during the group's initial sessions.

Nevertheless, even in a group where members share deep common interests and experiences, it is occasionally difficult to establish camaraderie and rapport. One technique to overcome this barrier is to encourage commentary from all the caregivers. In asking a question, for example, therapists should encourage all members to express their opinions and should be alert to members who dominate a session with lengthy dialogues or, in contrast, to those members who sit in silence, hesitant to participate in the discussion. In these instances, the dominant caregivers should be told courteously to confine their remarks so that others can comment, whereas reluctant caregivers should be encouraged to participate. It is the therapist's task to guide the group in its early sessions, in order to establish a working alliance.

Another aspect of the working alliance within caregiver–infant groups is the focus on developmental trends. One of the prime advantages of such groups is that they provide an unparalleled opportunity to observe infants at different developmental stages, manifesting diverse maturational trends that evoke varied interactional behaviors in their caregivers. The group environment is uniquely suitable for exploring interactional behaviors, for developing caregiver skill in previewing imminent changes in development, and for evaluating and resolving any conflict that threatens the dyadic exchange. As a result, therapists must reinforce in group members that the treatment setting is an arena for enhancing these skills.

For these reasons, therapists' styles will be crucial not only in guiding the group toward a productive working alliance but also in determining the overall direction of the group. As a consequence, therapists should, from the outset, establish themselves as being highly knowledgeable about interactional styles, about the trends of infant development, and about the use of previewing to enhance the dyadic rapport. This is not to suggest that therapists portray themselves as a dogmatic authority. Rather, group members should feel confident about the clinician's skill in discerning problems between caregivers and their infants and should also feel that he or she is experienced in handling a wide variety of interactional difficulties. Nevertheless, it is also important to convey that the group should resolve problems together. This approach is particularly significant. By requesting that members rely on one another for support and guidance, therapists not only foster interaction but also enhance the evolution of group identity and cohesion. This approach encourages the development of each member's transference to the group as an entity. The therapist's main purpose is not to solve the caregivers' problems but to provide the members with the confidence to resolve their own problems adaptively.

Therapists should also use every available opportunity to interact with the infant. Such interaction provides the therapist with the infant's perspective on interaction with the caregiver and also allows the therapist to model adaptive behaviors to the caregiver in a nonthreatening fashion. Subsequently, the caregiver herself can imitate these behaviors with the infant. This form of modeling is also helpful when the therapist wants to demonstrate previewing behaviors to the group as a whole.

STAGES IN THE THERAPEUTIC RELATIONSHIP INVOLVING A GROUP

Because the relationship between caregiver and infant tends to be highly intimate, it is wise for the therapist to proceed cautiously when probing the dyadic relationship. At the beginning of treatment, most caregivers will prefer to focus on the more superficial aspects of infant care. For example, changes in the infant's developmental status from week to week are common topics of conversation during the earlier sessions. Chapter 10 discussed the stages of therapeutic treatment with dyads. These same stages occur with groups. Thus, it is likely that during initial sessions caregivers will be either resistant or encyclopedic in their willingness to discuss perceptions of the infant. With time, as the caregivers become more comfortable about sharing deeper emotions, feelings of intimacy toward other group members and the therapist will evolve. Thus, as treatment progresses, caregivers become more inclined to focus on intimate concerns. One such subject is the father's response to the infant. Many caregivers feel that the birth of the child has alienated their marital relationship. Other caregivers begin to disclose feelings of depression, anger, and frustration toward the infant that they have been unable to express previously. Frequently, caregivers of new infants wish to attend a group so they can share their experiences with new mothers and learn more about the trends of infant development. Such caregivers usually have no history of psychiatric disturbance, nor have they ever engaged in the therapeutic group format before. Indeed, caregivers of this type may be the most common who seek out a group format.

Therapists should be aware, however, that even highly adaptive caregivers may still experience *intermittent minor depression* throughout the course of caring for the infant. Ironically enough, such depression may surface precisely because the caregiver has ordinarily been highly adaptive in her relationship with the child. In these situations the gratification the caregiver has derived from the exchange with the infant tends to create a unique bond of intimacy. When the forces of development inevitably propel the infant toward independence and autonomy, however, the caregiver is often ambivalent. By continuing to engage in adaptive interactions, she will accelerate the infant's development away from her and thus, she mistakenly believes, lose the intimacy of a cherished relationship. On the other hand, the caregiver's genuine affection for the infant motivates her to encourage development to help him master his environment. These ambivalent feelings can create conflict leading to episodes of depression each time the infant achieves a new developmental transition.

It is not unusual for ambivalence about the infant's development to cause mild depression in the caregiver. By working in the group format, however, the caregiver can often alleviate some of the more debilitating symptoms, and she can learn that fostering the infant's development will not necessarily disrupt the intimate relationship she shares with him. Sharing her feelings with other mothers who have had similar experiences offers the caregiver persuasive evidence about how she can overcome the depression and also shows her that although development continues, it will not diminish the intimacy she has known with the infant. Further, the therapist, who acts as both a supporter and educational guide, can reinforce the notion that developmental progress does not threaten the dyadic relationship. In fact, development enhances the rapport between infant and caregiver because they can share more complex skills and experiences. Among groups I have been involved with, members surmounted intermittent depression when their infants faced such developmental events as weaning, learning to walk, learning to say "no," and attending a preschool. Thus, the group format can serve as a highly beneficial therapeutic model for caregivers whose general background indicates the ability to engage in mature interaction.

The transition in family life caused by the infant's arrival can also cause conflict in the caregiver. Worthington (1989) notes that there are three significant variables to evaluate when assessing the effect of *transitions* on the family: the degree to which the transition has disrupted the routines of family members; the degree to which the transition has required new decisions that have provoked initial disagreement among family members; and the level of pretransitional conflict aroused in family members as a result of anticipating the transition. Danish, Smyer, and Nowak (1980) have identified six characteristics of transition that affect the individual's response:

1. The timing of the event (whether early or late).
2. The duration of the transition in relation to expectations.

3. The occurrence of the event with respect to social expectations.
4. Cohort specificity.
5. The probability of occurrence of the event.
6. The manner in which the event has occurred.

All of these factors can be explored with caregivers in the group setting. Worthington (1989) notes that some events promote intimacy, whereas others generate distance. Transitions require a readjustment in time schedules and a shifting in the roles played by family members. In addition, transition can also lead to change, which may cause feelings of uncontrollability in some family members. The therapist can ask about the response of the caregiver's spouse and other family members to the birth. This inquiry generally opens discussion to family issues. *Pretransitional* conflict, the third variable articulated by Worthington, also needs evaluation. Has the wife's pregnancy and her subsequent self-absorption caused the father to experience feelings of alienation that are later transferred to the infant in the form of resentment?

In applying this assessment of transition variables to the family context, Worthington recommends assessing disruption in time schedules by inquiring about the activities of each family member after the transition in comparison with activities prior to the occurrence of the transition. New disagreements caused by the transition generally emerge during discussion in therapy, as does evidence of pretransitional conflict. Worthington's directives are particularly useful for dyadic therapy because the advent of an infant is perhaps the greatest transition a family can experience. Analyzing the event as a transition that has provoked disruption, conflict, and anxiety may be one of the most useful means of resolving dysfunctional patterns within the family unit and in the relationship between the parents and infant.

Cognitive group psychotherapy is useful for depressive episodes. The primary goal of this treatment is helping patients achieve a relatively rapid and long-lasting alleviation of their depression (Roth & Covi, 1984). If the treatment is successful, the patient will be able to identify, evaluate, and modify self-defeating facets of his personal mode of interaction and will have incorporated cognitive skills into his daily life that enable successfully circumventing or alleviating potentially serious depressive episodes.

This type of group treatment, whereby members analyze the roots of their affective dysphoria with one another and acquire cognitive skills for staving off depressive feelings, may be especially helpful for parents who are experiencing a mild postpartum episode after the birth of their child. According to Roth and Covi, the group format encourages such caregivers to deal with feelings of low motivation. Consistent support and social reinforcement from less depressed members of the group often assist the patient in resuming a previously productive life-style. Veteran group members who describe their improved emotional status and its relationship to treatment can also provide impetus and a support network for patients entering the group. These findings suggest that therapists considering a group for depressed caregivers strive to include caregivers at various stages of their depression. Once again, this model enables each caregiver to derive her own resolution to the issue. For example, several caregivers who have overcome a postpartum affective disorder should be encouraged to continue in treatment to serve as models for those caregivers more deeply entrenched in the negative feelings that accompany the disorder.

Roth and Covi recommend organizing the therapeutic format around the concept of both short- and long-term goals. *Long-term goals* include the alleviation of depressive symptomatology and the patient's acquisition of skills that enable her to administer her own cognitive therapy program. *Short-term goals* represent the concrete steps to achieve the long-term relief. Both of these goals must be individualized to account for each patient's unique problems and conflicts. Every session begins with a "go-around" that encourages patients to report on their individual status. Next, patients share significant experiences of the past week, including events that have triggered depression and efforts to overcome these debilitating feelings through positive cognitions. The therapist then asks each patient to articulate an agenda for the upcoming week as well as a strategy for enhancing interaction with the infant.

Using cognitive approaches whenever depressive affect tinges the relationship can be productive for a variety of reasons. First, the group format exposes caregivers to others who have undergone similar experiences. Reinforcing the notion that the caregiver is not the only one undergoing these feelings is especially helpful with new mothers because such patients often feel that their postpartum "blues" are somehow unnatural, unwarranted, or inappropriate, or will somehow impair their future ability to interact adaptively with the infant. By encountering other parents who have experienced similar depressions, the caregiver becomes better able to place her own depression in perspective. Second, fostering cohesion with other caregivers who have surmounted the depressive episode helps caregivers recognize that affective disorder is generally a temporary condition. Third, sharing experiences and feelings with others in a similar situation provides a support network for caregivers who may feel isolated from their families. Caregivers who are undergoing mild-to-moderate depressive episodes may, therefore, find the group format efficacious.

Glick and Kessler (1974) have delineated three main stages for treatment in the group format. During the first stage, the therapist strives to achieve a better understanding of the overall family situation and the status of interaction while establishing a therapeutic alliance and promoting empathy and communication. Green (1981) has proposed a series of guidelines that include, first of all, taking a comprehensive family history and inquiring about the function that problematic behavior patterns serve within the family system. Next, the therapist should explore repetitive interactional patterns that contribute to the problem formation. For example, did the caregiver encounter the same problem with other children in the family, or were these problems common in her own childhood experience? As a third factor, the therapist should investigate the parental models and internalized relationship patterns the spouses are using to guide their own marital and caregiving actions. Fourth, current dysfunctional patterns should be put in the perspective of earlier deprivations the caregiver has experienced. For example, were the caregiver's own parents divorced or separated? Finally, the therapist should articulate the current crisis that has motivated the entrance into treatment within the context of past successes and strengths. Exploring each of these factors with the caregivers as the group progresses will expose some major conflicts. If scapegoating of particular family members is apparent, the therapist should strive to understand such behaviors. Eventually, the focus of attention begins to shift from the caregivers to the infant.

As the second phase of treatment begins, persistent interpersonal patterns and attitudes begin to emerge. For instance, caregivers begin to speak directly about interactions with the child and to question old, nonfunctional coalitions and alignments. It now becomes the therapist's task to formulate a series of treatment goals. Among the most common goals might be involving all members of the nuclear family as well as those outside the nuclear family who may be involved in the etiology of the problem; establishing more accurate communication and greater acknowledgment of problems in communication; facilitating self-differentiation among the caregivers and devising a strategy for a collaborative family effort in resolving the conflict (Green, 1981).

After articulating these goals, the therapist should conduct the first few months of treatment with the goal of observing how these interactional problems emerge during dyadic exchange. Videotaping is often of great assistance during such group therapy because it enables all group members to confront their own contributions to interactional failure, as well as to understand how the problem is the result of an impaired dynamic involving both the caregiver and the infant. Indeed, when the caregiver consents, videotaping is highly advantageous for all forms of dyadic therapy because it allows the caregiver to see palpable evidence of the infant's development and to cope with the emotional changes she has undergone during such development.

In the third and final stage of treatment, the therapist reviews the goals that have been achieved and those that have not been accomplished. Often it is helpful to review the entire course of therapy; for those therapists who have videotaped sessions, now is the time to replay earlier tapes to elicit comment and to stimulate an emotional response. Another task during this phase of treatment is to formulate strategies the caregivers can use in solving future conflict. It is important to acknowledge that some behavior cannot be changed and that the interaction between caregiver and infant will still raise problems. What is important, however, is that group members recognize strategies for coping with these future problems.

In reporting on the experience with dyads, Holman (1985) has also segmented the therapy into three phases: the initial, middle, and final phase. The initial phase was characterized by intense resistance and ambivalence. The caregivers discussed but could not arrive at a consensus or overriding goal to accomplish during the therapy. They noted repeatedly that they were looking for "advice" but commented that the recommendations they received from the therapist were "bad" and "disruptive." During this period the caregivers were sensitive to comparisons and differences among themselves and expressed anxiety and doubt about their practices with their children. The impact of the group was felt as negative. Dependency, coupled with ambivalence toward the therapist, was prominent. These caregivers also voiced concern about sharing perceptions with the therapist and seemed angry at her much of the time. The therapist addressed this anger and tried to be emotionally available to the mothers.

During the middle phase of treatment resistance diminished, and the caregivers resolved the issue of the benefits they wanted to obtain from the group. "Working through" the issues relevant to therapy characterized the middle phase. Caregivers discussed relationships with their own mothers extensively. They also discussed difficulties in separating from their toddlers as well as their feelings of jealousy and anger at being abandoned by the toddler during periods of developmental advancement. There was a sharing of affect, coupled with feelings of group cohesiveness. The emphasis was on differentiation among group members. Intramember relationships gradually became more important than the relationship with the therapist.

Finally, Holman noted that the terminating phase of the group was considered the most important period. The therapist focused actively on the pending separation from therapy, and during discussion the group members dealt overtly with reactions to this separation and loss. It was felt that greater autonomy and self-esteem would come with the mastery of this separation. The members tried to avoid termination by talking about continuing the group after the formal termination. Their denial of the termination of the group ended, however, with the suicidal gesture of one member. This woman required a brief period of hospitalization, during which she continued to attend the group. The members' relationship with the therapist became important again, and the group achieved some resolution of anger about the impending termination. There were assertions of growing independence from the therapist.

Holman's descriptions vividly illustrate the principle that a group composed of members from a homogeneous background or a group in which members share a similar goal or have undergone an identical experience is often the most effective treatment model. Nevertheless, occasionally groups with caregivers from diverse backgrounds or with less universal goals may also be effective. The therapeutic task here is twofold. First, therapists must create the group by selecting members they believe will benefit from exposure to one another. Second, therapists must guide the treatment so that those characteristics they initially believed would blend among the group members actually do emerge to enhance the group's development.

THE TRANSFERENCE RELATIONSHIP

Within the context of dyadic therapy, the emergence of the transference is a unique phenomenon. In traditional treatment involving one patient and a therapist, the transference generally occurs with the therapist. In dyadic treatment, however, no less than four different types of transference relationships may occur:

1. The traditional transference relationship that customarily occurs between the patient—here the caregiver—and therapist.
2. The transference relationship between the caregiver and infant.
3. A peer transference, whereby group members will transfer unresolved conflict to other group members.
4. A transference by individual group members to the group as an entity.

In addition, as with virtually all forms of treatment, the therapist will be prone to experience countertransference reactions to the patient(s). Depending on how the therapist evaluates and manages these emotions, such countertransference feelings can either facilitate or impede the resolution of conflict in the caregiver–infant relationship.

Because these diverse types of transference are seminal to treatment progress, each will be discussed separately.

Transference Between Caregiver and Therapist

As with most forms of treatment, a strong transferential bond is likely to evolve between each caregiver in the group and the therapist. This transference enables the caregiver to transfer unresolved feelings, generally stemming from her own childhood and the experiences with her primary caregiver, onto the person of the therapist. The therapist is then transformed into a paradigm for the "good" or "bad" mother or the "good" or "bad" father. Indeed, in dyadic therapy the therapist's frequent interaction with the infant enhances his or her status as a parental or authority figure. In other instances, the caregiver may view the therapist as a spouse or even as another one of her children. Regardless of the nature of the caregiver's transference to the therapist, the emotional reaction itself will provide the therapist with insights into how that particular caregiver interacts with others and introduces unresolved conflict into the relationship.

Transference Between Caregiver and Infant

As a treatment model, interventions with caregivers and infants, which continually contrast the parent's past and present, may be particularly effective for exploring whether transferential feelings affect the caregiver's relationship with the infant. Indeed, the infant may become a symbol for a figure in the caregiver's own past or may signify a representation of the parental self that she either repudiates or negates. During the therapeutic process, however, the therapist must guard against attributing too much emphasis to the caregiver's role as a provocateur of the dysfunctional symptomatology manifested with the infant. Thus, the therapist must advance explorations with the utmost caution. The etiology of interactional failure often lies buried deep within the caregiver's earliest experiences, which need to be revived and discussed in the therapeutic context. The gradual interpretation of the caregiver's ambivalent attitude toward the infant should accompany disclosure of such attitudes. Observing caregiver–infant interaction firsthand can offer the therapist further insight into the dynamics of this transference. Such observation should be followed by cautious, but probing inquiry.

Peer Transference Among the Caregivers

Peer transference occurs when the caregiver displaces feelings onto other caregivers whom she perceives to be in the same situation. Significantly, the therapist should explore whether the members of the group assume a dependent role or a dominant, leadership position, and whether they are receptive to helpful advice. Have specific alliances between certain group members been established and if so, what factors or similarities of experience motivated these alliances? Moreover, the therapist should also note how particular caregivers respond to the infants of the other caregivers. Does one caregiver praise another infant while criticizing her own or is the caregiver disdainful of the other infants? All of these behaviors reveal how the caregiver views her own situation and suggest the nature of the interpersonal skills she will eventually impart to the infant.

Transference to the Group as an Entity

The emotional response of the caregiver to the group as an entity also yields significant information about the caregiver's interpersonal skills. Some caregivers will view attendance at the group as a chore and will use time in the sessions to express this grievance. In other cases caregivers may accuse other members of not providing support or of "ganging up" with too much criticism. The therapist must evaluate each such reaction because it offers further insight into the kinds of conflict the caregiver brings to interpersonal relationships and, particularly, to her role in her family.

CONCLUSION

This chapter has explored the techniques of group therapy and applied these techniques to dyadic treatment involving caregivers and their infants. Group therapy is a highly flexible and adaptive treatment mode that enables group members to learn from and share common experiences and perceptions with one another. This treatment format is particularly appropriate to dyadic treatment because it enables caregivers to observe infants at different developmental stages and to share knowledge and perceptions with other caregivers who have undergone similar experiences and encountered similar obstacles in the developmental process.

As with other forms of group treatment, therapists working with caregivers and their infants need to select group members who will be compatible and who will benefit from sharing common experiences. A careful screening process, of the type described in this chapter, needs to be performed. The therapist should interview caregivers individually, determine their goals for entering such a treatment group, and attempt to find individuals with compatible demographic and psychological backgrounds. Once the group has been organized, therapists should be aware of the specific stages in this therapeutic relationship. The group undergoes three main stages during treatment. During the first stage the therapist's goal is to achieve a better understanding of the overall family situation and status of interaction within each group member's family. Other goals include establishing a therapeutic alliance and promoting empathy and communication among group members. During this stage observation and inquiry represent the therapist's two main tools. Subsequently, as treatment moves to the second stage, persistent interpersonal patterns and attitudes begin to emerge. Caregivers speak directly about interactions with the child, and the therapist evaluates coalitions and alliances within the family while formulating treatment goals and helping the caregivers work through conflict. Videotaping and modeling techniques are helpful during this time. It is also useful to explore the group members' skills in handling various developmental transitions, such as the adjustment of the family to the infant's arrival, the response of family members to various developmental milestones achieved by the infant, and potential conflicts from the caregiver's past that threaten to impede dyadic interaction. The third and final stage of treatment represents a time for evaluating the therapy. During this period therapists should help group members formulate strategies for dealing with future conflict.

Therapists should also be aware that four transference reactions will become apparent during group therapy: the transference between caregiver and therapist, between caregiver and infant, the peer transference between group members, and the transference to the group as an entity. Each of these reactions needs evaluation for the group members to derive optimal benefits from the treatment.

Chapter 16

Applying Previewing Exercises During Group Therapy

INTRODUCTION

Although previewing behavior is essential for promoting adaptive interactions between a caregiver and infant, it is also an effective intervention mode in the group format. As with treatment involving a single caregiver–infant dyad, group previewing techniques encourage group members to become more attuned to their infants' developmental processes and more sensitive to the implications of such developmental change for the dyadic rapport.

This chapter explains how to integrate previewing behaviors into the group format. Therapists working with dyadic groups should initially strive to ascertain the caregivers' perceptions about infant development. Several sessions should focus on this goal, with caregivers sharing their insights; all caregivers in the group should participate. Subsequently, the therapist should work with the caregivers to enhance their representational skills. It is often beneficial to go around the group and have each caregiver describe her infant's current developmental achievements as well as his previous developmental level. Emphasis here is on how the infant has changed, the caregiver's response to the change, and the common experiences of the caregivers. Eventually, the therapist can turn attention to the infant's future development by asking each caregiver to predict the developmental skills she believes are imminent for her infant. At this time the therapist should introduce the use of previewing behaviors to help the caregivers anticipate developmental trends and subsequently devise behavioral exercises that aid the infant in acquiring these new skills. A readily apparent benefit of the group format is that the differing ages of the infants in the group make it probable that some caregivers will already have previewed these behaviors for their infants. As a result, sharing experiences during this phase of the group treatment is particularly advantageous and will result in exposure to diverse previewing behaviors and styles.

Because the performance of previewing behaviors will occur when the infant is approaching a developmental milestone, this is also when the caregiver is likely to experience potential conflict because she may awaken earlier, unresolved conflict. Such group members may benefit from concurrent group and individual treatment at this time.

Other issues raised in this chapter include appropriate strategies for introducing the issue of termination and addressing the conflict that may arise from ending the group. Overall, this chapter reinforces the advantages of using previewing in a group setting.

PREVIEWING AS A FORM OF INTERVENTION IN GROUP THERAPY

An aspect of group therapy unique to mother–infant dyads is that it facilitates the conceptualization, modeling, and enactment of previewing behaviors. As noted in Chapter 1, previewing encompasses all of the caregiver's behaviors that predict both the infant's imminent developmental growth and the interpersonal implications that such change will evoke in the relationship. When the therapist is treating one dyad, such behaviors will tend to emerge gradually. However, when treatment involves a group of dyads, each of whom has an infant at a different developmental phase, previewing behaviors tend to become more prolific.

As an example of the proliferation of previewing in the group context, when caregivers are encouraged to relate changes in infant development they have encountered recently, virtually all caregivers will be able to share some information. One caregiver being treated in such a group format raised the issue of weaning, for instance. Almost immediately, every caregiver in the group had some experience to share about the event. Those caregivers who had undergone the weaning process with their infants contributed instructive insights for the other caregivers who had not yet confronted that maturational event. These more experienced caregivers answered questions about what had precipitated the weaning, how they experienced the event emotionally, and what infant feeding was like now that the weaning was complete. Sharing these experiences achieved two goals. First, the caregivers who had not yet engaged in weaning had an opportunity to explore how they would feel when their infants began to demonstrate weaning behaviors. These caregivers were motivated to *represent and predict* both the infant's future development and their own emotional response to it. They were, in other words, inevitably propelled to preview imminent developmental achievement. Second, those caregivers who had already undergone the weaning experience were able to reflect on their response and to review how they had coped with this aspect of infant development.

The group format further stimulates previewing behaviors by providing caregivers with diverse examples of how the other members deal with their infants' burgeoning development. It is inevitable, as the group progresses, for caregivers to begin playing with their infants during the session. As a result, each caregiver has palpable models of how other parents soothe, hold, vocalize to, and play with their infants. This display of the full spectrum of intuitive behaviors enables group members to become accustomed to how others in a similar situation are providing somatic, socio-affective, cognitive, and motivational cues to the infant. These diverse models provide each caregiver with a rich psychological stimulus to engage in these behaviors herself and, further, to experiment with various ways of interacting with the infant. Imitation of the other group members liberates the caregiver to practice her previewing skills with the infant and to observe how the infant responds to such cues. Although it is certainly possible to teach and enhance caregiver previewing skills during therapy with one dyad, there is virtually no substitute for the stimulation and encouragement a caregiver receives by observing others who are engaged in these behaviors.

The group format also encourages caregivers to verbalize and share their perceptions about infant development in a manner that stimulates representational abilities. One useful exercise is to have caregivers describe the infant's developmental progress during the previous week, comment on how this change is affecting their relationship, and then state what they predict will happen as other changes begin to develop and crystallize. As this exercise occurs, caregivers are encouraged to share their memories about their own development. For example, the caregiver of a 9-month-old daughter reported concern because the infant had not yet begun to show walking gestures, although her own mother had said that the infant's crawling was appropriate for her developmental stage. When the other mothers questioned this caregiver about her anxiety, she disclosed that her mother had also told her that she (the caregiver) had walked at an extremely early age and that this accomplishment had been a particular point of pride with her mother. The other caregivers then suggested that although the behavior may have been appropriate for her, such a rapid time frame of development might not be appropriate for her infant. In fact, they noted that the infant appeared to be a happy, healthy, well-adjusted child whose development would most likely proceed at a normal pace. Once the caregiver had received this feedback, she reflected on it deeply. At the next session, she seemed much calmer and revealed to the group that for the first time, she had seen her daughter as others saw her, from a different and independent perspective divorced from her own feelings, and had begun to recognize that perhaps she was communicating inappropriate messages to the infant. The communications that occurred within the group helped this caregiver to remove distortions and incorrect attributions that were affecting her previewing behaviors. During the following weeks, she was able to engage in more adaptive previewing that demonstrated her awareness of her infant as a unique individual with distinct developmental needs.

The group context also promotes caregivers' previewing skills because it provides a panorama of overall development in diverse infants. Exposure to many mothers undergoing the same developmental journey with their infants demonstrates to caregivers that the processes of development are continual and that various milestones can be predicted and prepared for. One caregiver commented to me after 6 months in such a group that one of the most fascinating aspects of attending was witnessing how four different infants began to speak their first words. The caregiver reported that this experience had resulted in a form of exhilaration. "I came to understand that all babies undergo the same developmental events but that each baby's ability to deal with those events is different, and that the mother's behaviors play a key role in helping the infant mature according to his own personality and needs," she reported.

This caregiver's remarks capture group therapy's prime advantage in enhancing caregiver previewing behaviors. By providing caregivers with varied and diverse illustrations of how development unfolds and how a nurturing figure can help stimulate such growth, the group serves as a paradigm for awakening and bolstering the caregiver's previewing skills as well as her sensitivity to her own infant's unique development.

A MODEL OF GROUP THERAPY INTERVENTION FOR PARENT–INFANT DYADS

The following is a suggested intervention model of a 10-session group to enhance caregiver perceptions of developmental phenomena. This model has been used with a group of adaptive caregivers who wished to acquire more general information about their infant's development and with a group of caregivers whose previous histories contained diverse psychiatric maladies. Obviously, the clinician should incorporate flexibility into this model, which can serve as a basic blueprint for integrating previewing behaviors into the dyadic group therapy format.

Sessions 1–2: Ascertaining Caregiver Perceptions About Development

The first two sessions of the clinical program are devoted to obtaining a diagnostic profile of the caregiver and infant in the context of the group as well as to assessing dyadic interaction. Each caregiver describes her knowledge of infant developmental status and provides as best as she can an overview of the basic achievements that her infant has already accomplished or "might be expected" to accomplish during the first 30 months of life.

The therapist initiates the discussion by asking the caregivers to volunteer information about developmental progress they have witnessed in their infants in the week prior to the initiation of treatment. Each parent is encouraged to give her own report. Because it is important to ascertain how sophisticated the caregiver's capacities are for integrating infant perceptions, the therapist should ask the caregivers to elaborate on their descriptions by offering insights into the four primary domains of infant perception—the somatic, the socio-affective, the cognitive, and the motivational. For example, how did the infant manifest the change through body movement, how did the infant feel emotionally, what intellectual processes did the infant experience, and was the infant enthusiastic, neutral, or hesitant about the change? Caregivers receive encouragement to volunteer information when they have encountered a situation similar to that of another caregiver in the group.

After acquiring a general diagnostic profile of each caregiver, the therapist should assume a didactic role and provide an overview of the basic developmental milestones of the first 2 years of life. At this juncture of the treatment many group members may be resistant to the therapist's insights and information, whereas other caregivers will adopt an authoritative role with respect to their own knowledge. Such caregivers may feel that their own role is being threatened or usurped, and so the therapist should be careful not to be overly assertive. Nevertheless, he or she should strive to depict the typical milestones of infancy, such as the acquisition of psychomotor skills (e.g., sucking, sitting, crawling, walking) (see Gesell & Amatruda, 1974); the acquisition of affective skills (e.g., the social smile) and other discrete affective displays (e.g., stranger anxiety and the security of attachment); the acquisition of cognitive skills (e.g., discrepancy and contingency awareness, intersubjectivity, social referencing, affect attunement); and other achievements with which caregivers may not be as familiar. Caregivers should be informed of such phenomena as infant imitation (Field, 1982) and the advent of play behaviors (Fein, 1979a, 1979b; McCune-Nicolich, 1981a, 1981b). The therapist should explain developmental milestones in a nontechnical fashion that the caregiver can readily understand and should avoid jargon. After hearing a description of these discrete milestones, each caregiver should be asked whether she has encountered any such developmental phenomena in her infant. If the answer is "yes," the caregiver should share with the group members the various behaviors her infant has displayed that illustrate the acquisition of such milestones; if the answer is "no," the caregiver should predict when the infant will display these behaviors.

When the caregivers have identified a particular developmental achievement, the therapist should encourage the caregivers to elaborate on its implications for their infants' future achievements and for the dyadic relationship. Caregivers here should describe their perceptions of how a particular milestone may affect and influence other achievements. It is advisable for the caregiver, when describing a milestone, to explain how attaining it affects all the domains of functioning (e.g., somatic, socio-affective, cognitive, and motivational).

In addition to offering caregivers a basic overview of developmental achievement during the years of infancy, the therapist should provide structure for the future sessions by articulating specific goals for each session. These goals include the following expectations:

1. Each caregiver will provide the group members with a summary of infant development relating to somatic, socio-affective, cognitive, and motivational perceptions during the previous week.
2. Each caregiver will share with the group a series of expectations about the infant's upcoming developmental achievements.
3. Each caregiver will provide the group with an interpretation of the meaning of such developmental change within the interpersonal domain.

The following is a group discussion that might occur during early treatment sessions:

THERAPIST: I would like to propose that each of you share your goals for coming to the group.

CAREGIVER 1: What I'm looking for from this group is a lot of information and feedback about my infant's growth, development, and personality.

THERAPIST: (To Caregiver 2) What about you?

CAREGIVER 2: Since I learned that I was pregnant, I always wanted to be part of a group. I was seeing someone individually, and it was very frustrating. I wanted to be in a group with other mothers and their babies. I wanted to see what they go through and share with them what I go through.

THERAPIST: (To Caregiver 3) Can you share your goals?

CAREGIVER 3: In addition to my twins, I also have a 3-year-old. Now I stay at home full-time because of all the responsibilities involved in caring for three young children, two of whom are infants, and I've had to make a lot of adjustments. I wanted to have an experience where I would be able to focus on the twins and their developing personalities. This group is a good opportunity for me to do that.

THERAPIST: What are some of the developmental changes in your infants that you have noticed in the last couple of weeks?

CAREGIVER 2: I switched him from breast-feeding to formula. I wasn't comfortable breast-feeding anymore. I've started to go out again, and it's easier just to take a bottle. My baby didn't want to take the bottle at first, but now he does.

CAREGIVER 1: (To Caregiver 2) It's very hard to travel when you're still breast-feeding. That's why I decided to introduce the bottle early— when my baby was 2½ months. Now she takes both. My husband and I both have allergies and we were afraid she would have a reaction to the formula. That's why I started breast-feeding. I got a lot of information about it from other mothers before I decided to mix both. But now after she has her bottle she looks for more. She says, "O.K., I'm ready to begin nursing now" (smiles).

THERAPIST: (To Caregiver 3) How was the switch from breast-feeding to formula for you?

CAREGIVER 3: It wasn't an issue for me this time around because the twins were born prematurely and they had to stay in the hospital. I expressed my milk and gave it to both of them in bottles. Even after they came home, it was very difficult to nurse them because they were so small. (To Caregiver 2) I have to admire you for giving up breast-feeding because there's pressure to be a "natural" mother and to breast-feed. I never really got into it either. I also expressed milk for my 3-year-old.

THERAPIST: Can you tell the members of the group how old your baby is now?

CAREGIVER 1: She is now 4½ months old.

THERAPIST: (To Caregiver 2) And yours?

CAREGIVER 2: He's 6 weeks old.

THERAPIST: (To Caregiver 3) How about your twins?

CAREGIVER 3: Sheila and Jenny are 3 months old.

CAREGIVER 1: Happy birthday, Sheila and Jenny (smiles).

Sessions 3–5: Instilling Skill in Representational Exercises

The next three sessions should foster the caregiver's *representational capacities* with the infant. Representational capacities here refer to the caregiver's ability to predict or anticipate specific trends in development and to verbalize how their infants will manifest these developmental events and how new acquisitions will affect their dyadic relationship with the infant. To do this, the therapist needs to engage in a series of inquiries with each caregiver.

The primary task here is to enhance the caregiver's appreciation of both the diversity and the sophistication of the infant's discrete capacities. The first representational exercise requires the caregiver to envision an integrated picture of the infant's behavior, in which she views somatic, socio-affective, cognitive, and motivational perceptions in a coordinated fashion. One caregiver in treatment responded to this inquiry by observing, "I think he *feels* happy and excited, because he is curious about the new toy" (socio-affective characterization); "He is probably *thinking* about how the qualities of this toy are different from his other toy (cognitive characterization); "He likes to *sit up* to see the toy and is using his fingers to stroke the fur on the toy" (somatic characterization); "He is *trying* to operate the toy on his own" (motivational characterization). Although such descriptions may seem simplistic, they help the caregiver to represent or perceive experiences from the infant's point of view and to appreciate the infant's multidimensional capacities for integrating experience. Having each caregiver voice these impressions facilitates this representational exercise.

Other representational exercises to encourage during this period include having the caregiver represent boundaries within the interaction. Representation of such structure refers to the caregiver's ability to provide appropriate boundaries to differentiate, channel, and/or contain the infant's affects and cognitions. To provide this degree of organization, caregivers need to differentiate the source of each message they share with the infant. By doing this, the infant not only will be able to validate communicative messages but will also be able to establish clear boundaries between internal demands and external realities. These exercises also enable the therapist to discern how the caregiver distinguishes her own identity from that of the infant. The caregiver should further envision how the infant synthesizes the dyadic interaction, how he perceives an intended act, and what responses it evokes in him.

Mastering these skills will enhance the caregiver's ability to adopt *the perspective of the infant*. At this point, the therapist can introduce other representational exercises that make the ability to adopt the infant's perspective even more imperative. For example, by the fourth session, group members should be able to represent sequences during which infant and caregiver *share* an object, an experience, or an emotion. Such representational exercises necessitate adopting the infant's perspective almost entirely. Caregivers should be able to represent sharing sequences with the infant and to describe how the infant *feels* during such interludes. From these comments, the therapist will be able to formulate a diagnostic profile that accurately charts the level of intimacy within the dyad. At this time the caregiver should also describe the infant's drive for mastery over the environment and the coordination of precursory developmental skills. Indeed, by this point in the treatment, the caregiver's grasp of the relationship between achievement and developmental transition will be keen. Characterizing the intricate perceptions of the infant in detail during this period should be relatively easy for her.

The representational exercises that the caregiver engages in during this phase of the clinical treatment challenge the caregiver to orient thought patterns in a way that heightens awareness of the infant's developmental capacities. Beyond this, however, the exercises themselves encourage the emergence of unconscious perceptions about the infant. In other words, as the representational exercises become more sophisticated, the caregiver must rely on more profound and, indeed, primitive perceptions of the infant that implicate her own deep-seated expectations and wishes. Moreover, by this point in the treatment it is likely that the various transference reactions described in Chapter 10 have been established. The emergence of these transference reactions will make it easier for the therapist to assess the caregiver's representations. In addition, the therapist will be able to detect any unresolved conflict that is intruding on the caregiver's perceptions and thereby preventing her from relating adaptively to her infant. The therapist should assess each category of the transference for each individual caregiver. Has the caregiver developed a peer transference and a transference to the group as an entity? If so, what is the nature of these transference responses? Therapists should also assess any residual emotion the caregivers have aroused in the form of a countertransference reaction.

Representation at this juncture of the treatment actually functions as a form of psychotherapy that strives to identify unconscious conflict. Because discussion of conflict encountered with the infant encourages the caregiver to explore earlier stages of her own development, this technique tends to intensify the transference relationship between the caregiver and therapist, providing the therapist with even greater insights into the roots of any unresolved conflict that may be impeding optimal dyadic interaction. Finally, because the caregivers share these exercises in a group setting, they have the opportunity to acquire diverse perspectives on infant development. This experience has two significant outcomes. First, the caregiver communicates her unique perceptions of her infant with clarity, and second, the caregiver acquires insight into how her perceptions of the infant resemble or diverge from the perceptions of other mothers.

THERAPIST: (Smiling at Caregiver 1's baby) I've noticed that she has gained more control over her body than when we began working 2 months ago.

CAREGIVER 1: She has developed a lot of motor skills during these last 2½ weeks. Her ability to roll over goes in both directions. She can go anywhere she wants (baby on her back, kicks with both legs). She also pulls herself up on her knees and rocks.

THERAPIST: Can you describe this more?

CAREGIVER 1: Well, at this point, I think crawling. I am beginning to realize that things have to be moved a lot faster because she can roll anywhere. She also entertains herself a lot more because she can reach for objects herself. It used to be that she would see something and look at me and look at the toy and then reach for it, but then would lose interest because she couldn't grab it without my help. Now she can work her way to getting anything she wants.

THERAPIST: Have you noticed any changes with her mouthing of toys or other objects?

CAREGIVER 1: (Thinks) The way she puts things in her mouth is different (becomes silent).

THERAPIST: Is she more coordinated?

CAREGIVER 1: (Picks toy out of bag) Instead of going like this (smacks forehead with toy), she can go like this now (puts her toy in mouth). Depending on what it is, she can get it in her mouth instead of smacking it against her face trying to figure out how to get it in. That's different.

THERAPIST: How do you feel about what is going on?

CAREGIVER 1: I feel very good. It is just happening so fast!

THERAPIST: Do you wish something would be different?

CAREGIVER 1: Hmmm . . . Not really. When you compare what your child does with what the books say, you realize that they all develop differently. (Other mothers nod.) I have always thought that she is doing better than what the books predicted anyway.

THERAPIST: (Turns to Caregiver 2) What experiences have you had with your baby?

CAREGIVER 2: (Baby is 6 weeks old.) He is more watchful. A lot more.

THERAPIST: What was it like before?

CAREGIVER 2: He just stared into space. Now he'll really look at you and follow the sound of your voice (looks at baby). (Baby looks at her.) And the bottle. (Baby looks at bottle; caregiver smiles.) I don't know if I'm imagining it, but I feel like he can see the bottle; he knows when it's coming. He's making faces. Do you see them?

CAREGIVER 3: (To Caregiver 2) Is he 6 weeks now?

CAREGIVER 2: Yes (trying to maintain eye contact with the baby, who is fussing).

CAREGIVER 3: I noticed that with my twins—with the fine motor coordination—the older one, one minute older—was the heavier one when she was born. I put her in a walker, and she works diligently on her eye–hand coordination—hand-to-mouth with a cracker or something like that. The younger one is not as aggressive when she moves.

THERAPIST: Could some of you share your experiences about predicting an emotional reaction in your baby, a response that you were sensitive to but that others may not have noticed? (Caregivers nod at each other.)

CAREGIVER 1: Absolutely. I think I've never seen anything like the ability of mothers to hear their babies while no one else in the room could. I had a baby shower for my sister on Saturday, and we had 30 people in the house. I had the intercom on, but I had it on very low. I heard something, and everybody was like, "You're crazy." It turned out she was sitting up in the crib when she was waking up from her nap and everybody—even my husband didn't hear. When she started teething, she started waking up a lot. I would wake up and it would be dead silent, and sure enough, 10 seconds later, I would hear her fussing because of the pain. My husband is a lighter sleeper than I am. But he wouldn't wake up. It was as if only I could hear the baby . . . like I was specially "tuned in."

CAREGIVER 2: That's mother's intuition.

CAREGIVER 3: I think it's more a question of just being really in tune with your baby. I think there's two different things that we're talking about. I kind of blew the whole thing with my 3-year-old when I was in the hospital with him. I had a roommate, and they wheeled a baby in, and I said, "Oh, there she is." It was the other woman's baby. I said, "Oh well, so much for bonding, I guess!" (Laughs) It sure looked like my kid. But I think it's more a question of just getting in tune with your baby and being able to figure out her schedule or kind of knowing, having been through a couple of episodes, a cold, sleeping, or eating habits.

THERAPIST: (To Caregiver 2) Are you beginning to notice the same kinds of things with your baby?

CAREGIVER 2: Oh yes!

THERAPIST: Can you share with us one of your experiences?

CAREGIVER 3: (To Therapist and Caregiver 2) It's difficult in the beginning because they still don't have much of a routine. They're just getting used to being out of the womb and getting used to their own environment so that they're changing everyday. That's tough on you because unpredictability sets you over the edge sometimes.

CAREGIVER 2: (Nods) That is absolutely true.

THERAPIST: (Back to Caregiver 2) What developmental changes have you predicted before they happened?

CAREGIVER 2: Well, now he's not just sleeping and eating. I know when he wants to play.

THERAPIST: How do you know when he wants to play?

CAREGIVER 2: When he's up and he won't go to sleep, I know he wants to play.

THERAPIST: What kinds of things do you do when you play?

CAREGIVER 2: I hold him and bounce him around, walk around, that sort of thing.

THERAPIST: Have you noticed that his attention span has increased as he likes to do more things?

CAREGIVER 2: Yes, exactly. He spends more time doing and seeing things.

THERAPIST: Do you sometimes find yourself using your child as the vehicle to communicate with your husband when you don't feel that good about him? If he did something that you did not like very much, how did you use the baby to begin conversing, to get back to the right track?

CAREGIVER 1: Repeat the question?

THERAPIST: Have you had an experience where you might have used your baby to communicate to your husband that you don't feel very good about him? Let's say you had an argument with him before he left in the morning. When he comes home, you don't communicate in the regular way with him. You use the baby to start a conversation with him. You use the baby as a vehicle for communication.

CAREGIVER 1: That's very interesting. No . . .

THERAPIST: (To Caregiver 2) Have you had any experiences?

CAREGIVER 2: (Shakes head)

THERAPIST: (To Caregiver 3) And you?

CAREGIVER 3: Yes. (Group laughs.) We used our 3-year-old quite a bit to deal with the tension right after our twins were born. We didn't want him to feel the turmoil that was going on so we would just be pleasant—and really nice people—to Steven and just nasty to each other. But we would communicate that we still cared about each other by demonstrating that we cared for our son. We had a lot of hurt and a lot of anger that we took out directly on the other person, but we were completely different people to Steven.

THERAPIST: How did you come to that very insightful formulation?

CAREGIVER 3: It was obvious because we knew each other. We knew it was a difficult time, and it was obvious what we were doing.

THERAPIST: You were able to sit down and talk about it.

CAREGIVER 3: It was one thing to talk about it and another thing to adapt it to life to deal with the change. We didn't have any other outlets for our anger and our hurt. We still had to take that out on the other one to a certain extent.

THERAPIST: When did you notice that this was not taking place anymore?

CAREGIVER 3: When . . . (Baby on floor rolls over.) Whoopie! When the babies came home . . . (Baby laughs.) Hi! That was funny (to the therapist). When the babies came home and they began to settle down. It was having them at home and having them out of danger that brought the change. I think maybe we had just been anxious about what it would be like to care for twins in addition to Steven.

Sessions 6–8: Previewing Exercises

As the caregiver's competence over the infant's development becomes more acute, it is likely to awaken a desire to practice these skills with the infant. *Previewing exercises* apply the insights gained from the representational exercises. An advantage of using the group format with new mothers is that from the first session on, caregivers will tend to play with, comfort, or minister to their infants during the group. Thus, the transition to previewing exercises, which entail direct interaction with the infant, will be a natural outgrowth of the group dynamic.

Previewing behaviors capture the caregiver's enhanced awareness of development and enable the infant to experience this new awareness in a supportive fashion during the interaction with the caregiver. To introduce the caregivers to the notion of previewing, the therapist should ask all the group members to describe an imminent developmental milestone that they anticipate their infant will soon be experiencing in full-fledged form. Each caregiver should then relate a developmental phenomenon that she has perceived briefly or intermittently. Incipient crawling behaviors or the infant's fine motor gestures while grasping for a utensil are two examples of behaviors that signify the onset of a new developmental acquisition.

After a caregiver has articulated a specific example, the therapist should ask her to envision the infant's gestures when he fully experiences and manifests the milestone on his own. (Precursory milestones refer to those incipient or rudimentary changes that have begun to emerge and indicate the imminent attainment of a new developmental function. In contrast, full-fledged milestones refer to changes that will be fully consolidated in the future, but for which there is at present only precursory evidence.) The therapist should also ask other group members to describe their experience with this milestone and, for the precursory changes, should ask the caregiver to interact supportively by gradually introducing the infant to the full-fledged sensation of the particular milestone. For example, the caregiver might help the infant grasp a spoon, might exercise his legs to simulate crawling, or might help him to sit in an erect position while offering him bodily support.

Because previewing depends on the caregiver's sensitivity to the infant's developmental status, it is not surprising that another aspect of this skill is the ability to allow the infant to return gradually to his previous level of development after the previewing exercise. Therapists should observe caregivers during these exercises to ensure that this form of well-paced and rhythmic transition between states occurs. Once again, other group members should be encouraged to volunteer their perceptions of these behaviors.

In some cases, caregivers may be reluctant to engage in previewing behaviors with the infant. This reluctance can stem from a wide variety of sources. First, some caregivers may possess a representational deficit that impedes their ability to predict or envision the infant's future development. Other caregivers may perceive previewing exercises as threatening because they trigger unresolved conflict from their own earlier developmental histories. Still other caregivers may have physical disabilities that hinder them from fully manifesting previewing behaviors with the infant.

However, the therapist can overcome many of these problems and much of the caregiver's reluctance by engaging in the modeling strategies mentioned in Chapter 13. Modeling requires that the therapist interact with the infant and graphically demonstrate how to perform a particular behavior competently and adaptively. Once modeling has occurred, the therapist can encourage the caregiver to imitate the behavior in a nonthreatening manner. Such modeling also enables the therapist to experience the infant's responses in vivo and thus allows better evaluation of any unresolved conflict impeding adaptive dyadic interaction. Another advantage of the group format is that the caregiver will have a wide variety of models for imitating appropriate previewing behaviors.

THERAPIST: What do you think will be the next developmental milestone or skill your infant will manifest?

CAREGIVER 1: I think the next milestone she will show is an ability to understand what is being communicated verbally. I think she's going to use more vocabulary words and I think this will make her more responsive.

THERAPIST: What are some of the things she says now?

CAREGIVER 1: She says "Mama," "Dada," "button."

THERAPIST: What changes do you think she is going to show next?

CAREGIVER 1: I think she will want me to start teaching her more important words so that she can tell me how she feels or what she doesn't want to do or what she wants me to start teaching her.

THERAPIST: If she could speak right now, what do you think she would ask you to teach her?

CAREGIVER 1: I think she would tell me that she wants to learn more abstract vocabulary words like "society" or "man." She would want to learn words that help her describe herself in relation to others.

THERAPIST: (To Caregiver 2) Has your baby started to say anything yet?

CAREGIVER 2: He makes a lot of noises, and sometimes we can pick out a "Mama" or "Dada." My husband speaks to him in silly voices, and he seems to enjoy that.

THERAPIST: When do you anticipate that he will begin talking?

CAREGIVER 2: Maybe in another couple of months. I am using exercises to help him with his speech.

THERAPIST: Can you give us an example?

CAREGIVER 2: Yes. When I point things out to him I also talk to him, repeating the name of the object.

THERAPIST: How has he responded?

CAREGIVER 2: Great! He smiles a lot. I like it!

THERAPIST: (To Caregiver 3) How do you think your twins will respond when you begin pointing things out to them?

CAREGIVER 3: They will probably try to repeat what I'm saying.

THERAPIST: And what do you think will be the next milestone they are going to demonstrate?

CAREGIVER 3: They will probably try to sit up by themselves.

THERAPIST: When do you think they will be able to do this by themselves?

CAREGIVER 3: (Caregiver 3 cuddles her babies.) Probably in a couple of weeks.

THERAPIST: Are you doing anything to help them sit up on their own?

CAREGIVER 3: Yes. When I notice one of them making motions to try to sit up, I prop her up in my lap so she's sitting up.

Sessions 9–10: Integration of Skills and Termination

The final two sessions of the therapeutic regimen should be devoted to ensuring that caregivers can rely on their newly gained representational and previewing skills in their daily lives. To accomplish this goal, the therapist should advise the caregivers to discuss some representational skills that they will use daily to foster a more sensitive understanding of the infant's development. The caregiver should also be encouraged to integrate previewing behaviors into daily interactions with the infant.

Another aspect of these final sessions is the issue of termination. It is particularly important to explore caregiver perceptions of treatment termination, because this event serves as an analogue for caregiver separation from the infant, which occurs with the consolidation of each milestone. Developmental achievement implicates both separation and differentiation because each acquisition propels the infant in the direction of autonomy. If the prospect of termination distresses the caregiver, the therapist should work through this conflict thoroughly because it may foreshadow future conflict that will arise when the infant attempts to separate from the caregiver. During this time, the therapist may also wish to explore issues of separation directly with the caregivers. For example, how will each caregiver cope with the infant's attendance in school? Forecasting and focusing on such future development helps caregivers resolve potential conflict before it surfaces to threaten the relationship with the infant.

The time constraints of this short-term model may prevent therapists from encouraging members to deal with individual issues or to interact fully with the other group members. Researchers such as Roth (1980) and Roth and Covi (1984) have thus outlined some advantages of a more open-ended format that lacks a preestablished termination date: (a) It enhances the opportunity to offer and consider constructive feedback nondefensively; (b) from the patient's viewpoint, it encourages disclosure of highly personal experiences; and, (c) it facilitates the development of stable cohesive relationships. In addition, a longer treatment format allows working through transference phenomena at a more leisurely pace. This last factor has special value in dealing with caregivers and their infants because establishing cohesive bonds between group members or between the therapist and group members helps caregivers transfer adaptive behavior patterns to their infants. The decision to use a particular therapeutic framework should be based on an evaluation of the patient's needs and available resources.

THERAPIST: When infants reach a certain age, they start manifesting different skills. What kinds of feelings do you experience in response to your infant's new developments?

CAREGIVER 1: Most mothers I've spoken to agree that by 8 or 9 o'clock they are exhausted and need some time to themselves.

THERAPIST: (to Caregiver 2) Do you agree?

CAREGIVER 2: (Emphatically) Yes!

CAREGIVER 1: I have a very full day, and sometimes I get cranky. When my baby is crying after I put her in the crib, sometimes I feel like I want to cry! When I put my baby to bed, I want to make sure she is comfortable. After I'm sure that she's comfortable, I want to minimize the amount of time that it takes for her to fall asleep. I don't want to feel angry, but I really believe that I need some time to myself or with my husband.

THERAPIST: How do you deal with your feelings when your baby makes a demand on you?

CAREGIVER 1: I try to appease her a little bit. I let her cry for about 15 minutes, and then I come and take her out of her crib for 15 minutes. Then I put her back to bed and try again.

THERAPIST: (To Caregiver 2) Have you felt anything similar when your baby wants you, but you would prefer to have some time to yourself?

CAREGIVER 2: He's pretty good about sleeping. He usually sleeps from 8 at night until 8 the next morning. I don't really feel like he needs me that much. During the day, I put him down on the living room floor and he'll play by himself.

THERAPIST: It looks like he's doing that now. (Infant lies on his stomach on the floor occupying himself with a toy.)

CAREGIVER 2: Yes. Sometimes he'll make a whimpering noise. I go into the living room and check to see if he is all right. I never felt like he needed me to be there for him all of the time. A friend of mine had a baby who was about the same age as my baby. Her baby screams when she's not around. I feel a little self-conscious because I think that maybe my baby doesn't need me. Does he know I'm his mother? Why doesn't he cling to me like her baby does to her? In a way, I would like that, but it could eventually become a nuisance. Why doesn't he feel that attachment? Or if he does feel it, why doesn't he express it in the same way?

THERAPIST: The two babies we have here are very different. Tyler makes whimpering noises while you're in the other room, but Carlie cries from her crib when she wants attention.

CAREGIVER 1: I don't think of Carlie as a very needy baby either, though. She is starting to tell us when she wants attention and is becoming more demanding, but in a selective way. She doesn't need to be held all of the time or always need me to be with her in her room.

CAREGIVER 2: She's probably just being very sociable. She wants somebody to play with.

COMBINED INDIVIDUAL AND GROUP THERAPY

As has been pointed out previously, dyadic therapy involving a caregiver and infant bears some resemblance to individual therapy. In dyadic therapy, the caregiver generally communicates emotional experiences to the therapist verbally and behaviorally during interaction with the infant in the therapist's presence. A therapeutic alliance is gradually established that encourages the disclosure of unresolved conflict.

Nevertheless, dyadic therapy also bears some resemblance to group therapy, because the caregiver's interactions with the infant will enable the therapist to draw some inferences about how the caregiver functions in an interpersonal arena. Despite this unique aspect of dyadic therapy, however, there may be times when both individual and group therapy are warranted for a caregiver and infant. Some mothers are eager to share their daily experiences with other mothers in similar circumstances and also benefit from observing how other mothers cope with the dilemmas that are an ordinary component of raising an infant. Other mothers are unfamiliar with developmental phenomena and wish to observe the varieties of individual maturation offered by a group format. Moreover, the group format focuses attention on development as an overriding issue in the relationship between mother and infant. The therapist may feel that the caregiver will benefit from exposure to other mothers who will serve as models for appropriate, adaptive interaction or whose interaction with their infants may evoke conflict that the caregiver has been unable to discuss or confront previously.

To effectively respond to the unique needs of each mother–infant pair, dyadic therapy must be flexible, which may involve providing concurrent individual and group therapy with the same patient (Schachter, 1987). As is apparent, both understanding the individual caregiver and the way that her personality manifests in a group setting are crucial for dyadic therapy. The caregiver's personality will affect her attitudes and attributions toward the infant as well as any unresolved conflict she brings to the relationship. It is best to explore these issues during individual, insight-oriented psychotherapy. On the other hand, the techniques of interpersonal rapport used by the caregiver may only fully manifest themselves during interactions with others, such as the infant or other caregivers in a similar situation. As a result, group sessions with other mothers and their infants may reveal interactional patterns that may either be disguised during individual treatment or may only emerge after a prolonged period. Therapists should use flexibility, therefore, in recommending group or individual therapy for each caregiver and, when the circumstances are appropriate, should consider combining these formats.

Certain dilemmas may arise when instituting these formats simultaneously. One such problem concerns the use of the same or a different therapist for the varying formats (Alonso & Rutan, 1990). Traditionally, the transference relationship that develops with a single therapist has been viewed as a paramount motivation to progress in the treatment, and it is through the transference interpretation that the patient ultimately works through conflict. As a consequence, one school of thought advocates using the same therapist for both the individual and group formats to maintain the integrity of the transference. In addition, maintaining the same therapist provides a unified portrait of the patient as both an individual and a participant in the interpersonal arena. With caregiver–infant dyadic therapy, using the same therapist will also enable direct observation of how the caregiver's interactions with the infant may change in different settings.

Caligor (1990), who advocates a model that uses individual therapy from the outset and then supplements it with group therapy, emphasizes the value of the transference relationship for effective change within the patient. According to Caligor, the beginning phases of treatment are most effectively managed within a format of individual therapy. During the middle phase of treatment, however—the so-called "working-through" phase of confronting and resolving conflict—the combination of individual and group treatment is preferable. Caligor notes that by the time the patient is ready to enter the group, a therapeutic relationship with a particular transference has been established, and the therapist has an intimate familiarity with the individual's history. The patient's entrance into the group, however, always expands understanding of the patient's inner psychological mechanisms because the therapist can observe the patient's interactions with others. Within the group, different personalities will interact with the patient and evoke different aspects of the transference. Significantly, the therapy has moved from the relative safety of the dyad to the anxiety-generating atmosphere of the group, with its potential for evoking competitiveness and jealousy. When the therapist is dealing with a caregiver and infant, this group context may have added benefits. The therapist is able to compare the infant's development and interactional style with those of other infants and to observe first-hand how the caregiver responds to other mothers in similar situations. These other mother–infant pairs also serve as models who motivate the caregiver to overcome her own deficiencies of interaction with her infant.

Alonso and Rutan propose, though, that in cases where the intensity of the transference is counterproductive, as is the case with some patients who feel vulnerable and exposed in the therapeutic environment, it may be beneficial to offer a different group therapist as a target for transference. Additionally, a very vulnerable patient may be unable to tolerate sharing the individual therapist in a group and this will jeopardize the treatment. Other issues that arise if both individual and group formats are used include the problem of privacy versus secrecy, the ability of the patient to leave one format and maintain the other, and the problem of "acting-out" behaviors in one format. Privacy versus secrecy refers to whether intimate disclosures given in the individual format may also be disclosed in the group format. The therapist who contemplates treating a patient in both formats should discuss this issue with the patient thoroughly before commencing group therapy. For patients whose treatment may be jeopardized, different therapists may be advisable for the individual and group formats. Another reason for using different therapists in the individual and group formats— especially therapists of different genders—is to activate a range of transference-related affects and fantasies.

Another issue that relates to the combined format is whether the individual and group therapy should occur simultaneously or sequentially. Some patients will experience a strong bond with the therapist in individual treatment which in itself represents an aspect of the transference relationship. By beginning group therapy later, these patients may experience loss or rejection, as if the individual therapist is somehow displeased with them. On the other hand, patients whose transference with the individual therapist is overly intense may benefit from diffusing this intensity in a subsequent group experience. The therapist must therefore carefully evaluate the patient's status before recommending the appropriate format.

Amaranto and Bender (1990) have advocated another format of combined therapy, in which the individual therapy is used as an adjunct to the group therapy. This model consists of once-a-week group therapy sessions lasting for 110 minutes and weekly individual sessions of 50 minutes. Patients who adapted well to this format and demonstrated progress in treatment included those who had initially reported interpersonal problems as a catalyst to entering therapy and those who had at least a minimal understanding of psychological functioning. In addition, those patients with strong motivation for changing their behavior also did well. It is worth keeping these criteria in mind when determining whether a caregiver and infant would benefit from a combined treatment regimen.

COMBINED FAMILY THERAPY AND GROUP THERAPY

Combining family therapy with group therapy can also provide further valuable insight for the therapist working with caregiver–infant dyads. In adapting these techniques to the dyadic treatment, it is advisable to keep in mind that any conflict between the caregivers is likely to have repercussions on the infant. In fact, whether the caregiver is receiving treatment individually with the infant, in a group, or in the context of a family setting, the significance of this message cannot be underscored enough. Moreover, helping the caregiver to understand the conflicts of her own childhood and to recognize how these conflicts are reenacted during interactive sequences with the infant is a vital form of intervention. The all-encompassing philosophy of group and family principles, then, can be incorporated into a model of dyadic treatment in order to achieve optimal interaction between infant and caregiver and to replicate such behavior within the home environment.

Brief family interventions can be beneficial within the group dyadic milieu. For example, Breit, Im, and Wilner (1983) have reported that brief therapy, consisting of 10 sessions that utilize a variety of treatment strategies, often helps dysfunctional families. It is necessary to monitor these strategies carefully because the caregiver's interactions with the infant can have an enduring effect on family life and the relationships among family members. *Reframing* is one technique that these researchers recommend. This strategy requires giving the patient another perspective for viewing certain behavior. For example, one caregiver in group treatment was particularly depressed because she viewed her infant's weaning behavior as a rejection of her nurturing. When the other caregivers in the group persuaded the caregiver that the infant had not rejected her but was rather seeking to acquire a new sense of independence and mastery, the caregiver was able to view the weaning with less trepidation. Another technique these researchers advocate as a further strategy for dramatically modifying dysfunctional behavior is *role-playing*. This technique is particularly advantageous for caregivers of new infants because it heightens their sensitivity to the infant's perceptions as well as to the perceptions of spouses and other family members. The group members and the therapist can then discuss the effect of these interventions.

TERMINATION

Ascertaining when group members are ready to leave treatment can be a formidable task. The therapist, nevertheless, should be alert to some key phenomena. Has the caregiver acquired a terminology to describe the infant's development objectively? Has she enhanced her skills in perceiving reality from the infant's point of view, in terms of somatic, socio-affective, cognitive, and motivational awareness? Does the caregiver share her perceptions freely with other group members? Is she optimistic about the infant's future? Has the caregiver learned to represent and preview imminent developmental change and to integrate such skills into her daily routine? Most significantly, has she been able to resolve any conflicts aroused by the infant's imminent separation as a consequence of developmental growth? Finally, do the caregiver's responses to the infant's perceptions promote and enhance optimal development and facilitate the adaptive previewing of imminent maturational change?

If the therapist can answer these questions affirmatively and observes frequent episodes of adaptive interaction within the dyad, then more likely than not it is appropriate to terminate the therapy if the caregiver concurs. Caregivers who want to continue the sessions should be encouraged to do so.

CONCLUSION

Clearly, the phenomena of interaction that emerge during group therapy are particularly useful for fostering the goals of dyadic therapy. Each dyad, in and of itself, represents a paradigm of interpersonal exchange and of a distinctive relationship. As a consequence, whether the therapist is treating an individual dyad or several dyads in a group format, he or she should be familiar with the advantages of techniques offered by the group and family treatment models. The group format presents both caregivers and therapists with many models of interaction to use for experimentation, for the exploration of conflict, and for the sharing of common experiences.

In addition, the therapist should use the dyad's replication of familial behavior patterns to diagnose domains of familial conflict. Because the infant is present during these sessions, it is also possible to institute modeling techniques that offer caregivers a palpable example of how to enhance interaction with the infant. The presence of other caregivers who have undergone similar experiences with their infants serves to inspire group members, motivating them to resolve interpersonal conflict with the infant adaptively. This feature of the group dynamic also stimulates the caregiver's previewing capacities, by introducing her to the full panorama of developmental growth during the years of infancy and by establishing that the ability to predict growth in her infant can facilitate the adaptive emergence of such behaviors, resulting in enhanced intimacy between mother and infant. Indeed, by seeing how other caregivers preview and by learning how they overcame problems or conflicts stemming from developmental growth and the changing relationship with the infant, caregivers receive encouragement to construct their own style of adaptive interaction under the guidance and support of the therapist.

Chapter 17

Applying the Principles of Short-Term Psychotherapy to Dyadic Intervention

INTRODUCTION

Psychotherapy has undergone a dramatic transformation in the past few decades that has resulted in innovative diagnostic and intervention techniques, as well as in a changed perception of the therapist's role. Traditionally, the psychotherapeutic approach mandated that treatment would last for an indeterminate period. The therapist's role was that of a neutral observer who witnessed the patient's gradual recognition and resolution of conflict. In turn, the patient was expected to be ruminative, painstakingly working through layers of resistance to expose and ultimately resolve conflict. But in recent years a new, more pragmatic approach has advocated effecting alterations in the patient's interactional patterns in a relatively brief period. Moreover, the therapist's role has changed; it is now proposed that rather than function as a nonintrusive recipient of the patient's disclosures, the therapist become a more active participant in the treatment.

These new attitudes toward psychotherapy are embodied in the model of *short-term* treatment that has been reported on in the literature with increased frequency. The short-term model is distinctive in several respects. First, the model recommends rigorous patient selection. Patients who are suitable for this form of treatment should possess the following characteristics: a high degree of insight into their own behavior patterns, a mature ego structure, motivation to change, the ability to withstand criticism, and a specific and circumscribed problem involving interpersonal issues. In contrast to patients who require long-term treatment, candidates for the short-term approach need not reconstruct their entire history. Rather, these patients will benefit from subjecting only *discrete areas* of past experience to analysis. Patient selection is also crucial in the short-term model because the patient must be capable of recognizing that the treatment will terminate within a specific time frame.

A second feature of the short-term approach is its *pragmatic orientation*. The emphasis on specific and discernible changes in behavior patterns is exemplified by "plan of action" or "task implementation" techniques. Task implementation requires the patient, with the guidance of the therapist, to develop pragmatic schemes of action for accomplishment prior to the next session. Self-defeating behavior patterns must be replaced with more adaptive strategies within the limited time imposed by the model.

The short-term approach also recommends an aggressive stance for handling patient *resistance*. In this regard, the therapist addresses resistance immediately after it surfaces. Although the therapist remains highly empathic and supportive of the patient's needs, issues of resistance are pursued with vigor, so that the patient confronts the resistance and overcomes it quickly. This pragmatic, almost "no-nonsense" approach to patient defense structure distinguishes the short-term model from traditional models that rely on such techniques as free association.

Despite its apparent break with tradition, on closer examination the short-term model shares many roots with traditional psychotherapy and, in particular, views patient conflict as being *developmental* in origin. Conflict becomes manifest at a particular stage of the patient's development. One goal of short-term psychotherapy is to determine at which period of development the patient encountered conflict. Advocates of the short-term approach have noted that the patient must reenact earlier stages of development to catalyze the emergence and resolution of conflict. Moreover, as the termination of treatment nears, the primary issue revolves around ending the treatment and separating from the therapist, an issue reminiscent of the patient's earlier separation experiences. Thus, short-term psychotherapy shares a goal with more traditional techniques—the evocation and ultimate resolution of developmental conflict.

As a result of the emphasis of short-term psychotherapy on the developmental roots of conflict, the application of *previewing* principles to this model may be beneficial. Moreover, previewing strategies may be especially advantageous when the treatment involves a caregiver–infant dyad. As has been discussed, previewing in the dyadic relationship helps the infant to predict developmental change and to achieve new skills that result in control and mastery over both internally experienced demands and external challenges. The mother's empathic role when introducing the infant to these trends reinforces the dyadic rapport, such that the infant comes to view dyadic change as an arena from which he can relate to others in an adaptive manner. Previewing also validates infant expectation that the caregiver will manifest continuity between her past, present, and future interactions, and will remain a supportive and nurturing partner. Because both the short-term model and the previewing paradigm between caregiver and infant emphasize pragmatic and adaptive change, the application of previewing principles to this form of treatment will likely result in a highly compatible match.

This chapter discusses the application of previewing to enhance the short-term model of psychotherapy, particularly when treatment involves a caregiver–infant dyad. Subsequently, a case history involving a caregiver and infant illustrates the use of previewing techniques during short-term treatment.

THE TECHNIQUES OF SHORT-TERM PSYCHOTHERAPY

As its name suggests, short-term psychotherapy differs from other forms of intervention because treatment lasts for a relatively brief and circumscribed period. The brief duration of the treatment requires using rigorous patient selection and adopting assertive intervention strategies to expedite the emergence of adaptive behavior patterns. In keeping with these more aggressive therapeutic strategies, the therapist assumes an assertive role in motivating new behavior and challenging ingrained patterns and resistances. Nevertheless, this form of treatment also requires the therapist to show substantial empathy in supporting the patient as she confronts and resolves conflict.

Patient Selection

Rigorous patient selection criteria are essential. As with traditional forms of treatment, the premise of the short-term model is that the patient's problem stems from developmental conflict. Mann (1973) comments that the treatment rests on the substantive base of the patient's early life separation–individuation crisis. Gustafson and Dichter (1983a, 1983b) refer to conflict as the "unsolved family problem," and Davanloo (1986) speaks of the patient's long-forgotten conflict.

To access conflict from a developmental point of view most efficaciously, the short-term model seeks patients with high levels of ego adaptation, the ability to become actively engaged in the therapeutic process, and a strong motivation for change (Alexander & French, 1946). Short-term candidates have a circumscribed chief complaint, the capacity to interact flexibly with the therapist, and the ability to express emotions candidly (Sifneos, 1972). Moreover, they should have the capacity to understand the psychological roots of problems, to respond positively to criticism and interpretation, and to withstand the anxiety aroused by the intensity of this form of treatment (Malan, 1979, 1986).

Because the treatment is so intense, Mann (1973) and Mann and Godlman (1982) caution that the therapist should select patients who either do not resort to resistance or are able of recognizing and overcoming resistance rapidly. Moreover, the patient should be able to negotiate the termination of the therapeutic relationship. Davanloo (1984, 1986), who views the short-term approach as a means of unlocking the unconscious and providing a direct view of the multifocal core of neurotic structure, stresses that the therapist should assess ego functioning, affective regulation, and the quality of the patient's relationships before accepting a patient for this form of treatment.

Moreover, short-term psychotherapy is not recommended for patients suffering from certain disorders; for example, borderline personalities, whose complex defensive operations (e.g., splitting, primitive idealization, devaluation) may require a long-term approach to work through structural conflict. Similarly, patients with separation anxiety, psychotic episodes, or suicidal tendencies are inappropriate candidates because of their need for a long-term relationship with the therapist (Gustafson, Dichter, & Kaye, 1983). The ideal psychological profile of a short-term patient describes a highly motivated individual capable of understanding the origins of his or her conflict, of withstanding rigorous and critical scrutiny of behavior, and of being able to expose interpersonal problems.

The prime reason for these stringent criteria is that intensive therapeutic work must occur in a relatively short period. To expedite the resolution of conflict, the therapist must promote a rapid rapport and therapeutic alliance, and transference feelings must be interpreted as soon as they surface. In essence, the therapist will be actively pursuing and confronting the patient, occasionally to the point of anger. According to Malan (1979), this active pursuit leads to the disclosure of the patient's true feelings and the eventual resolution of conflict.

The Therapist's Empathic Approach

The emblematic technique used in short-term psychotherapy is the rigorous handling of the patient's resistance. To help the patient withstand this intervention, the therapist must instill an *empathic* atmosphere early in the treatment. Malan (1986) and Rosenberg (1988) have emphasized that the emergence of transference feelings should be interpreted early during the short-term process and that an effort should be made to relate these feelings to the patient's relationship with the parents. Because of the rigorous nature of these techniques, the therapist must use every opportunity to sustain an empathic relationship with the patient.

Sifneos (1972) has developed a short-term model that relies on forced choice questions, the therapist's rapid interpretation of transference reactions, active confrontation with conflict rooted in childhood, and the continual pointing out of neurotic behavior patterns. This assertive protocol requires establishing a durable rapport with the patient from the outset of treatment. Mann (1973) and Mann and Godlman (1982) recommend that the therapist continually use empathy and support to encourage the patient.

The empathic attitude that short-term psychotherapy requires of the therapist may best be described as aggressive or "tough." Gustafson, Dichter, and Kaye (1983) have characterized the short-term approach as having a "loaded beginning," in the sense that once the patient enters the treatment, assertive strategies begin to overcome resistance. These theorists caution, however, that the active pursuit of the patient's resistance must be tempered with an equally active degree of empathy that convinces the patient of the therapist's consistent support. In other words, the therapist must maintain a delicate balance between active pursuit of the patient's resistance and the provision of a supportive and nurturing environment.

Plan of Action Implementation

Another distinctive quality of short-term psychotherapy is *plan of action implementation*. This technique involves assigning specific tasks that the patient must complete by the next session. Often the short-term approach focuses on a particular problem that the patient has deemed as being crucial. The therapist and patient then collaborate on a strategy for resolving the problem. For example, the therapist would assist the patient in generating and evaluating alternative courses of action for handling conflict-laden episodes likely to occur in the imminent future. The patient would be asked to implement one such plan by the next session. Although the therapist may occasionally suggest or assign tasks, the goal is to help the patient conceive problem-solving methods, develop alternatives, and enact these strategies during future interactions.

A specific plan of action is then articulated. In some instances, the plan may be very specific, whereas in other cases the plan may be open and flexible. Regardless of the structure, however, it is vital that the patient understand the plan, predict its outcome, and express a commitment to its implementation. The patient's ability to predict the outcome is especially important here, because both patient and therapist can subsequently evaluate the patient's skill in formulating and achieving an adaptive resolution for conflict. As a result, unilateral directives by the therapist should be avoided. When tasks involve anxiety-provoking behaviors, practice sessions or rehearsals may be necessary. Helping the patient preview future obstacles that are likely to interfere with task performance is also helpful.

At the beginning of each session, there should be a review of the patient's progress, covering developments in the problem and describing the accomplished tasks. If the patient has completed a task, the therapist may formulate another task with the patient concerning either the same or a different problem. If the task has not been successfully completed, the patient and therapist should discuss obstacles and devise a different plan for achieving the task. In some cases they may reformulate the task or the problem itself.

According to Reid (1990), during the review of tasks, obstacles to achievement often emerge in the patient's narrative. Although obstacles block progress, resources facilitate it. Resources include the strengths and competencies of the patient, significant relationships in the patient's life, and the patient's social support systems. The therapist helps the patient identify and resolve obstacles, as well as locate and utilize resources. In addition, during a task implementation report, the therapist assists the patient in modifying distorted perceptions and unrealistic expectations. Maladaptive interpersonal patterns may be clarified through the development of new predictions and strategies for a more adaptive outcome.

The Realignment of Behavior Patterns

The temporal limitations of short-term psychotherapy force the patient to recognize that the sessions will eventually end, that the relationship with the therapist will be terminated, and that the results of therapy will be evaluated within a specific amount of time. Moreover, to be successful, the treatment must not only resolve the patient's symptoms but also replace maladaptive interpersonal patterns with adaptive patterns. By the time of termination, the patient should possess both cognitive and emotional insight into the structure of the conflict that motivated the entrance into therapy. Beyond this, the patient should now possess some practical strategies for overcoming future problems.

Essentially, this means that during the relatively short duration of the treatment, the patient should learn new strategies for engaging in more adaptive interactional patterns and should understand why old patterns of interaction were unsuccessful. This result requires relinquishing old models of interaction based on flawed developmental patterns and replacing them with new models of interaction that enable the patient to deal more adaptively with conflict.

Pursuing the Resistance

The rigorous management and eventual surmounting of the patient's resistance has become emblematic of short-term psychotherapy. Davanloo (1984) comments that overcoming the patient's resistance is the sine qua non of the short-term approach and recommends that the therapist's assertive behavior focus on challenging the signs of resistance as soon as they surface. In addition, Davanloo (1989) has referred to this approach as achieving a "head-on collision" with the transference resistance. According to Davanloo, the therapist first mobilizes the therapeutic alliance and then maximizes the tension between the alliance and the patient's resistance. For Davanloo, short-term therapy has two phases—the *preinterpretive* phase, when the therapist interprets the patient's resistance, and the *interpretive* phase, which begins when the resistances are overcome and the therapeutic alliance is activated. Moreover, the therapist works on two psychological triangles of the patient—the triangle of conflict and the triangle of the person. The triangle of conflict refers to the patient's impulses, anxieties, and defenses, whereas the triangle of the person alludes to the source of the conflict in the patient's intrapsychic structure. For example, in exploring conflict, the therapist would identify significant persons from the patient's past with whom unresolved conflict existed and significant persons in the patient's current life with whom these conflicts are being contemporaneously reenacted.

Davanloo's techniques for challenging the patient's resistances are representative of those used in short-term psychotherapy. Initially, Davanloo recommends rapid identification and clarification of the patient's defenses. Next, the therapist applies pressure to the patient's experience of impulses and strong emotions, by questioning the patient about the presence and meaning of these emotions. As a result of this tactic, the patient may experience a surge of transferential feelings along with an intensification of resistance. Eventually, Davanloo comments, a direct collision occurs between the transference resistance and the transference feelings. The patient may then experience anger at the therapist, which, in turn, unlocks the unconscious. This systematic interpretation of the transference continues until the patient's resistance abates and entry into the unconscious is achieved (Davanloo, 1989).

SHORT-TERM PSYCHOTHERAPY INVOLVING CAREGIVER–INFANT DYADS

The short-term model may be particularly beneficial for mother–infant dyads seeking treatment. As a preliminary matter, the rapid pace of developmental processes calls for treatment protocols capable of yielding insights into the dynamics that affect the mother–infant relationship sooner rather than later. Provided the caregiver is an appropriate candidate for the short-term approach, this format may be the preferred method of treatment because of its limited duration.

The short-term model may be particularly useful in the dyadic context because it emphasizes changes in behaviors in an ongoing intimate relationship that is often the centerpiece of the patient's life. Cramer and Stern (1988) reported on one such case that explored the correlations between the mental representations or subjective descriptions of the mother and her behavioral displays toward her infant. The researchers noted that three processes occur during this form of treatment involving mothers and their newborns. First, through the mother's description of her infant's symptoms and their meaning to her, the therapist perceives interactional patterns that reveal conflicts and anxieties. Second, these configurations are related to the mother's past and current history and to her own repressed unconscious conflicts. Third, when the mother has liberated her mental representations of the infant from these interfering representations from her own history, new paths for growth and development become available to both mother and infant.

Cramer and Stern (1988) also report on a case in which the caregiver and infant seemed to be continually engaged in a physical struggle. After a few initial sessions, the therapists became convinced that the conflicted behavior stemmed from the mother's own conflicts during her childhood. This caregiver had been sickly and had undergone several painful operations in her youth. She had come to associate physical touch with pain and avoided unnecessary contact with her infant by thrusting him away from her, a response that led the infant to experience frustration and to respond with distress. After several sessions during which the caregiver described her representations of the infant and the therapist modeled appropriate holding behaviors for the mother, she began to modify her actions and was able to acknowledge that some of her own behaviors may have caused the infant's unmanageable physical manifestations.

The researchers noted that the focus of their treatment was limited to representational themes that were clearly relevant to the mother–infant relationship or to the infant's symptoms. According to Cramer and Stern, the mother has a representational world that embodies numerous conflictual themes from her past and present life, such as "I am not loved" or "I am not lovable because . . ." These representational themes, composed of specific generalized memories and expectations, originate at many points in the mother's life, beginning with her own childhood. If these representational themes become activated, the theme is enacted and reexperienced in the specific actions and perceptions that make up the mother–infant interaction. In this fashion, the caregiver converts the themes into interactive behavioral patterns. The therapist must first identify those themes in the mother's life history that form conflicted memories and expectations. Next, the therapist must interpret how the theme has infiltrated the parent–child content. Cramer and Stern then recommend that the therapist, through observation and inquiry, determine how the mother enacts the theme during her interaction with the infant. Enactment, according to Cramer and Stern, refers to the caregiver's actions toward and responses to the infant with attributed meanings that emanate from the caregiver's representations disclosed in treatment.

The short-term approach used by Cramer and Stern during dyadic therapy represents a technique that may be applied to many caregivers who seek treatment for a particular problem with the infant. Often this circumscribed problem emanates not from the caregiver–infant interaction per se, but rather from some earlier caregiver conflict that is being transferred to the interaction with the infant. In such cases the therapist should focus the caregiver on her representations and subjective perceptions of the infant to discern patterns that may suggest a past conflict. In addition, the therapist should attempt previewing exercises with the caregiver and encourage her to express her subjective insights about the infant's growth. By combining Cramer and Stern's representational approach with previewing exercises, the therapist is apt to discern in a relatively short period any potential or actual conflict that threatens dyadic interaction.

Moreover, other aspects of the short-term approach are also compatible with the status and psychological position of the new mother. For example, much of the new mother's daily routine will focus on interpersonal activities with the infant. The short-term model advocates that problem-solving occurs within the patient's interactional arena. As a result, the plan-of-action implementations that are a seminal part of the short-term technique may actually take place during sessions as the mother enacts behavioral sequences with the infant. In addition, the element of empathy between caregiver and infant can be related to the empathic approach of the therapist during short-term treatment. In cases where the caregiver already shares an empathic relationship with the infant, this base can rapidly solidify a rapport with the therapist; in cases where the caregiver lacks empathy with her infant, the therapist can help the mother establish this bond of affection by emulating with the infant the empathic atmosphere that prevails in the therapeutic alliance. Short-term therapy places the patient in a supportive interactional relationship with the therapist, analogous to the relationship between mother and infant, that enables the rapid development of strategies for exploring and dealing with conflict.

Perhaps the most compelling parallel that can be drawn between short-term techniques and dyadic intervention, however, concerns the caregiver's resistance. The short-term approach, as noted earlier, adopts an active and rigorous posture when attempting to overcome resistance. The therapist questions the patient repeatedly, points out instances of resistance, and requires the patient to confront and overcome the resistance. The method is highly interactional and achieves rapid behavioral changes. Similarly, dyadic treatment focuses attention on the relationship between caregiver and infant and attempts to effect change in the caregiver's approach that she can immediately transfer to her interactions with the infant.

The final premise of short-term psychotherapy is that the patient's conflict is developmental in origin. Although the conflict may not be as pervasive as the type encountered in patients more suited to long-term treatment (e.g., personality disorders), it is present nonetheless and may be viewed as deriving from the patient's early life experience. As a result, the developmental principles used during dyadic therapy are particularly compatible with the strategies of short-term psychotherapy. Both forms of treatment seek patients who are motivated to change and are receptive to techniques that require the representation of upcoming interactions, the anticipation of interpersonal behavior during these episodes, and the formulation of an adaptive outcome.

In general terms, previewing conveys to the infant that the caregiver's supportive ministrations will help him master future developmental change. These changes relate to discrete developmental skills and are often very specific. In fact, they resemble the circumscribed conflicts confronting patients in short-term psychotherapy.

Previewing strategies complement the techniques of short-term psychotherapy in four specific ways:

1. The previewing process provides opportunities for diagnosing conflict more rapidly than is possible with traditional techniques and thus is allied with the technique of rigorously handling the patient's defenses and resistances.

2. Previewing strategies result in interpersonal manifestations that are compatible with the task implementation methods of short-term treatment.

3. Previewing techniques provide the infant with skills for coping adaptively with upcoming change and therefore coincide with the short-term goal of helping the patient realign internal structures. As an example, short-term treatment teaches patients pragmatic skills for predicting future behavior in order to avoid conflict.

4. The empathy encountered during previewing can be used analogously by the therapist engaged in short-term treatment to foster a therapeutic alliance.

Previewing and Resistance

How does previewing facilitate overcoming resistance during short-term treatment? Previewing adopts a *prospective* approach. If the caregiver cannot predict the future, conflict is probably impeding the representation of imminent events. It is necessary to work through this conflict before the caregiver can predict and subsequently rehearse imminent development with the infant.

Previewing techniques perform a similar diagnostic function during therapy. Short-term therapy requires that the patient be able to describe the problem that precipitated the need for therapy. Thereafter, the therapist explains the process of *representation* to the patient and asks the patient to engage in a series of representations concerning upcoming events. Representation here refers to the patient's internal imagery about life events and incorporates her full emotional experience. When the patient is unable to formulate such representations, it is likely that conflict is present and is interfering with the ability to formulate images.

As noted earlier, short-term therapy relies on a rigorous handling of patient resistance and confrontational techniques to overcome defenses. Traditional retrospective techniques that mandate an examination of the patient's past are more likely to evoke defensive operations. In contrast, previewing techniques defuse the power of the defenses by continually motivating the patient to represent future experiences. Because these representations involve future events, the patient is free to explore in an arena that has not yet been contaminated by the defenses. Moreover, because the level of resistance is lower when the patient previews, the therapist can adopt more assertive strategies than would be the case with retrospective techniques. Thus, the therapist's role is analogous to that of the caregiver who motivates the infant to explore imminent developmental events through previewing exercises. Previewing also helps the therapist delineate the scope of the patient's interpersonal patterns. These patterns emerge because the kinds of experience being predicted have not yet been subjected to the defensive operations. For the therapist engaging in short-term therapy, then, previewing offers a dynamic method of diagnosing and clarifying the patient's conflict, as well as a strategy for using the patient's inherent motivation for change.

Previewing and Plan of Action Implementation

Once the nature of the patient's conflict has been identified, the working-through phase of treatment begins. In short-term therapy, however, pragmatic plans of action designed to be implemented, rather than intensive retrospective analysis, characterize the working-through phase. For example, the therapist will ask the patient to devise specific tasks for enactment before the next session. After the patient and therapist have decided on a task, the patient will be asked to represent alternative plans of action for achieving that particular goal.

Task implementation is reminiscent of the caregiver–infant previewing process. During the initial stages of previewing, the caregiver represents imminent developmental milestones the infant will soon achieve. Subsequently, the caregiver devises behaviors to enact with the infant that help him experience the developmental event in an adaptive fashion. The caregiver selects the most suitable action for sharing imminent change with the infant.

The process the caregiver undergoes in preparing and implementing a previewing exercise for the infant resembles the process of developing a plan of action during short-term psychotherapy. In fact, the therapist can borrow facets of the previewing process to help the patient formulate and implement a task. For example, during previewing, the representation of an upcoming event or experience is essential for introducing the infant to a new developmental milestone. Similarly, during short-term treatment, the patient can use representation to achieve a plan of action strategy. Thus, the patient should be encouraged to use representational skills to predict future interpersonal outcome and to anticipate the effect of these actions on the relationship with others. Subsequently, the patient should formulate alternative strategies for enacting the plan. In discussing these possibilities with the patient, the therapist should focus on alternatives that are most likely to achieve the immediate goal in a psychologically adaptive manner. The patient should also be encouraged to predict several scenarios for the upcoming event and the implications of each scenario, just as the caregiver who formulates previewing exercises for the infant envisions how future behavior will affect the infant in terms of his social, cognitive, emotional, and physiological experience. As a result, applying previewing to the task-implementation aspect of short-term therapy is likely to enhance the results of the treatment.

Previewing and the Realignment of Behavior Patterns

Because short-term treatment is so brief, it is essential that the patient leave therapy with a repertoire of skills for overcoming future conflict and engaging adaptively in interpersonal relationships. The techniques of caregiver–infant previewing provide a useful paradigm for helping the patient to relinquish old behavior patterns and formulate new ones.

During previewing exercises, the caregiver represents and predicts the contours of imminent developmental change for the infant. In turn, the infant internalizes these predictions of imminent developmental change and eventually begins to coordinate developmental achievement on his own. At that point, the caregiver's predictions have been confirmed because the infant has incorporated this model of predictive ability.

Previewing strategies can achieve a similar function in short-term psychotherapy. These strategies teach the patient how to predict upcoming events and experiences and subsequently enable her to test the accuracy of the predictions during implementation exercises. By reviewing the results of the plan of action and the degree to which the patient has accurately predicted outcome, the therapist validates the patient's experience. With practice, the patient will eventually develop models of adaptive interaction that replace maladaptive ones. Moreover, previewing fosters the ability to develop behavioral alternatives and to evaluate which alternatives will best achieve adaptive goals. Thus, the application of previewing techniques to the process of short-term psychotherapy enables the patient to complete treatment with a repertoire of adaptive skills for dealing with future conflict and formulating adaptive models.

Previewing and Empathy

Previewing strategies incorporate a particular form of empathic exchange that is compatible with the model of short-term psychotherapy. The caregiver's acute sensitivity to the infant's developmental trends enables her to determine an appropriate time for introducing the infant to a previewing episode and acquainting him with imminent developmental change. At the same time, however, adaptive caregivers are also sensitive to signals that the infant wishes to cease the previewing activity and return to his earlier level of mastery.

Sensitivity to behavioral and affective rhythms resembles, in a number of respects, the empathic sensitivity demonstrated by the therapist engaged in short-term psychotherapy. As Gustafson, Dichter, and Kaye (1983) have noted, the therapist involved in short-term treatment must be attuned both to the "dangers of activity" that occur when the treatment attempts to overcome the patient's resistance too rigorously and to the "dangers of passivity" that enable the patient to procrastinate and impede progress with defensive operations. Malan (1979) has characterized the empathic attitude of the therapist during short-term treatment by noting that the therapist must continually predict the themes and direction of the treatment. At the same time, Malan cautions that the therapist must nurture the patient by monitoring the effect of interpretations and of the patient's behavior outside sessions. This pattern of sustained monitoring resembles the astute observational skill the caregiver uses for previewing exercises with the infant, and so the therapist engaged in short-term treatment should utilize the previewing model of empathy. Sensitivity to patient cues will indicate when the patient is ready for an active assault on resistance and when it is appropriate to adopt a more supportive, less confrontational stance.

Previewing and the Countertransference

Just as the therapeutic encounter awakens transference feelings in the patient, so too does traditional psychotherapy posit that the patient will evoke a countertransference response in the therapist. Traditional treatment has taken the position that the therapist should serve as a neutral recipient of the patient's narrative and that countertransference feelings should be eliminated either through self-analysis or more formal therapy (Epstein & Feiner, 1979).

Perhaps because the therapist adopts a more assertive role in short-term psychotherapy, this model of treatment has often ignored the countertransference or has emphasized its negative aspects. These aspects include interference with rapport and motivation for treatment (Davanloo, 1978) and obstruction of therapeutic focusing (Malan, 1979). Binder, Strupp, and Schacht (1983), however, have suggested that the countertransference warrants more attention in short-term therapy.

In this regard, it may be helpful to turn to the previewing model. Previewing requires that the caregiver be continually vigilant to the infant's rhythms and simultaneously share her perceptions so that a mutual goal-oriented partnership emerges, enabling both dyadic members to achieve the full benefits of developmental progress. This model may also be applied to short-term psychotherapy. During short-term treatment the therapist not only must be attuned to the patient's needs but also must analyze countertransference feelings so that his own emotions do not interfere with the treatment process. Unless this procedure is followed, it will be difficult to establish the intensive rapport essential for progress in the short-term model.

CASE HISTORY

The following case history illustrates the application of short-term psychotherapy to the treatment of a mother and infant. Both caregiver and therapist "contracted" during their first meeting to limit the treatment to ten weekly sessions. The caregiver's focal complaint on entering into treatment was her concern that her infant son had been "damaged" during the process of delivery.

Laura G was a 37-year-old mother. Her 14-month-old son, Teddy, was her first child. Laura had been referred to treatment by Teddy's pediatrician for an evaluation of possible hyperactivity. During the first session, Laura described her son as being "tense" and "different from other children." She confided to the therapist that she feared his hyperactive behavior might be due to some "brain damage" he had suffered at birth, but then she noted that she knew her concerns were just "silly" because the doctors had given Teddy a clean bill of health. In addition, she told the therapist that she wished her husband, Clark, would be more responsive to her concerns.

The therapist reminded Laura that the short-term model would require her to examine all facets of her problem, including her own possible contribution to her son's behavior. The therapist also noted that Laura would have to be willing to examine rigorously her own motivations in having a "damaged" son and to explore the effects of Teddy's behavior on her relationship with her husband. When the therapist asked Laura if she was willing to undergo this intensive psychological scrutiny, she agreed to work hard to get to the root of her problem because she sensed that she had somehow provoked many of her family's maladaptive behaviors. She also expressed an understanding that this process of examination might, at times, be emotionally painful.

During the next few sessions, the therapist asked Laura to explain her concerns about her son. Why did she have the impression that he was somehow damaged? Laura began by saying that her own mother had yelled at her "all the time" and that consequently she wanted to "be a better mother for Teddy than my own mother was for me." Apparently, Laura meant that she was concerned about meeting Teddy's needs in an adaptive manner that contrasted with her own mother's behavior when she was growing up. Laura's attitude was reflected in the overly enmeshed relationship she had with her son. She said she sometimes felt that Teddy had received less than optimal care at his delivery and that, as a result, she felt a strong sense of identification with her son. Laura's belief that her son was damaged was also bolstered by her fear that an abortion she had had in college might have compromised her ability to bear children. She and Clark had experienced difficulty when Laura had attempted to conceive, and she had had two prior miscarriages. Nonetheless, Laura was also able to concede that many of her fears regarding her son's health lacked a medical basis.

In fact, Teddy had experienced some medical complications at the time of his delivery. There was meconium-stained amniotic fluid, and it was necessary to suction the baby. Within 6 hours after the birth, rapid respiration had been noted and he had been transferred to an intensive care nursery. Teddy was placed on pure oxygen for a short period of time and given antibiotics. However, after being weaned from the oxygen and discharged from the hospital within 8 days of his birth, Teddy experienced no other physical ailments. During his first year of life, his pediatrician reported him to be in good health.

During these first sessions, the therapist carefully monitored Laura's behavior during interaction with Teddy. Laura appeared attuned to her infant's needs, anticipating his desire for feeding, play episodes, and rest times. During play episodes, she interacted with him affectionately. Nevertheless, she appeared uneasy when Teddy interacted with the therapist and seemed reluctant to encourage the infant's exploratory activities. Teddy manifested age-appropriate fine and gross motor and language skills, but his reactions seemed overly intense, his attention span low, his distractibility high, and his ability to contend with new stimuli minimal. He would only play with the therapist if his mother joined in the game. Laura, however, failed to act as a supportive partner encouraging Teddy's development because each developmental gain made her doubt her belief that her son was abnormal. She seemed to cling to the view that he was abnormal because it allowed her to perpetuate her enmeshment with the child.

During these first few sessions, the therapist conveyed empathy for Laura's concerns about her son but simultaneously challenged some of her assumptions in a rigorous manner. For example, after observing Laura's interaction with Teddy, the therapist asked whether transforming the infant into a damaged object would allow Laura to remain close to him. In addition, the therapist suggested that because Laura's own caregiving experience has been less than optimal, perhaps she felt inadequate about her caregiving skills. Saying that Teddy was flawed developmentally enabled Laura to evade her own feelings of inadequacy. "After all," the therapist suggested, "you can just blame it on Teddy." Laura initially protested the therapist's comments but then stopped and lapsed into deep thought. When several minutes had passed, she admitted that the therapist might have made some valid points, but she said she was unable to extricate herself from her behavior patterns. "They have become a sort of convenient habit," she said bitterly.

The therapist then began explaining the techniques of developmental representation to Laura and asked her to focus on some of the positive trends she had observed in Teddy. Initially, Laura professed inability to do this, but as the therapist persisted, she began identifying various developmental achievements Teddy had undergone. The therapist also asked Laura to describe both her own and her husband's responses to these achievements. Laura then began to admit ruefully that she tended to discount Teddy's achievements, whereas her husband was always more enthusiastic and optimistic.

Next, the therapist suggested that Laura attempt to predict some of the upcoming developmental skills that Teddy would soon be manifesting. Initially, Laura was resistant to this suggestion. Her resistance was manifested by an effort to discount what the therapist was saying through laughter, intellectual challenge, and finally anger. As each of these obfuscating tactics emerged, the therapist continued to challenge Laura's motives. Finally, Laura agreed that she would attempt to engage in these representational exercises concerning Teddy's imminent development. Her assignment was to engage in the exercises during the following week and report on her impressions of Teddy's progress at the next session.

The therapist's goal here focused on encouraging the momentum in Laura and Teddy's relationship so as to curtail the enmeshment that threatened to stifle Laura's adaptive behavior. To further disassemble the closely fused bond between mother and infant, the therapist challenged Laura's notions of her son's abnormality. It had become clear to the therapist that Teddy's hyperactive symptoms were due, in part, to Laura's emotional state. During her initial interview Laura had reported that she had brought Teddy to the doctor for a neurological checkup because she believed he was impaired. "I think Teddy is tense because he had such a bad experience at birth with the doctor and nurses. I just want him to relax." Laura grew agitated when she had discussed the "horrible whining sound" Teddy sometimes made and said it reminded her of her own "horrible childhood."

When Laura sometimes recounted these memories during treatment, Teddy's behavior would become frantic; he would race around the room darting from one activity to another, returning frequently to his mother, but never lingering for more than a couple of seconds. However, when Laura became less agitated and spoke more calmly, Teddy began to play more quietly. Noticing this pattern, the therapist pointed out to Laura that Teddy might be picking up on her tension, Laura at first would claim that Teddy's real tension had resulted from his traumatic birth. The therapist, however, would repeat this point and eventually Laura's attitude began to change.

At the next session, Laura was more reflective about the past and its implications for Teddy. She reported that when she, Teddy, and Clark had visited Clark's mother over the weekend, her mother-in-law had lectured the entire time about the necessity for more discipline. "I know her kind of discipline," Laura said. "It's the kind I had when I was a kid and it's not what I want for Teddy." As Laura's voice rose in pitch while discussing the difficulty she was having in setting limits for Teddy, and as she began to imitate Teddy's whine for the therapist, the child ran to her and climbed in her lap. Laura tried to soothe him. At this juncture, the therapist suggested to Laura that her behavior was a perfect example of how Teddy sensed the tension in her voice and had come to her seeking reassurance, and that his so-called hyperactive behavior was actually a response to her own fears about his poor developmental progress despite clear-cut evidence that he was physically normal. Laura nodded, and said she was now coming to recognize that this was the case, given what she had learned from the previous therapy sessions. Meanwhile, Teddy had returned to the toy area to play quietly.

The therapist also used this opportunity to ask Laura how she had progressed with her assignment of representing Teddy's imminent development. Laura then perked up and began explaining how she was predicting aspects of Teddy's speech patterns, which were slowly maturing. Suddenly, however, she paused. Then she said, "It's hard, though, because I feel that to a certain extent his development is out of my hands and that's when I start to feel inadequate." The therapist then began to discuss previewing with Laura, explaining that she could learn to interact with Teddy in such a way as to encourage his skill, while enhancing her own feelings of mastery and guidance over his development. The therapist suggested some previewing enactments concerning speech and requested that Laura attempt these behaviors with Teddy in the coming week.

At subsequent sessions, Laura discussed how Teddy's crying disturbed her because her own mother had cried throughout Laura's childhood. "It's like I am making my baby into my mother," she said. It also became increasingly evident to both Laura and the therapist that her interaction with Teddy was influenced by her relationship with her husband. Laura reported that Clark ignored her fears about Teddy's development. "It really bothers me sometimes," she said. "I wish he would be more concerned." At previous sessions, Teddy had responded to Laura's agitated tone with frantic behaviors and high-pitched vocalizations. However, as the therapist encouraged Laura to vocalize her feelings and reassured her that Teddy's behavior was normal, the child's behavior became more relaxed and his vocalizations were less pressured. At the end of the session, Laura made a visible effort to remain calm, even when discussing some of her frustrations with her husband.

Laura also discussed her attempts at previewing behavior with Teddy. "At first," she said, "it was difficult—it was very scary." But with practice, she had begun to feel a new sense of mastery over her caregiving skills. "I'm starting to focus more on Teddy, and now I recognize so many more aspects of his behaviors. It's really incredible. I also feel closer to him, and I'm starting to be happier about all the new skills he is displaying."

Clark came to the next session with Laura and Teddy. His manner was calm and deliberate. At one point during the session, Laura became irritated with Clark, and her face contorted into a frown. Clark attempted to ignore his wife's anger by playing with his son. Teddy, however, ran back and forth between his mother and father, his agitated vocalizations mimicking his staccato and jerky movements. Finally, as his mother's outburst reached a peak, Teddy ran to his father and buried his head in his lap. He then grabbed and pulled on his father's hand, taking him out into the hall.

After several minutes, when everyone had calmed down considerably, Teddy returned to the room, approached his mother, and took her out into the hall. During this time, Clark reported that Teddy seemed to be developing normally, although he believed Teddy sensed the tension between himself and Laura. When Teddy returned to the room, his parents remained calm for the rest of the session. Teddy also remained calm and played with some toys.

At the next session, Laura explained that she was finally beginning to understand Teddy's sensitivity to her fights with Clark, and as a result both she and Clark were trying to minimize fighting in front of Teddy. Moreover, for the first time Laura agreed with the therapist that Teddy probably had a "difficult" temperament, that his behavior was age appropriate, and that his development was normal.

At the therapist's suggestion, Clark attended the next session. Both parents remained calm while they spoke about how previewing exercises had enhanced their sensitivity to and rapport with their son. They also mentioned some slight anxiety about terminating treatment but said that they hoped the continued use of previewing would result in more optimal family interaction.

During the remaining few therapy sessions, the therapist noted distinct changes in Teddy's and Laura's behavior. Teddy was able to play happily for the duration of the session while both of his parents interacted with the therapist. Laura and Clark also appeared more calm and relaxed. Each expressed an intention to be more optimistic about their marriage and each other. The final session focused more on Laura's marriage than on Teddy, but even when the discussion became slightly tense, Teddy proved capable of dealing with the tension by playing and engaging in positive interactions with his mother during peaceful interludes.

CONCLUSION

This chapter has described a model of short-term psychotherapy and has discussed the application of previewing techniques to this therapeutic model. Because short-term psychotherapy premises the patient's awareness of a developmental conflict, previewing strategies may augment the benefits of the short-term approach in several respects. First, previewing offers the therapist a strategy for diagnosing unresolved conflict at a more preliminary phase of treatment than is offered by traditional diagnostic strategies. The benefits of rapid diagnostic accuracy are of particular advantage because short-term psychotherapy aims to accomplish definitive goals within a limited time. Expediting the diagnosis therefore facilitates the treatment. Second, previewing is also adaptable to the intervention techniques that have become emblematic of short-term psychotherapy, in particular, the vigorous overcoming of the patient's resistance, the subsequent analysis of the transference, confrontational methods, and task or plan-of-action implementation. Previewing fosters competence in the areas of prediction, the formulation of behavioral alternatives, and interpersonal skills, all of which help the patient withstand the rigors of confrontation and engage in plan-of-action implementation. The circumscribed nature of the short-term method dictates that patients leave treatment with an armamentarium of techniques that will enable them to deal with upcoming life events adaptively, devoid of conflict. In this respect as well, previewing behaviors are advantageous, because they provide patients with the skills necessary to represent and devise behaviors for mastering imminent changes. Finally, empathy demonstrated by the caregiver engaged in previewing techniques—an empathy sensitive to cycles of activity and passivity, and based on the infant's needs—is also appropriate to the short-term model. Because short-term treatment is intensive and brief, it is essential that the therapist acclimate rapidly to the patient's ability to withstand confrontation as well as to her needs for rest and passivity. The case history indicated how previewing techniques may be integrated into short-term psychotherapy with a mother and infant.

Chapter 18

Applying the Principles of Social Support to Dyadic Intervention

INTRODUCTION

This chapter addresses the issue of *social support,* a topic that is to a certain extent beyond the usual scope of psychotherapy. Social support is a phrase that is generally associated with such disciplines as sociology, social work, and political science. In the broadest sense, social support is the constellation of services and programs created by society as an interface between the family and society, the parent and society, and the parent and child. Thus, social support encompasses all of those institutions that facilitate the individual's effective integration into society, including schools, hospitals, day care centers, social service agencies run by the government or private sector, and the like. In a more circumscribed sense, however, social support means those social networks that individuals create to provide meaning and guidance in their lives. Social support in this latter sense refers to the cluster of individuals and agencies to which a particular individual turns during times of crisis, stress, or difficulty. All social support systems, whether created by the society or the individual, augment, enhance, or otherwise supplement insufficiencies in family and individual function.

Regardless of the services encompassed, though, many therapists believe that social support remains an area beyond their training and experience. Nevertheless, recent studies have reinforced the notion that individuals manifest increased productivity and adaptation in their lives because of their associations with social services and programs. The adeptness with which an individual forges these social connections and is able to rely on them during times of crisis and upheaval often underscores the degree of psychological health. In addition, individuals who are able to find support from diverse social organizations will be better equipped to weather psychological crises.

The therapist must also recognize that modern society is in a state of rapid and dramatic transition. For example, the configuration of the family has undergone remarkable transformation during the past few decades. We no longer live in a society where one parent functions as an economic provider while the other parent remains at home to care for the children. Instead, the dual-income family, in which both parents work, has become the norm. Accompanying this change has come a pressing need for day care services and other facilities that provide surrogate parenting for children when the parents are absent. Rampant marital separation and divorce have also left their imprints on the modern family. Studies have shown that these events, which irrevocably alter the structure of the family, can leave enduring psychological scars on the children from these homes, who experience feelings of rejection and abandonment long after the actual event has occurred (Einstein, 1985; Goetting, 1985; Pepernow, 1984). Other families confront a readjustment period because of remarriage and the introduction of stepparents and stepsiblings into the family.

These revisions in family structure are compounded further by the social and political events that enter our awareness, sometimes very forcefully, through television and other media. Substance and alcohol abuse, teenage sexual activity, and the pervasive specter of violence in modern life are intrusions that even the most adaptive families must somehow confront.

Given these stark realities, it becomes incumbent upon therapists, particularly those involved in treating caregiver–infant dyads, to gain familiarity with the services offered by *social support networks.* Such familiarity enables the therapist to better respond to the caregiver's needs, particularly those needs that lie beyond the scope of psychotherapy. Moreover, an awareness of social support provides the therapist with access to resources and techniques that can bolster the individual's sense of mastery and competence, and instill feelings of optimism about the future. This chapter acquaints therapists with the concept of social support and describes specific strategies that may be integrated into dyadic therapy to enhance the status of social support.

DEFINING SOCIAL SUPPORT

One reason it is vital for the therapist dealing with dyads to understand the meaning and implications of social support is that research has determined a correlation exists between impaired social support and the incidence of both adult and child psychiatric disorders, particularly depression (Puig-Antich et al., 1985). Other studies have demonstrated that social support promotes health maintenance and prevents disease etiology, suggesting that individuals with stronger and more intact psychological and material resources enjoy better physical health than those with fewer social contacts and less access to support systems (Caplan, 1974; Lin, Dean, & Ensel, 1986). Because research has also demonstrated the high sensitivity of infants to the psychological and physical status of their caregivers, it becomes especially important for therapists to be well versed in methods that bolster access to social support resources. With a thorough knowledge of social support, therapists can offer caregivers further strategies for deterring the debilitating effects that depression and other psychiatric conditions can exert on the dyadic relationship during the first years of life.

In recent years researchers have proposed several definitions of social support. Lin (1986) has been instrumental in providing two general definitions of the concept. The first definition views *social support* as the combination of resources that the community, social networks, and confiding partners offer in terms of perceived and actual support to individuals and families. The degree to which the individual has access to and use of societal resources that reinforce mastery and competence represents that person's level of social support. Dolgoff and Feldstein (1984) adopt a similar definition, observing that social support encompasses the nonprofit facilities available in society that are clearly designed to alleviate distress and poverty or to ameliorate crisis situations. Lin explains that the community represents the individual's broadest type of social relationship, providing the person with a sense of belonging to the greater society. The *social network,* on the other hand, constitutes those more intimate relationships that bind the individual to others through kinship, friendships, and a shared working environment. From this network the individual receives feelings of bonding and unity, enabling him or her to depend on others during times of stress. For example, Tinsley and Parke (1984) have found that extended family relationships, such as ties to grandparents and other relatives, often function as an important support system for parents. The third tier of social support, referred to as *confiding partners,* encompasses relationships that anticipate reciprocal interaction and accept responsibility for the well-being of the other. Individuals can compare their perceptions about infant and child development with these confiding partners as well as learn ways to preview imminent development and the impending changes in their lives that parenthood entails. Under this definition both the objective and subjective dimensions of social support are highly significant to the individual (Caplan, 1979).

When these definitions are combined, it becomes apparent that social support embodies two distinct systems: (a) the social institutions designed to assist individuals in an altruistic fashion; and (b) the interactive patterns of individuals, ranging from the most intimate coupling of husband and wife or mother and infant to the most formal and perfunctory of human relationships. These definitions provide insight into how therapists working with caregiver–infant dyads can become active participants in a caregiver's social support systems and can enhance her ability to deal more effectively with them. On a very fundamental level, the therapist strives to portray a model of adaptive behavior that the caregiver can replicate during interaction with the infant. In particular, the therapist's efforts to promote adaptive previewing behaviors within the dyad help mother and infant to become "confiding partners." In turn, this relational model may be replicated in other relationships, fostering links with social networks and ultimately an adaptive connection to the greater community. The adaptive behaviors that the therapist instills in the caregiver will reverberate into other social arenas and relationships affecting mother and infant. This role in establishing previewing behaviors in the dyad has further implications for social support as well. By engaging in previewing, caregivers enhance their ability to perceive and predict infant development and to respond appropriately to upcoming trends. As a result, the caregiver acquires the sense that she can regulate her relationship with the infant and prepare herself for the future. This enhanced sense of expectation and prediction generates optimism about the upcoming relationship of the dyad, the family, and the ability of family members to function effectively in the society.

On another level, however, the therapist serves as a societal resource for the caregiver during a time of stress and turbulence. As a consequence, the therapist's attitude is likely to exert a strong influence on the caregiver's attitude toward social support services. If she experiences the therapeutic relationship as being predictable, supportive, and encouraging, the caregiver will incorporate these behaviors and come to associate them with the potential benefits of social support resources. Similarly, the therapist's condescension or overly critical approach may not only stifle the development of a transference relationship but can drive the caregiver away from other sources of social support. Therapists must, therefore, continually remember the two roles they are enacting: On one level, therapists are paradigms of adaptive interaction; simultaneously, they serve as symbols of the mental health care system and the services it has to offer the caregiver. By understanding the intricacy of these roles, therapists can better facilitate the emergence of adaptive behavior patterns toward both the infant and society.

THE RELATION OF STRESSFUL EVENTS TO SOCIAL SUPPORT

As mentioned earlier, we live in an era of rapid social, political, and psychological transition. Nowhere are these perpetual transitions more evident and alarming than within the family structure. Traditionally, the family consisted of one parent who served as an economic provider, one parent who remained at home to care for the children, and the children themselves. Previously, it was common for families also to include the extended generations of grandparents who lived with the nuclear family. But the past few decades have witnessed a dramatic alteration in this structure, as the family has undergone several metamorphoses in its composition, alignments, and relationships to society as a whole.

Sussman (1977), for example, examined six traditional forms of family structure and the percentage of the total population each such structure comprised. The researcher found that the standard nuclear intact family, consisting of two married parents and at least one child, represented only 37% of the population; nuclear remarried families made up 11% of the population; and single-parent families represented 12% of all families. In addition to these basic configurations, other family structures have arisen that suggest the demise of the traditional family unit. Among these trends are two-career families, in which both husband and wife work outside the home for prolonged periods of time. Gertsel and Gross (1983) have reported on the "commuter marriage," in which one or both partners experience opposing pulls from commitment to individual careers on the one hand and commitment to family life on the other. "Empty nest syndrome," investigated by Swenson (1985), occurs when children grow up and leave the home at earlier ages than in the past. An even more recent occurrence is the phenomenon of empty nest syndrome in reverse, whereby older children who have completed college, return to live with their parents because of depleted financial resources.

Other dynamic trends that have wreaked havoc with the customary patterns of family life include divorce, remarriage, stepfamilies, and a shocking ascendance in abusive and violent behavior patterns among family members. Another notable change is the degree to which the two-income household has required families to find substitute caregivers for the children. Full-time babysitters, nannies, and day care workers now often fulfill the function of surrogate parent. In many cases, a child may be exposed to several such surrogates during childhood. These issues need exploration to achieve a full understanding of the effects of surrogate parenting.

Family violence—in the form of child abuse and neglect, spouse abuse, incest, and sexual molestation—has also altered the landscape of the American family. Although some researchers hypothesize that such trends always existed but were somehow eclipsed from public awareness and consciousness, others have suggested that the prevailing trends of violence among our families have erupted because of the vacillating patterns of family structure, coupled with the drug culture and the disintegration of religious, educational, and social institutions that previously tied families together and required them to share activities and experiences. A common reason for social support intervention is the subjection of a child to unrelenting physical or sexual abuse that endangers his physical or mental well-being. Crittenden (1985) has offered evidence of the advantages social support networks play in forging a mother–infant attachment. This researcher studied abusive and nonabusive mothers and infants using both the Strange Situation Paradigm (Ainsworth & Wittig, 1969) and various indexes of the mother's social networks. It was found that nonabusive mothers had a more enriched and complex social network as well as a more satisfying interaction with their infants than the abusive mothers. Colletta (1981), in a report on adolescent mothers, found that mothers who received a high level of support from their families manifested less hostility, indifference, and rejection toward their infants and toddlers than mothers who received a low level of family support. This finding was particularly evident when the mothers received social support in the form of emotional encouragement. Colletta's findings were confirmed by those of Mercer, Hackley, and Bostrom (1983), who examined adolescent mothers at 1 month postpartum and found that emotional support was related to enhanced feelings of affection for their infants and an overall greater gratification in the mothering role.

Howard and Kropenske (1990) conducted a study of mothers being seen for prenatal care. These expectant mothers were poly-drug abusers, 55% of whom provided a history of intravenous drug use. Socially, 75% of the mothers had grown up in households with a history of parental drug or alcohol abuse, and 40% had experienced physical and/or sexual abuse. Fully 80% of the women had chosen a spouse or partner who also abused drugs and alcohol. The infants born to these mothers exhibited a variety of medical and neurobiological complications, including tremors, lethargy, irritability, and abnormal eye movements.

Assessment in this program consisted of meetings with social workers, pediatricians, and a public health nurse. The areas of assessment moved progressively from the interpersonal to the social realms. Following these assessments, a 6-month intervention plan was designed for each caregiver. A target individual, generally a nurse, was designated as the coordinator of information. Intervention efforts focused on enhancing functioning in four distinct areas: the caregiver's mental status and representational abilities; environmental inconsistency, particularly of the type that would expose the infant to noncontingency experiences; extensive involvement of community-based systems; and the overall safety of the child. At the end of the program the researchers reported stabilization in all key areas.

Rothenberg (1990) notes that as a result of our mass media culture, the average American child will witness approximately 18,000 murders on television by the time he has graduated from high school and will also be exposed to countless episodes of robbery, beatings, arson, and rapes. According to Rothenberg, children as young as 5 years old learn about drinking alcohol from television by observing actors who can consume unbelievable amounts of liquor and gorge themselves on huge quantities of food. Yet, the characters on television are almost universally attractive, conveying the message that unhealthy behavior is not harmful. Rothenberg is equally scathing in his attack on the American educational system, citing results of a 1987 study that revealed that one in eight Americans graduating from high school is functionally illiterate. Episodes of child abuse and neglect have by this time become an unshocking part of our society, and the epidemic of missing or abducted children shows no signs of abating.

Regardless of the source, the documentary evidence indicates that the American family is currently at a crossroads of crisis. Moreover, the disintegration of the family exerts a particularly chilling effect on those family members most vulnerable to unexpected change—the infants. For infants, who are just beginning to experience the vast fluctuations that exist in the external world as well as the startling transformations occurring within their own bodies, unpredictable and uncontrollable events can be terrifying and can lead to withdrawal from the world and, eventually, depression. The most vital catalyst for adaptive development is the presence of a consistent, nurturing caregiver figure who gradually guides the infant in surmounting the challenges posed by both internal and external arenas. Previewing behaviors that acquaint the infant with developmental skills in a supportive manner provide the most effective introduction to these phenomena. Given the inordinate amount of stress that virtually all families encounter, however, even highly adaptive caregivers may become distracted by the demands of the environment. As an exquisitely sensitive organism, the infant will be attuned to the caregiver's change of mood, and in particular to the way in which the caregiver's behaviors lack a consistent, contingent, and nondiscrepant rhythm.

Unfortunately, no therapist—no matter how skilled—can reverse the societal trends eroding the fabric of the family. Nevertheless, therapists can reinforce for caregivers the preeminent importance of an attitude of consistent nurturance that enables the infant to begin formulating predictions about the world around himself. Such predictive skills will allow the infant to anticipate upcoming change and assert mastery and control over developmental change. To do this, the therapist must instill feelings of stability within the caregiver herself. That is, the caregiver's perspective on the world must be optimistic and must envision the future as a place where the infant will continue to develop as the dyadic relationship grows increasingly more complex and intimate. If the caregiver lacks this perspective, the therapist must serve as a stable paradigm and must emphasize that controllable and predictable events will govern the future. By adopting these attitudes, the therapist will alleviate at least some of the stress confronting the family and, in particular, the unique tensions that threaten to end the relationship between mother and infant before it has an opportunity to flourish.

ENHANCING THE ROLE OF SOCIAL SUPPORT AS A FORM OF INTERVENTION

In addition to functioning as a paradigm of individual behavior, the therapist may also rely on the intervention techniques derived from social support theory. In this context, the therapist will often be acting as a liaison figure who initiates the caregiver and infant into other networks and forms of treatment that provide unique social support services. The therapist's responsibility is to ascertain whether the caregiver is adhering to the social support regime, whether the caregiver's problems are being adequately addressed, and whether additional services are necessary. In this capacity the therapist facilitates access to services.

Visiting 34 mothers and their 3- to 6-month-old infants on five different occasions, Hann (1989) found that both independent and combined positive ratings of infant temperament, maternal personality, and social support correlated with the overall level of infant responsivity, as manifested by longer sequences of positive affect during caregiver–infant interaction. Moreover, families were especially apt to rely on external social support systems under conditions of high stress or family crisis. Recent data suggest that parents are more prone to rely on social support systems when their infants are born prematurely than when infants are born at term. Crnic, Greenberg, Ragozin, Robinson, and Basham (1983) examined and compared samples of both preterm and full-term 4-month-old infants and reported positive relationships between informal social support systems and a variety of measures of parenting attitudes and behavior—regardless of the birth status of the infant. Crockenberg (1981) has found that the utilization of social support correlated with the quality of the attachment bond between mother and infant. This was particularly evident with infants who were categorized as having difficult temperaments. A number of studies have examined the impact of informal social support on parent–infant interaction in both preterm and full-term infants. Especially with infants who displayed an irritable disposition, the use of increased social support services was associated with the development of a secure attachment to the caregiver. These kinds of outcomes may indicate that social support can help a parent manifest behaviors that better fit the child's temperamental disposition.

Programs for chemically dependent caregivers are another example of a social support intervention model. In the majority of cases these women are unable to surmount their addictions, even with the assistance of drug and alcohol treatment programs. Moreover, as the pattern of prenatal drug use has escalated, hospitals throughout the country have documented a disturbing increase in infants exposed prenatally to drugs. In fact, in some areas of the country legal authorities have attempted to intervene by bringing charges of child abuse against mothers who have given birth to drug-addicted infants.

In cases of extreme family dysfunction, professionals may recommend removing the child from the home. Among the placement options are family foster care, residential treatment programs, and psychiatric hospitalization (Schachter, 1989). Often a therapist must evaluate the severity of the case and make a recommendation. Besides considering the child's immediate physical safety, Schachter recommends reviewing the following criteria:

1. Whether the continued presence of the child in the family milieu indicates ongoing obstruction of development or deterioration that would not be altered by existing outpatient therapeutic possibilities.
2. Whether there is an adequate community-based school or alternative daytime environment that can tolerate the child's behavior and provide for cognitive social learning; or, alternatively, whether there is an antagonistic community that cannot tolerate the child's behavior or presence.

3. Whether the child's disturbed behavior patterns are not conducive to effective fostering by naturally selected surrogates.

For severely disturbed, maltreated children, psychiatric hospitalization may be the program of choice. Obviously, placement outside the home represents a dramatic disruption in the child's development and should only be considered as an alternative in dire situations. Child preventive service agencies may sometimes be able to avert removal of the child in less serious maltreatment cases by providing homemaker services and other forms of assistance. The therapist's task is to serve as a consistent figure who guides the child to a more adaptive environment that will allow a sense of competence and mastery to emerge. Of course, this can only happen in a nurturing environment that predictably meets the child's needs.

All of these studies indicate that therapists involved with dyads need to investigate closely the nature of the social support network sustaining the family in treatment. Is the network formal or informal and how does the network coalesce to provide emotional support, particularly in times of crisis? Are the caregivers willing to accept help from outsiders or do they resist social support efforts as being intrusive? It is vital for the therapist to ascertain the answers to these questions, because the developmental process can often trigger crises that will require outside support.

In addition to knowing the specific areas of social support intervention, health care professionals should become *child advocates* by being particularly alert to social phenomena that can affect children's lives (Rothenberg, 1990). Among these phenomena are the overwhelming influence of the mass media; the educational system and, especially, the common use of corporal punishment in the schools; the epidemic of child abuse and neglect; and the need for adequate day care facilities.

In each of the preceding intervention models therapists must adopt unique roles and attitudes. As a liaison who links children and their parents to social support systems, therapists should be vigilant in follow-up meetings; as administrators of the treatment and as advocates, therapists must work within already existing systems to promote environments conducive to childhood development. Although each of these roles is distinct, it is also incumbent on therapists to continually promote the phenomenon of previewing. This means that therapists must strive to instill optimism about the future in the parents and children they treat and to convey the notion that the world is a predictable place with challenges that may be daunting but are nevertheless capable of being mastered.

Case Management

The strategy of *case management* helps families at risk obtain the necessary social support services they need to establish an adaptive environment. This approach is an outgrowth of the realization that many families have multiple disabilities that require attention and have a difficult time negotiating complex and fragmented health and social service delivery systems. As Austin (1990) has commented, families who require services from a number of different social agencies often need assistance with the difficult task of coordinating those services.

In explaining the role of the case manager, who integrates these diverse services for the family, Austin notes that most case managers do not purchase services for their clients. Rather, they function primarily as "brokers," making referrals and following up with both providers and the families receiving the services. The case manager seeks to circumvent the fragmentation in delivery systems and to assist clients with multiple and frequently chronic disabilities in locating the services they need. This role encompasses two important functions: the coordination of services, and the interaction between the client and the case manager. As advocates, case managers monitor their clients' rights to services (Altschuler & Forward, 1978). The case manager should have the most comprehensive information on services available to the client and, as that client's auxiliary, should provide a familiarity with the system that allows the client to exercise choice in accessing needed services. Researchers have observed that each family has a host of emotional needs, whether conscious or unconscious, as well as a host of external needs for concrete environmental services. Because most families requiring multiple social services are poor and suffer from many problems, there may be a tendency to become overly involved in attempting to manage outer needs without responding to the family's inner difficulties. The tendency to focus on the delivery of coordinated concrete services may result in part from the case manager's own difficulties in listening to or empathizing with a family's fear, despair, anger, or other intense feelings. This is one reason it is advantageous to have an individual trained in psychotherapy function in the role of a case manager.

The therapist not only can address both the family's external stresses and more internal psychological needs but also can offer strategies to help the members prepare for the future in an adaptive fashion, in particular, by continually reinforcing principles of previewing. To do this, the case manager must evaluate the family's future on a continual basis and strive to identify realistic possibilities that the family may optimistically achieve.

Placement

In some family situations, however, the child's protection may warrant more radical intervention. Immediate removal of the child is likely to be necessary in cases of suspected physical or sexual abuse or in circumstances that suggest extreme neglect has led to a deterioration of the child's developmental processes. The latter situation is often found with parents who suffer from severe mental disturbance or substance abuse. The primary responsibility of therapists working with maltreated children and their families, however, is to prevent placement outside the home whenever possible (Schachter, 1989) because it signifies one of the most radical interventions that can occur in a child's life. Nevertheless, when the child appears to be in serious danger and the family circumstances cannot be ameliorated, the therapist may be called upon to facilitate the placement. It is important to point out, however, that the danger must be verifiable and convincing to court personnel who have the ultimate responsibility for making decisions about placement. Once it becomes apparent that removal from the home is the only feasible alternative, the therapist must also determine what type of placement would be appropriate. According to Schachter, differential criteria for selecting placement options are necessary to ensure that these critical decisions are not determined arbitrarily, colored by agency bias, or controlled by the availability of community resources. Among the most common placement options are *foster care* in a family or group home, for infants, and *residential treatment* or *psychiatric hospitalization,* for parents.

Infants suitable for family foster care should be emotionally capable of meeting the normal expectable requirements of family life. Often infants who have received some exposure to good parenting and are being temporarily placed in foster care because of a family crisis will do well. On the other hand, children who come out of an atmosphere of extreme abuse may be so developmentally damaged and distrustful that they are incapable of receiving or giving affection. Such children may need specialized programs. Foster parents, it should be remembered, seek some form of emotional reward for their investment. They seek to obtain appreciation and love from the foster children they care for and are likely to experience feelings of defeat if the child is not responsive. Fish (1984), for example, considered family foster care inappropriate for children whose severe and unpredictable aggressive behavior would not be tolerated in the community.

For teenaged parents who display aggressive behavior, a residential treatment program may be appropriate. Schachter reports that such a residential treatment facility should offer a controlled living environment geared to the growth and therapeutic needs of the parent and infant. The element of control or structure is of special significance because many of these teens come from environments that did not reinforce developmental acquisition and mastery. The structured approach therefore exposes the teen, perhaps for the first time, to an environment that appreciates his individual needs and encourages his unique skills. Residential treatment programs should also provide individual, family, and group therapy in various combinations, a flexible educational program with strong remedial features, and a professional staff with the training to tolerate disturbing behavior and the sensitivity to avoid becoming ensnared in the cycle of rejecting-abandoning behavior that severely abused infants tend to provoke in their caregivers.

Therapists should consider placement in such a residential program based on a variety of criteria. For example, has the infant or child failed to gain from earlier exposure to nonresidential treatment? Does his continued presence in the family indicate ongoing deterioration of his development or deterioration that only residential treatment can alter? Has the community, particularly the school, found the child unacceptable and rejected him? Is the child's behavior so disturbed that effective nurturing by surrogates without special qualifications is inadequate?

Finally, there may be some cases in which psychiatric hospitalization is necessary to ensure that optimal development gets back on track. This option is appropriate for parents who are unable to handle even the most minimal demands of natural family and community life. Hospitalization should also be initiated for patients who are suicidal or homicidal or in those cases where extreme aggressive and assaultive behavior may require an even more structured and less pressured environment than residential treatment programs provide.

It often falls to the therapist to recommend the appropriate form of care. Although the preceding guidelines offer some insight into how the therapist should proceed, each case will present a unique constellation of factors that require evaluation. In particular, the therapist should always ascertain the level of the child's development and the degree to which his environment promotes the attainment of future maturational skills in a supportive and nurturing atmosphere.

It is clear that we live in a society that, at best, takes its children for granted and fails to comprehend the extraordinary sensitivity required to raise an infant in an adaptive, growth-enhancing environment. Therapists involved in treating young children and their families cannot, of course, be expected to reverse the trends of society. But therapists do have the capacity to change lives one at a time. Ensuring that each child and family being treated receives access to optimal social support services is a step in that direction.

Day Care

Certainly during the past decade, infant *day care* has become an increasingly popular option for families in which both parents work or for single parent families in which the sole caregiver is employed. For some families, economic realities mandate that both parents work outside of the home, making day care a necessity; in other cases, both parents choose to work, viewing day care as a viable alternative to nurturing the infant during the hours when they are away from the home.

Because institutionalized day care is a relatively new phenomenon, there is not a great deal of data concerning its effects on the infant's development, attachment bond to significant others, and overall ability to mature in a socially adaptive fashion. Nonetheless, one researcher, Belsky (1986), recently summarized some tentative findings concerning the effect of day care environment on the infant's development and, in particular, on the attachment relationship the infant forms with the caregiver. Belsky has written that early infant care may be associated with increased avoidance of the mother, possibly to the point of insecurity in the attachment relationship and that, as such, day care may be associated with diminished compliance with adults, increased aggressiveness, and possibly social maladaptation in the preschool and early school years. Researchers who have investigated Belsky's tentative findings have come up with diverse conclusions. Of the research currently available, however, Berger (1990) notes that several studies include infants from various socioeconomic groups as well as comparisons of care across different child-rearing settings. In Berger's view, these investigations taken together represent a trend that indicates that early out-of-home care is a factor, although not necessarily an independent factor, that may *predict risk* in attachment relationships. Berger notes that although alternative interpretations of the meaning of attachment behavior evaluated by the Strange Situation with day-care-reared children can and have been advanced (Clarke-Stewart & Fein, 1983), such research, for the most part, demonstrates a probabilistic connection between day care attendance and *insecurity in attachment* classification as well as a deviation from anticipated norms for development in this culture during infancy.

Other researchers have, however, questioned whether exposure to day care has a detrimental or indeed any notable effect on the infant or on his attachment behavior. Caruso (1990), for example, questions whether early entry to out-of-home care is a risk factor for later developmental difficulties, observing that researchers know very little about similarities and differences across day care settings or about how infants' experiences in this range of environments differ from typical experiences infants have at home.

Clearly, this difference of opinion concerning the effect of day care exposure on young infants and their future attachment patterns remains unsettled. Nonetheless, therapists treating young infants and their caregivers must often confront the issue of day care. Because of economic realities day care for many families is not a choice, but rather a necessity. Under these circumstances, the therapist should explore the caregiver's attitude toward day care services. In addition, therapists should recommend that the caregiver visit the day care facility to determine whether it provides a supportive environment. Parents should be encouraged to meet with the day care workers to discuss their infant's special needs and to observe sessions during which the day care workers are attending to other children.

The therapist should also remind caregivers that even if the day care provides an optimal environment, it still represents a form of separation between mother and infant. As a result, it becomes especially important for the caregiver to set aside a certain amount of quality time with the infant to establish an appropriate attachment bond. Some caregivers may also experience guilt because their work situations necessitate that they must be separated from the infant for lengthy periods. The therapist should help the caregiver find the most supportive day care facility available and work with the caregiver to optimize the time that she does spend with the infant. Perhaps she should set aside time during weekends or vacations to spend with the child. During treatment sessions the therapist should attempt to promote representational and previewing patterns that promote attachment within the dyad.

CONCLUSION

Beyond purveying treatment, the therapist also has the capacity to ensure that children in treatment receive essential social support services to enhance their development. Providing social support may require therapists to act as liaisons with other agencies or may necessitate more direct intervention in the form of recommending whether the child is a candidate for foster care, a residential treatment program, or psychiatric hospitalization. Therapists, then, must understand that they will frequently exert influence beyond the arena of the child's immediate family.

The therapist, in determining an appropriate stance toward social support systems, must recognize that American society has undergone dramatic changes in the past few decades and that these changes have particularly affected the structure of the family. Not only are divorces and remarriages far more prevalent than in earlier decades but disturbed and dysfunctional behaviors, such as abuse and neglect, have become rampant and even commonplace. In addition, substance and alcohol abuse and exposure to violence unfortunately have also become recognized parts of the American fabric.

On a very fundamental level, all of these phenomena conspire to undermine the infant's adaptation. Development in this context refers to the capacity to attain increasingly more sophisticated skills that, with mastery and control, meet the challenges of the environment and of inner psychological needs. When the child witnesses apparently uncontrollable violence or a drug epidemic that seemingly cannot be stopped or hears stories of child abuse in which well-meaning adults seem unable to stop the destructive behavior, feelings of hopelessness begin to permeate his consciousness. Eventually, these feelings can become exacerbated and emerge as full-fledged depression. To counter these debilitating feelings, health care professionals must generate optimism for the future by helping children and their caregivers acquire the skills they need to predict and master future challenge. Previewing is one way of achieving this goal, but therapists can also use the resources of social support systems to enhance the child's development.

References

Aaron, N. A., Calkins, S., & Fox, N. A. (1990). *Infant temperament and attachment predict behavioral inhibitions at 24 months.* In C. Rovee-Collier (Ed.), Abstracts of papers presented at the Seventh International Conference on Infant Studies (p. 235), Montreal. Norwood, NJ: Ablex.

Abelin, E. L. (1975). Some further observations and comments on the earliest role of the father. *International Journal of Psychoanalysis, 56,* 293–302.

Abramson, L. (1990). *Facial affect and self-regulation in failure to thrive and normal infants.* In C. Rovee-Collier (Ed.), Abstracts of papers presented at the Seventh International Conference on Infant Studies (p. 236), Montreal. Norwood, NJ: Ablex.

Ackerman, N. (1953). Selected problems in supervised analysis. *Psychiatry, 16,* 283–290.

Ackerman, N. (1966). *Treating the troubled family.* Boston: Little, Brown.

Adams-Hillard, P. J. (1985). Physical abuse in pregnancy. *Obstetrics and Gynecology, 16,* 185–190.

Adamson, L. B., & Bakeman, R. (1985). *Infant's conventionalized acts with mothers and peers.* Paper presented at the biennial meeting of the Society for Research in Child Development, Toronto.

Ainsworth, M. D. S. (1973). The development of infant–mother attachment. In B. M. Caldwell & H. R. Ricciuti (Eds.), *Review of Child Development Research* (pp. 1–94). Chicago: University of Chicago Press.

Ainsworth, M. D. S., & Wittig, B. (1969). Attachment and exploratory behavior of one year olds in a strange situation. In B. M. Foss (Ed.), *Determinants of infant behavior,* IV. London: Metheun.

Alessandri, S. M., & Sullivan, M. W. (1990). *Stability and change in infant emotion expressions.* In C. Rovee-Collier (Ed.), Abstracts of papers presented at the Seventh International Conference on Infant Studies (p. 238), Montreal. Norwood, NJ: Ablex.

Alexander, F., & French, T. M. (1946). *Psychoanalytic therapy.* New York: Ronald Press.

Alger, I. (1973). Audio-visual techniques in family therapy. In D. Bloch (Ed.), *Techniques of Family Psychotherapy* (pp. 65–75). New York: Grune & Stratton.

Alger, I. (1978). Freeze-frame video in psychotherapy. In M. M. Berger (Ed.), *Videotape Techniques in Psychiatric Training and Treatment* (pp. 244–252). New York: Brunner/Mazel.

Al Naquib, N., & Sadek, A. (1990). *Child development & iron deficiency anemia. A screening study on Middle Eastern children using the Denver Developmental Screening Test.* In C. Rovee-Collier (Ed.), Abstracts of papers presented at the Seventh International Conference on Infant Studies (p. 239), Montreal. Norwood, NJ: Ablex.

Alonso, A., & Rutan, J. S. (1990). Common dilemmas in combined individual and group treatment. *Group, 14,* 5–12.

Als, H., Duffy, F. H., & McAnulty, G. B. (1990). *Neurobehavioral regulation disorder of prematurity.* In C. Rovee-Collier (Ed.), Abstracts of papers presented at the Seventh International Conference on Infant Studies (p. 159), Montreal. Norwood, NJ: Ablex.

Altman, J. (1974). Observational study of behavior: Sampling methods. *Behaviour, 49,* 227–267.

Altschuler, S. C., & Forward, J. (1978). The inverted hierarchy: A case management approach to mental health services. *Administration in Mental Health, 6,* 57–68.

Amaranto, E. A., & Bender, S. S. (1990). Individual psychotherapy as an adjunct to group psychotherapy. *International Journal of Group Psychotherapy, 40,* 91–101.

Ambrose, S., & Poulsen, M. (1990). *Characteristics of inner-city mothers who use drugs during pregnancy.* In C. Rovee-Collier (Ed.), Abstracts of papers presented at the Seventh International Conference on Infant Studies (p. 82), Montreal. Norwood, NJ: Ablex.

Anders, T. F. (1990). *Falling asleep and waking up during the night: Developmental patterns.* In C. Rovee-Collier (Ed.), Abstracts of papers presented at the Seventh International Conference on Infant Studies (p. 162), Montreal. Norwood, NJ: Ablex.

Anderson, J. R. (1978). Arguments concerning representations for mental imagery. *Psychological Review, 85,* 249–277.

Anderson, S. (1990). *Turn exchange patterns between babies and adults: Are they inconsistent with rules of turn-taking in adult conversation?* In C. Rovee-Collier (Ed.), Abstracts of papers presented at the Seventh International Conference on Infant Studies (p. 241), Montreal. Norwood, NJ: Ablex.

Andersson, B.-E. (1990). *Socio-emotional competence in Swedish schoolchildren related to early child care and mother's employment rate.* In C. Rovee-Collier (Ed.), Abstracts of papers presented at the Seventh International Conference on Infant Studies (p. 242), Montreal. Norwood, NJ: Ablex.

Anzieu, D. (1986). Paradoxical transference: From paradoxical communication to negative therapeutic reaction. *Contemporary Psychoanalysis, 22,* 520–547.

Aponte, H. J. (1976). Underorganization in the poor family. In P. J. Guerin (Ed.), *Family therapy: Theory and practice.* New York: Gardner.

Aponte, H. J., & Van Deusen, J. M. (1981). Structural family therapy. In A. S. Gurman & D. P Kniskern (Eds.), *Handbook of family therapy* (pp. 310–360). New York: Brunner/Mazel.

Appelbaum, S. A. (1973). Psychological-mindedness: Word, concept, and essence. *International Journal of Psychoanalysis, 54,* 35–46.

Apprey, M. (1987). Projective identification and maternal misconception in disturbed mothers. *British Journal of Psychotherapy, 4,* 5–20.

Araoz, D. L. (1982). *Hypnosis and sex therapy.* New York: Brunner/Mazel.

Arlow, J. A. (1963). The supervisory situation. *Journal of the American Psychoanalytic Association, 11,* 576–594.

Arterberry, M. E. (1990). *Integration skills in 8-, 10- and 12-month-old infants.* In C. Rovee-Collier (Ed.), Abstracts of papers presented at the Seventh International Conference on Infant Studies (p. 246), Montreal. Norwood, NJ: Ablex.

Ascher, M. (1985). Conjoint treatment of a mother and her 16-month-old toddler. *International Journal of Psychoanalytic Psychotherapy, 11,* 315–337.

Ashmead, D. H. (1990). *Posture and prehension in infants.* In C. Rovee-Collier (Ed.), Abstracts of papers presented at the Seventh International Conference on Infant Studies (p. 185), Montreal. Norwood, NJ: Ablex.

Austin, C. D. (1990). Case management: Myths and realities. *Families in Society: The Journal of Contemporary Human Services*, 398–405.

Bakeman, R., & Adamson, L. B. (1984). Coordinating attention to people and objects in mother–infant and peer–infant interaction. *Child Development, 55*, 1278–1289.

Bakeman, R., & Gottman, J. M. (1987). Applying observational methods: A systematic view. In J. D. Osofsky (Ed.), *Handbook of Infant Development* (2nd ed., pp. 818–854). New York: Wiley.

Baldwin, D. A. (1990). *Infants' contribution to joint reference*. In C. Rovee-Collier (Ed.), Abstracts of papers presented at the Seventh International Conference on Infant Studies (p. 253), Montreal. Norwood, NJ: Ablex.

Ballinger, C. B., Smith, A. H., & Hobbs, P. R. (1985). Factors associated with psychiatric morbidity in women: A general practice survey. *Acta Psychiatrica Scandinavica, 71*, 272–280.

Ballou, J. (1978). The significance of reconciliative themes in the psychology of pregnancy. *Bulletin of the Menninger Clinic, 42*, 383–413.

Ban, P. L., & Lewis, M. (1974). Mothers and fathers, girls and boys: Attachment behavior in the one-year-old. *Merrill Palmer Quarterly-Journal of Developmental Psychology, 20*, 195–204.

Bandler, R., & Grinder, J. (1975). *The structure of magic*. Palo Alto, CA: Science & Behavior Books.

Bandura, A. (1977a). Self-efficacy: Toward a unifying theory of behavioral change. *Psychological Review, 84*, 191–215.

Bandura, A. (1977b). *Social learning theory*. Englewood Cliffs, NJ: Prentice-Hall.

Bandura, A. (1982a). The self and mechanisms of agency. In J. Suls (Ed.), *Social Psychological Perspectives on the Self*. Hillsdale, NJ: Erlbaum.

Bandura, A. (1982b). Self-efficacy mechanism in human agency. *American Psychologist, 37*, 122–147.

Bardwick, J. M. (1971). *Psychology of women: A study of bio-cultural conflicts*. New York: Harper & Row.

Barnett, D., Ganiban, J., Martin, R., Cicchetti, D., & Carlson, V. (1990). *Affect regulation among maltreated infants with disorganized attachments*. In C. Rovee-Collier (Ed.), Abstracts of papers presented at the Seventh International Conference on Infant Studies (p. 256), Montreal. Norwood, NJ: Ablex.

Barnhill, L. (1979). Healthy family stems. *The Family Coordinator, 28*, 94–100.

Barrerra, M., & Kitching, K. (1990). *Preschool performance of VLBW, HBW, and FT children*. In C. Rovee-Collier (Ed.), Abstracts of papers presented at the Seventh International Conference on Infant Studies (p. 257), Montreal. Norwood, NJ: Ablex.

Barton, C., & Alexander, J. F. (1981). Functional family therapy. In A. S. Gurman & D. P. Kniskern (Eds.), *Handbook of family therapy* (pp. 403–443). New York: Brunner/Mazel.

Baxter, A., Knieps, L. J., & Walden, T. A. (1990). *Social referencing and affective shifts in down syndrome infants*. In C. Rovee-Collier (Ed.), Abstracts of papers presented at the Seventh International Conference on Infant Studies (p. 260), Montreal. Norwood, NJ: Ablex.

Beaumont, S., & Bloom, K. (1990). *Does the quality of infant vocalization signal intentionality?* In C. Rovee-Collier (Ed.), Abstracts of papers presented at the Seventh International Conference on Infant Studies (p. 261), Montreal. Norwood, NJ: Ablex.

Beckmann, C. (1990). *Effects of postterm pregnancy on neurobehavioral responsiveness and mother–infant interaction.* In C. Rovee-Collier (Ed.), Abstracts of papers presented at the Seventh International Conference on Infant Studies (p. 264), Montreal. Norwood, NJ: Ablex.

Beckwith, L. (1990). *Responsive parenting from infancy to age 12.* In C. Rovee-Collier (Ed.), Abstracts of papers presented at the Seventh International Conference on Infant Studies (p. 265), Montreal. Norwood, NJ: Ablex.

Beebe, B., & Stern, D. N. (1977). Engagement-disengagement and early object experiences. In N. Freedman & S. Grand (Eds.), *Communicative structures and psychic structures: A psychoanalytic interpretation of communication* (pp. 35–55). New York: Plenum.

Beeghly, M., Vo, D., Burrows, E., & Brazelton, T. B. (1990). *Social and task-related behavior of fullterm small-for-gestational-age (SGA) infants at two years.* In C. Rovee-Collier (Ed.), Abstracts of papers presented at the Seventh International Conference on Infant Studies (p. 266), Montreal. Norwood, NJ: Ablex.

Behrends, R. S., & Blatt, S. J. (1985). Internalization and psychological development throughout the life cycle. *Psychoanalytic Study of the Child, 40,* 11–39.

Bell, J. (1961). *Family therapy group therapy* (Public Health Monograph No. 64). Washington, DC: U. S. Department of Health, Education, and Welfare.

Bell, N. W., & Vogel, E. F. (1968). *A modern introduction to the family.* New York: Free Press.

Bell, S. M. (1970). The development of the concept of object as related to infant-mother attachment. *Child Development, 41,* 291–313.

Belsky, J. (1984). The determinants of parenting: A process model. *Child Development, 55,* 83–96.

Belsky, J. (1985). Experimenting with the family in the newborn period. *Child Development, 56,* 407–414.

Belsky, J. (1986). Infant day care: A cause for concern? *Zero to Three, 6,* 1–7.

Belsky, J., Goode, M. K., & Most, R. K. (1980). Maternal stimulation and infant exploratory competence: Cross-sectional, correlational, and experimental analyses. *Child Development, 51,* 1163–1178.

Bem, S. (1974). The measurement of psychological androgyny. *Journal of Consulting and Clinical Psychology, 42,* 155.

Benedek, T. (1959a). Parenthood as a developmental phase. A contribution to the libido theory. *Journal of the American Psychoanalytic Association, 7,* 389–417.

Benedek, T. (1959b). Sexual functions in women and their disturbance. In S. Arieti (Ed.), *American handbook of psychiatry* (Vol. 1, pp. 727–748). New York: Basic Books.

Benedek, T. (1970a). Fatherhood and providing. In E. J. Anthony & T. Benedek (Eds.), *Parenthood: Its psychology and psychopathology* (pp. 167–183). Boston: Little, Brown.

Benedek, T. (1970b). Parenthood during the life cycle. In E. J. Anthony & T. Benedek (Eds.), *Parenthood: Its psychology and psychopathology* (pp. 185–206). Boston: Little, Brown.

Benedek, T. (1970c). The psychobiology of pregnancy. In E. J. Anthony & T. Benedek (Eds.), *Parenthood: Its psychology and psychopathology* (pp. 137–151). Boston: Little, Brown.

Benoit, D., Zeanah, C., & Barton, M. (1989). Maternal attachment disturbances in failure to thrive. *Infant Mental Health Journal, 10,* 185–202.

Benson, J. B. (1990). *Great expectations: How infants anticipate the future.* In C. Rovee-Collier (Ed.), Abstracts of papers presented at the Seventh International Conference on Infant Studies (p. 13), Montreal. Norwood, NJ: Ablex.

Berger, M. M. (1978a). Confrontation through videotape. In M. M. Berger (Ed.), *Videotape techniques in psychiatric training and treatment.* New York: Bruner/Mazel.

Berger, M. M. (Ed.) (1978b). *Videotape techniques in psychiatric training and treatment.* New York: Bruner/Mazel.

Berger, S. P. (1990). Infant day care, parent-child attachment, and developmental risk: A reply to Caruso. *Infant Mental Health Journal, 11,* 365–373.

Bergman, P., & Escalona, S. K. (1949). Unusual sensitivities in very young children. *The Psychoanalytic Study of the Child, 3–4,* 333–352.

Berlin, B. (1978). Ethnobiological classification. In E. Rosch & B. B. Lloyd (Eds.), *Cognition and categorization* (pp. 9–26). Hillsdale, NJ: Erlbaum.

Berlin, L. J., & Cassidy, J. (1990). *Infant–mother attachment and the ability to be alone in early childhood.* In C. Rovee-Collier (Ed.), Abstracts of papers presented at the Seventh International Conference on Infant Studies (p. 274), Montreal. Norwood, NJ: Ablex.

Bernheim, K. F., & Lehman, A. F. (1985). Teaching mental health trainees to work with families of the chronic mentally ill. *Hospital and Community Psychiatry, 36,* 1109–1111.

Bertenthal, B., & Fischer, K. (1978). Development of self-recognition in the infant. *Developmental Psychology, 14,* 44–50.

Bigelow, A. (1990). *Locomotion and search behavior in blind infants.* In C. Rovee-Collier (Ed.), Abstracts of papers presented at the Seventh International Conference on Infant Studies (p. 279), Montreal. Norwood, NJ: Ablex.

Bills, B. (1980). Enhancement of paternal-newborn affectional bonds. *Journal of Nurse-Midwifery, 25,* 21–25.

Binder, J. L., & Smokler, I. (1980). Early memories: A technical aid to focusing in time limited dynamic psychotherapy. *Psychotherapy: Theory, Research, & Practice, 17,* 52–62.

Binder, J. L., Strupp, H. H., & Schacht, T. E. (1983). Countertransference in time-limited dynamic psychotherapy. *Contemporary Psychoanalysis, 19,* 605–622.

Blanck, R., & Blanck, G. (1986). *Beyond ego psychology: Developmental object relations theory.* New York: Columbia University Press.

Blass, E., Ganchrow, J. R., & Steiner, J. E. (1984). Classical conditioning in newborn humans 2–48 hours of age. *Infant Behavior & Development, 7,* 223–235.

Blass, E., & Smith, B. (1990). *Psychobiology of pain and coping in human newborns.* In C. Rovee-Collier (Ed.), Abstracts of papers presented at the Seventh International Conference on Infant Studies (p. 16), Montreal. Norwood, NJ: Ablex.

Blicharski, T., & Feider, H. (1990). *Mother-toddler discourse: Towards an ethnolinguistic analysis of language development.* In C. Rovee-Collier (Ed.), Abstracts of papers presented at the Seventh International Conference on Infant Studies (p. 43), Montreal. Norwood, NJ: Ablex.

Blitzsten, N. L., & Fleming, J. (1953). What is supervisory analysis? *Bulletin of the Menninger Clinic, 17,* 117–129.

Bloom, K. (1979). Evaluation of infant vocal conditioning. *Journal of Experimental Child Psychology, 27,* 60–70.

Bloom, K. (1990). *Infant vocal quality affects adult attitudes.* In C. Rovee-Collier (Ed.), Abstracts of papers presented at the Seventh International Conference on Infant Studies (p. 281), Montreal. Norwood, NJ: Ablex.

Bollas, C. (1983). Expressive uses of the countertransference. *Contemporary Psychoanalysis, 19,* 1–34.

Bornstein, M. H. (1981). Psychological studies of color perception in human infants. In L. P. Lipsitt (Ed.), *Advances in infancy research* (Vol. 1, pp. 1–4). Norwood, NJ: Ablex.

Bornstein, M. H. (1985). How infant and mother jointly contribute to developing cognitive competence in the child. *Proceedings of the National Academy of Sciences, 82,* 7470–7473.

Bornstein, M. H., & Tamis-LeMonda, C. S. (1989). Maternal responsiveness and cognitive development in children. *New Directions for Child Development, 43,* 49–61.

Boss, P. G. (1983). Normative family stress. In D. H. Olson & B. C. Miller (Eds.), *Family studies review yearbook* (Vol. 1). Beverly Hills, CA: Sage Publications.

Boszormenyi-Nagy, I., & Ulrich, D. N. (1981). Contextual family therapy. In A. S. Gurman & D. P. Kniskern (Eds.), *Handbook of family therapy* (pp. 159–186). New York: Brunner/Mazel.

Bowen, M. (1978). *Family therapy in clinical practice.* New York: Jason Aronson.

Bower, T. G. R. (1972). Object perception in infants. *Perception, 1,* 15–20.

Bower, T. G. R. (1974). *Development in infancy.* San Francisco: Freeman.

Bower, T. G. R., & Patterson, J. G. (1973). The separation of place, movement, and object in the world. *Journal of Experimental Child Psychology, 15, 161–168.*

Bowlby, J. (1969). *Attachment and loss: Vol. 1. Attachment.* New York: Basic Books.

Bowlby, J. (1973). *Attachment and loss: Vol. 2. Separation.* New York: Basic Books.

Bowlby, J. (1980). *Attachment and loss: Vol. 3. Loss.* New York: Basic Books.

Bowlby, J. (1982). *Attachment and loss: Vol. 3. Attachment* (2nd ed.). New York: Basic Books.

Boyd, H. S., & Sisney, V. V. (1967). Immediate self-image confrontation and changes in self-concept. *Journal of Consulting Psychology, 31,* 291–294.

Brackbill, Y., White, M., Wilson, M., & Kitch, D. (1990). Family dynamics as predictors of infant disposition. *Infant Mental Health, 11,* 113–126.

Bradlow, P. A. (1973). Depersonalization, ego splitting, non-human fantasy and shame. *International Journal of Psycho-Analysis, 54,* 487–492.

Bradt, J. O. (1988). Becoming parents: Families with young children. In B. Carter & M. McGoldrick (Eds.), *The changing family life cycle: A framework for family therapy* (2nd ed., pp. 235–254). New York: Gardner.

Brazelton, T. B., & Als, H. (1979). Four early stages in the development of mother-infant interaction. *The Psychoanalytic Study of the Child, 34,* 349–369.

Brazelton, T. B., Als, H., Tronick, E., & Lester, B. (1979). Specific neonatal measures: The Brazelton neonatal behavioral assessment scale. In J. Osofsky (Ed.), *Handbook of infant development.* New York: Wiley.

Brazelton, T. B., Koslowski, B., & Main, M. (1974). The origins of reciprocity: The early mother–infant interaction. In M. Lewis & L. A. Rosenblum (Eds.), *The effect of the infant on its caregiver* (pp. 49–76). New York: Wiley.

Brazelton, T. B., & Yogman, M. W. (Eds.) (1986). *Affective development in infancy.* Norwood, NJ: Ablex.

Breit, M., Im, W., & Wilner, R. S. (1983). Strategic approaches with resistant families. *American Journal of Family Therapy, 11,* 51–58.

Bremner, G. J. (1978a). Egocentric versus allocentric coding in nine-month-old infants: Factors influencing the choice of code. *Developmental Psychology, 14,* 346–355.

Bremner, G. J. (1978b). Spatial errors made by infants: Inadequate spatial cues or evidence of egocentrism? *British Journal of Psychology, 69,* 77–84.

Bretherton, I. (1990). Communication patterns, internal working models, and the intergenerational transmission of attachment relationships. *Infant Mental Health Journal, 11,* 237–252.

Bretherton, I. (1987). New perspective on attachment relations: Security, communication and internal working models. In J. Osofsky (Ed.), *Handbook of Infant Development* (pp. 1061–1100). New York: Wiley.

Bretherton, I., & Bates, E. (1979). The emergence of intentional communication. In I. Uzigris (Ed.), *New directories for child development* (Vol. 4). San Francisco: Jossey-Bass.

Brodey, W. M. (1968). *Changing the family.* New York: Potter.

Bruner, J. S. (1977). Early social interaction and language acquisition. In H. R. Schaffer (Ed.), *Studies in mother–infant interaction.* New York/London: Academic Press.

Budman, S. H., & Gurman, A. S. (1988). *Theory and practice of brief therapy.* New York: Guilford.

Busnel, M. C., Granier-Deferre, C., & Lecanuet, J.-P. (1990). *Fetal audition, known facts and their consequences.* In C. Rovee-Collier (Ed.), Abstracts of papers presented at the Seventh International Conference on Infant Studies (p. 298a), Montreal. Norwood, NJ: Ablex.

Buss, A. H., & Plomin, R. (Eds.) (1975). *A temperament theory of personality development.* New York: Wiley.

Butterworth, G. (Ed.) (1977). *The child's representation of the world.* New York: Plenum.

Byng-Hall, J. (1990). Attachment theory and family therapy: A clinical view. *Infant Mental Health Journal, 11,* 228–236.

Caldera, Y. M. (1990). *Attachment to mother and father, family characteristics, and the role of father in families of home care and day care infants.* In C. Rovee-Collier (Ed.), Abstracts of papers presented at the Seventh International Conference on Infant Studies (p. 301), Montreal. Norwood, NJ: Ablex.

Caligor, L. (1981). Parallel and reciprocal processes in psychoanalytic supervision. *Contemporary Psychoanalysis, 17,* 1–27.

Caligor, J. (1990). A current look at transference in combined analytic therapy. *Group, 14,* 16–24.

Camli, O., & Wachs, T. D. (1990). *Ecological and physical environment influences upon mother–infant interaction.* In C. Rovee-Collier (Ed.), Abstracts of papers presented at the Seventh International Conference on Infant Studies (p. 303), Montreal. Norwood, NJ: Ablex.

Campos, J. J., Barrett, K., Lamb, M. E., & Stenberg, C. (1983). Socioemotional development. In M. M. Haith & J. J. Campos (Eds.), *Handbook of child psychology: Vol. 2. Infancy and developmental psychobiology* (pp. 783–916). New York: Wiley.

Campos, J. J., Qi, D., Li, P., Fleener, M., & Tu, C. H. (1990). *Changes in the family system following crawling onset: A comparison of U.S. and Chinese families.* In C. Rovee-Collier (Ed.), Abstracts of papers presented at the Seventh International Conference on Infant Studies (p. 221), Montreal. Norwood, NJ: Ablex.

Caplan, G. (1959). *Concept of mental health and consultation: Their application in public health social work* (Publication No. 373, pp. 65–66). Washington, DC: U. S. Government Printing Office.

Caplan, G. (1974). *Social systems and community mental health.* New York: Behavioral Publications.

Caplan, R. D. (1979). Social support, person–environment fit, and coping. In L. A. Ferman & J. P. Gordus (Eds.), *Mental health and the economy* (pp. 89–138). Kalamazoo, MI: Upjohn Institute for Employment Research.

Caruso, D. A. (1990). Infant day care and the concept of developmental risk. *Infant Mental Health Journal, 11,* 358–364.

Charlesworth, W. R. (1978). Ethology: Its relevance for observational studies of human adaptation. In G. P. Sackett (Ed.), *Observing behavior: Vol. 1. Theory and applications in mental retardations* (pp. 7–32). Baltimore: University Park Press.

Chase-Lansdale, P. L., & Owen, M. T. (1987). Maternal employment in a family context: Effects of infant–mother and infant–father attachments. *Child Development, 58,* 1505–1512.

Chethick, L., Burns, K. A., Burns, W. J., & Clark, R. (1990). *The assessment of early relationship dysfunction in cocaine abusing mothers and their infants.* In C. Rovee-Collier (Ed.), Abstracts of papers presented at the Seventh International Conference on Infant Studies (p. 312), Montreal. Norwood, NJ: Ablex.

Chiodo, L., & Mann, J. (1990). *Stimulation and reciprocal interaction among extremely-low-birth-weight preterm infants and their mothers.* In C. Rovee-Collier (Ed.), Abstracts of papers presented at the Seventh International Conference on Infant Studies (p. 313), Montreal. Norwood, NJ: Ablex.

Chomsky, N. (1965). *Aspects of the theory syntax.* Cambridge, MA: MIT Press.

Clarke-Stewart, K. A. (1973). Interactions between mothers and their young children: Characteristics and consequences. *Monographs of the Society for Research in Child Development, 38*(6–7, Serial No. 153).

Clarke-Stewart, K. A. (1978). And daddy makes three: The father's impact on mother and young child. *Child Development, 49,* 466–478.

Clarke-Stewart, K. A., & Fein, G. (1983). Early childhood programs. In M. M. Haith & J. J. Campos (Eds)., *Handbook of child psychology: Vol 2. Infancy and developmental psychobiology* (pp. 917–999). New York: Wiley.

Clarkson, M. G., Swain, I. U., Clifton, R. K., & Cohen, K. (1990). *Newborns' head orientation toward trains of very brief sounds.* In C. Rovee-Collier (Ed.), Abstracts of papers presented at the Seventh International Conference on Infant Studies (p. 314), Montreal. Norwood, NJ: Ablex.

Cohen, L. B., & Salapalek, P. (Eds.) (1975). *Infant perception: From sensation to cognition.* New York: Academic Press.

Cohen, S. E. (1990). *Antecedents during infancy of self perception.* In C. Rovee-Collier (Ed.), Abstracts of papers presented at the Seventh International Conference on Infant Studies (p. 316), Montreal. Norwood, NJ: Ablex.

Coleman, J. S. (1974). Youth: Transition to adulthood. *School Review, 83,* 176.

Coles, C. D., Platzman, K. A., James, M., & Herbert, S. (1990). *Prenatal phenothiazine exposure and neonatal behavior.* In C. Rovee-Collier (Ed.), Abstracts of papers presented at the Seventh International Conference on Infant Studies (p. 320), Montreal. Norwood, NJ: Ablex. .

Coles, C. D., Platzman, K. A., Smith, I. E., & James, M. (1990). *Effects of maternal use of cocaine and alcohol on neonatal behavior.* In C. Rovee-Collier (Ed.), Abstracts of papers presented at the Seventh International Conference on Infant Studies (p. 321), Montreal. Norwood, NJ: Ablex.

Colletta, N. D. (1981). Social support and the risk of maternal rejection. *Journal of Psychology, 109,* 191–197.

Condon, J. T. (1986). The spectrum of fetal abuse in pregnant women. *Journal of Nervous and Mental Disorders, 174,* 509–516.

Condon, J. T. (1987a). Altered cognitive functioning in pregnant women: A shift towards primary process thinking. *British Journal of Medical Psychology, 60,* 329–334.

Condon, J. T. (1987b). The battered fetus syndrome. Preliminary data on the incidence of the urge to physically abuse the unborn child. *Journal of Nervous and Mental Disease, 175,* 722–725.

Condon, J. T., & Dunn, D. J. (1988). Nature and determinants of parent-to-infant attachment in the early postnatal period. *Journal of the American Academy of Child Adolescent Psychiatry, 27,* 293–299.

Cooper, A. (1989). Working through. *Contemporary Psychoanalysis, 25,* 34–61.

Cooper, R. P. (1990). *Preference for infant-directed speech in newborn infants.* In C. Rovee-Collier (Ed.), Abstracts of papers presented at the Seventh International Conference on Infant Studies (p. 324), Montreal. Norwood, NJ: Ablex.

Corman, H. H., & Escalona, S. K. (1969). Stages of sensorimotor development: A replication study. *Merrill-Palmer Quarterly, 15,* 351–361.

Cossette, L., Pomerleau, A., Malcuit, G., & Brault, M. (1990). *Emotional reactions to various contexts at 2 ½ and 5 months of age.* In C. Rovee-Collier (Ed.), Abstracts of papers presented at the Seventh International Conference on Infant Studies (p. 325), Montreal. Norwood, NJ: Ablex.

Courage, M., Adams, R., & Mercer, M. (1990). *Using color cards to assess the development of color vision.* In C. Rovee-Collier (Ed.), Abstracts of papers presented at the Seventh International Conference on Infant Studies (p. 326), Montreal. Norwood, NJ: Ablex.

Cowan, P. A., & Cowan, C. P. (1984). To have and to hold: Marriage, the 1st baby and preparing couples for parenthood. *Social Science & Medicine, 18,* 802–803.

Cowan, P. A., & Cowan, C. P. (1987). Men's involvement in parenthood: Identifying the antecedents and understanding the barriers. In P. W. Berman & F. A. Pederson (Eds.), *Men's transitions to parenthood: Longitudinal studies of early family experience* (pp. 145–174). Hillsdale, NJ: Erlbaum.

Coysh, W. S. (1983). Men's role in caring for their children: Predictive and concurrent correlates of father involvement. *Dissertation Abstracts International, 45* (6–B).

Coysh, W. S. (1984, August). *Predictive and concurrent factors related to fathers' involvement in childrearing.* Paper presented at the meeting of the American Psychological Association, Anaheim, CA.

Cramer, B. G., & Stern, D. N. (1988). Evaluation of changes in mother-infant brief psychotherapy: A single case study. *Infant Mental Health Journal, 9,* 20–45.

Crittenden, P. M. (1985). Social networks, quality of child rearing, and child development. *Child Development, 56,* 1299–1313.

Crnic, K. A., Greenberg, M. T., Ragozin, A. S., Robinson, N. M., & Basham, R. B. (1983). Effects of stress and social support on mothers and premature and full-term infants. *Child Development, 54,* 209–217.

Crockenberg, S. (1981). Infant irritability, mother responsiveness, and social influences on the security of infant-mother attachment. *Child Development, 52,* 857–865.

Crockenberg, S. (1990). *Predicting mental development at two years from early mother-infant interaction.* In C. Rovee-Collier (Ed.), Abstracts of papers presented at the Seventh International Conference on Infant Studies (p. 330), Montreal. Norwood, NJ: Ablex.

Crowther, J. H. (1985). The relationship between depression and marital maladjustment. *Journal of Nervous and Mental Disease, 173*(4), 227–231.

Culp, A. M., Culp, R. E., & Friese, S. (1990). *Language delay in infants born to adolescent mothers.* In C. Rovee-Collier (Ed.), Abstracts of papers presented at the Seventh International Conference on Infant Studies (p. 331), Montreal. Norwood, NJ: Ablex.

Daitzman, R. J. (1977). Methods of self-confrontation in family therapy. *Journal of Marriage and Family Counseling, 3*(4), 3–9.

Danish, S. J., Smyer, M. A., & Nowak, C. A. (1980). Developmental intervention: Enhancing life-event processes. In P. B. Bates & O. G. Brim, Jr. (Eds.), *Life-span development and behavior* (Vol. 3, pp. 336–339). New York: Academic Press.

Davanloo, H. (Ed.) (1978). *Basic principles and techniques in short-term dynamic psychotherapy*. New York: Spectrum.

Davanloo, H. (1984). Intensive short-term dynamic psychotherapy. In H. Kaplan and B. Sadock (Eds.), *Comprehensive textbook of psychiatry* (4th ed., pp. 1460–1467). Baltimore: Williams & Wilkins.

Davanloo, H. (1986). Intensive short-term psychotherapy with highly resistant patients. *International Journal of Short-Term Psychotherapy, 1*(4), 107–133.

Davanloo, H. (1989). The central dynamic sequence in the unlocking of the unconscious and comprehensive trial therapy. Part I. Major unlocking. *International Journal of Short-Term Psychotherapy, 4*, 1033.

Davenport, Y. B., & Adland, M. L. (1985). Issues in the treatment of the married bipolar patient: Denial and dependency. In M. Lansky (Ed.), *Family approaches to major psychiatric disorders* (pp. 47–65). Washington, DC: American Psychiatric Press.

Davis, A. L. (1990a). *Clarifying and refining video replay methodology: Improving self-efficacy via self-modeling*. In C. Rovee-Collier (Ed.), Abstracts of papers presented at the Seventh International Conference on Infant Studies (p. 336), Montreal. Norwood, NJ: Ablex.

Davis, A. L. (1990b). *Clarifying the role of maternal self-confidence in interactional competence*. In C. Rovee-Collier (Ed.), Abstracts of papers presented at the Seventh International Conference on Infant Studies (p. 335), Montreal. Norwood, NJ: Ablex.

Davis, D. (1989). Resistance and transference in intensive short-term dynamic psychotherapy (IS-TDP) and classical psychoanalysis: Similarities and differences. Part 1. *International Journal of Short-Term Psychotherapy, 4*, 313–331.

DeBaryshe, B. D. (1990). *What a bedtime story may mean: Effects of literacy exposure and maternal reading style on children's oral language ability*. In C. Rovee-Collier (Ed.), Abstracts of papers presented at the Seventh International Conference on Infant Studies (p. 338), Montreal. Norwood, NJ: Ablex.

DeBoysson, B., Sagart, L., & Durand, C. (1984). Discernible differences in the babbling of infants according to target language. *Journal of Child Language, 11*(1), 1–15.

DeCarie, T. G., & Simineau, K. (1979). Cognition and perception in the object concept. *Canadian Journal of Psychology, 33*, 396–407.

DeCasper, A. J. (1979). The mommy tapes. *Science News, 115*(4), 56.

DeCasper, A. J., & Carstens, A. A. (1981). Contingencies of stimulation: Effects on learning and emotion in neonates. *Infant Behavior & Development, 4*, 19–35.

DeGangi, G. A. (1990). *A longitudinal study of sensory and developmental functions in normal and regulatory disordered infants*. In C. Rovee-Collier (Ed.), Abstracts of papers presented at the Seventh International Conference on Infant Studies (p. 209), Montreal. Norwood, NJ: Ablex.

Deutsch, H. (1944). *The psychology of women: A psychoanalytic interpretation*. New York: Grune & Stratton.

Diamond, A. (1990). *Why studies find earlier evidence of memory in looking than in reaching*. In C. Rovee-Collier (Ed.), Abstracts of papers presented at the Seventh

International Conference on Infant Studies (p. 342), Montreal. Norwood, NJ: Ablex.

Dichtelmiller, M., Meisels, S. J., Plunkett, J. W., & King, C. (1990). *The relationship of parental knowledge of the development of extremely low birth weight infants.* In C. Rovee-Collier (Ed.), Abstracts of papers presented at the Seventh International Conference on Infant Studies (p. 345), Montreal. Norwood, NJ: Ablex.

Dolgoff, R., & Feldstein, D. (1984). *Understanding social welfare.* Green, NY: Longmans.

Donovan, W. L., Leavitt, L. A., & Walsh, R. O. (1990). *The effects of perception of control and infant temperament on maternal physiologic response.* In C. Rovee-Collier (Ed.), Abstracts of papers presented at the Seventh International Conference on Infant Studies (p. 351), Montreal. Norwood, NJ: Ablex.

Doussard-Roosevelt, J. A., Walker, P. S., Portales, A. L., Greenspan, S. I., & Porqes, S. W. (1990). *Vagal tone and the fussy infant: Atypical vagal reactivity in the difficult infant.* In C. Rovee-Collier (Ed.), Abstracts of papers presented at the Seventh International Conference on Infant Studies (p. 352), Montreal. Norwood, NJ: Ablex.

Dowling, S. (1987). *The interpretation of dreams in the reconstructions of trauma.* In A. Rothstein (Ed.), The interpretations of dreams in clinical work (pp. 27–36). New York: International Universities Press.

Dowrick, P. W. (1983). Self-modelling. In P. W. Dowrick & S. J. Biggs (Eds.), *Using video* (pp. 105–124). New York: Wiley.

Duhl, F. J., Kantor, D., & Duhl, B. S. (1973). Learning, space and action in family therapy: A primer of sculpture. *Seminars in Psychiatry, 5*(2), 167–183.

Dunst, C. J., & Trivette, C. M. (1990). *Family-systems determinants of poor and positive outcomes.* In C. Rovee-Collier (Ed.), Abstracts of papers presented at the Seventh International Conference on Infant Studies (p. 147), Montreal. Norwood, NJ: Ablex.

Echols, C. H. (1990). *An influence of labeling on infants' attention to objects and consistency: Implications for word-referent mappings.* In C. Rovee-Collier (Ed.), Abstracts of papers presented at the Seventh International Conference on Infant Studies (p. 354), Montreal. Norwood, NJ: Ablex.

Edelson, M. (1973). Language and dreams: The interpretation of dreams revisited. *Psychoanalytic Study of the Child, 27,* 203–282.

Einstein, S. (1985). Considering roles for beliefs, explainability, and obviousness in the planned treatment of drug misusers. *International Journal of the Addictions, 20*(9), iii–iv.

Eisen, L. N. (1990). *Effects of perinatal cocaine exposure on neonatal behavior and withdrawal symptoms.* In C. Rovee-Collier (Ed.), Abstracts of papers presented at the Seventh International Conference on Infant Studies (p. 356), Montreal. Norwood, NJ: Ablex.

Eisenhart, C. E., & Hrncir, E. J. (1990). *Reciprocity between mothers and infants with cerebral palsy during interactive play.* In C. Rovee-Collier (Ed.), Abstracts of papers presented at the Seventh International Conference on Infant Studies (p. 357), Montreal. Norwood, NJ: Ablex.

Eisnitz, A. J. (1987). The perspective of the self representation in dreams. In A. Rothstein (Ed.), *The interpretations of dreams in clinical work* (pp. 27–36). New York: International Universities Press.

Ekman, P., & Friesen, W. V. (1978). *Facial action coding system.* Palo Alto, CA: Consulting Psychologists Press.

Elderkin, J. B. (1975). *Family therapy.* New York: Jason Aronson.

Elliot, C., & Ozolins, M. (1983). Use of imagery and imagination in treatment of children. In C. E. Walker & M. C. Roberts (Eds.), Handbook of clinical child psychology. New York: Wiley.

Ellis, A. E. (1990). *Infants' recognition of the categories of "dog" and "cat."* In C. Rovee-Collier (Ed.), Abstracts of papers presented at the Seventh International Conference on Infant Studies (p. 359), Montreal. Norwood, NJ: Ablex.

Emde, R. N. (1980). Emotional availability: A reciprocal reward system for infant and parents with implications for prevention of psychosocial disorders. In P. Taylor (Ed.), *Parent–infant relationships* (pp. 87–115). Orlando, FL: Grune & Stratton.

Emde, R. N. (1984). The affective self: Continuities and transformations from infancy. In J. D. Call, E. Galenson, & R. L. Tyson (Eds.), *Frontiers in child development* (Vol. 2., pp. 38–54). New York: Basic Books.

Emde, R. N., Gaensbauer, T. J., & Harmon, R. J. (1976). Emotional expression in infancy: A biobehavioral study. *Psychological Issues, 10,* 1–200.

Emde, R. N., Kligman, D. H., Reich, J. H., & Wade, T. (1978). Emotional expression in infancy. 1. Initial studies of social signalling and an emergent model. In M. Lewis & L. Rosenblum (Eds.), *The development of affect.* New York: Plenum.

Epstein, L. and Feiner, A. H. (Eds.) (1979). *Countertransference.* New York: Jason Aronson.

Epstein, N. B., & Bishop, D. S. (1981). Problem-centered systems therapy of the family. In A. S. Gurman & D. P. Kniskern (Eds.), *Handbook of family therapy* (pp. 444–482). New York: Brunner/Mazel.

Erikson, E. (1954). The dream specimen of psychoanalysis. *Journal of the American Psychoanalytic Association, 2,* 5–56.

Evans, B., Pederson, D. R., Bento, S., Chance, G. W., & Fox, A. M. (1990). *Do premature infants have difficult temperaments?* In C. Rovee-Collier (Ed.), Abstracts of papers presented at the Seventh International Conference on Infant Studies (p. 364), Montreal. Norwood, NJ: Ablex.

Fagen, J. W., Morrongiello, B. A., Rovee-Collier, C., & Gekoski, M. J. (1984). Expectancies and memory retrieval in three-month-old infants. *Child Development, 55,* 936–943.

Fagen, J. W., & Ohr, P. S. (1985). Temperament and crying in response to the violation of a learned expectancy in early infancy. *Infant Behavior and Development, 8,* 157–166.

Feagans, L., McGhee, S., Kipp, E., & Blood, I. (1990). *Attention to language in daycare attending children: A mediating factor in the developmental effects of otitis media.* In C. Rovee-Collier (Ed.), Abstracts of papers presented at the Seventh International Conference on Infant Studies (p. 368), Montreal. Norwood, NJ: Ablex.

Fein, G. (1979a). Echoes from the nursery: Piaget, Vygotsky, and the relationship between language and play. *New Directions for Child Development, 6,* 1–14.

Fein, G. (1979b). Play and the acquisition of symbols. In L. E. Katz (Ed.), *Current topics in early childhood education.* Baltimore: University Park Press.

Feldman, L. B. (1979). Strategies and techniques of family therapy. In J. G. Howells (Ed.), *Advances in family psychiatry* (Vol. 1). New York: International Universities Press.

Feldman, S. S., Nash, S. C., & Aschenbrenner, B. G. (1983). Antecedents of fathering. *Child Development, 54,* 1628–1636.

Feldstein, S., DiGregorio, I., Crown, C. L., & Jasnow, M. D. (1990). *Infant temperament and coordinated interpersonal timing.* In C. Rovee-Collier (Ed.), Abstracts of papers presented at the Seventh International Conference on Infant Studies (p. 369), Montreal. Norwood, NJ: Ablex.

Fenson, L., Dale, P., Reznick, S., Hartung, J., & Burgess, S. (1990). *Norms for the Macarthur communicative development inventories.* In C. Rovee-Collier (Ed.), Abstracts of papers presented at the Seventh International Conference on Infant Studies (p. 370), Montreal. Norwood, NJ: Ablex.

Fenson, L., Kagan, J., Kearsley, R. B., & Zelazo, P. R. (1976). Developmental progression of manipulative play in 1st 2 years. *Child Development, 47,* 232–236.

Fenson, L., & Ramsay, D. S. (1980). Decentration and integration of the child's play in the 2nd year. *Child Development, 51,* 171–178.

Fernald, A. (1990a). *From preference to reference: Affective and linguistic functions of prosody in speech to infants.* In C. Rovee-Collier (Ed.), Abstracts of papers presented at the Seventh International Conference on Infant Studies (p. 50), Montreal. Norwood, NJ: Ablex.

Fernald, A. (1990b). *Themes and variations: Cross-cultural comparisons of melodies in mothers' speech.* In C. Rovee-Collier (Ed.), Abstracts of papers presented at the Seventh International Conference on Infant Studies (p.137), Montreal. Norwood, NJ: Ablex.

Fernald, A., & Dorado, J. (1990). *Young children's use of prosody in their speech to infant siblings: Is it really "motherese"?* In C. Rovee-Collier (Ed.), Abstracts of papers presented at the Seventh International Conference on Infant Studies (p. 371), Montreal. Norwood, NJ: Ablex.

Fernald, A., & Kuhl, P. K. (1987). Acoustic determinants of infant preference for motherese speech. *Infant Behavior and Development, 10,* 279–293.

Field, T. M. (1982). Affective displays of high-risk infants during early interaction. In T. Field & A. Fogel (Eds.), *Emotion and early interactions.* Hillsdale, NJ: Erlbaum.

Field, T. M. (1990). *Behavior states and rhythms of depressed mother–infant dyads.* In C. Rovee-Collier (Ed.), Abstracts of papers presented at the Seventh International Conference on Infant Studies (p. 58), Montreal. Norwood, NJ: Ablex.

Field, T. M., Woodson, R., Greenberg, R., & Cohen, D. (1982). Discrimination and imitation of facial expression by neonates. *Science, 218,* 179–181.

Fiese, B. H. (1990). *Family Stories.* In C. Rovee-Collier (Ed.), Abstracts of papers presented at the Seventh International Conference on Infant Studies (p. 372), Montreal. Norwood, NJ: Ablex.

Fish, M. (1990). *Early family origins of boundary violation behavior in families with four-year-olds.* In C. Rovee-Collier (Ed.), Abstracts of papers presented at the Seventh International Conference on Infant Studies (p. 373), Montreal. Norwood, NJ: Ablex.

Fish, S. (1984). Casework to foster parents. In F. Maidman (Ed.), *Child welfare: A sourcebook of knowledge and practice* (pp. 235–262). New York: Child Welfare League of America.

Fletcher, K., & Averill, J. (1984). A scale for the measurement of role-playing ability. *Journal of Research in Personality, 18,* 131–149.

Fogel, A., & Hannan, T. E. (1985). Manual actions of nine- to fifteen-week-old human infants during face-to-face interaction with their mothers. *Child Development, 56,* 1271–1279.

Fosshage, J. L. (1987). A revised psychoanalytic approach. In J. L. Fosshage & C. A. Loew (Eds.), *Dream interpretation: A comparative study* (rev. ed.). New York: PMA Publishing.

Foulkes, D. (1985). *Dreaming: A cognitive-psychological analysis.* New Jersey: Erlbaum.

Fraiberg, S. (Ed.) (1980). *Clinical studies in infant mental health.* New York: Basic Books.

Fraiberg, S. (1982). Pathological defenses in infancy. *Psychoanalytic Quarterly, 51,* 612–635.

Fraiberg, S., Shapiro, V., & Cherniss, D. P. (1980). Treatment modalities. In S. Fraiberg (Ed.), *Clinical studies in infant mental health: The first year of life* (pp. 49–77). New York: Basic Books.

Freud, A. (1965). *Normality and pathology in childhood: Assessments of development.* New York: International Universities Press.

Freud, A. (1966). *The ego and the mechanisms of defense.* New York: International Universities Press.

Freud, S. (1893). Some points for a comparative study of organic and hysterical motor paralyses. *Standard Edition* (Vol. 1, p. 157). London: Hogarth Press.

Freud, S. (1894). The neuro-psychoses of defence. *Standard Edition* (Vol. 3, pp. 45–61). London: Hogarth Press.

Freud, S. (1895a). Obsessions and phobias: Their physical mechanism and their aetiology. *Standard Edition* (Vol. 3, pp. 71–86). London: Hogarth Press.

Freud, S. (1895b). On the grounds for detaching a particular syndrome from neurasthenia under the description of 'Anxiety Neurosis.' *Standard Edition* (Vol. 3, pp. 87–115). London: Hogarth Press.

Freud, S. (1895c). A reply to criticism of my paper on anxiety neurosis. *Standard Edition* (Vol. 3, pp. 121–140). London: Hogarth Press.

Freud, S. (1900). The interpretation of dreams. *Standard Edition* (Vols. 4 and 5). London: Hogarth Press.

Freud, S. (1905). Three essays on the theory of sexuality. *Standard Edition* (Vol. 7, pp. 173–206). London: Hogarth Press.

Freud, S. (1915). The unconscious. Standard Edition (Vol. 12, pp. 3–82). London: Hogarth Press.

Freud, S. (1917). General theory of neurosis. *Standard Edition* (Vol. 16, pp. 358–377). London: Hogarth Press.

Freud, S. (1918). From the history of an infantile neurosis. *Standard Edition* (Vol. 17, pp. 29–81). London: Hogarth Press.

Freud, S. (1923). The ego and the id. *Standard Edition* (Vol. 19, pp. 57–59). London: Hogarth Press.

Freud, S. (1930). Civilization and its discontents. *Standard Edition* (Vol. 21, pp. 64–132). London: Hogarth Press.

Freud, S. (1931). Female sexuality. *Standard Edition* (Vol. 21, pp. 223–240). London: Hogarth Press.

Freud, S. (1933). New introductory lectures on psychoanalysis. *Standard Edition* (Vol. 22, pp. 81–111). London: Hogarth Press.

Freud, S. (1938). An outline of psychoanalysis. *Standard Edition* (Vol. 23, pp. 145–207). London: Hogarth Press.

Fried, C. (1971). Icarianism, masochism, and sex differences in fantasy. *Journal of Personality Assessment, 35,* 38–55.

Friedlander, S. R., & Watkins, C. E. (1985). Therapeutic aspects of support groups for parents of the mentally retarded. *International Journal of Group Psychotherapy, 35,* 65–78.

Fries, M. E. (1937). Factors in character development, neuroses, psychoses and deliquency. *American Journal of Orthopsychiatry, 7,* 142–181.

Fries, M. E. (1944). Psychosomatic relationships between mother and infant. *Psychosomatic Medicine, 6,* 159–162.

Fries, M. E., & Lewis B. (1938). Interrelated factors in development: A study of pregnancy, labor, delivery, lying-in period, and childhood. *American Journal of Orthopsychiatry, 8,* 726–752.

Fries, M. E., & Woolf, P. J. (1953). Some hypotheses on the role of the congenital activity type in personality development. *Psychoanalytic Study of the Child, 8,* 48–62.

Fromm-Reichmann, F. (1960). *Principles of intensive psychotherapy.* Chicago: University of Chicago Press.

Fuchs, S. H. (1937). On introjection. *International Journal of Psycho-Analysis, 18,* 269–293.

Gable, S., & Isabella, R. A. (1990). *Infant–mother face-to-face interaction: Maternal predictors of infant avoidance.* In C. Rovee-Collier (Ed.), Abstracts of papers presented at the Seventh International Conference on Infant Studies (p. 379), Montreal. Norwood, NJ: Ablex.

Gaffney, K. F. (1986). Maternal-fetal attachment in relation to self-concept and anxiety. *Maternal-Child Nursing Journal, 15,* 91–101.

Gardner, J. M., Magnano, C. L., & Karmel, B. Z. (1990). *Arousal effects on visual preferences and cortisol levels in neonates prenatally exposed to cocaine/crack.* In C. Rovee-Collier (Ed.), Abstracts of papers presented at the Seventh International Conference on Infant Studies (p. 124), Montreal. Norwood, NJ: Ablex.

Garmezy, N. (1983). Stressors of childhood. In N. Garmezy & M. Rutter (Eds.), *Stress, coping, and development in children* (pp. 43–84). New York: McGraw-Hill.

Gelles, R. (1975). Violence and pregnancy: A note on the extent of the problem and needed services. *Family Coordinator, 24,* 81–86.

George, C., & Solomon, J. (1989). Internal working models of caregiving and security of attachment at age six. *Infant Mental Health Journal, 10,* 222–237.

Gerstel, N., & Gross, H. (1983). Commuter marriage: Couples who live apart. In E. Macklin & R. H. Rubin (Eds.), *Contemporary families and alternative lifestyles*. Beverly Hills, CA: Sage Publications.

Gesell, A., & Amatruda, A. (Eds.) (1974). *Developmental diagnosis: The evaluation and management of normal and abnormal neuropsychologic development in infancy and early childhood*. New York: Harper & Row.

Gewirtz, J. L., & Peláez-Nogueras, M. (1990). *Complications of uncontrolled mother/ stranger contingencies in maternal departures and in the strange situation: A functional analysis*. In C. Rovee-Collier (Ed.), Abstracts of papers presented at the Seventh International Conference on Infant Studies (p. 75), Montreal. Norwood, NJ: Ablex.

Gewirtz, J. L., & Stingle, K. G. (1972). Learning of generalized imitation as the basis for identification. In C. S. Lavatelli & F. Stendler (Eds.), *Readings in child behavior and development* (pp. 355–364). New York: Harcourt Brace Jovanovich.

Gibson, J. J. (1979). *The ecological approach to visual perception*. Boston: Houghton Mifflin.

Gillman, R. D. (1987). Dreams as resistance. In A. Rothstein (Ed.), *The interpretations of dreams in clinical work* (pp. 27–36). New York: International Universities Press.

Gilman, I. P. (1986). Student responses to two literary passages and two paintings as they relate to the perception of stylistic complexity and the dimension of extraversion-introversion: I and II. *Dissertation Abstracts International, 47*(4–A), 1223.

Glick, I. D., Clarkin, J. F., & Kessler, D. R. (1987). *Marital and family therapy*. New York: Grune & Stratton.

Glick, I. D., & Kessler, D. R. (1974). *Marital and family therapy*. New York: Grune & Stratton.

Goetting, A. (1985). The six stages of remarriage: Developmental tasks of remarriage and divorce. In L. Cargan (Ed.), *Marriage and family: Coping with change*. Belmont, CA: Wadsworth Publishing.

Gold, D., Andres, D., & Glorieux, J. (1979). The development of francophone nursery-school children with employed and nonemployed mothers. *Canadian Journal of Behavioral Science, 11*, 169–173.

Goldberg, S. (1977). Social competence in infancy: A model of parent-infant interaction. *Merrill-Palmer Quarterly, 23*, 163–177.

Goodyear, R. K., & Parish, T. S. (1978). Perceived attributes of the terms client, patient, and typical person. *Journal of Counseling Psychology, 25*, 356–358.

Gordon, S. B., & Davidson, N. (1981). Behavioral parent training. In A. S. Gurman & D. P. Kniskern (Eds.), *Handbook of family therapy* (pp. 517–555). New York: Bruner/Mazel.

Gratch, G., Appel, K. J., Evans, W. F., LeCompte, G. K., & Wright, N. A. (1974). Piaget's Stage IV object concept error: Evidence of forgetting or object conception? *Child Development, 45*, 71–77.

Graziano, A. M. (1977). Parents as behavior therapists. In M. Hersen, R. M. Eisler, & P. M. Miller (Eds.), *Progress in behavior modification*. New York: Academic Press.

Green, R. J. (1981). An overview of major contributions to family therapy. In R. J. Green and J. L. Framo (Eds.), *Family therapy: Major contributions.* New York: International Universities Press.

Greenberg, M., & Morris, N. (1974). Engrossment: The newborn's impact upon the father. *American Journal of Orthopsychiatry, 44,* 520–531.

Greenson, R. R. (1954). The struggle against identification. *Journal of the American Psychoanalytical Association, 2,* 200–217.

Greenson, R. R. (1960). Empathy and its vicissitudes. *International Journal of Psychoanalysis, 41,* 418–424.

Greenson, R. R. (1967). *The technique and practice of psychoanalysis.* New York: International Universities Press.

Gross-Doehrman, M. J. (1976). Parallel processes in supervision and psychotherapy. *Bulletin of the Menninger Clinic, 40*(1), 1–104.

Grotstein, J. S. (1985). The evolving and shifting trends in psychoanalysis and psychotherapy. *Journal of the American Academy of Psychoanalysis, 13,* 423–452.

Gunnar, M. R. (1990). *Emotion regulation in infancy: Relations between regulatory behavior, affect and physiological responses to stressful events.* In C. Rovee-Collier (Ed.), Abstracts of papers presented at the Seventh International Conference on Infant Studies (p. 107), Montreal. Norwood, NJ: Ablex.

Gunnar, M. R., Kopp, C. B., Tronick, E., & Rothbart, M. K. (1990). *Emotion regulation in infancy.* In C. Rovee-Collier (Ed.), Abstracts of papers presented at the Seventh International Conference on Infant Studies (p. 104), Montreal. Norwood, NJ: Ablex.

Gurwitt, A. R. (1976). Aspects of prospective fatherhood: A case report. *Psychoanalytic Study of the Child, 31,* 237–271.

Gustafson, G. E., Brady, K. L., & Hinse, L. M. (1990). *Caregiving experience and prototypic social responses to infants' cries.* In C. Rovee-Collier (Ed.), Abstracts of papers presented at the Seventh International Conference on Infant Studies (p. 112), Montreal. Norwood, NJ: Ablex.

Gustafson, J. P., & Dichter, H. (1983a). Winnicott and Sullivan in the brief psychotherapy clinic: Part I. *Contemporary Psychoanalysis, 19,* 625–637.

Gustafson, J. P., & Dichter, H. (1983b). Winnicott and Sullivan in the brief psychotherapy clinic: Part II. *Contemporary Psychoanalysis, 19,* 638–652.

Gustafson, J. P., Dichter, H., & Kaye, D. (1983). Winnicott and Sullivan in the brief psychotherapy clinic: Part III. *Contemporary Psychoanalysis, 19,* 653–672.

Guy, J. D., Guy, M. P., & Liaboe, G. P. (1986). First pregnancy: Therapeutic issues for both female and male psychotherapists. *Psychotherapy, 23,* 297–302.

Haekel, M. (1985, July). *Greeting behavior in 3-month-old infants during mother-infant interaction.* Presentation at the Eighth Biennial Meeting of the International Society for the Study of Behavioral Development, Tours, France. Abstracted in *Cahiers de psychologie cognitive, 5,* 275–276.

Haith, M. M. (1980). *Rules that babies look by.* Hillsdale, NJ: Erlbaum.

Haith, M. M. (1990). *Great expectations: How infants anticipate the future: The formation of visual expectations in early infancy.* In C. Rovee-Collier (Ed.), Abstracts of papers presented at the Seventh International Conference on Infant Studies (p. 11), Montreal. Norwood, NJ: Ablex.

Haith, M. M., Bergman, T., & Moore, M. J. (1977). Eye contact and face scanning in early infancy. *Science, 198,* 853–855.

Haley, J. (1976). *Problem-solving therapy.* San Francisco: Jossey-Bass.

Hann, D. (1989). A systems conceptualization of the quality of mother–infant interaction. *Infant Behavior and Development, 12,* 251–263.

Hans, S. L., Bernstein, V. J., & Henson, L. G. (1990). *Interaction between drug-using mothers and their toddlers.* In C. Rovee-Collier (Ed.), Abstracts of papers presented at the Seventh International Conference on Infant Studies (p. 190), Montreal. Norwood, NJ: Ablex.

Harris, P. L. (1975). Development of search and object permanence during infancy. *Psychological Bulletin, 82,* 332–344.

Harrison, L. L. (1990). *Effects of early parent touch on preterm infants.* In C. Rovee-Collier (Ed.), Abstracts of papers presented at the Seventh International Conference on Infant Studies (p. 410), Montreal. Norwood, NJ: Ablex.

Hårsman, I. (1990). *Infants' cognitive development during the first five months in day care centers.* In C. Rovee-Collier (Ed.), Abstracts of papers presented at the Seventh International Conference on Infant Studies (p. 411), Montreal. Norwood, NJ: Ablex.

Hartmann, H. (1939). *Ego psychology and the problem of adaptation.* New York: International Universities Press.

Hartmann, H., & Lowenstein, R. M. (1962). Comments on the formation of psychic structure. *Psychological Issues, 14,* 144–181.

Hartup, W. W. (1979). The social worlds of childhood. *American Psychologist, 34,* 944–950.

Hayne, H., Rovee-Collier, C., & Perris, E. E. (1987). Categorization and memory retrieval by three-month-olds. *Child Development, 58,* 750–767.

Heckhausen, J. (1987). Balancing for weaknesses and challenging developmental potential: A longitudinal study of mother–infant dyads. *Developmental Psychology, 23,* 762–770.

Heilveil, I. (1983). *Video in mental health practice.* New York: Springer.

Heim, L., & Mangelsdorf, S. (1990). *Associations between life events, social support and attachment.* In C. Rovee-Collier (Ed.), Abstracts of papers presented at the Seventh International Conference on Infant Studies (p. 413), Montreal. Norwood, NJ: Ablex.

Heinicke, C. M. (1990). *Patterns of husband-wife adaptation.* In C. Rovee-Collier (Ed.), Abstracts of papers presented at the Seventh International Conference on Infant Studies (p. 414), Montreal. Norwood, NJ: Ablex.

Hendrick, I. (1951). Early development of the ego: Identification in infancy. *Psychoanalytic Quarterly, 20,* 44–61.

Hersen, M., & Bellack, A. S. (1976). A multiple-baseline analysis of social-skills training for chronic psychiatric patients: Rationale, research findings, and future directions. *Comprehensive Psychiatry, 17,* 559–580.

Hertsgaard, L., Wanner, M. B., Jodl, K., & Mason, L. (1990). *Group versus individual care: Effects on adrenocortical responses to brief maternal separation in human infants.* In C. Rovee-Collier (Ed.), Abstracts of papers presented at the Seventh International Conference on Infant Studies (p. 417), Montreal. Norwood, NJ: Ablex.

Herzog, J. (1982). Patterns of expectant fatherhood. In S. Cath, A. Gurwitt, & J. Ross (Eds.), *Father and child* (pp. 85–92). Boston: Little, Brown.

Hetherington, E. M. (1989). Coping and family transitions: Winners, losers, survivors. *Child Development, 60,* 1–14.

Hetherington, E. M., Cox, M., & Cox, R. (1982). Effects of divorce on parents and children. In M. Lamb (Ed.), *Nontraditional families* (pp. 233–288). Hillsdale, NJ: Erlbaum.

Hirshberg, L. (1990). *Infants response to conflicting parental emotional signals.* In C. Rovee-Collier (Ed.), Abstracts of papers presented at the Seventh International Conference on Infant Studies (p. 117), Montreal. Norwood, NJ: Ablex.

Hirshberg, L., Solomon, J., Buschsbaum, H., Stern, D., & Emde, R. (1990). *Conflict in infancy and early childhood: A symposium.* In C. Rovee-Collier (Ed.), Abstracts of papers presented at the Seventh International Conference on Infant Studies (p. 116), Montreal. Norwood, NJ: Ablex.

Hoffman, H. J., Bartlett, G. S., Hillman, L., & Orr, W. C. (1990). *Results from the NICHD SIDS cooperative epidemiological study.* In C. Rovee-Collier (Ed.), Abstracts of papers presented at the Seventh International Conference on Infant Studies (p. 418), Montreal. Norwood, NJ: Ablex.

Hoffman, M. L. (1975). Developmental synthesis of affect and cognition and its implications for altruistic motivation. *Developmental Psychology, 11,* 607–622.

Hoffman, M. L. (1977). Empathy, its development and prosocial implications. *Nebraska Symposium on Motivation, 25,* 169–217.

Hoffman, M. L. (1982). The measurement of empathy. In C. E. Izard (Ed.), *Measuring emotions in infants and children* (pp. 279–296). Cambridge, England: Cambridge University Press.

Hoffman, M. L. (1984). Interaction of affect and cognition in empathy. In C. E. Izard, J. Kagan, & R. B. Zajonc (Eds.), *Emotions, cognition and behavior* (pp. 103–131). Cambridge, England: Cambridge University Press.

Holman, S. L. (1985). A group program for borderline mothers and their toddlers. *International Journal of Group Psychotherapy, 35,* 79–93.

Holt, S. A. (1990). *Toddler smile characteristics: Type and context similarities, sex and age differences.* In C. Rovee-Collier (Ed.), Abstracts of papers presented at the Seventh International Conference on Infant Studies (p. 422), Montreal. Norwood, NJ: Ablex.

Hopkins, B., & van Wufften Palthe, T. (1985). Staring in infancy. *Early Human Development, 12,* 261–267.

Hopkins, B., & Westra, T. (1988). Maternal handling and motor development: An intracultural study. *Genetic, Social, and General Psychology Monographs, 114,* 377–408.

Hopkins, B., & Westra, T. (1989). Maternal expectations of their infant's development: Some cultural differences. *Developmental Medicine and Child Neurology, 31,* 384–390.

Hopkins, B., & Westra, T. (1990). Motor development, maternal expectations and the role of handling. *Infant Behavior and Development, 13,* 117–122.

Hosford, R. E., & Mills, M. E. (1983). Video in social skills training. In P. W. Dowrick & S. J. Biggs (Eds.) *Using video: Psychological and social applications* (pp. 125–150). New York: Wiley.

Houck, G. M., Booth, C. L., & Barnard, K. E. (1990). *Maternal depression and control orientation in relation to dyadic play behavior.* In C. Rovee-Collier (Ed.), Abstracts of papers presented at the Seventh International Conference on Infant Studies (p. 425), Montreal. Norwood, NJ: Ablex.

Howard, J., & Kropenske, V. (1990). A preventive intervention model for chemically dependent parents. In S. Goldston, J. Yager, C. Heinicke, & R. Pynoos (Eds.), *Preventing mental health disturbances in childhood* (pp. 71–84). Washington: American Psychiatric Press.

Howes, C., & Rodning, C. (1990). *Attachment security and social pretend play negotiations.* In C. Rovee-Collier (Ed.), Abstracts of papers presented at the Seventh International Conference on Infant Studies (p. 426), Montreal. Norwood, NJ: Ablex.

Hron-Stewart, K. M., Lefever, G. B., & Weintraub, D. (1990). *Correlates and predictors of mastery motivation.* In C. Rovee-Collier (Ed.), Abstracts of papers presented at the Seventh International Conference on Infant Studies (p. 427), Montreal. Norwood, NJ: Ablex.

Huntington, L., & Hans, S. L. (1990). *Perceptual ratings of the cries of methadone-exposed and comparison infants.* In C. Rovee-Collier (Ed.), Abstracts of papers presented at the Seventh International Conference on Infant Studies (p. 429), Montreal. Norwood, NJ: Ablex.

Imber, S. D., Lewis, P. M., & Loiselle, R. H. (1979). Uses and abuses of the brief intervention group. *International Journal of Group Psychotherapy, 29,* 39–49.

Isabella, R. A. (1990). *Origins of attachment: Infant–mother interaction across the first year of life.* In C. Rovee-Collier (Ed.), Abstracts of papers presented at the Seventh International Conference on Infant Studies (p. 431), Montreal. Norwood, NJ: Ablex.

Izard, C. E. (1978). On the ontogenesis of emotions and emotion-cognition relationship in infancy. In M. Lewis & L. A. Rosenblum (Eds.), *The development of affect.* New York: Plenum Press.

Jacobson, E. (1954). Contribution to the metapsychology of psychotic identifications. *Journal of the American Psychoanalytic Association, 2,* 239–262.

Jacobson, E. (1964). *The self and the object world.* New York: International Universities Press.

Jacobson, N. S. (1987). *Psychotherapists in clinical practice: Cognitive and behavioral perspectives.* New York: Guilford.

Jensen, J. L., & Thelen, E. (1990). *Regulation of muscle stiffness in the leg movements of prewalking infants.* In C. Rovee-Collier (Ed.), Abstracts of papers presented at the Seventh International Conference on Infant Studies (p. 438), Montreal. Norwood, NJ: Ablex.

Jernberg, A. M. (1979). *Theraplay: A new treatment using structured play for problem children and their families.* Washington: Josey-Bass.

Johnson, E. J. (1990). *Role of knowledge of child development in adolescent and adult teaching interactions.* In C. Rovee-Collier (Ed.), Abstracts of papers presented at the

Seventh International Conference on Infant Studies (p. 439), Montreal. Norwood, NJ: Ablex.

Jones, D., & Emde, R. N. (1990). *Temperament and walking onset.* In C. Rovee-Collier (Ed.), Abstracts of papers presented at the Seventh International Conference on Infant Studies (p. 442), Montreal. Norwood, NJ: Ablex.

Jones, S., Raag, T., Collins, K., & Hong, H.-W. (1990). *Smiling: Physical form and maternal response.* In C. Rovee-Collier (Ed.), Abstracts of papers presented at the Seventh International Conference on Infant Studies (p. 444), Montreal. Norwood, NJ: Ablex.

Josselyn, I. M. (1956). Cultural forces, motherliness and fatherliness. *American Journal of Orthopsychiatry, 26,* 264–271.

Kagan, J. (1958). The concept of identification. *Psychological Review, 65,* 296–305.

Kagan, J., Kearsley, R. B., & Zelazo, P. R. (1978). *Infancy: Its place in human development.* Cambridge, MA: Harvard University Press.

Katona, F. (1990). *Development of central control: Neuroanatomical and clinical evidence.* In C. Rovee-Collier (Ed.), Abstracts of papers presented at the Seventh International Conference on Infant Studies (p. 233), Montreal. Norwood, NJ: Ablex.

Kauffman, E., & Kauffmann, P. (1979). *Family therapy of drug and alcohol abuse.* New York: Gardner.

Kaye, K. (1982). Construction of the person. In K. Kaye (Ed.), *The mental and social life of babies: How parents create persons.* Chicago: University of Chicago Press.

Kaye, K., & Fogel, A. (1980). The temporal structure of face-to-face communication between mothers and infants. *Developmental Psychology, 16,* 454–464.

Kazdin, A. (1979). Imagery and self efficacy in the covert modeling treatment of unassertive behavior. *Journal of Consulting and Clinical Psychology, 47,* 725–733.

Kazdin, A. (1974). Covert modelling, model similarity, and reduction of avoidance behavior. *Behavior Therapy, 5,* 325–340.

Kemple, K., & Hazen, N. (1990). *Attachment and shyness.* In C. Rovee-Collier (Ed.), Abstracts of papers presented at the Seventh International Conference on Infant Studies (p. 452), Montreal. Norwood, NJ: Ablex.

Kennedy-Caldwell, C., & Lipsitt, L. (1990). *Effect of early feeding methods on premature infants.* In C. Rovee-Collier (Ed.), Abstracts of papers presented at the Seventh International Conference on Infant Studies (p. 453), Montreal. Norwood, NJ: Ablex.

Kermoian, R. (1990). *Locomotor experience and psychological development.* In C. Rovee-Collier (Ed.), Abstracts of papers presented at the Seventh International Conference on Infant Studies (p. 222), Montreal. Norwood, NJ: Ablex.

Kernberg, O. F. (1984). Projection and projective identification: Development and clinical aspects. *Journal of the American Psychoanalytic Association, 35,* 795–819.

Kerr, M. E. (1981). Family systems theory and therapy. In A. S. Gurman & D. P. Kniskern (Eds.), *Handbook of family therapy* (pp. 226–266). New York: Brunner/Mazel.

Kerr, M. E., & Bowen, M. (Eds.) (1988c). *Family evaluation: An approach based on Bowen theory.* New York: Norton.

Kerr, M. E., & Bowen, M. (1988a). Multigenerational emotional process. In M. E. Kerr & M. Bowen (Eds.), *Family evaluation: An approach based on Bowen theory* (pp. 221–255). New York: Norton.

Kerr, M. E., & Bowen, M. (1988b). Triangles. In M. E. Kerr & M. Bowen (Eds.), *Family evaluation: An approach based on Bowen theory* (pp. 134–163). New York: Norton.

Kestenbaum, R., & Nelson, C. A. (1990). *On what basis do infants recognize emotional expressions?* In C. Rovee-Collier (Ed.), Abstracts of papers presented at the Seventh International Conference on Infant Studies (p. 454), Montreal. Norwood, NJ: Ablex.

Kestenberg, J. (1956). On the development of maternal feelings in early childhood. *Psychoanalytic Study of the Child, 11,* 257–291.

Klein, M. (1952). *Developments in psychoanalysis* London: Hogarth Press.

Klinger, E. (1981). *Structure and functions of fantasy* (pp. 227–278). New York: Wiley-Interscience.

Klinnert, M., Campos, J., Sorce, J., Emde, R., & Svejda, M. (1983). Emotions as behavior regulators: Social referencing in infancy. In R. Plutchik & H. Kellerman (Eds.), *Emotions in early development* (pp. 57–86). New York: Academic Press.

Knight, R. P. (1943). Functional disturbances in the sexual life of women: Frigidity and related disorders. *Bulletin of the Menninger Clinic, 7,* 25–35.

Kohut, H. (1959). Introspection, empathy, and psychoanalysis. An examination of the relationship between mode of observation and theory. *Journal of the American Psychoanalytic Association, 7,* 459–483.

Kohut, H. (1977). *The analysis of self.* New York: International Universities Press.

Kolstad, V. T., & Baillargeon, R. (1990). *Functional and perceptual categorization by young infants.* In C. Rovee-Collier (Ed.), Abstracts of papers presented at the Seventh International Conference on Infant Studies (p. 459), Montreal. Norwood, NJ: Ablex.

Koopmans-van-Deinun, F. J., & van der Stelt, B. (1985). Early stages in the development of speech movements. In B. Lindblom & R. Zetterstrom (Eds.), *Precursors of early speech.* Basingstrake, Hampshire: MacMillan.

Kopp, C. B. (1982). Antecedents of self-regulation: A developmental perspective. *Developmental Psychology, 18*(2), 199–214.

Kopp, C. B. (1990). *Language, toddlers and emotion regulation.* In C. Rovee-Collier (Ed.), Abstracts of papers presented at the Seventh International Conference on Infant Studies (p. 105), Montreal. Norwood, NJ: Ablex.

Korner, A. F. (1972). State as variable, as obstacle, and as mediator of stimulation in infant research. *Merrill-Palmer Quarterly, 18,* 77–94.

Koss, M. P., & Butcher, J. N. (1986). Research on brief psychotherapy. In S. L. Garfield & A. E. Bergin (Eds.), *Handbook of psychotherapy and behavior change* (pp. 627–670). New York: Wiley.

Kotelchuck, M. (1975, August). *Father caretaking characteristics and their influence on infant-father interaction.* Paper presented at the annual meeting of the American Psychological Association, Chicago, IL.

Kotelchuck, M. (1981). The infant's relationship to the father: Experimental evidence. In M. E. Lamb (Ed.), *The role of the father in child development* (pp. 329–345). New York: Wiley.

Kuhl, P., & Meltzoff, A. N. (1982). The bimodal perception of speech in infancy. *Science, 218,* 1138–1141.

Kurzweil, S. R. (1990). *Newborns' recognition of mother.* In C. Rovee-Collier (Ed.), Abstracts of papers presented at the Seventh International Conference on Infant Studies (p. 463), Montreal. Norwood, NJ: Ablex.

Lagerspetz, K., Nygard, M., & Strandvik, C. (1971). The effects of training in crawling on the motor and mental development of infants. *Scandinavian Journal of Psychology, 12,* 192–197.

Lalonde, C. W., & Werker, J. F. (1990). *Cognitive/perceptual integration of three skills at 9 months.* In C. Rovee-Collier (Ed.), Abstracts of papers presented at the Seventh International Conference on Infant Studies (p. 464), Montreal. Norwood, NJ: Ablex.

Lamb, M. E. (1976). Twelve-month-olds and their parents: Interactions in a laboratory playroom. *Developmental Psychology, 12,* 237–244.

Lamb, M. E. (1981). Fathers and child development: An integrative overview. In M. E. Lamb (Ed.), *The role of the father in child development* (pp. 329–345). New York: Wiley.

Lamb, M. E., & Sherrod, L. R. (1981). *Infant social cognition.* Hillsdale, NJ: Erlbaum.

Lamb, M. E., Sternberg, K. J., & Prodromidis, M. (1990). *On the attachment between daycare and attachment.* In C. Rovee-Collier (Ed.), Abstracts of papers presented at the Seventh International Conference on Infant Studies (p. 465), Montreal. Norwood, NJ: Ablex.

Landry, S. H., Richardson, M. A., & Garner, P. (1990). *Effects of joint attention interactions on low birth weight (LBW) infants' exploratory behavior actions.* In C. Rovee-Collier (Ed.), Abstracts of papers presented at the Seventh International Conference on Infant Studies (p. 469), Montreal. Norwood, NJ: Ablex.

Langs, R. (1973). *The technique of psychoanalytic psychotherapy* (Vol. 1). New York: Jason Aronson.

Langs, R. (1989). Reactions of supervisees (and supervisors) to new levels of psychoanalytic discovery and meaning. *Contemporary Psychoanalysis, 25,* 76–97.

LaPlanche, J., & Pontalis, J.-B. (1973). *The language of psycho-analysis.* New York: Norton.

Lask, B. (1982). The child within the family. In J. Apley & C. Ounsted (Eds.), *One child* (pp. 166–174). Philadelphia: Lippincott.

Lavatelli, C. S., & Stendler, F. (1972). *Readings in child behavior and development.* New York: Harcourt Jovanovich.

Lazarus, A. A. (1971). *Behavior therapy and beyond.* New York: McGraw-Hill.

Lederman, R. P. (1984). *Psychosocial adaptation in pregnancy: Assessment of seven dimensions of maternal development.* Englewood Cliffs, NJ: Prentice-Hall.

Legerstee, M., & Moore, C. (1990). *Three-month-old infants selectively imitate vowel sounds.* In C. Rovee-Collier (Ed.), Abstracts of papers presented at the Seventh International Conference on Infant Studies (p. 477), Montreal. Norwood, NJ: Ablex.

Legerstee, M., Pomerleau, A., Malcuit, G., & Feider, H. (1987). The development of infants' responses to people and a doll: Implications for research in communication. *Infant Behavior & Development, 10,* 81–95.

Lein, L. (1979). Male participation in home life: Impact of social supports and breadwinner responsibility on the allocation of tasks. *Family Coordinator, 29,* 489–496.

Lester, B. M., Hoffman, J., & Brazelton, T. (1985). The rhythmic structure of mother-infant interaction in term and preterm infants. *Child Development, 56,* 15–27.

Levenson, E. (1972). *The fallacy of understanding.* New York: Basic Books.

Levitt, M. J., & Coffman, S. (1990). *Close relationships, maternal well-being and infant difficulty: An expectancy model.* In C. Rovee-Collier (Ed.), Abstracts of papers presented at the Seventh International Conference on Infant Studies (p. 482), Montreal. Norwood, NJ: Ablex.

Levy, J., & McGee, R. (1975). Childbirth as a crisis: A test of Janis' theory of communication and stress resolution. *Journal of Personality and Social Psychology, 31,* 171.

Lewis, M. (1979). *Social cognition and the acquisition of self.* New York: Plenum.

Lewis, M., & Brooks, J. (1978). Self-knowledge and emotional development. In M. Lewis & L. A. Rosenblum (Eds.), *The development of affect* (pp. 205–226). New York: Plenum.

Lewis, M., Wolan-Sullivan, M., & Brooks-Gunn, J. (1985). Emotional behavior during the learning of a contingency in early infancy. *British Journal of Developmental Psychology, 3,* 307–316.

Lewkowicz, D. J., & Turkewitz, G. (1980). Cross-modal equivalence in early infancy: Auditory-visual intensity matching. *Developmental Psychology, 16,* 597–607.

Libet, J. M., & Lewinsohn, P. M. (1973). Concept of social skill with special reference to the behavior of depressed persons. *Journal of Consulting and Clinical Psychology, 40,* 304–312.

Lin, N. (1986). Conceptualizing social support. In N. Lin, A. Dean, & W. Ensel (Eds.), *Social support, life events, and depression* (pp. 17–30). Orlando, FL: Academic.

Lin, N., Dean, A., & Ensel, W. (Eds.) (1986). *Social support, life events, and depression.* Orlando, FL: Academic.

Lipsitt, L. P. (1983). *Advances in infancy research,* Vol. 2. Norwood, NJ: Ablex.

Loewald, H. (1962). Internalization, separation, mourning, and the superego. *Psychological Quarterly, 31,* 483–504.

Lövaas, O. (1961). Effect of exposure to symbolic aggression on aggressive behavior. *Child Development, 32,* 37–44.

Luborsky, L. (1984). *Principles of psychoanalytic psychotherapy: A manual for supportive-09expressive treatment.* New York: Basic Books.

Mahler, M. S. (1958). Autism and symbiosis: Two extreme disturbances of identity. *International Journal of Psychoanalysis, 29,* 77–83.

Mahler, M. S., & McDevitt, J. B. (1968). Observations on adaptation and defense in statu nascendi: Developmental precursors in the first two years of life. *Psychoanalytic Quarterly, 37,* 1–21.

Mahler, M. S., Pine, F., & Bergman, A. (1975). *The psychological birth of the human infant: Symbiosis and individuation.* New York: Basic Books.

Main, M., Kaplan, K., & Cassidy, J. (1985). Security in infancy, childhood and adulthood. A move to the level of representation. In I. Bretherton & E. Waters (Eds.), Growing points of attachment theory and research. *Monographs of the Society for Research in Child Development, 50*(1–2, Serial No. 209), 66–104.

Malan, D. H. (1979). *Individual psychotherapy and the science of psychodynamics.* London: Butterworths.

Malan, D. H. (1986). Beyond interpretation, initial evaluation and technique. *Short-Term Dynamic Psychotherapy* (Parts I & II), 1(2), 59–106.

Mann, J. (1973). *Time-limited psychotherapy.* Cambridge, MA: Harvard University Press.

Mann, J., & Godlman, R. (1982). *A case book on time-limited psychotherapy.* New York: McGraw-Hill.

Mast, V. K., Fagen, J. W., Rovee-Collier, C. K., & Sullivan, M. V. (1980). Immediate and longterm memory for reinforcement context: The development of learned expectancies in early infancy. *Child Development, 51,* 700–707.

McCall, R. B., & Kagan, J. (1970). Individual differences in the infant's distribution of attention to stimulus discrepancy. *Developmental Psychology, 2,* 90–98.

McCall, R. B., & McGhee, P. E. (1977). The discrepancy hypothesis of attention and affect in infants. In I. C. Uzgiris & F. Weizmann (Eds.), *The structuring of experience* (pp. 179–210). New York: Plenum.

McComas, J., & Field, J. (1990). *Locomotion and infant social referencing.* In C. Rovee-Collier (Ed.), Abstracts of papers presented at the Seventh International Conference on Infant Studies (p. 512), Montreal. Norwood, NJ: Ablex.

McCune-Nicolich, L. (1981a). The cognitive bases of relational words in the single word period. *Journal of Child Language, 8,* 15–34.

McCune-Nicolich, L. (1981b). Toward symbolic functioning: Structure of early pretend games and potential parallels with language. *Child Development, 52,* 785–797.

McCune-Nicoloch, L., & Carroll, S. (1981). Development of symbolic play: Implications for the language specialist. *Topics in Language Disorders, 21,* 1–15.

McDonough, L., & Mandler, J. (1990). *Very long-term recall in two-year-olds.* In C. Rovee-Collier (Ed.), Abstracts of papers presented at the Seventh International Conference on Infant Studies (p. 514), Montreal. Norwood, NJ: Ablex.

McGoldrick, M., & Carter, E. A. (1982). The family life cycle. In F. Walsh (Ed.), *Normal family processes* (pp. 167–195). New York: Guilford.

McGurk, H., & MacDonald, J. (1976). Hearing lips and seeing voices. *Nature, 264*(5588), 746–748.

McHale, S. M., & Huston, T. L. (1984). Men and women as parents: Sex role orientations, employment, and parental roles with infants. *Child Development, 55,* 1349–1361.

McLaughlin, F. J., Altemeier, W. A., Sherrod, K. B., & Christensen, M. J. (1990). *Comprehensive prenatal care and birthweight: Preventing prematurity or promoting fetal growth?* In C. Rovee-Collier (Ed.), Abstracts of papers presented at the Seventh

International Conference on Infant Studies (p. 519), Montreal. Norwood, NJ: Ablex.

McRea, C. (1983). Impact on body-image. In P. W. Dowrick & S. J. Biggs (Eds.), *Using video* (pp. 95–103). New York: Wiley.

Medin, D. L. (1983). Structural principles in categorization. In B. Shepp & T. Tighe (Eds.), *Interaction: Perception, development and cognition* (pp. 203–230). Hillsdale, NJ: Erlbaum.

Meerloo, J. A. M. (1952). *Conversation and communication: A psychological inquiry into language and human relations*. New York: International Universities Press.

Meissner, W. W. (1971). Notes on identification. *Psychoanalytic Quarterly, 40,* 277–302.

Meltzoff, A. N. (1981). Imitation, intermodal coordination, and representation in early infancy. In G. Butterworth (Ed.), *Infancy and epistemology* (pp. 85–114). London: Harvester Press.

Meltzoff, A. N. (1988). Infant imitation after 1–week delay: Long-term memory for novel acts and multiple stimuli. *Developmental Psychology, 24,* 470–476.

Meltzoff, A. N., & Borton, W. (1979). Intermodal matching by human neonates. *Nature, 282,* 403–404.

Meltzoff, A. N., & Moore, M. K. (1983). The origins of imitation in infancy: Paradigm, phenomena, and theories. In L. P. Lipsitt (Ed.), *Advances in infancy* (Vol. 2, pp. 265–301). Norwood, NJ: Ablex.

Meltzoff, A. N., & Moore, M. K. (1977). Imitation of facial and manual gestures by human neonates. *Science, 198,* 75–78.

Mercer, R. T., Hackley, K. C., & Bostrom, A. (1983). Social support of teenage mothers. *Birth Defects: Original Article Series, 20*(5), 245–290.

Miller, W. H. (1975). *Systematic parent training*. Champaign, IL: Research Press.

Minde, K., Popiel, K., Leos, N., & Falkner, S. (1990). *Are sleep disturbances in young children a sign of behavioral dysregulation?* In C. Rovee-Collier (Ed.), Abstracts of papers presented at the Seventh International Conference on Infant Studies (p. 160), Montreal. Norwood, NJ: Ablex.

Minuchin, S. (1974). *Families and family therapy*. Cambridge, MA: Harvard University Press.

Moore, B. E., & Fine, B. D. (Eds.) (1967). *A glossary of psycho-analytic terms and concepts*. New York: American Psychoanalytic Association.

Moore, B. E., & Fine, B. D. (Eds.) (1968). *A glossary of psychoanalytic terms and concepts*. New York: American Psychoanalytic Association.

Moore, M. K., & Meltzoff, A. N. (1978). Object permanence, imitation, and language development in infancy: Toward a neo-Piagetian perspective on communicative and cognitive development. In F. D. Minifie & L. L. Lloyd (Eds.), *Communicative and cognitive abilities: Early behavioral assessment* (pp. 151–183). Baltimore: University Park Press.

Moran, G., Pederson, D. R., Petit, P., & Krupka, A. (1990). *Maternal sensitivity and infant attachment in a high-sample*. In C. Rovee-Collier (Ed.), Abstracts of papers presented at the Seventh International Conference on Infant Studies (p. 531), Montreal. Norwood, NJ: Ablex.

Morris, W. (Ed.) (1970). *American Heritage dictionary of the English language*. Boston: Houghton Mifflin.

Mosier, C., & Rogoff, B. (1990). *Infants' instrumental use of mothers*. In C. Rovee-Collier (Ed.), Abstracts of papers presented at the Seventh International Conference on Infant Studies (p. 535), Montreal. Norwood, NJ: Ablex.

Myers, W. A. (1987). Dreams of mourning and separation in older individuals. In A. Rothstein (Ed.), *The interpretations of dreams in clinical work* (pp. 27–36). New York: International Universities Press.

Nagera, H., & Baker, S. (1969). *Basic psychoanalytic concepts on the theory of dreams*. London: Allen & Unwin.

Naud, J., & Manikouska, M. (1990). *The observation of interpersonal regulation during mother–child interaction*. In C. Rovee-Collier (Ed.), Abstracts of papers presented at the Seventh International Conference on Infant Studies (p. 540), Montreal. Norwood, NJ: Ablex.

Needham, A. (1990). *3–5 month-old infants' knowledge of support relations*. In C. Rovee-Collier (Ed.), Abstracts of papers presented at the Seventh International Conference on Infant Studies (p. 541), Montreal. Norwood, NJ: Ablex.

Nelson, K., & Gruendel, J. M. (1981). Generalized event representations: Basic building blocks to cognitive development. In E. Lamb & A. L. Brown (Eds.), Advances in developmental psychology (Vol. 1). Hillsdale, NJ: Erlbaum.

New, R. S., Richman, A. L., & Welles-Nystrom, B. (1990). *Moder, madre, mother: The maternal role in Sweden, Italy and the U.S.* In C. Rovee-Collier (Ed.), Abstracts of papers presented at the Seventh International Conference on Infant Studies (p. 545), Montreal. Norwood, NJ: Ablex.

Ninio, A. (1979). The naive theory of the infant and other maternal attitudes in two subgroups in Israel. *Child Development, 50,* 976–980.

Ninio, A. (1990). *The relation of children's single-word utterances to the input*. In C. Rovee-Collier (Ed.), Abstracts of papers presented at the Seventh International Conference on Infant Studies (p. 45), Montreal. Norwood, NJ: Ablex.

Ninio, A., & Rinott, N. (1988). Fathers' involvement in the care of their infants and their attributions of cognitive competence to infants. *Child Development, 59,* 652–663.

Novick, J., & Kelly, K. (1970). Projection and externalization. *Psychoanalytic Study of the Child, 25,* 69–95.

Nugent, J. K., & Greene, S. (1990). *Effects of prenatal alcohol exposure on newborn cry*. In C. Rovee-Collier (Ed.), Abstracts of papers presented at the Seventh International Conference on Infant Studies (p. 549), Montreal. Norwood, NJ: Ablex.

Nwokah, E., Hsu, H.-C., & Fogel, A. (1990). *The role of imitation and laughter in discourse: The dynamics of shared laughter in mother–infant interaction*. In C. Rovee-Collier (Ed.), Abstracts of papers presented at the Seventh International Conference on Infant Studies (p. 69), Montreal. Norwood, NJ: Ablex.

Oates, R. K., & Forrest, D. (1984). Reliability of mothers' reports of birth data. *Australian Paediatric Journal, 20,* 185–186.

O'Connor, M. J. (1980). A comparison of preterm and full-term infants on auditory discrimination at four months and on Bayley Scales of infant development at eighteen months. *Child Development, 51,* 81–88.

O'Connor, M. J., Kasari, C., & Sigman, M. (1990). *The influence of mother–infant interaction of attachment behavior of infants exposed to alcohol prenatally.* In C. Rovee-Collier (Ed.), Abstracts of papers presented at the Seventh International Conference on Infant Studies (p. 189), Montreal. Norwood, NJ: Ablex.

Oehler, J. (1990). *Maternal views of interaction with their premature infants.* In C. Rovee-Collier (Ed.), Abstracts of papers presented at the Seventh International Conference on Infant Studies (p. 555), Montreal. Norwood, NJ: Ablex.

Olson, S. L., Bates, J. E., & Bayles, K. (1984). Mother–infant interaction and the development of individual differences in children's cognitive competence. *Developmental Psychology, 20,* 166–179.

Osofsky, J. D., Hann, D., Biringen, Z., Emde, R., Robinson, J., & Little, C. (1990). *Emotional availability: Strengths and vulnerabilities in development.* In C. Rovee-Collier (Ed.), Abstracts of papers presented at the Seventh International Conference on Infant Studies (p. 164), Montreal. Norwood, NJ: Ablex.

Owen, M. T., & Cox, M. J. (1990). *Maternal employment and marital quality during the first year of parenthood.* In C. Rovee-Collier (Ed.), Abstracts of papers presented at the Seventh International Conference on Infant Studies (p. 562), Montreal. Norwood, NJ: Ablex.

Owen, M. T., Easterbrooks, M. A., Chase-Lansdale, L., & Goldberg, W. A. (1984). The relation between maternal employment status and the stability of attachments to mother and to father. *Child Development, 55,* 1894–1901.

Oyemade, U. J. (1990). *Prenatal correlates of prenatal and infant development.* In C. Rovee-Collier (Ed.), Abstracts of papers presented at the Seventh International Conference on Infant Studies (p. 30), Montreal. Norwood, NJ: Ablex.

Pan, B. A., & Snow, C. E. (1990). *Shared definitions of communicative activity in early mother–infant interaction.* In C. Rovee-Collier (Ed.), Abstracts of papers presented at the Seventh International Conference on Infant Studies (p. 44), Montreal. Norwood, NJ: Ablex.

Paolino, Jr., T. J. (1981). Analyzability: Some categories for assessment. *Contemporary Psychoanalysis, 17,* 321–340.

Papousek, H., & Papousek, M. (1979). Early ontogeny of human social interaction: Its biological roots and social dimensions. In M. Von Cranach, K. Foppa, W. Lepnies, & D. Ploog (Eds.), *Human ethology: Claims and limits of a new discipline* (pp. 456–490). Cambridge, England: Cambridge University Press.

Papousek, H., & Papousek, M. (1987). Intuitive parenting: A dialectic counterpart to the infant's integrative competence. In J. D. Osofsky (Ed.), *Handbook of infant development* (2nd ed.). New York: Wiley.

Papousek, M. (1990). *Infant cry and non-cry vocalizations as signals in early parent–infant interactions.* In C. Rovee-Collier (Ed.), Abstracts of papers presented at the Seventh International Conference on Infant Studies (p. 114), Montreal. Norwood, NJ: Ablex.

Parke, R. D., Grossman, K., & Tinsley, B. R. (1981). Father–mother–infant interaction in the newborn period: A German-American comparison. In T. M. Field, A. M. Sostek, P. Vietze, & P. H. Leiderman (Eds.), *Culture and early interactions.* Hillsdale, NJ: Erlbaum.

Parke, R. D., & O'Leary, S. E. (1976). Father–mother–infant interaction in the newborn period: Some findings, some observations and some unresolved issues. In K. Riegel & J. Meacham (Eds.), *The developing individual in a changing world: Vol. 2. Social and environmental issues.* The Hague: Mouton.

Parke, R. D., O'Leary, S. E., & West, S. (1972). Mother–father–newborn interaction: Effects of maternal medication, labor and sex of infant. *Proceedings of the American Psychological Association, 7,* 85–86.

Parke, R. D., & Sawin, D. B. (1975, April). *Infant characteristics and behavior as elicitors of maternal and paternal responsibility in the newborn period.* Paper presented at the biennial meeting of the Society for Research in Child Development, Denver.

Parke, R. D., & Tinsley, B. R. (1981). The father's role in infancy: Determinants of involvement in caregiving and play. In M. E. Lamb (Ed.), *The role of the father in child development* (2nd. ed., pp. 429–457). New York: Wiley.

Parke, R. D., & Tinsley, B. R. (1987). Family interaction in infancy. In J. D. Osofsky (Ed.), *Handbook of infant development* (2nd ed., pp. 579–641). New York: Wiley.

Parker, K., & Popiel, K. (1990). *Development of a scale measuring biological and psychological sleep disorders.* In C. Rovee-Collier (Ed.), Abstracts of papers presented at the Seventh International Conference on Infant Studies (p. 161), Montreal. Norwood, NJ: Ablex.

Parsons, T. (1954). The father symbol: An appraisal in the light of psychoanalytic and sociological theory. In L. Bryson, L. Finkelstein, R. M. MacIver, & R. McKeon (Eds.), *Symbols and values.* New York: Harper & Row.

Patterson, G. R. (1982). *Coercive family process.* Eugene, OR: Castalia Publishing.

Pedersen, F. A. (1975, August). *Mother, father and infant as an interactive system.* Paper presented at the Annual Convention of the American Psychological Association, Chicago.

Pedersen, F. A., & Robson, K. S. (1969). Father participation in infancy. *American Journal of Orthopsychiatry, 39,* 466–472.

Pepernow, P. L. (1984). The stepfamily cycle: An experiential model of stepfamily development. *Family Relations, 33,* 355–363.

Piaget, J. (1937). Principal factors determining intellectual evolution from childhood to adult life. In E. D. Adrian (Ed.), *Factors determining human behavior* (pp. 32–48). Cambridge, MA: Harvard University Press.

Piaget, J. (1952). *The origins of intelligence in children.* New York: International Universities Press.

Piaget, J. (1954). *The construction of reality in the child.* New York: Basic Books. (Original work published 1937)

Piaget, J., & Inhelder, B. (1971). *Mental imagery in the child.* New York: Basic Books.

Pick, I. B. (1985). Working through in the countertransference. *International Journal of Psychoanalysis, 66,* 157–166.

Pines, D. (1972). Pregnancy and motherhood: Interaction between fantasy and reality. *British Journal of Medical Psychology, 45,* 333–343.

Pipp, S., Fischer, K. W., & Jennings, S. (1987). Acquisition of self and mother knowledge in infancy. *Developmental Psychology, 23,* 86–96.

Poey, K. (1985). Guidelines for the practice of brief, dynamic group therapy. *International Journal of Group Psychotherapy, 35,* 331–354.

Portales, A. L., Porqes, S. W., & Greenspan, S. I. (1990). *Parenthood and the difficult child*. In C. Rovee-Collier (Ed.), Abstracts of papers presented at the Seventh International Conference on Infant Studies (p. 573), Montreal. Norwood, NJ: Ablex.

Poulsen, M., & Ambrose, S. (1990). *Characteristics of 50 drug exposed infants in the foster care system*. In C. Rovee-Collier (Ed.), Abstracts of papers presented at the Seventh International Conference on Infant Studies (p. 81), Montreal. Norwood, NJ: Ablex.

Power, T. G. (1985). Mother– and father–infant play: A developmental analysis. *Child Development, 56*, 1514–1524.

Power, T. G., & Parke, R. D. (1981). Play as a context for early learning: Lab and home analyses. In L. M. Laosa & I. E. Sigel (Eds.), *The family as a learning environment*. New York: Plenum.

Puig-Antich, J., Lukens, E., Davies, M., Goetz, D., Quatrode, J. B., & Toback, G. (1985). Psychosocial functioning in prepubertal major depressive disorders. *Archives of General Psychiatry, 42*, 500–507.

Racker, H. (1954). *Transference and countertransference* (pp. 71–78). London: Hogarth Press.

Racker, H. (1957). The meanings and uses of countertransference. *Psychoanalytic Quarterly, 26*, 303–357.

Radin, N. (1982). Primary caregiving and role-sharing fathers of pre-schoolers. In M. E. Lamb (Ed.), *Nontraditional families: Parenting and child development*. Hillsdale, NJ: Erlbaum.

Radin, N. (1985, February). *Antecedents of stability in high father involvement*. Paper presented at Conference on Equal Parenting: Families of the future, University of California, Chico, CA.

Ramsay-Douglas, S., & Campos, J. J. (1978). The onset of representation and entry into stage 6 of object permanence development. *Developmental Psychology, 14*, 79–86.

Raphael-Leff, J. (1980). Psychotherapy with pregnant women. In B. L. Blum (Ed.), *Psychosocial aspects of pregnancy, birthing and bonding* (pp. 174–205). New York: Human Sciences.

Reid, W. J. (1990). An integrative model for short-term treatment. In R. A. Wells & V. J. Giannetti (Eds.), *Handbook of the brief psychotherapies* (pp. 55–77). New York: Plenum.

Reilly, J. S. (1990). *Child-directed language in ASL: Taking expressions at face value*. In C. Rovee-Collier (Ed.), Abstracts of papers presented at the Seventh International Conference on Infant Studies (p. 51), Montreal. Norwood, NJ: Ablex.

Reiss, D. (1989). The represented and practicing family: Contrasting visions of family continuity. In A. Sameroff & R. Emde (Eds.), *Relationship disturbances in early childhood: A developmental approach* (pp. 191–220). New York: Basic Books.

Reissland, N. (1988). Neonatal imitation in the first hour of life: Observations in rural Nepal. *Developmental Psychology, 24*, 464–469.

Resnick, J. S., & Kagan, J. (1983). Category detection in infancy. In L. P. Lipsitt (Ed.), *Advances in infancy research* (Vol. 2, pp. 79–111). Norwood, NJ: Ablex.

Richards, M. P. M., Dunn, J. F., & Antonis, B. (1977). Caretaking in the first year of life: The role of fathers, and mother's social isolation. *Child: Care, Health and Development, 3,* 23–36.

Ricks, S. S. (1985). Father–infant interactions: A review of empirical research. *Family Relations: Journal of Applied Family & Child Studies, 34,* 505–511.

Riese, M. L., & Matheny, A. P. (1990). *Nurses' ratings of mother–infant dyads: Prediction of "poorness of fit" and developmental risk.* In C. Rovee-Collier (Ed.), Abstracts of papers presented at the Seventh International Conference on Infant Studies (p. 586), Montreal. Norwood, NJ: Ablex.

Rimm, D. C., & Masters, J. C. (1979). *Behavior therapy: Techniques and empirical findings.* New York: Academic Press.

Roberts, R. N., & Wasik, B. (1990). *Survey of home visiting programs.* In C. Rovee-Collier (Ed.), Abstracts of papers presented at the Seventh International Conference on Infant Studies (p. 590), Montreal. Norwood, NJ: Ablex.

Robertson, J., & Bowlby, J. (1952). Responses of young children to separation from their mothers. *Courrier du Centre International de l'Enfance, 2,* 131–142.

Rosenberg, P. E. (1988). Transference in psychoanalysis and intensive short-term dynamic psychotherapy. *International Journal of Short-Term Psychotherapy, 3,* 47–76.

Rosenstein, D., & Oster, H. (1988). Differential facial responses to four basic tastes in newborns. *Child Development, 59,* 1555–1568.

Ross, S. A., & Kay, D. A. (1980). The origins of social games. *New Directions for Child Development, 9,* 17–31.

Roth, D. (1980). Suggestions for behavioral group therapy of depression. In D. Upper & A. M. Ross (Eds.), *Behavioral group therapy.* Champaign, IL: Research Press.

Roth, D., & Covi, L. (1984). Cognitive group psychotherapy of depression: The open-ended group. *International Journal of Group Psychotherapy, 34,* 67–82.

Rothbart, M. K., & Derryberry, D. (1981). Development of individual differences in temperament. In M. E. Lamb & A. L. Brown (Eds.), *Advances in developmental psychology* (Vol. 1, pp. 37–86). Hillsdale, NJ: Erlbaum.

Rothbart, M. K., Halsted, L., & Posner, M. I. (1990). *Orienting and soothing in infancy.* In C. Rovee-Collier (Ed.), Abstracts of papers presented at the Seventh International Conference on Infant Studies (p. 106), Montreal. Norwood, NJ: Ablex.

Rothenberg, M. B. (1990). Child advocacy: Using public policy to prevent mental illness. In S. E. Goldston, J. Yager, C. M. Heinicke, & R. S. Pynoos (Eds.), *Preventing mental health disturbances in childhood* (pp. 25–36). Washington DC: American Psychiatric Press.

Rothstein, A. (1983). *The structural hypothesis: An evolutionary perspective.* New York: International Universities Press.

Rovee-Collier, C., & Fagen, J. W. (1981). The retrieval of memory in early infancy. *Advances in Infancy Research, 1,* 225–254.

Rubin, J. A. (1984). *Child art therapy: Understanding and helping children grow through art.* New York: Van Nostrand Reinhold.

Ruddy, M. G., & Bornstein, M. H. (1982). Cognitive correlates of infant attention and maternal stimulation over the first year of life. *Child Development, 53,* 183–188.

Ruff, H. A. (1990). *Great expectations: How infants anticipate the future.* In C. Rovee-Collier (Ed.), Abstracts of papers presented at the Seventh International Conference on Infant Studies (p. 12), Montreal. Norwood, NJ: Ablex.

Russell, G. (1983). *The changing role of fathers?* St. Lucia, Queensland: University of Queensland Press.

Rutter, M. (1975). *Helping troubled children.* New York: Plenum.

Rutter, M. (1983). Stress, coping, and development: Some issues and some questions. In N. Garmezy & M. Rutter (Eds.), *Stress, coping, and development in children* (pp. 1–42). New York: McGraw-Hill.

Rutter, M. (1987). Psychosocial resilience and protective mechanisms. *American Journal of Orthopsychiatry, 57,* 316–331.

Saal, D. R. (1975). A study of the development of object conception in infancy: Varying the degree of discrepancy between the disappearing and reappearing object. *DAI, V36*(07), 3582.

Sackett, G. P. (1978). Measurement in observational research. In G. P. Sackett (Ed.), *Observing behavior: Vol. 2. Data collection and analysis methods.* Baltimore: University Park Press.

Sagi, A. (1982). Antecedents and consequences of various degrees of parental involvement in childrearing: The Israeli project. In M. E. Lamb (Ed.), *Nontraditional families: Parenting and child development.* Hillsdale, NJ: Erlbaum.

Salzman, L. (1984). Change and the therapeutic process. In J. M. Myers (Ed.), *Cures by psychotherapy: What effects change?* New York: Praeger.

Sandler, L. (1973). A multiprofessional approach to the early detection and treatment of developmentally disordered preschool children. *School Psychology Digest, 2*(4), 41–46.

Satir, V. (1967). *Conjoint family therapy.* Palo Alto, CA: Science & Behavior Books.

Scafidi, F. A., Field, T. M., Schanberg, S. M., Bauer, C. R., Tucci, K., Roberts, J., Morrow, C., & Kuhn, C. M., (1990). Massage stimulates growth in preterm infants: A replication. *Infant Behavior and Development, 13,* 167–188.

Schachere, K. (1990). Attachment between working mothers and their infants: The influence of family processes. *American Journal of Orthopsychiatry, 60,* 19–34.

Schachter, B. (1989). Out-of-home care: Family foster care and residential treatment. In S. M. Ehrenkranz, E. G. Goldstein, L. Goodman, & J. Seinfeld (Eds.), *Clinical social work with maltreated children and their families: An introduction to practice* (pp.104–127). New York: New York University Press.

Schachter, J. (1987). Concurrent individual and individual-in-a-group psychoanalytic psychotherapy. *Journal of the American Psychoanalytic Association, 36,* 455–480.

Schafer, R. (1981). Narration in the psychoanalytic dialogue. In W. J. T. Mitchell (Ed.), *On narrative.* Chicago: University of Chicago Press.

Schafer, R. (1968). *Aspects of internalization.* New York: International Universities Press.

Schafer, R. (1959). Generative empathy in the treatment situation. *Psychoanalytic Quarterly, 28,* 347–373.

Schechter, D. E., & Corman, H. H. (1979). The birth of a family: Some early developments in parent-child interaction. *Contemporary Psychoanalysis, 15,* 380–406.

Schlessinger, N. (1966). Supervision of psychotherapy. *Archives of General Psychiatry, 15,* 129–134.

Schmidt, C. (1990). *Ostensive naming: Language from context.* In C. Rovee-Collier (Ed.), Abstracts of papers presented at the Seventh International Conference on Infant Studies (p. 610), Montreal. Norwood, NJ: Ablex.

Searles, H. (1955). The informational value of the supervisor's emotional experiences. *Psychiatry: Journal for the Study of Interpersonal Processes, 18,* 135–146.

Seligman, M. E. P. (1972). Learned helplessness. *Annual Review of Medicine, 23,* 407–412.

Seligman, S. P., & Pawl, J. H. (1983). Impediments to the formation of the working alliance in infant–parent psychotherapy. In J. D. Call, E. Galenson, & R. L. Tyson (Eds.), *Frontiers of infant psychiatry.* New York: Basic Books.

Sheehy, G. (1979). Introducing the postponing generation. *Esquire, 92*(4), 25–33.

Sherman, M. H. (1990). Family narratives: Internal representations of family relationships and affective themes. *Infant Mental Health Journal, 11,* 253–258.

Sherman, R., & Fredman, N. (1986). *Handbook of structured techniques in marriage and family therapy.* New York: Brunner/Mazel.

Sherwen, L. N. (1981). Fantasies during the third trimester of pregnancy. *MCN, American Journal of Maternal Child Nursing, 6,* 398–401.

Sherwen, L. N. (1986). Third trimester fantasies of first-time expectant fathers. *Maternal-Child Nursing Journal, 15(3),* 153–170.

Shields, M. M. (1978). The child as psychologist: Contriving the social world. In A. Lock (Ed.), *Action, gesture and symbol.* New York: Academic Press.

Shotter, J. (1983). On viewing videotape records of oneself and others: A hermeneutical analysis. In P. W. Dowrick & S. J. Biggs (Eds.), *Using video* (pp. 199–210). New York: Wiley.

Shultz, N. W. (1980). A cognitive-developmental study of the grandchild–grandparent bond. *Child Study Journal, 10,* 7–26.

Shyi, G. C.-W., Schecter, A., & Shields, P. (1990). *Contextual alterations and memory retrieval at six months.* In C. Rovee-Collier (Ed.), Abstracts of papers presented at the Seventh International Conference on Infant Studies (p. 617), Montreal. Norwood, NJ: Ablex.

Sifneos, P. E. (1972). *Short-term psychotherapy and emotional crisis.* Cambridge, MA: Harvard University Press.

Singer, D. L. (1968). Aggression, arousal, hostile humor, catharsis. *Journal of Personality and Social Psychology, 8*(1), Suppl, 1–14.

Singer, J. L. (1971). Theoretical implications of imagery and fantasy techniques. *Contemporary Psychoanalysis, 8,* 82–96.

Singer, J. L. (1974). *Imagery and daydreaming methods in psychotherapy and behavior modification.* New York: Academic Press.

Singer, J. L., & Antrobus, J. A. (1972). Daydreaming, imaginal processes and personality: A normative study. In P. Sheehan (Ed.), *The function and nature of imagery* (pp. 175–202). New York: Academic Press.

Slater, A. (1990). *The origins of visual competence.* In C. Rovee-Collier (Ed.), Abstracts of papers presented at the Seventh International Conference on Infant Studies (p. 622), Montreal. Norwood, NJ: Ablex.

Solomon, J., & George, C. (1990). *Conflict and attachment: The experience of disorganized/controlling children and their mothers.* In C. Rovee-Collier (Ed.), Abstracts of papers presented at the Seventh International Conference on Infant Studies (p. 119), Montreal. Norwood, NJ: Ablex.

Sosa, R., Kennell, J., Klaus, M., Robertson, S., & Urrutia, J. (1980). The effect of a supportive companion on perinatal problems, length of labor, and mother–infant interaction. *New England Journal of Medicine, 303,* 597–600.

Spanos, N. P. (1971). Goal-directed fantasy and the performance of hypnotic test suggestions. *Psychiatry, 34,* 86–96.

Spelke, E. S., & Breinlinger, K. (1990). *Early conceptions of object motion: Continuity and solidity.* In C. Rovee-Collier (Ed.), Abstracts of papers presented at the Seventh International Conference on Infant Studies (p. 625), Montreal. Norwood, NJ: Ablex.

Spitz, R. A. (1959). *A genetic field theory of ego formation: Its implications for pathology.* New York: International Universities Press.

Spitz, R. A. (1965). *The first year of life.* New York: International Universities Press.

Spitz, R. A., & Wolf, K. M. (1946). Anaclitic depression. *Psychoanalytic Study of the Child, 2,* 313–342.

Stanton, M. D. (1981). Strategic approaches to family therapy. In A. S. Gurman & D. P. Kniskern (Eds.), *Handbook of family therapy* (pp. 361–402). New York: Brunner/Mazel.

Stern, D. N. (1985). *The interpersonal world of the infant.* New York: Basic Books.

Stern, D. N. (1989). The representation of relational patterns: Developmental considerations. In A. J. Sameroff & R. N. Emde (Eds.), *Relational disturbances in early childhood* (pp. 52–69). New York: Basic Books.

Stern, D. N., Beebe, B., Jaffe, J., & Bennett, S. L. (1977). The infant's stimulus world during social interaction: A study of caregiver behaviors with particular reference to repetition and timing. In H. R. Schaffer (Ed.), *Studies in mother–infant interaction.* London: Academic Press.

Stern, D. N., & Gibbon, J. (1978). Temporal expectancies of social behaviors in mother–infant play. In E. Thoman (Ed.), *Origins of the infant's social responsiveness* (pp. 409–429). New York: Erlbaum.

Stevenson, M. B., & Roach, M. A. (1990). *Determinants of maternal vocalization to 4-month-old infants.* In C. Rovee-Collier (Ed.), Abstracts of papers presented at the Seventh International Conference on Infant Studies (p. 629), Montreal. Norwood, NJ: Ablex.

Stevenson-Hinde, J. (1990). Attachment within family systems: An overview. *Infant Mental Health Journal, 11,* 218–227.

Stifter, C. A. (1990). *General issues in infant irritability.* In C. Rovee-Collier (Ed.), Abstracts of papers presented at the Seventh International Conference on Infant Studies (p. 206), Montreal. Norwood, NJ: Ablex.

St. James-Roberts, I., & Wolke, D. (1988). Convergences and discrepancies among mothers' and professionals' assessments of difficult neonatal behavior. *Journal of Child Psychology and Psychiatry, 29,* 21–42.

Stolorow, R. D., Brandchaft, B., & Atwood, G. E. (1987). *Psychoanalytic treatment: An intersubjective approach.* Hillsdale, NJ: Erlbaum.

Stolorow, R. D., Brandchaft, B., Atwood, G. E., & Lachmann, F. M. (1987). Transference: The organization of experience. In R. Stolorow, B. Brandchaft, & G. E. Atwood (Eds.), *Psychoanalytic treatment: An intersubjective approach* (pp. 28–179). Hillsdale, NJ: Erlbaum.

Streri, A., Molina, M., & Millet, G. (1990). *Tactual representation in 2-month-old infants.* In C. Rovee-Collier (Ed.), Abstracts of papers presented at the Seventh International Conference on Infant Studies (p. 634), Montreal. Norwood, NJ: Ablex.

Stuckey, M. F., McGhee, P. E., & Bell, N. J. (1982). Parent–child interaction: The influence of maternal employment. *Developmental Psychology, 18,* 635–644.

Sullivan, H. S. (1953). *The interpersonal theory of psychiatry.* New York: Norton.

Sullivan, H. S. (1954). *The psychiatric interview.* New York: Norton.

Summerfield, A. B. (1983). Recording social interaction. In P. W. Dowrick & S. J. Biggs (Eds.), *Using video* (pp. 3–11). New York: Wiley.

Sussman, M. B. (1977). Family. In *Encyclopedia of social work* (17th ed., pp. 357–368). Washington, DC: National Association of Social Workers.

Swenson, W. M. (1985). The development of automated personality assessment in medical practice. *Psychiatric Annals, 15,* 549–553.

Szapocznik, J., Perez-Vidal, A., Hervis, O., Brickman, A. L., & Kurtines, W. M. (1990). Innovations in family therapy: Strategies for overcoming resistance to treatment. In R. A. Wells & V. J. Giannetti (Eds.), *Handbook of the brief psychotherapies* (pp. 93–114). New York: Plenum.

Tamis-Lemonda, C., & Bornstein, M. H. (1989). Habituation and maternal encouragement of attention in infancy as predictors of toddler language, play, and representational competence. *Child Development, 60,* 738–751.

Tamis-LeMonda, C., & Bornstein, M. H. (1990). Language, play, and attention at one year. *Infant Behavior and Development, 13,* 85–98.

Tansey, M. J., & Burke, W. F. (1985). Projective identification and the empathic process. *Contemporary Psychoanalysis, 21,* 42–69.

Tauber, E. S. (1954). Exploring the therapeutic use of countertransference data. *Psychiatry, 17,* 331–336.

Telzrow, R. (1990). *Effects of locomotor handicap on cognition and communication.* In C. Rovee-Collier (Ed.), Abstracts of papers presented at the Seventh International Conference on Infant Studies (p. 218), Montreal. Norwood, NJ: Ablex.

Tenzer, A. (1984). Piaget and psychoanalysis, II: The problem of working through. *Contemporary Psychoanalysis, 20,* 421–436.

Terkelsen, K. G. (1980). Toward a theory of the family life cycle. In E. Carter & M. McGoldrick (Eds.), *The family life cycle: A framework for family therapy* (pp. 21–53). New York: Gardner Press.

Termine, I., & Izard, C. E. (1988). Infant's responses to their mother's expressions of joy and sadness. *Developmental Psychology, 24,* 223–229.

Teti, D. M., & Gelfand, D. M. (1990). *Maternal depression and infant development: Preliminary results of an early intervention program.* In C. Rovee-Collier (Ed.), Abstracts of papers presented at the Seventh International Conference on Infant Studies (p. 55), Montreal. Norwood, NJ: Ablex.

Teti, D. M., Gelfand, D. M., & Pompa, J. (1990). *Differences in depressed mothers' ability to parent: Maternal, infant, and environmental correlates.* In C. Rovee-Collier (Ed.), Abstracts of papers presented at the Seventh International Conference on Infant Studies (p. 640), Montreal. Norwood, NJ: Ablex.

Tharp, R. G., & Wetzel, R. J. (1969). *Behavior modification in the natural environment.* New York: Academic Press.

Thelen, E. (1990). *Motor development and the reconstruction of the infant.* In C. Rovee-Collier (Ed.), Abstracts of papers presented at the Seventh International Conference on Infant Studies (p. 232), Montreal. Norwood, NJ: Ablex.

Thoman, E. B., & Acebo, C. (1990). *Crys in their social and behavioral contexts: Crying when baby and mother are together.* In C. Rovee-Collier (Ed.), Abstracts of papers presented at the Seventh International Conference on Infant Studies (p. 111), Montreal. Norwood, NJ: Ablex.

Thomas, A., & Chess, S. (1977). *Temperament and development.* New York: Brunner/ Mazel.

Thomas, A., Chess, S., & Birch, H. G. (1968). *Temperament and behavior disorders.* New York: New York University Press.

Thomas, A., Chess, S., & Birch, H. G. (1970). The origin of personality. *Scientific American, 223,* 102–109.

Tinsley, B. J., & Parke, R. D. (1984). The contemporary impact of the extended family on the nuclear family: Grandparents as support and socialization agents. In M. Lewis (Ed.), *Beyond the dyad.* New York: Plenum.

Tower, R. B., & Singer, J. L. (1981). The measurement of imagery: How can it be clinically useful? In P. C. Kendall & S. Hollon (Eds.), *Assessment methods for cognitive-behavioral interventions.* New York: Academic Press.

Trad, P. V. (1986). *Infant depression: Paradigms and paradoxes.* New York: Springer-Verlag.

Trad, P. V. (1987). *Infant and childhood depression: Developmental factors.* New York: Wiley.

Trad, P. V. (1989). *The preschool child: Assessment, diagnosis, and treatment.* New York: Wiley.

Trad, P. V. (1990). *Infant previewing.* New York: Springer-Verlag.

Trevarthen, C. (1980). The foundations of intersubjectivity: Development of interpersonal and cooperative understanding in infants. In D. R. Olson (Ed.), *The social foundations of language and thought: Essays in honor of Jerome S. Bruner* (pp. 316–342). New York: Norton.

Trevarthen, C. (1985). Facial expressions of emotion in mother-infant interaction. *Human Neurobiology, 4*, 21–32.

Trevarthen, C., & Hubley, P. (1978). Secondary intersubjectivity: Confidence, confiding and acts of meaning in the first year. In A. Lock (Ed.), *Action, gesture and symbol: The emergence of language.* London: Academic Press.

Tronick, E. Z., Als, H., Adamson, L., Wise, S., & Brazelton, T. B. (1978). The infant's response to entrapment between contradictory messages in face-to-face interaction. *Journal of American Academy of Child Psychiatry, 17*, 1–13.

Tronick, E. Z., & Weinberg, M. K. (1990). *Emotion regulation in infancy: Stability of regulatory behaviors.* In C. Rovee-Collier (Ed.), Abstracts of papers presented at the Seventh International Conference on Infant Studies (p. 108), Montreal. Norwood, NJ: Ablex.

Tulkin, S. R., & Kagan, J. (1972). Mother–child interaction in the first year of life. *Child Development, 43*, 31–41.

Urdang, L., & Flexner, S. B. (Eds.) (1972). *Random House College Dictionary.* New York: Random House.

Uzgiris, I. C. (1990). *Imitation in mother–child conversations.* In C. Rovee-Collier (Ed.), Abstracts of papers presented at the Seventh International Conference on Infant Studies (p. 67), Montreal. Norwood, NJ: Ablex.

Vygotsky, L. S. (1962). *Thought and language.* Cambridge, MA: MIT Press.

Vygotsky, L. S. (1978). *Mind in society: The development of higher psychological processes.* Cambridge, MA: Harvard University Press.

Vyt, A. (1990). *Parental differences in play with toddlers: Being sensitive to cognitive needs.* In C. Rovee-Collier (Ed.), Abstracts of papers presented at the Seventh International Conference on Infant Studies (p. 658), Montreal. Norwood, NJ: Ablex.

Wachs, T. D. (1987). Specificity of environmental action as manifest in environmental correlates of infant's mastery motivation. *Developmental Psychology, 23*, 782–790.

Waelder, R. (1956). Introduction to the discussion on problems of transference. *International Journal of Psycho-Analysis, 37*, 367–368.

Walden, T., & Johnson, K. (1990). *Infant attention and social referencing.* In C. Rovee-Collier (Ed.), Abstracts of papers presented at the Seventh International Conference on Infant Studies (p. 659), Montreal. Norwood, NJ: Ablex.

Wallerstein, R. S. (1976). *Psychoanalysis as a science: Its present status and its future tasks.* (Psychological Issues, Monograph No. 36). New York: International University Press.

Ward, M. J., Brinckerhoff, C. B., Lent, L. A., Gruber, S. K., Carlson, L. S., & Kessler, D. B. (1990). *Adolescent mother–infant attachment: Continuity in adaptation from 12 to 14 months.* In C. Rovee-Collier (Ed.), Abstracts of papers presented at the Seventh International Conference on Infant Studies (p. 662), Montreal. Norwood, NJ: Ablex.

Ward, M. J., Carlson, E. A., Altman, S. C., Levine, L., Greenburg, R. H., & Kessler, D. B. (1990). *Predicting infant–mother attachment from adolescents' prenatal working models of relationships.* In C. Rovee-Collier (Ed.), Abstracts of papers presented at the Seventh International Conference on Infant Studies (p. 661), Montreal. Norwood, NJ: Ablex.

Ward, W. D., & Bendak, S. (1964). The response of psychiatric patients to photographic self-image experience. *Newsletter for Research in Psychology* (Veterans Administration), 6, 29–30.

Watson, J. S. (1966). The development of and generalization of "contingency awareness" in early infancy. *Merrill Palmer Quarterly, 18,* 323–339.

Watson, J. S. (1971). Cognitive-perceptual development in infancy: Setting for the Seventies. *Merrill Palmer Quarterly, 12,* 123–125.

Watson, J. S. (1972). Smiling, cooing, and "the game." *Merrill Palmer Quarterly, 18,* 323–339.

Watson, J. S., & Ramey, C. T. (1972). Reactions to response contingent stimulation in early infancy. *Merrill Palmer Quarterly, 18,* 219–227.

Watzlawick, P., Beavin, J., & Jackson, D. (1967). *Pragmatics of human communication.* New York: Norton.

Waxer, P. H. (1977). Short-term group psychotherapy: Some principles and techniques. *International Journal of Group Psychotherapy, 27*(10), 33–42.

Welles-Nystrom, B. (1990). *Radical fathering: Infant caretaking in Swedish and American men.* In C. Rovee-Collier (Ed.), Abstracts of papers presented at the Seventh International Conference on Infant Studies (p. 667), Montreal. Norwood, NJ: Ablex.

Werner, H. (1948). *The comparative psychology of mental development.* New York: International Universities Press.

Werner, H., & Kaplan, B. (1963). *Symbol formation.* New York: Wiley.

Whitaker, C. A. (1976). A family is a four-dimensional relationship. In P. J. Guerin, Jr. (Ed.), *Family therapy: Theory and practice* (pp. 182–191). New York: Gardner Press.

Whitaker, C. A., & Keith, D. V. (1981). Symbolic-experiential family therapy. In A. S. Gurman & D. P. Kniskern (Eds.), *Handbook of family therapy* (pp. 187–225). New York: Brunner/Mazel.

Wolff, P. H. (1966). *The causes, controls, and organization of behavior in the neonate.* New York: International Universities Press.

Wolstein, B. (1964). *Transference: Its structure and function in psychoanalytic therapy.* New York: Grune & Stratton.

Wood, D., Bruner, J. S., & Ross, G. (1976). The role of tutoring in problem solving. *Journal of Child Psychology & Psychiatry & Allied Disciplines, 17*(2), 89–100.

Worchel, J. (1986). Transference in intensive short-term dynamic psychotherapy: I. Technique of handling initial transference. *International Journal of Short-Term Psychotherapy, 1,* 135–146.

Worchel, J. (1990). Short-term dynamic psychotherapy. In R. A. Wells & V. J. Giannetti (Eds.), *Handbook of the brief psychotherapies* (pp. 193–215). New York: Plenum.

Worobey, J., & Thomas, D. A. (1990). *Intrauterine exposure to toxins and cognitive outcomes.* In C. Rovee-Collier (Ed.), Abstracts of papers presented at the Seventh International Conference on Infant Studies (p. 679), Montreal. Norwood, NJ: Ablex.

Worthington, E. L. (1989). Matching family treatment to family stressors. In S. R. Figley (Ed.), *Treating stress in families* (pp. 44–63). New York: Brunner/Mazel.

Yalom, I. D. (1975). *The theory and practice of group psychotherapy.* New York: Basic Books.

Yarrow, L. J., Morgan, G. A., Jennings, K. D., Harmon, R. J., & Gaiter, J. L. (1982). Infants' persistence at tasks: Relationships to cognitive functioning in early experience. *Infant Behavior and Development, 5,* 131–141.

Yogman, M. J., Dixon, S., Tronick, E., Als, H., & Brazelton, T. B. (1977). *The goals and structure of face-to-face interaction between infants and fathers.* Paper presented at the biennial meeting of the Society for Research in Child Development, New Orleans.

Yogman, M. W. (1981). Development of the father–infant relationship. In H. Fitzgerald, B. Lester, & M. W. Yogman (Eds.), *Theory and research in behavioral pediatrics* (Vol. 1). New York: Plenum.

Zaslow, M. J., Pedersen, F. A., Suwalsky, J. T. D., Rabinovich, B., & Cain, R. L. (1986). Fathering during the infancy period: Implications of the mother's employment role. *Infant Mental Health Journal, 7,* 225–234.

Zeanah, C. H., & Barton, M. L. (1989). Introduction: Internal representations and parent-infant relationships. *Infant Mental Health Journal, 10,* 135–141.

Zeanah, C. H., Benoit, D., & Barton, M. L. (1986). *Working model of the child interview.* Unpublished manuscript, Brown University.

Zelazo, P. R. (1990). *Central and peripheral influences on early motor development.* In C. Rovee-Collier (Ed.), Abstracts of papers presented at the Seventh International Conference on Infant Studies (p. 230), Montreal. Norwood, NJ: Ablex.

Zelazo, P., Zelazo, N., & Kolb, S. (1972). "Walking" in the newborn. *Science, 177,* 1058–1059.

Zuk, G. (1971). Family therapy. In J. Haley (Ed.), *Changing families* (pp. 212–226). New York: Grune & Stratton.

Author Index

Aaron, N. A., 80, 500
Abelin, E. L., 182, 500
Abramson, L., 69, 500
Acebo, C., 110, 536
Ackerman, N., 194, 402, 500
Adams, R., 73, 509
Adams-Hillard, P. J., 333, 500
Adamson, L., 142, 230, 231, 500, 502, 537
Adland, M. L., 410, 510
Ainsworth, M. D.S., 24, 83, 488, 500
Alessandri, S. M., 89, 500
Alexander, F., 466, 500
Alexander, J. F., 411, 502
Alger, I., 381, 382, 404, 500
Al Naquib, N., 106, 500
Alonso, A., 459, 460, 500
Als, H., 49, 87, 106, 142, 500, 506, 537, 539
Altemeier, W. A., 104, 525
Altman, J., 229, 501
Altman, S. C., 537

Altschuler, S. C., 493, 501
Amaranto, E. A., 460, 501
Amatruda, A., 79, 86, 446, 516
Ambrose, S., 105, 501, 530
Anders, T. F., 113, 501
Anderson, J. R., 255, 501
Anderson, S., 83, 501
Andersson, B. -E., 501
Andres, D., 54, 516
Antonis, B., 42, 531
Antrobus, J. A., 38, 534
Anzieu, D., 356, 501
Aponte, H. J., 409, 410, 501
Appel, K. J., 73, 516
Appelbaum, S. A., 286, 501
Apprey, M., 148, 152, 501
Araoz, D. L., 259, 501
Arlow, J. A., 193, 194, 501
Arterberry, M. E., 73, 501
Aschenbrenner, B. G., 180, 513
Ascher, M., 339, 501
Ashmead, D. H., 79, 501

Atwood, G. E., 206, 209, 535
Austin, C. D., 493, 502
Averill, J., 40, 514

Baillargeon, R., 522
Bakeman, R., 229, 230, 231, 500, 502
Baker, S., 527
Baldwin, D. A., 83, 502
Ballinger, C. B., 429, 502
Ballou, J., 327, 502
Ban, P. L., 45, 502
Bandler, R., 260, 502
Bandura, A., 369, 383, 502
Bardwick, J. M., 326, 502
Barnard, K. E., 107, 520
Barnett, D., 80, 502
Barnhill, L., 177, 502
Barrerra, M., 106, 502
Barrett, K., 72, 507
Bartlett, G. S., 104, 519
Barton, C., 411, 502
Barton, M. L., 21, 24, 504, 539
Basham, R. B., 491, 509

Bates, E., 92, 506
Bates, J. E., 19, 528
Bauer, C. R., 532
Baxter, A., 128, 502
Bayles, K., 19, 528
Beaumont, S., 110, 503
Beavin, J., 31, 538
Beckmann, C., 106, 503
Beckwith, L., 106, 503
Beebe, B., 72, 92, 95, 117, 503, 534
Beeghly, M., 106, 503
Behrends, R. S., 140, 503
Bell, J., 403, 405, 503
Bell, N. J., 54, 535
Bell, N. W., 183, 184, 503
Bell, S. M., 73, 503
Bellack, A. S., 382, 518
Belsky, J., 19, 180, 182, 495, 496, 503
Bem, S., 38, 503
Bendak, S., 375, 538
Bender, S. S., 460, 501
Benedek, T., 327, 328, 503, 504
Bennett, S. L., 72, 534
Benoit, D., 21, 24, 504, 539
Benson, J. B., 74, 504
Bento, S., 512
Berger, M. M., 376, 378, 504
Berger, S. P., 496, 504
Bergman, A., 83, 525
Bergman, P., 391, 504
Bergman, T., 128, 518
Berlin, B., 26, 504
Berlin, L. J., 116, 504
Bernheim, K. F., 385, 386, 388, 504
Bernstein, V. J., 118, 518
Bertenthal, B., 132, 504
Bigelow, A., 504
Bills, B., 38, 504
Binder, J. L., 426, 476, 504
Birch, H. G., 89, 391, 536
Biringen, Z., 528
Bishop, D. S., 411, 512
Blanck, G., 206, 504
Blanck, R., 206, 504
Blass, E., 109, 263, 504, 505
Blatt, S. J., 140, 503
Blicharski, T., 120, 505

Blitzsten, N. L., 194, 505
Blood, I., 84, 512
Bloom, K., 71, 110, 503, 505
Bollas, C., 357, 505
Booth, C. L., 107, 520
Bornstein, M. H., 19, 20, 26, 505, 532, 535
Borton, W., 27, 526
Boss, P. G., 165, 505
Bostrom, A., 488, 526
Boszormenyi-Nagy, I., 412, 413, 505
Bowen, M., 171, 178, 505, 521, 522
Bower, T. G.R., 29, 73, 505
Bowlby, J., 22, 83, 86, 137, 138, 139, 161, 505, 531
Boyd, H. S., 382, 505
Brackbill, Y., 177, 505
Bradlow, P. A., 322, 505
Bradt, J. O., 181, 506
Brady, K. L., 110, 517
Brandchaft, B., 206, 209, 535
Brault, M., 69, 509
Brazelton, T. B., 49, 87, 95, 106, 112, 114, 142, 174, 176, 336, 503, 506, 524, 537, 539
Breinlinger, K., 73, 534
Breit, M., 461, 506
Bremner, G. J., 73, 506
Bretherton, I., 83, 92, 137, 138, 506
Brickman, A. L., 410, 535
Brinckerhoff, C. B., 116, 537
Brodey, W. M., 149, 506
Brooks, J., 83, 92, 95, 524
Brooks-Gunn, J., 92, 524
Bruner, J. S., 16, 26, 538
Budman, S. H., 168, 506
Burgess, S., 513
Burke, W. F., 157, 211, 212, 535
Burns, K. A., 105, 507
Burns, W. J., 105, 507
Burrows, E., 106, 503
Buschsbaum, H., 96, 519
Busnel, M. C., 80, 506
Buss, A. H., 89, 506

Butcher, J. N., 522
Butterworth, G., 73, 506
Byng-Hall, J., 414, 415, 416, 418, 506

Cain, R. L., 54, 539
Caldera, Y. M., 80, 507
Caligor, L., 193, 212, 459, 507
Calkins, S., 80, 500
Camli, O., 106, 507
Campos, J., 72, 73, 74, 79, 92, 507, 522, 530
Caplan, G., 327, 329, 485, 507
Caplan, R. D., 486, 507
Carlson, E. A., 116, 537
Carlson, L. S., 116, 537
Carlson, V., 80, 502
Carroll, S., 83, 525
Carstens, A. A., 72, 510
Carter, E. A., 171, 172, 525
Caruso, D. A., 496, 507
Cassidy, J., 21, 116, 504, 525
Chance, G. W., 512
Charlesworth, W. R., 66, 507
Chase-Lansdale, L., 53, 528
Chase-Lansdale, P. L., 54, 507
Cherniss, D. P., 16, 514
Chess, S., 89, 265, 391, 536
Chethick, L., 105, 507
Chiodo, L., 106, 507
Chomsky, N., 86, 507
Christensen, M. J., 104, 525
Cicchetti, D., 80, 502
Clark, R., 105, 507
Clarke-Stewart, K. A., 19, 46, 496, 508
Clarkin, J. F., 409, 516
Clarkson, M. G., 80, 508
Clifton, R. K., 80, 508
Coffman, S., 126, 524
Cohen, D., 69, 513
Cohen, K., 80, 508
Cohen, L. B., 26, 508
Cohen, S. E., 84, 508
Coleman, J. S., 328, 508
Coles, C. D., 105, 508
Colletta, N. D., 488, 508

Collins, K., 119, 521
Condon, J. T., 167, 328, 333, 334, 508
Cooper, A., 292, 508
Cooper, R. P., 83, 508
Corman, H. H., 72, 73, 177, 508, 533
Cossette, L., 69, 509
Courage, M., 73, 509
Covi, L., 433, 434, 456, 531
Cowan, C. P., 54, 181, 509
Cowan, P. A., 54, 181, 509
Cox, M., 187, 519
Cox, M. J., 106, 528
Cox, R., 187, 519
Coysh, W. S., 40, 509
Cramer, B. G., 470, 471, 509
Crittenden, P. M., 488, 509
Crnic, K. A., 491, 509
Crockenberg, S., 491, 509
Crown, C. L., 106, 513
Crowther, J. H., 166, 509
Culp, A. M., 110, 509
Culp, R. E., 110, 509

Daitzman, R. J., 381, 509
Dale, P., 513
Danish, S. J., 432, 509
Davanloo, H., 466, 469, 470, 476, 510
Davenport, Y. B., 410, 510
Davidson, N., 371, 372, 516
Davies, M., 530
Davis, A. L., 510
Davis, D., 349, 364, 510
Dean, A., 485, 524
DeBaryshe, B. D., 107, 510
DeBoysson, B., 83, 510
DeCarie, T. G., 73, 74, 510
DeCasper, A. J., 72, 140, 510
DeGangi, G. A., 113, 510
DeGregorio, I., 106, 513
Derryberry, D., 89, 531
Deutsch, H., 357, 510
Diamond, A., 73, 510
Dichtelmiller, M., 511
Dichter, H., 466, 467, 475, 517
Dixon, S., 49, 539
Dolgoff, R., 485, 511

Donovan, W. L., 106, 511
Dorado, J., 110, 513
Doussard-Roosevelt, J. A., 511
Dowling, S., 330, 511
Dowrick, P. W., 384, 511
Duffy, F. H., 106, 500
Duhl, B. S., 403, 511
Duhl, F. J., 403, 511
Dunn, D. J., 167, 328, 334, 508
Dunn, J. F., 42, 531
Dunst, C. J., 511
Durand, C., 83, 510

Easterbrooks, M. A., 53, 528
Echols, C. H., 85, 511
Edelson, M., 321, 511
Einstein, S., 484, 511
Eisen, L. N., 105, 511
Eisenhart, C. E., 87, 511
Eisnitz, A. J., 322, 512
Ekman, P., 231, 378, 512
Elderkin, J. B., 172, 512
Elliot, C., 254, 512
Ellis, A. E., 83, 512
Emde, R., 83, 89, 92, 95, 96, 111, 125, 512, 519, 521, 522, 528
Ensel, W., 485, 524
Epstein, L., 476, 512
Epstein, N. B., 411, 512
Erikson, E., 322, 411, 512
Escalona, S. K., 72, 73, 391, 504, 508
Evans, B., 512
Evans, W. F., 73, 516

Fagen, J. W., 72, 92, 95, 125, 142, 512, 525, 531
Falkner, S., 113, 526
Feagans, L., 84, 512
Feider, H., 83, 120, 505, 524
Fein, G., 446, 496, 508, 513
Feiner, A. H., 476, 512
Feldman, L. B., 180, 402, 403, 404, 513
Feldman, S. S., 513
Feldstein, D., 485, 511
Feldstein, S., 106, 513

Fenson, L., 83, 513
Fernald, A., 83, 110, 513
Field, J., 69, 89, 127, 142, 266, 446, 525
Field, T. M., 513, 532
Fiese, B. H., 107, 513
Fine, B. D., 205, 405, 526
Fischer, K., 92, 132, 504, 529
Fish, M., 80, 92, 514
Fish, S, 494, 514
Fleener, M., 79, 507
Fleming, J., 194, 505
Fletcher, K., 40, 514
Flexner, S. B., 411, 537
Fogel, A., 79, 83, 119, 121, 514, 521, 527
Forrest, D., 353, 527
Forward, J., 493, 501
Fosshage, J. L., 322, 514
Foulkes, D., 322, 514
Fox, A. M., 512
Fox, N. A., 80, 500
Fraiberg, S., 16, 93, 95, 145, 159, 204, 514
Fredman, N., 259, 533
French, T. M., 466, 500
Freud, A., 139, 514
Freud, S., 141, 148, 204, 205, 316, 319, 320, 321, 322, 349, 354, 514
Fried, C., 429, 515
Friedlander, S. R., 429, 515
Fries, M. E., 89, 391, 515
Friese, S., 110, 509
Friesen, W. V., 231, 378, 512
Fromm-Reichmann, F., 293, 515
Fuchs, S. H., 143, 515

Gable, S., 80, 515
Gaensbauer, T. J., 95, 512
Gaffney, K. F., 167, 515
Gaiter, J. L., 19, 539
Ganchrow, J. R., 263, 504
Ganiban, J., 80, 502
Gardner, J. M., 105, 515
Garmezy, N., 187, 515
Garner, P., 115, 523
Gekoski, M. J., 142, 512

Gelfand, D. M., 106, 118, 536
Gelles, R., 333, 515
George, C., 21, 22, 93, 515, 534
Gerstel, N., 487, 516
Gesell, A., 79, 86, 446, 516
Gewirtz, J. L., 120, 369, 516
Gibbon, J., 72, 92, 122, 534
Gibson, J. J., 27, 516
Gillman, R. D., 323, 324, 516
Gilman, I. P., 355, 516
Glick, I. D., 409, 417, 418, 434, 516
Glorieux, J., 54, 516
Godlman, R., 466, 467, 525
Goetting, A., 484, 516
Goetz, D., 530
Gold, D., 54, 516
Goldberg, S., 73, 516
Goldberg, W. A., 53, 528
Goode, M. K., 19, 503
Goodyear, R. K., 381, 516
Gordon, S. B., 371, 372, 516
Gottman, J. M., 229, 230, 502
Granier-Deferre, C., 80, 506
Gratch, G., 73, 516
Graziano, A. M., 371, 516
Green, R. J., 434, 435, 517
Greenberg, M., 41, 491, 509, 517
Greenberg, R., 69, 513, 537
Greene, S., 105, 527
Greenson, R. R., 143, 153, 346, 348, 349, 517
Greenspan, S. I., 116, 511, 530
Grinder, J., 260, 502
Gross, H., 487, 516
Gross-Doehrman, M. J., 193, 517
Grossman, K., 180, 528
Grotstein, J. S., 153, 155, 517
Gruber, S. K., 537
Gruendel, J. M., 22, 527
Gunnar, M. R., 109, 517
Gurman, A. S., 168, 506

Gurwitt, A. R., 181, 182, 517
Gustafson, G. E., 110, 517
Gustafson, J. P., 466, 467, 475, 517
Guy, J. D., 357, 517
Guy, M. P., 357, 517

Hackley, K. C., 488, 526
Haekel, M., 83, 120, 517
Haith, M. M., 28, 74, 128, 517, 518
Haley, J., 409, 411, 518
Halsted, L., 109, 531
Hann, D., 490, 518, 528
Hannan, T. E., 79, 514
Hans, S. L., 118, 518, 520
Harmon, R. J., 19, 95, 512, 539
Harris, P. L., 73, 518
Harrison, L. L., 109, 518
Håursman, I., 120, 518
Hartmann, H., 141, 149, 518
Hartung, J., 513
Hartup, W. W., 379, 518
Hayne, H., 26, 518
Hazen, N., 80, 521
Heckhausen, J., 20, 518
Heilveil, I., 376, 377, 378, 380, 518
Heim, L., 80, 518
Heinicke, C. M., 116, 518
Hendrick, I., 151, 518
Henson, L. G., 118, 518
Herbert, S., 105, 508
Hersen, M., 382, 518
Hertsgaard, L., 106, 518
Hervis, O., 410, 535
Herzog, J., 37, 38, 519
Hetherington, E. M., 187, 188, 189, 519
Hillman, L., 104, 519
Hinse, L. M., 110, 517
Hirshberg, L., 96, 519
Hobbs, P. R., 429, 502
Hoffman, H. J., 104, 519
Hoffman, J., 524
Hoffman, M. L., 32, 84, 87, 92, 153, 519
Holman, S. L., 429, 436, 519

Holt, S. A., 70, 519
Hong, H. -W., 119, 521
Hopkins, B., 17, 18, 19, 20, 21, 92, 519
Horsman, I., 518
Hosford, R. E., 382, 520
Houck, G. M., 107, 520
Howard, J., 489, 520
Howes, C., 80, 520
Hrncir, E. J., 87, 511
Hron-Stewart, K. M., 106, 520
Hsu, H. -C., 119, 527
Hubley, P., 153, 210, 537
Huntington, L., 520
Huston, T. L., 40, 525

Im, W., 506
Imber, S. D., 426, 520
Inhelder, B., 255, 529
Isabella, R. A., 80, 515, 520
Izard, C. E., 69, 520, 536

Jackson, D., 31, 538
Jacobson, E., 143, 520
Jacobson, N. S., 368, 520
Jaffe, J., 72, 534
James, M., 105, 508
Jasnow, M. D., 106, 513
Jennings, K. D., 19, 539
Jennings, S., 92, 529
Jensen, J. L., 97, 520
Jernberg, A. M., 391, 520
Jodl, K., 106, 518
Johnson, E. J., 128, 520
Johnson, K., 537
Jones, D., 521
Jones, S., 119, 521
Josselyn, I. M., 53, 521

Kagan, J., 18, 26, 83, 92, 123, 151, 513, 521, 525, 530, 537
Kantor, D., 403, 511
Kaplan, B., 88, 89, 538
Kaplan, K., 21, 525
Karmel, B. Z., 105, 515
Kasari, C., 105, 528
Katona, F., 73, 521
Kauffman, E., 409, 521
Kauffman, P., 409, 521
Kay, D. A., 83, 531

Kaye, D., 466, 467, 475, 517
Kaye, K., 16, 88, 121, 521
Kazdin, A., 254, 383, 521
Kearsley, R. B., 26, 83, 513, 521
Keith, D. V., 413, 538
Kelly, K., 148, 149, 527
Kemple, K., 80, 521
Kennedy-Caldwell, C., 106, 521
Kennell, J., 111, 534
Kermoian, R., 521
Kernberg, O. F., 154, 521
Kerr, M. E., 178, 405, 406, 521, 522
Kessler, D. B., 537
Kessler, D. R., 409, 434, 516
Kestenbaum, R., 128, 522
Kestenberg, J., 328, 522
King, C., 511
Kipp, E., 84, 512
Kitch, D., 177, 505
Kitching, K., 106, 502
Klaus, M., 111, 534
Klein, M., 152, 210, 522
Kligman, D. H., 92, 512
Klinger, E., 40, 522
Klinnert, M., 92, 128, 522
Knieps, L. J., 128, 502
Knight, R. P., 143, 522
Kohut, H., 153, 321, 322, 522
Kolb, S., 17, 539
Kolstad, V. T., 522
Koopmans-van-Deinun, F. J., 83, 522
Kopp, C. B., 52, 67, 83, 86, 92, 95, 517, 522
Korner, A. F., 231, 522
Koslowski, B., 87, 336, 506
Koss, M. P., 522
Kotelchuck, M., 46, 49, 522, 523
Kropenske, V., 489, 520
Krupka, A., 118, 526
Kuhl, P., 83, 86, 92, 513, 523
Kuhn, C. M., 532
Kurtines, W. M., 410, 535
Kurzweil, S. R., 130, 523

Lachmann, F. M., 209, 535
Lagerspetz, K., 16, 17, 523
Lalonde, C. W., 73, 523
Lamb, M. E., 26, 49, 53, 72, 80, 507, 523
Landry, S. H., 115, 523
Langs, R., 193, 234, 235, 236, 240, 241, 242, 244, 347, 349, 359, 361, 523
LaPlanche, J., 353, 523
Lask, B., 183, 355, 523
Lavatelli, C. S., 369, 523
Lazarus, A. A., 382, 523
Leavitt, L. A., 106, 511
Lecanuet, J. -P., 80, 506
LeCompte, G. K., 73, 516
Lederman, R. P., 40, 523
Lefever, G. B., 106, 520
Legerstee, M., 83, 86, 130, 523, 524
Lehman, A. F., 385, 386, 388, 504
Lein, L., 40, 524
Lent, L. A., 537
Leos, N., 113, 526
Lester, B., 87, 174, 506, 524
Levenson, E., 207, 524
Levine, L., 537
Levitt, M. J., 126, 524
Levy, J., 40, 524
Lewinsohn, P. M., 382, 524
Lewis, B., 89, 515
Lewis, M., 45, 83, 92, 95, 123, 502, 524
Lewis, P. M., 426, 520
Lewkowicz, D. J., 28, 524
Li, P., 79, 507
Liaboe, G. P., 357, 517
Libet, J. M., 382, 524
Lin, N., 485, 486, 524
Lipsitt, L., 26, 106, 521, 524
Little, C., 528
Loewald, H., 524
Loiselle, R. H., 426, 520
Lövaas, O., 369, 524
Lowenstein, R. M., 141, 518
Luborsky, L., 288, 289, 524
Lukens, E., 530

MacDonald, J., 28, 525
Magnano, C. L., 105, 515
Mahler, M., 83, 89, 92, 139, 524, 525
Main, M., 21, 87, 336, 506, 525
Malan, D. H., 351, 466, 467, 476, 525
Malcuit, G., 69, 83, 509, 524
Mandler, J., 122, 525
Mangelsdorf, S., 80, 518
Manikouska, M., 527
Mann, J., 106, 466, 467, 507, 525
Martin, R., 80, 502
Mason, L., 106, 518
Mast, V. K., 92, 122, 525
Masters, J. C., 382, 531
Matheny, A. P., 531
McAnulty, G. B., 106, 500
McCall, R. B., 71, 92, 123, 525
McComas, J., 89, 525
McCune-Nicolich, L., 83, 446, 525
McDevitt, J. B., 92, 524
McDonough, L., 122, 525
McGee, R., 40, 524
McGhee, P. E., 54, 71, 525, 535
McGhee, S., 84, 512
McGoldrick, M., 171, 172, 525
McGurk, H., 28, 525
McHale, S. M., 40, 525
McLaughlin, F. J., 104, 525
McRea, C., 375, 526
Medin, D. L., 26, 526
Meerloo, J. A.M., 194, 526
Meisels, S. J., 511
Meissner, W. W., 149, 526
Meltzoff, A. N., 27, 29, 73, 86, 92, 127, 266, 523, 526
Mercer, M., 73, 509
Mercer, R. T., 488, 526
Miller, W. H., 373, 526
Millet, G., 73, 535
Mills, M. E., 382, 520
Minde, K., 113, 526

Minuchin, S., 404, 409, 410, 526
Molina, M., 73, 535
Moore, B. E., 205, 405, 526
Moore, C., 86, 523
Moore, M. J., 128, 518
Moore, M. K., 29, 73, 92, 127, 266, 526
Moran, G., 118, 526
Morgan, G. A., 19, 539
Morris, N., 41, 517
Morris, W., 259, 527
Morrongiello, B. A., 142, 512
Morrow, C., 532
Mosier, C., 83, 527
Most, R. K., 19, 503
Myers, W. A., 329, 527

Nagera, H., 319, 320, 527
Nash, S. C., 180, 513
Naud, J., 114, 527
Needham, A., 73, 527
Nelson, C. A., 128, 522
Nelson, K., 22, 527
New, R. S., 116, 527
Ninio, A., 18, 51, 83, 527
Novick, J., 148, 149, 527
Nowak, C. A., 432, 509
Nugent, J. K., 105, 527
Nwokah, E., 119, 527
Nygard, M., 16, 523

Oates, R. K., 353, 527
O'Connor, M. J., 105, 527, 528
Oehler, J., 105, 528
Ohr, P. S., 72, 512
O'Leary, S. E., 41, 42, 529
Olson, S. L., 19, 528
Orr, W. C., 104, 519
Osofsky, J. D., 126, 528
Oster, H., 69, 531
Owen, M. T., 53, 54, 106, 507, 528
Oyemade, U. J., 104, 528
Ozolins, M., 254, 512

Pan, B. A., 110, 528
Paolino, T. J., Jr., 286, 528
Papousek, H., 83, 92, 108, 109, 111, 528

Papousek, M., 83, 92, 108, 109, 110, 111, 528
Parish, T. S., 381, 516
Parke, R. D., 41, 43, 49, 179, 180, 486, 528, 529, 530, 536
Parker, K., 113, 529
Parsons, T., 48, 529
Patterson, G. R., 419, 529
Patterson, J. G., 73, 505
Pawl, J. H., 348, 363, 364, 533
Pedersen, F. A., 44, 54, 180, 529, 539
Pederson, D. R., 118, 512, 526
Peláez-Nogueras, M., 120, 516
Pepernow, P. L., 484, 529
Perez-Vidal, A., 410, 535
Perris, E. E., 26, 518
Petit, P., 118, 526
Piaget, J., 71, 72, 79, 87, 148, 255, 266, 529
Pick, I. B., 357, 529
Pine, F., 83, 525
Pines, D., 328, 329, 529
Pipp, S., 92, 529
Platzman, K. A., 105, 508
Plomin, R., 89, 506
Plunkett, J. W., 511
Poey, K., 429, 529
Pomerleau, A., 69, 83, 509, 524
Pompa, J., 106, 536
Pontalis, J. -B., 353, 523
Popiel, K., 113, 526, 529
Porqes, S. W., 116, 511, 530
Portales, A. L., 116, 511, 530
Posner, M. I., 109, 531
Poulsen, M., 105, 501, 530
Power, T. G., 49, 50, 530
Prodromidis, M., 80, 523
Puig-Antich, J., 485, 530

Qi, D., 79, 507
Quatrode, J. B., 530

Raag, T., 119, 521
Rabinovich, B., 54, 539

Racker, H., 153, 157, 211, 212, 530
Radin, N., 37, 52, 530
Ragozin, A. S., 491, 509
Ramey, C. T., 142, 538
Ramsay, D. S., 83, 513
Ramsay-Douglas, S., 73, 74, 530
Raphael-Leff, J., 328, 530
Reich, J. H., 92, 512
Reid, W. J., 468, 530
Reilly, J. S., 125, 126, 530
Reiss, D., 416, 417, 530
Reissland, N., 266, 530
Resnick, J. S., 26, 530
Reznick, S., 513
Richards, M. P.M., 42, 531
Richardson, M. A., 115, 523
Richman, A. L., 116, 527
Ricks, S. S., 86, 531
Riese, M. L., 531
Rimm, D. C., 382, 531
Rinott, N., 51, 527
Roach, M. A., 110, 534
Roberts, J., 532
Roberts, R. N., 531
Robertson, J., 161, 531
Robertson, S., 111, 534
Robinson, J., 528
Robinson, N. M., 509
Robson, K. S., 44, 529
Rodning, C., 80, 520
Rogoff, B., 83, 527
Rosenberg, P. E., 467, 531
Rosenstein, D., 69, 531
Ross, G., 16, 538
Ross, S. A., 83, 531
Roth, D., 433, 456, 484, 531
Rothbart, M. K., 89, 109, 517, 531
Rothenberg, M. B., 489, 492, 531
Rothstein, A., 323, 531
Rovee-Collier, C., 26, 92, 95, 125, 142, 512, 518, 525, 531
Rubin, J. A., 40, 531
Ruddy, M. G., 19, 532
Ruff, H. A., 74, 532
Russell, G., 37, 40, 41, 532
Rutan, J. S., 459, 460, 500
Rutter, M., 188, 368, 532

Saal, D. R., 73, 532
Sackett, G. P., 229, 532
Sadek, A., 106, 500
Sagart, L., 83, 510
Sagi, A., 37, 52, 532
Salapalek, P., 26, 508
Salzman, L., 375, 532
Sandler, L., 347, 532
Satir, V., 172, 403, 532
Sawin, D. B., 43, 179, 529
Scafidi, F. A., 391, 532
Schachere, K., 55, 532
Schacht, T. E., 476, 504
Schachter, B., 491, 494, 532
Schachter, J., 458, 532
Schafer, R., 141, 143, 153, 532, 533
Schanberg, S. M., 532
Schechter, A., 92, 533
Schecter, D. E., 177, 533
Schlessinger, N., 213, 533
Schmidt, C., 85, 533
Searles, H., 193, 194, 533
Seligman, M. E.F., 52, 533
Seligman, S. P., 348, 363, 364, 533
Shapiro, V., 16, 514
Sheehy, G., 53, 533
Sherman, M. H., 416, 417, 418, 533
Sherman, R., 259, 533
Sherrod, K. B., 104, 525
Sherrod, L. R., 26, 523
Sherwen, L. N., 38, 40, 327, 533
Shields, M. M., 86, 533
Shields, P., 92, 533
Shotter, J., 384, 533
Shultz, N. W., 268, 533
Shyi, G. C.-W., 92, 533
Sifneos, P. E., 466, 467, 533
Sigman, M., 105, 528
Simineau, K., 73, 74, 510
Singer, D. L., 38, 293, 533
Singer, J. L., 255, 256, 533, 534, 536
Sisney, V. V., 382, 505
Slater, A., 73, 534
Smith, A. H., 429, 502
Smith, B., 109, 505
Smith, I. E., 105, 508
Smokler, I., 426, 504

Smyer, M. A., 432, 509
Snow, C. E., 110, 528
Solomon, J., 21, 22, 93, 96, 515, 519, 534
Sorce, J., 92, 522
Sosa, R., 111, 534
Spanos, N. P., 254, 534
Spelke, E. S., 73, 534
Spitz, R. A., 69, 87, 92, 534
St. James-Roberts, I., 353, 535
Stanton, M. D., 411, 534
Steiner, J. E., 263, 504
Stenberg, C., 72, 507
Stendler, F., 369, 523
Stern, D., 21, 22, 26, 27, 30, 72, 92, 95, 96, 117, 122, 125, 148, 153, 210, 336, 470, 471, 503, 509, 519, 534
Sternberg, K. J., 80, 523
Stevenson, M. B., 110, 534
Stevenson-Hinde, J., 414, 415, 416, 418, 534
Stifter, C. A., 106, 535
Stingle, K. G., 369, 516
Stolorow, R. D., 205, 209, 535
Strandvik, C., 16, 523
Streri, A., 73, 535
Strupp, H. H., 476, 504
Stuckey, M. F., 54, 535
Sullivan, H. S., 207, 216, 357, 535
Sullivan, M. V., 92, 525
Sullivan, M. W., 89, 500
Summerfield, A. B., 378, 379, 535
Sussman, M. B., 487, 535
Suwalsky, J. T.D., 54, 539
Svejda, M., 92, 522
Swain, I. U., 80, 508
Swenson, W. M., 488, 535
Szapocznik, J., 410, 535

Tamis-LeMonda, C., 19, 20, 505, 535
Tansey, M. J., 157, 211, 212, 535
Tauber, E. S., 207, 535
Telzrow, R., 535
Tenzer, A., 294, 535

Terkelsen, K. G., 165, 536
Termine, I., 69, 536
Teti, D. M., 106, 118, 536
Tharp, R. G., 371, 536
Thelen, E., 79, 97, 520, 536
Thoman, E. B., 110, 536
Thomas, A., 89, 265, 391, 536
Thomas, D. A., 92, 104, 538
Tinsley, B. J., 486, 536
Tinsley, B. R., 49, 179, 180, 528, 529
Toback, G., 530
Tower, R. B., 255, 256, 536
Trad, P., 37, 69, 86, 87, 96, 108, 118, 139, 165, 207, 266, 336, 536
Trevarthen, C., 32, 87, 92, 127, 153, 210, 536, 537
Trivette, C. M., 511
Tronick, E., 49, 89, 93, 142, 174, 506, 517, 537, 539
Tu, C. H., 79, 507
Tucci, K., 532
Tulkin, S. R., 18, 537
Turkewitz, G., 28, 524

Ulrich, D. N., 412, 413, 505
Urdang, L., 411, 537
Urrutia, J., 111, 534
Uzgiris, I. C., 119, 537

van der Stelt, B., 83, 522
Van Deusen, J. M., 409, 410, 501
van Wufften Palthe, T., 92, 519
Vo, D., 106, 503
Vogel, E. F., 183, 184, 503
Vygotsky, L. S., 16, 86, 537
Vyt, A., 118, 537

Wachs, T. D., 73, 87, 106, 507, 537
Wade, T., 92, 512
Waelder, R., 206, 537
Walden, T., 128, 502, 537
Walker, P. S., 511
Wallerstein, R. S., 159, 537
Walsh, R. O., 106, 511
Wanner, M. B., 106, 518

Ward, M. J., 116, 537
Ward, W. D., 375, 538
Wasik, B., 531
Watkins, C. E., 429, 515
Watson, J. S., 72, 142, 538
Watzlawick, P., 31, 538
Waxer, P. H., 426, 538
Weinberg, M. K., 93, 537
Weintraub, D., 106, 520
Welles-Nystrom, B., 106,
    116, 527, 538
Werker, J. F., 73, 523
Werner, H., 29, 88, 89, 538
West, S., 41, 529
Westra, T., 17, 18, 19, 20,
    519
Wetzel, R. J., 371, 536

Whitaker, C. A., 183, 185,
    413, 538
White, M., 177, 505
Wilner, R. S., 461, 506
Wilson, M., 177, 505
Wise, S., 142, 537
Wittig, B., 24, 488, 500
Wodan-Sullivan, M., 92
Wolan-Sullivan, M., 524
Wolf, K. M., 69, 534
Wolff, P. H., 230, 538
Wolke, D., 353, 535
Wolstein, B., 205, 206, 538
Wood, D., 16, 538
Woodson, R., 69, 513
Woolf, P. J., 89, 515
Worchel, J., 312, 313, 538

Worobey, J., 92, 104, 538
Worthington, E. L., 432,
    433, 539
Wright, N. A., 73, 516

Yalom, I. D., 427, 539
Yarrow, L. J., 19, 539
Yogman, M. J., 180, 539
Yogman, M. W., 49, 95,
    112, 114, 506, 539

Zaslow, M. J., 54, 539
Zeanah, C., 21, 24, 504, 539
Zelazo, N., 17, 539
Zelazo, P. R., 17, 26, 83,
    513, 521, 539
Zuk, G., 403, 539

Subject Index

Adaptive maternal attitude, 201
Affect attunement, 6, 32, 125–126
Affective processing, observing, 69–71
Alliances. *See* Therapeutic alliances
Amodal perception, 27–28, 29
Analogic communication mode, 31, 75, 88
Anger in infants, 70
Anticipatory imagery, 255
Assertiveness therapy stage, 284, 290, 297, 305, 311
Assessment therapy stage, 290–291, 297–298, 311
Attachment behaviors, 75
  case history, 55–59
  developmental list of, 81–83
  differences between parental figures, 44–48
  in dysfunctional families, 414–416
  effect of deprivation, 161
  effects of parental employment, 53–55
  emergence of, 119–120
  and families, 44–48, 53–55, 414–416
  insecure, 80, 161
  and internal working models, 22–23
  observing, 75, 79–80, 81–83

  predicting later development from, 46–48
Autonomy in infants
  awareness of, 129–130
  development of, 116–117
Avoidance, 93, 159
Avoidant maternal attitude, 202–203

Bem Sex Inventory, 38
Bills Affectional Relationship Questionnaire, 38
Body gestures, infant, 74–75
Boundaries, 272–273
  and autonomy, 129–130
  in families, 409

Canonical babbling, 83
Caregiver–infant relationship
  affect attunement in, 6, 32, 125–126
  assessing intuitive behavior in, 107–112
  vs. caregiver–therapist relationship, 192–203
  communication in, 80, 83–86, 110–111
  defense operations in, 136–161
  effect of caregiver–therapist relationship on, 222–224

Caregiver–infant relationship (*Continued*)
and infant's attachment behaviors,
119–120
and infant's autonomy, 116–117,
129–130
and infant's capacity for regulation,
112–116
and infant's contingency awareness, 72,
122–124, 263
and infant's core self, 125
and infant's defense operations,
159–161
and infant's discrepancy awareness,
122–124
and infant's engagement/disengagement,
117–118
and infant's expectancy awareness,
122–124
and infant's external reality, 140–144
and infant's greeting responses, 108,
120–121
and infant's identification, 143–144
and infant's internalization, 141–143,
149
and infant's internal reality, 144–159
and infant's internal working model,
137–140
and infant's self-recognition, 132
and infant's social referencing, 128–129
and infant's stranger reactions, 80,
130–132
neonatal factors in, 105–107
prenatal factors in, 104–105
short-term psychotherapy for, 470–476
transference in, 204–205, 313, 354, 355,
356, 438
treatment of. *See* Dyadic therapy
Caregivers. *See also* Fathers; Parents
and affect attunement, 6, 32, 125–126
assessing intuitive behaviors in, 107–112
attitude toward parents as, 52–60
depression of, 108
and duetting, 121–122
employment of, 53–55, 106
enhancing previewing in, 252–258
and externalization, 147–152
holding behavior of, 109–110
infant's imitating of, 118–119, 151
internal working models of, 22–23, 25
and intersubjectivity, 127–128
maladaptive, 296–304, 305–306
maternal attitudes of, 201–203

meaning attribution of, 111–112,
145–147
modeling strategies for, 371–375
neonatal factors, 105–107
parent training for, 371–375
playfulness of, 110–111
prenatal factors, 104–105
and previewing, 16–25, 97–98, 102,
252–253
and projection, 147–152, 158
psychoeducation for, 385–389
psychological mindedness of, 286
taking infant's perspective, 237–239
and visual cuing, 108–109
and vocalization, 80, 83–86, 110–111
Caregiver–therapist relationship, 2–4. *See
also* Dyadic therapy
building alliance, 104, 285–289,
306–313
vs. caregiver–infant relationship,
192–203
effect on caregiver–infant relationship,
222–224
exploring with dream imagery, 339–342
parallel processes in. *See* Parallel
processes
Stage 1, assertiveness, 290, 297, 305, 311
Stage 2, assessment, 290–291, 297–298,
305, 311
Stage 3, working through, 291–295,
298–300, 305, 311–312
Stage 4, perspective taking, 295–296,
300–302, 306
Stage 5, conflict resolution, 296,
301–304, 306
summary of stages in, 245–248,
289–296
transference in. *See* Transference
Caregiving, parental, changing attitudes
toward, 52–60
Case management, 492–493
Categorization, 26–27, 29
Children. *See also* Infants
effect of parental divorce on, 187–189
effect of parental remarriage on,
187–189
at risk, 487–490
social support for, 490–497
Clarification, 235–236, 362
Cognitive processing
and father–infant interaction, 51–52
observing, 71–74

Communication modes
    analogic, 31, 75, 88
    caregiver–infant, 80, 83–86, 110–111
    digital, 31, 84, 88
    unconscious, 351–352
Confrontation
    experiential, 403, 404
    in family therapy, 402–404
    as intervention strategy, 244–245
    when to avoid, 361
Contingency awareness, 72, 122–124, 263
Core behaviors. *See* Intuitive behaviors
Core self, 30, 125
Counterprojection as intervention strategy,
        243–244
Countertransference
    and previewing, 476
    in treating caregiver–infant dyads, 353,
        357–360
Cross-modal functioning, 266–267

Day care, 106, 495–497
Defense operations, 93, 95–96, 136–137
    avoidance, 93, 159
    externalization, 147–152
    fighting, 95, 159
    freezing, 93, 95, 159
    in infants, 93, 95–96, 159–161
    projection, 147–152, 158
    projective identification, 152–159
    relationship of internal working models
        to, 137–140
    and transference, 209
Depression, 108, 253, 304, 347, 431–434
Developmental dyssynchrony, 168–169
Didactic stimulation, maternal, 19, 20
Digital communication mode, 31, 84, 88
Discrepancy awareness, 122–124
Disgust in infants, 70
Distress in infants, 70
Divorce, parental, 187–188
Dreams, 316–319
    adaptive functions of, 319–323
    manifest *vs.* latent content of, 321, 322
    overcoming resistance to exploring,
        323–327
    postnatal, 334–339
    prenatal, 327–333
    and transference, 209, 339–342
    using to explore therapeutic
        relationship, 339–342
Drug abuse, 105, 489, 491

Duetting, 121–122
Dyadic relationships. *See also*
        Caregiver–infant relationship
    in families, 174–180
    group therapy for, 426–428
    regulatory capacities in, 112–116
Dyadic therapy, 2–9
    applying family therapy to, 398–401
    applying group therapy to, 424–440
    confrontation in, 244–245, 361
    conrasting past and present in, 239–240
    counterprojection in, 243–244
    features of, 2–3
    vs. group therapy, 2–3, 66, 198,
        284–285, 313, 346, 347, 351, 369,
        458
    vs. individual therapy, 458
    inquiry in, 233–237
    interpretation in, 241–243
    intervention by stage of, 245–248
    modeling in, 370–371
    observation in, 66–68, 229–233
    parallel processes in, 193–197, 217–222
    perspective taking in, 237–239
    previewing in, 14–16, 286–287
    reconstruction in, 240–241
    resistance during, 346–365
    and social support, 484–497
    stages in, 289–296
    transference in, 313, 350–356
    value of dreams in, 317–318
Dyssynchrony, developmental, 168–169

Empathy, 32, 87, 153, 467, 475–476
Employment, maternal, effects of, 53–55,
        106
Engagement/disengagement, 117–118
Enmeshed maternal attitude, 201–202
Enmeshment, 405, 407, 408
Episodic memory, 22
Ethology, 66–67
Expectancy awareness, 122–124
Experiential confrontation, 403, 404
Externalization, 147–152
External locus of control, 52
External reality, 140–144, 287

Facial Action Coding System (FACS), 231,
        378
Facial expressions, 69–71
Families. *See also* Family therapy; Parents
    boundaries in, 409

Families (*Continued*)
   dyadic relationships within, 174–180
   life cycles of, 171–172
   role of infants in, 164
   stress in, 165–169
   structural changes in, 487–490
   structure of, 174–180
   triadic relationships within, 174–180
   undifferentiated, 407
Family sculpture, 403–404
Family therapy, 398–399
   applying to dyadic intervention,
      398–401
   attachment approach, 414–416,
      418–419
   combined with group therapy, 461
   confrontation in, 402–404
   contextual approaches to, 412–413
   family narratives approach, 416–417,
      418
   family sculpture in, 403–404
   functional approach, 411–412
   insight–working through approach,
      402–405
   interpretation in, 404–405
   problem-centered approach, 411
   structural approach, 409–411
   summary of approaches to, 399–401
   symbolic–experiential approach,
      413–414
   systems approach, 405–409, 418
   video recording in, 404
Fantasies, 316. *See also* Dreams
   of expectant fathers, 37–40
   representations as, 254
Father–infant interaction, 36–37
   and attachment behavior, 44–48
   case history, 55–59
   and cognition, 51–52
   and developmental skills, 41–44
   and locus of control, 52
   and play behaviors, 48–51
   predictors of, 37–41
Fathers
   enhancing previewing abilities of, 59–60
   exclusion of, 180–182
   expectant, 37–40
   intuitive behaviors of, 41–44, 59
   mental representations of, 37–40
   role in parental caregiving, 52–60
   self-esteem of, 40–41
Fighting, 95, 159

Formal handling, 18, 19
Free association, 317, 321
Freezing, 93, 95, 159

Generalization, 148
Greeting responses, 108, 120–121
Group therapy
   combined with family therapy, 461
   combined with individual therapy,
      458–460
   contracting in, 429–430
   defining goals for groups of dyads,
      426–428
   in dyadic intervention, 424–440
   group composition in, 428–429
   model of, 442–458
   previewing in, 442–445, 453–456
   representational exercises in, 448–453
   stages in, 431–437
   termination issues in, 456–458, 461–462
   transference in, 424–425, 437–439
   universality in, 427
   video recording in, 435
   working alliances in, 429–431

Happiness in infants, 70
Holding behavior, 109–110

Idealized transference, 356
Identification, 143–144
Imagery
   in dreams *See* Dreams
   in representations, 254–256
Imaginal Processes Inventory (IPI), 38
Imitation, 118–119, 151
Individual therapy
   combined with group therapy, 458–460
   vs. dyadic therapy, 2–3, 66, 198,
      284–285, 313, 346, 347, 351, 369,
      458
Individuation, 185
Infants. *See also* Children
   and affect attunement, 6, 32, 125–126
   affective processing by, 69–71
   amodal perception in, 27–28, 29
   assessing by observing, 66–68
   attachment behaviors of, 75, 79–80,
      81–83, 119–120
   and autonomy, 116–117, 129–130
   body gestures of, 74–75
   capacity to symbolize, 88
   categorization of events, 26–27, 29

cognitive processing by, 51–52, 71–74
contingency awareness in, 72, 122–124
and core self, 30, 125
defense operations of, 93, 95–96,
    159–161
discrepancy awareness in, 122–124
and duetting, 121–122
effect on marriages, 169–173
emerging sense of self, 25–30
emotional expressions of, 69–71
engagement/disengagement of, 117–118
expectancy awareness in, 122–124
and external reality, 140–144
facial expressions of, 69–71
and family stress, 165–169
and fathers, 37–48
greeting responses of, 108, 120–121
and identification, 143–144
and imitation, 118–119, 151
and internalization, 141–143, 149
and internal reality, 144–159
internal working models of, 30,
    137–140
and intersubectivity, 127–128
language development of, 80, 83–86,
    110–111
massaging, 390–391
mental representations of, 127–128
motor processing by, 74–75, 76–79
object permanence in, 72–74
regression in, 74–75
response to conflict, 95–96
roles as family members, 164
as scapegoats, 167, 183–187, 407
self-recognition in, 132
and self-regulation, 89, 92–93, 94–95,
    112–116, 142–143
sense of self, 25–32, 86–89
and social referencing, 128–129
startle behavior of, 74
and stranger reactions, 80, 130–132
subjective development in, 31–32,
    86–89, 90–92
taking perspective of, 237–239
and temperament, 89, 92–93, 115–116,
    160–161, 188, 265–266
in triadic systems, 176–179
Inquiry
    assessing caregiver–infant relationship
        by, 200–203
    assessing parallel processes by, 217–222
    as intervention strategy, 233–237

and transference, 207
Intentionality, 268–270
Internalization, 141–143, 149
Internal locus of control, 52
Internal reality, 144–159, 288
Internal working models, 22, 137–140
    and attachment security, 22–23
    and external reality, 140–144
    of infants, 30, 137–140
    and internal reality, 144–159
Interpretation. *See also* Counterprojection
    in family therapy, 404–405
    as intervention strategy, 241–243
Intersubjectivity, 32, 87–88, 127–128
    and transference, 210
    as variation of projective identification,
        153–154
Intervention strategies, 4–5, 228–229
    confrontation, 244–245, 361
    counterprojection, 243–244
    group therapy model for dyads,
        445–458
    inquiry, 233–237
    interpretation, 241–243
    observation, 229–233
    perspective taking, 237–239
    reconstruction, 240–241
    social support as, 490–497
    by stage of dyadic therapy, 245–248
Introspection, vicarious. *See* Empathy
Intuitive behaviors, 4, 5, 8, 252
    assessing, 107–112
    in father–infant interactions, 42, 43
    holding, 109–110
    and infant's sense of self, 86–87
    meaning attribution, 111–112, 145–147
    parental, 107–112
    playfulness, 110–111
    and previewing skills, 59
    visual cuing, 108–109
    vocal communication, 110–111

Language development
    observing, 80, 83–86
    vocalization of caregivers, 110–111
Locus of control, 52

Marriage, effect of newborn on, 169–173
Massage, infant, 390–391
Mastery, 270–271
Maternal caregiving. *See also* Caregivers
    alternative attitudes in, 201–203
    changing attitudes toward, 52–60

Maternal didactic stimulation, 19, 20
Meaning attribution, 111–112, 145–147
Mechanisms of interaction, 232
Memory
    episodic, 22
    prototype, 22
Mental representation. *See* Representation
Mirroring, 32, 388–389
Mirror transference, 355–356
Modeling, 8, 103, 318, 368–371
    interventive techniques, 375–385
    strategies for caregivers, 371–375
    use of video recording, 375–385
Models. *See* Internal working models
Mothers. *See* Caregivers; Parents
Motor processing
    developmental skills list, 76–79
    observing, 74–75, 76–79

Neonatal phase, 105–107
Newborns, effect on marriages, 169–173

Objective reality. *See* External reality
Object permanence, 72–74
Observation, 66–68
    of affective processing, 69–71
    of attachment behaviors, 75, 79–80,
        81–83
    case history, 98–100
    of cognitive processing, 71–74
    of defensive operations, 93, 95–96
    of differences in self-regulation, 89,
        92–93, 94–95
    of infant's subjective experience, 86–89,
        90–92
    as intervention strategy, 229–233
    of language development, 80, 83–86
    of motor processing, 74–75, 76–79
    of parallel processes, 200–203, 217–
        222
    video recording as tool for, 231, 233,
        375–380
One-step-ahead model, 20–21
Overstimulation, 117

Parallel processes
    assessing, 200–203, 217–222
    in dyadic therapy, 192–203
    effect of therapist's reactions to,
        212–217
    effect of transference phenomena on,
        204–212

reciprocity in, 195
Parental mirroring, 32, 388–389
Parenthood as developmental phase,
        176–177
Parents. *See also* Caregivers; Families
    changing caregiving attitudes, 52–60
    cultural differences among, 17–18
    differences in infant attachment, 44–48
    divorce/remarriage of, 187–188
    effects of employment on caregiving,
        53–55, 106
    psychoeducation for, 385–389
    training of, 371–375
Pauses. *See* Therapeutic pause
Peer transference, 425, 438
Perspective taking, 237–239, 295–296,
        300–301, 306, 449
Placement, 493–495
Plan of action, 467–468, 474
Play behaviors
    differences between parents, 48–51
    and vocal communication, 110–111
Postnatal phase
    dream imagery during, 334–339
    variables in, 105–107
Pregnancy. *See* Prenatal phase
Prenatal phase
    dream imagery during, 327–333
    variables in, 104–105
Previewing, 6–7, 8, 14–16, 252
    assessing, 96–98
    caregiver's perspective, 16–25
    and countertransference, 476
    and dream material, 318
    and empathy, 475–476
    enhancing behavior of, 7
    enhancing fathers' abilities, 59–60
    exercises for, 252–279
    in family therapy, 399, 408, 417–418,
        419
    in group therapy, 442–445, 453–456
    infant's perspective, 25–33
    key components of, 15
    overcoming resistance with, 473–474
    paternal, 59–60
    and plan of action implementation,
        474
    in psychoeducation, 387–388
    and realignment of behavior patterns,
        475
    in short-term psychotherapy, 472–476

Projection, 147–152, 158. *See also*
Counterprojection
vs. projective identification, 152,
210–211
and transference, 209
Projective identification
in caregiver–infant dyad, 152–159
in caregiver–therapist dyad, 156
interactional fit in, 157–158
manifestations of, 154–157
vs. projection, 152, 210–211
Prototype memory, 22
Psychoeducation, 385–391
Psychomotor development. *See* Motor
processing
Psychotherapy, short–term
case history, 476–481
empathic approach in, 467, 475–476
exploratory, 389–390
involving caregiver–infant dyads,
470–476
overcoming resistance with previewing
in, 473–474
patient selection in, 466–467
plan of action implementation in,
467–468, 474
pursuing resistance in, 469–470, 472
realignment of behavior patterns in,
468–469, 475
techniques of, 465–470

Questions, 234–235

Reality
external, 140–144
internal, 144–159
Reciprocity, 6, 87, 195
Reconstruction
dream material in, 330–331
as intervention strategy, 240–241
Referencing. *See* Social referencing
Reframing, 409, 461
Regression, 74–75, 316
Regulation, 89, 92–93, 94–95
in dyadic relationships, 112–116
internal *vs.* external, 142–143
Rehearsals, 96–97, 252
Relationships. *See* Caregiver–infant
relationship; Caregiver–therapist
relationship; Families
Remarriage, parental, 187–188

Replication
in group therapy, 427
parallel processes as, 192, 193, 194
Representation, 7, 15, 252–258
association exercises in, 259
caregiver deficits in, 360
completion exercises in, 259
construction exercises in, 259
deletion process in, 260
distortion process in, 260
expression exercises in, 259
as fantasies, 254
of the future, 260
generalization process in, 260
imagery in, 254–256
by infants, 25, 127–128
internal, evolution of, 21–25
maladaptive, 258
maternal, classification of, 24–25
paternal, 37–40
strategies for, 259–261
Representational exercises, 258–261
boundaries, 272–273
caregiver's past interactions, 272
cognitive dimensions, 262–265
cross-modal abilities, 266–267
developmental transitions, 271–272
feelings after separation, 273–275
in group therapy, 448–453
infant in his absence, 275–277
infant's arrival, 261–262
infant's temperament, 265–266
instilling skill in, 448–453
intentionality, 268–270
mastery, 270–271
motivational dimensions, 262–265
reunion, 277–279
socio-affective dimensions, 262–265
somatic dimensions, 262–265
transitions, 267–268
Reproductive imagery, 255
Resistance
confronting, 244–245, 361, 362
emergence of, 346–349
to exploring dreams, 323–327
manifestations of, 349–360
overcoming with previewing, 473–474
in short–term psychotherapy, 469–470
therapeutic approaches to, 361–364
Resolution therapy stage, 284, 296,
301–304, 306
Reunion, 277

Rhythmicity, 87, 114–115
Role playing, 461

Sadness in infants, 70
Scaffolding, 16
Scapegoats, infants as, 167, 183–187, 407
Scripts, 22
Self-esteem and father–infant interactions,
    40–41
Self-recognition, 132
Self-regulation, 89, 92–93, 94–95
    in dyadic relationships, 112–116
    internal *vs.* external, 142–143
Separation, 103, 273–275, 329
Short-term psychotherapy
    case history, 476–481
    empathic approach in, 467, 475
    involving caregiver–infant dyads,
        470–476
    overcoming resistance with previewing
        in, 473–474
    patient selection in, 466–467
    plan of action implementation in,
        467–468
    previewing in, 472–476
    pursuing resistance in, 469–470, 472
    realignment of behavior patterns in,
        468–469, 475
    techniques of, 465–470
Sibling rivalry, 182
Soberness in infants, 70
Social referencing, 79, 128–129
Social support
    case management for, 492–493
    for children of divorce, 188–189
    day care as, 495–497
    definition of, 485–487
    and dyadic intervention, 484–497
    as intervention, 490–497
    placement for, 493–495
    relation of stressful events to, 487–490
Startle behavior, 74
Stranger reactions, 80, 130–132
Subjective reality. *See* Internal reality
Subjectivity, 87. *See also* Intersubjectivity
Substance abuse, 105, 489, 491
Surprise in infants, 70

Temperament, 89, 92–93, 115–116,
    160–161, 188, 265–266
Termination, 456–458, 461–462

Therapeutic alliances, 66, 104
    building, 285–289
    case history, 306–311
    in group therapy, 429–431
    parallel processes in, 197–203
    stages in, 311–313
Therapeutic pause, 236–237
Therapists. *See also* Caregiver–therapist
    relationship
    in dyadic therapy, 2–5
    reaction to parallel processes, 212–217
    role in transference, 206–209
Theraplay, 391–392
Therapy. *See* Dyadic therapy; Family
    therapy; Group therapy
Training, parent, 371–375
Transference, 204, 312–313, 350–356
    caregiver–infant, 204–205, 313, 354,
        355, 356, 438
    definition of, 353–355
    dream material in, 209, 339–342
    effect of inquiry on, 207
    effect on parallel processes, 204–212
    encouragement of, 424–425
    in groups of dyads, 424–425, 437–
        439
    idealized, 356
    mirror, 355–356
    signs of, 207–209
    therapist's role in, 206–209
    variations of, 355–356
Transitions
    in autonomous functioning, 116–117
    in family life, 432–433
    representing, 267–268, 271–272
Triadic relationships
    in families, 174–180
    in therapy, 196
Triangulation, 178, 355, 405–407

Unconscious communication, 351–352
Unconscious defense processes. *See* Defense
    operations
Undifferentiated families, 407
Universality, 427

Vicarious introspection. *See* Empathy
Video recording
    assessing infant motor behaviors by, 74
    in family therapy, 404
    in group therapy, 435
    model videotapes as alternative to, 383

as observation tool, 231, 233
role of, 8, 375–380
self-modeling in, 383–385
techniques for, 380–385
Visual checking. *See* Social referencing
Visual cuing, 108–109
Vitality affects, 29
Vocal communication of caregivers, 80,
    83–86, 110–111

Working models. *See* Internal working
    models
Working through therapy stage, 284,
    291–295, 298–300, 305, 311–
    312

Zone of proximal development, 16